Signs and Symptoms
in Family Medicine

Signs and Symptoms in Family Medicine
A Literature–Based Approach

PAUL M. PAULMAN, MD
Assistant Dean for Clinical Skills and Quality
Professor and Predoctoral Director
University of Nebraska College of Medicine
Department of Family Medicine
Omaha, Nebraska

JEFFREY HARRISON, MD
Associate Professor and Residency Program Director
Department of Family Medicine
University of Nebraska Medical Center
Omaha, Nebraska

AUDREY PAULMAN, MD
Clinical Assistant Professor
Department of Family Medicine
University of Nebraska Medical Center
Omaha, Nebraska

LAETH S. NASIR, MD
Professor
Chairman of the Department of Family Medicine
Creighton University School of Medicine
Family Medicine Physician
Creighton Medical Associates
Omaha, Nebraska

DEAN S. COLLIER, PHARMD, BCPS
Assistant Professor
University of Nebraska College of Pharmacy
Department of Pharmacy Practice
Omaha, Nebraska

SARAH BRYAN, BA
Department of Family Medicine
University of Nebraska College of Medicine
Omaha, Nebraska

Series Editor
MARK ALAN DAVIS, MD, MS
Director
International Emergency Medicine and Health
Brigham and Women's Hospital
Department of Emergency Medicine
Boston, Massachusetts

ELSEVIER
MOSBY

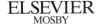

ELSEVIER
MOSBY

1600 John F. Kennedy Blvd.
Ste 1800
Philadelphia, PA 19103-2899

Signs and Symptoms in Family Medicine   ISBN: 978-0-323-04981-8

ISBN: 978-0-323-04981-8

Acquisitions Editor: James Merritt
Developmental Editor: Nicole DiCicco
Publishing Services Manager: Jeff Patterson
Project Manager: Jeanne Genz
Design Direction: Steve Stave

Printed in the United States of America

Last digit is the print number: 9 8 7 6 5 4 3 2 1

Contributors

IVAN ABDOUCH, MD
Associate Professor, Associate Residency Program Director
Department of Family Medicine
University of Nebraska Medical Center
Omaha, Nebraska

DEBRA A. AHERN, DO
Assistant Professor of Medicine
Department of Community and Family Medicine
University of Missouri-Kansas City
Kansas City, Missouri

ELISABETH L. BACKER, MD
Clinical Associate Professor
Department of Family Medicine
University of Nebraska Medical Center
Omaha, Nebraska

ELLEN BAJOREK, PHD
Director of Behavioral Sciences
Coordinator of Research
Department of Family Medicine
Family Medicine Residency Program
CHRISTUS Santa Rosa Health Care
San Antonio, Texas

GINA M. BASELLO, DO
Assistant Clinical Professor
Department of Family Medicine
Albert Einstein College of Medicine
Bronx, New York;
Program Director
Family Medicine Residency Program
Jamaica Hospital Medical Center
Jamaica, New York

DAVID M. BERCAW, MD
Vice Chair of Clinical Programs
Department of Family and Community Medicine
Christiana Care Health System
Newark, Delaware

KAYE B. CARSTENS, MD
Clinical Associate Professor
Department of Family Medicine
University of Nebraska Medical Center
Omaha, Nebraska

JOHN C. CHENG, MD
Clinical Associate Professor
Department of Family Medicine
David Geffen School of Medicine at UCLA
Los Angeles, California;
Clinic Director
Department of Family Medicine
Harbor – UCLA Medical Center
Torrance, California

DANIEL S. CLARK, MD, FACC
Assistant Clinical Professor
Department of Family Medicine
David Geffen School of Medicine at UCLA
Los Angeles, California;
Director of Medicine and Cardiology
Ventura County Medical Center
Ventura, California

DEBORAH S. CLEMENTS, MD
Program Director
Associate Professor
Department of Family Medicine
University of Kansas Medical Center
Kansas City, Kansas

STEPHEN W. COBB, MD, FAAFP
Medical Director
Exempla Physician Network
Denver, Colorado

DEAN S. COLLIER, PHARMD, BCPS
Assistant Professor
Department of Pharmacy Practice
University of Nebraska College of Pharmacy
Omaha, Nebraska

MARY CORRIGAN, MD
Assistant Professor
Department of Family Medicine
Case Western Reserve University
Cleveland, Ohio

W. SCOTT CRAIG, PSYD
Clinical Psychologist
Department of Psychological and Behavioral Health
Cabarrus Family Medicine
Condord, North Carolina

DAN F. CRISWELL, MD
Faculty
Southwest Oklahoma Family Medicine
Residency Clinical Professor
Department of Family and Preventive Medicine
University of Oklahoma Health Science Center
Oklahoma City, Oklahoma

D. TODD DETAR, DO
Clinical Professor
Department of Family Medicine
Medical University of South Carolina
Charleston, South Carolina

SHARON L. DIAMOND-MYRSTEN, MD
Visiting Assistant Professor of Family Medicine
Department of Family Medicine
University of Virginia
Charlottesville, Virginia;
Community Physician
Department of Family Medicine
Centra Health
Lynchburg, Virginia

GRETCHEN DICKSON, MD
University of Missouri-Kansas City School of Medicine
Department of Community and Family Medicine
Kansas City, Missouri

ELIZABETH EDDY–BERTRAND, MD
Family Practice
Northridge, California

RICHARD B. ENGLISH, MD, MHA
Associate Dean for Regional Campus Development
Department of Family Medicine and Community Medicine
The Commonwealth Medical College
Scranton, Pennsylvania;
Active Staff
Department of Family Medicine
Wilkes Barre General Hospital
Wilkes Barre, Pennsylvania

JOSEPH S. ESHERICK, MD, FAAFP
Associate Professor of Family Medicine
Department of Family Medicine
David Geffen School of Medicine at UCLA
Los Angeles, California;
Associate Director of Medicine/Medical ICU Director
Department of Internal Medicine
Ventura County Medical Center
Ventura, California

T. EDWIN EVANS, MD
Associate Professor
Department of Family Medicine
Medical University of South Carolina
Charleston, South Carolina;
Chair
Department of Family Medicine
Oconee Medical Center
Seneca, South Carolina

EVELYN FIGUEROA, MD
Assistant Professor of Clinical and Family Medicine
University of Illinois at Chicago
Chicago, Illinois

ALAN FISCHLER, MD
Martinsburg Veterans Administration
Martinsburg, West Virginia

TINA M. FLORES, MD
Assistant Professor
Department of Family Medicine
University of Nebraska Medical Center
Omaha, Nebraska

DEAN GIANAKOS, MD
Associate Director
Lynchburg Family Medicine Residency
Centra Health
Lynchburg, Virginia

HEATH A. GRAMES, PhD
Assistant Professor and Program Director
Marriage and Family Therapy Program
Department of Child and Family Studies
University of Southern Mississippi
Hattiesburg, Mississippi

DAVID S. GREGORY, MD, FAAFP
Assistant Clinical Professor
Department of Family Medicine
University of Virginia
Charlottesville, Virginia;
Faculty Physician
Department of Family Medicine
Lynchburg General Hospital
Lynchburg, Virginia

SAMUEL NEIL GRIEF, MD
Associate Professor of Clinical Family Medicine
Faculty Attending
Department of Family Medicine
University of Illinois at Chicago
Chicago, Illinois

GEORGE D. HARRIS, MD, MS
Professor
Assistant Dean Year 1 and 2 Medicine
Sports Medicine Fellowship Faculty
University of Missouri-Kansas City School of Medicine
Kansas City, Missouri

JEFFREY D. HARRISON, MD
Professor and Program Director
Department of Family Medicine
Assistant Dean for Admissions and Student Affairs
College of Medicine
University of Nebraska Medical Center
Omaha, Nebraska

JOEL J. HEIDELBAUGH, MD
Clinical Assistant Professor
Department of Family Medicine
University of Michigan Medical School
Ann Arbor, Michigan;
Medical Director
Ypsilanti Health Center
Ypsilanti, Michigan

CHRISTINE CRISCUOLO HIGGINS, MD
Family Medicine Residency Program
CHRISTUS Santa Rosa – City Center
San Antonio, Texas

SHERRY HUANG, MD
Department of Family Medicine
Palo Alto Medical Foundation
Palo Alto, California

MARK K. HUNTINGTON, MD, PhD, FAAFP
Associate Professor
Department of Family Medicine
Sanford School of Medicine
The University of South Dakota;
Assistant Director
Sioux Falls Family Medicine Residency Program
Center for Family Medicine
Sioux Falls, South Dakota

ROGENA JOHNSON, MD
Department of Family Medicine
The University of Kansas School of Medicine
Kansas City, Kansas

CRYSTAL L. JONES, MD
Senior Medical Officer
Department Head of Family Medicine
Department Head of Military Medicine
Naval Station Ingleside
Ingleside, Texas

SUNITA KALRA, MD
Private Practice
Mesa, Arizona

SHAILENDRA KAPOOR, MD
Family Medicine
Bon Secours Richmond Health System
Aylett, Virginia

LARRY KARRH, MD, FAAFP
Family Medicine Residency Program
CHRISTUS Santa Rosa Health Care
San Antonio, Texas

MARY PARKS LAMB, MD
Private Practice
Canonsburg, Pennsylvania

MARK LEPORE, MD
Hospitalist, Family, Physician
Ventura County Medical Center
Ventura, California

MARCIA M. LU, MD
Clerkship Director, Assistant Professor
Department of Family and Community Medicine
University of Nevada School of Medicine
Department of Family Medicine
Renown Regional Medical Center
Department of Family Medicine
Saint Mary's Regional Medical Center
Reno, Nevada

PAUL LYONS, MD
Associate Chair
Family and Community Medicine
Temple University School of Medicine;
Associate Chair
Family and Community Medicine
Temple University Hospital
Philadelphia, Pennsylvania

ROBERT MALLIN, MD
Professor
Department of Family Medicine, Psychiatry
   and Behavioral Science
Medical University of South Carolina
Charleston, South Carolina

DAVID MCBRIDE, MD
Assistant Professor
Department of Family Medicine
Director
Department of Student Health Services
Boston University;
Attending Physician
Department of Family Medicine
Boston Medical Center
Boston, Massachusetts

CATHERINE McCARTHY, MD
Associate Professor
Department of Family and Community Medicine
University of Nevada School of Medicine
Reno, Nevada

KARL E. MILLER, MD
Private Practice
Chattanooga, Tennessee

SHERRI L. MORGAN, MD, MPH, ABFM
Clinical Faculty
Department of Family Medicine
Wright State University Boonshooft School of Medicine
Dayton, Ohio;
Chair
Department of Family Medicine
Assistant Program Director
Mount Carmel Family Medicine Residency Program
Mount Carmel St. Ann's Hospital
Westerville, Ohio;
Clinical Faculty
Department of Family Medicine
The Ohio State University College of Medicine
Columbus, Ohio

ARWA NASIR
Department of Emergency Medicine—Pediatrics
Children's Hospital & Medical Center
Omaha, Nebraska

LAETH NASIR, MD
Professor; Chairman of the Department of Family
Creighton University School of Medicine
Family Medicine Physician
Creighton Medical Associates
Omaha, Nebraska

JENNIFER M. NATICCHIA, MD
Department of Family Medicine
Christiana Care Family Medicine Center
Wilmington, Delaware

KATHLEEN NURENA, MD
Family Medicine Clerkship Director/Faculty
Department of Family Medicine
Columbia College of Physicians and Surgeons
New York, New York;
Department of Family Medicine
Stamford Hospital
Stamford, Connecticut;
Clinical Instructor
Department of Family Medicine
University of Connecticut
Farmington, Connecticut

DEEPAK PATEL, MD, FAAFP
Assistant Professor
Department of Family Medicine
Rush Medical College
Chicago, Illinois;
Director of Sports Medicine
Rush-Copley Family Medicine Residency
Aurora, Illinois;
Family Medicine and Sports Medicine
Yorkville Primary Care
Yorkville, Illinois

HIMADRI M. PATEL, DO
Attending Physician
Department of Family Medicine
Northridge Hospital Medical Center
Northridge, California

ILABEN BHAGUBHAI PATEL, MD
Assistant Professor
Department of Family Medicine
Meharry Medical College
Staff Medical Doctor
Department of Family Medicine
Metro General Hospital
Nashville, Tennessee

PRITESH PATEL, DC
Private Practice
Lombard, Illinois

AUDREY PAULMAN, MD
Clinical Associate Professor
Department of Family Medicine
University of Nebraska Medical Center
Omaha, Nebraska

PAUL M. PAULMAN, MD
Assistant Dean for Clinical Skills and Quality
Professor and Predoctoral Director
University of Nebraska College of Medicine
Department of Family Medicine
Omaha, Nebraska

ROGER PAULMAN, MD
Pulmonary Fellow
Department of Pulmonary and Critical Care
University of Nebraska Medical Center
Omaha, Nebraska

STEPHANUS PHILIP, MD
Clinical Instructor
Department of Family Medicine
University of California
Los Angeles School of Medicine
Los Angeles, California;
Staff Hospitalist Physician
Department of Medicine
Ventura County Medical Center
Ventura, California

YVES-MARIO PIVERGER, MD
Department of Family Practice
MetroSouth Health Center at South Holland
South Holland, Illinois

PATRICIA PLETKE, MD
Clinical Assistant Professor
Department of Family Medicine
University of Virginia
Charlottesville, Virginia;
Medical Director
Centra Hospice of the Hills
Centra Health
Lynchburg, Virginia

MICHAEL J. POLIZZOTTO, MD
Medical Director
Family Medicine Residency Program
University of Illinois College of Medicine – Rockford
Rockford, Illinois

DAVID D. PROUM, MD
Staff Physician
Department of Family Medicine
U.S. Naval Hospital Camp Pendleton
Oceanside, California

STEPHANIE S. RICHARDS, MD
Clinical Instructor
Department of Psychiatry
University of Pittsburgh School of Medicine
Attending Psychiatrist
Department of Family Medicine
UPMC Shadyside
Pittsburgh, Pennsylvania

ROBERTO RODRIGUEZ
Private Practice
Miami, Florida

ALAN R. ROTH, DO, FAAFP
Assistant Clinical Professor
Department of Family Medicine
Albert Einstein College of Medicine
Bronx, New York;
Chairman
Department of Family Medicine
Jamaica Hospital Medical Center
Jamaica, New York

SETH RUBIN, MD, MSCP
Department of Family Medicine
University of Pittsburgh School of Medicine
Pittsburgh, Pennsylvania

TED C. SCHAFFER, MD
Clinical Associate Professor
Family Medicine
University of Pittsburgh School of Medicine
Director of Family Medicine Residency Program
UPMC St. Margaret Hospital
Pittsburgh, Pennsylvania

L. PETER SCHWEIBERT, MD
Professor
Department of Family Medicine
University of Oklahoma Health Sciences Center
Oklahoma City, Oklahoma

DEAN THOMAS SCOW, MD
Clinical Assistant Professor
Department of Family Medicine
University of Colorado School of Medicine
Denver, Colorado
Faculty
St. Mary's Family Medicine Residency
Grand Junction, Colorado

KATHRYN A. SEITZ, MD
Associate Director
Family Medicine Residency Program
Exempla Saint Joseph Hospital
Denver, Colorado

VANATHI A. SIDDAIAH, MD
Assistant Professor
Department of Family Medicine
University of Mississippi
Jackson, Mississippi

EVAN SIHOTANG, MD
Resident Family Physician
Department of Family Medicine
Northridge Hospital Medical Center
Family Medicine Residency Program
Northridge, California

AMANPREET SINGH, MD
Urgent Care
Casa Grande Regional Medical Center
Casa Grande, Arizona

DAN SONTHEIMER, MD, MBA
Vice President Medical Affairs
Family Medicine
CoxHealth, Inc.
Springfield, Missouri

TRAVIS STEPHENSEN, MD
Private Practice
Nebraska

RICHARD STRINGHAM, MD
Assistant Professor Clinical Family Medicine
Department of Family Medicine
College of Medicine
University of Illinois at Chicago
University of Illinois Medical Center
Chicago, Illinois

JEREMY W. SZETO, DO
Private Practice
Family Medicine
Sugar Land, Texas

TODD A. THAMES, MD
Program Director and Chair
Family Medicine Residency Program
CHRISTUS Santa Rosa Health Care
Clinical Assistant Professor of Family Medicine
Family and Community Medicine
University of Texas Health Sciences Center at San Antonio
San Antonio, Texas

TERRY J. THOMPSON, MD
Assistant Clinical Professor of Family Medicine
University of Virginia School of Medicine
Virginia Commonwealth University School of Medicine
Lynchburg Family Medicine Residency
Family Medicine
Centra Health
Lynchburg, Virginia

MONTY VANBEBER, MD
Staff Physician
Department of Family Medicine
Colmery-O'Neil VA Medical Center
Topeka, Kansas

BRADFORD S. VOLK, MD
Physician
Department of Family Medicine
U.S. Naval Hospital Yokosuka
Yokosuka, Japan

JACQUELINE WEAVER-AGOSTONI, DO, MPH
Family Medicine
University of Pittsburgh
Director of Pediatric Education
Family Medicine Residency
UPMC Shadyside Hospital
Pittsburgh, Pennsylvania

MICHELLE WHITEHURST-COOK, MD
Associate Professor of Family Medicine
Associate Dean for Admissions
Virginia Commonwealth University School of Medicine
Associate Professor of Family Medicine
Virginia Commonwealth University Health Systems
Richmond, Virginia

JAMILA WILLIAMS, MD, MPH
Associate Program Director Preventive Medicine Residency
Assistant Professor
Department of Family and Community Medicine
Division of Preventive and Occupational Medicine
Meharry Medical College
Nashville, Tennessee

STEVEN R. WOLFE, DO, MPH
Program Director
Osteopathic Graduate Medical Education
Director of Undergraduate Medical Education
Forbes Family Medicine Residency Program
The Western Pennsylvania Hospital
Monroeville, Pennsylvania

BRYAN WONG, MD
Clinical Instructor
Family Medicine
University of California
Los Angeles, California;
Faculty
Family Medicine
Ventura County Medical Center
Ventura, California

ROGER ZOOROB, MD, MPH, FAAFP
Professor and Chair of Family Medicine
Meharry Medical College
Nashville, Tennessee

Contents

CHAPTER 1

Abdominal Pain
Joel J. Heidelbaugh

The most widely accepted recommendations for the management of acute abdominal pain in the office and emergency department settings are summarized in a consensus statement from the American College of Emergency Physicians (ACEP), a clinical policy for the initial evaluation and management of patients presenting with a chief complaint of nontraumatic acute abdominal pain. These guidelines recommend against restricting the differential diagnosis solely by the location of pain, as well as not using the presence or absence of a fever to distinguish potential surgical from medical etiologies of abdominal pain. In cases in which the diagnosis is unclear, serial abdominal examinations over several hours or ancillary testing may help improve the diagnostic accuracy in patients with unclear causes of abdominal pain. Stool for occult blood testing, as well as a pelvic examination in females, should be strongly considered in all patients.

The ACEP statement recommends that patients at a high risk for atypical presentations of acute abdominal pain should be identified early in their presentation to avoid potential misdiagnosis. An electrocardiogram (ECG) should be considered in older adult patients, in those with cardiac risk factors, and in diabetic patients with upper abdominal pain of unclear etiology. A pregnancy test should be obtained in women of childbearing potential. The diagnosis of appendicitis should be considered (though testing may not be required) in women with pelvic inflammatory disease or urinary tract infections because occasionally pelvic examination findings and urinalysis may be positive in patients whose pain is caused by an inflamed appendix. Appropriate narcotic analgesia should be provided to patients being evaluated for abdominal pain in the emergency department.

This chapter focuses on several of the most common conditions related to the gastrointestinal (GI) system. Conditions that may cause significant abdominal pain include cardiovascular, gynecologic, pulmonary, renal, and other various etiologies.

GASTROINTESTINAL

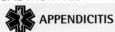 **APPENDICITIS**

Symptoms
- Right lower quadrant (RLQ) migratory abdominal pain +++++
- Fever ++++

- Anorexia +++
- Nausea +++
- Vomiting +++
- Tenesmus ++

Signs

- Abdominal tenderness and guarding (may indicate peritoneal irritation) +++++
- Tenderness at McBurney's point (two thirds of the distance from the umbilicus along a straight line to the anterior superior iliac spine of the pelvis) ++++
- Rovsing's sign (referred tenderness from the left lower quadrant [LLQ] to the RLQ during palpation) +++
- Psoas sign (pain elicited by extending the hip posteriorly with the patient lying prone) ++
- Obturator sign (pain elicited by abducting the right hip with the patient lying supine) ++

Note: No sign or symptom has been shown to be completely reliable in predicting acute appendicitis.

Workup

- The patient may walk in a flexed or guarded fashion, alerting the clinician to consider peritoneal irritation due to ruptured appendix.
- Auscultation of bowel sounds is not considered to be helpful in examining a child for potential appendicitis because they tend to be hypoactive or absent once peritonitis occurs after appendiceal perforation.
- Rectal examination should be performed to rule out anorectal pathology (e.g., abscess).
- In the past, it was thought that pain medications should not be administered prior to surgical evaluation. Recent literature demonstrates the safety of this practice, which may in fact improve the reliability of abdominal examination.
- No laboratory studies have been proven to be adequately predictive of acute appendicitis. Complete blood count with platelets and differential (CBCPD) do not have adequate sensitivity or specificity to be particularly useful. Urinalysis may be helpful, but may be falsely positive or negative.
- A urine pregnancy test should be performed to rule out complications of pregnancy such as ectopic pregnancy in women of childbearing age.
- Recent advances in computed tomography (CT) scan technology and accuracy have led to increased reliance on CT for diagnosis. Diagnostic imaging is not necessarily required when there is either a high or low probability of appendicitis, when a clinical diagnosis can be made.
- Plain film radiographs of the abdomen may reveal a fecalith in the appendix in 10% of cases, but are not routinely ordered because they are almost never diagnostic.
- Ultrasound (US) may be advantageous in thin patients. CT is the preferred choice in obese patients.

- If the abdominal CT does not show evidence of acute appendicitis, the patient may either be admitted for observation or discharged at the discretion of the examiner and/or parents with instructions for follow-up if symptoms worsen.

Comments and Treatment Considerations

In major U.S. hospital centers, the incidence of appendiceal perforation in the general pediatric population ranges from 20% to 40%. These patients are often dehydrated and toxic appearing with obvious physical signs of peritonitis, and should be immediately fluid resuscitated and treated with broad-spectrum antibiotics prior to being taken to the operating room.

There is a small subgroup of patients with appendiceal perforations in whom the diagnosis is missed or who do not present for medical evaluation until late in the course of the illness. In these patients who may have been ill for a period of 7 to 10 days, radiographic studies often reveal a walled-off abscess or phlegmon in the RLQ. These patients can often be treated medically and have their abscesses drained percutaneously by an interventional radiologist, then sent home to convalesce when stable. After 6 weeks, surgeons may opt to perform an interval appendectomy.

After completion of a careful history and physical examination and equivocal laboratory and imaging studies, there are still patients in whom a diagnosis of appendicitis remains unclear. A diagnostic laparoscopy is an acceptable procedure in this group of patients, and during the procedure the appendix should generally be resected, regardless of appearance, and sent to pathology.

Whether an appendectomy should be performed via traditional open laparotomy or via laparoscopy is debatable. Guidelines recommend that the primary modality should be the surgeon's choice because equivalent success and complication risks are seen following both procedures. In obese patients the laparoscopic approach may have an advantage, yielding decreased operating time and a shorter hospital stay.

Preoperative antibiotics should be routinely administered as soon as possible after presentation in all patients with appendicitis. Evidence to support the use of any specific antibiotic or combination of antibiotics is lacking. Broad-spectrum antibiotics may provide effective coverage but may also increase the risk of susceptibility to multidrug-resistant organisms.

Infectious complications related to appendicitis include intraabdominal abscesses, peritonitis, and wound infection. Rates of postoperative wound infection vary between 6% and 50% based primarily on antibiotic coverage and perforated versus nonperforated appendicitis. Antibiotics should be discontinued once the patient is afebrile, tolerates a regular diet, and demonstrates a normal white blood cell (WBC) count without a leftward shift to band neutrophils.

Feeding the patient after perforated appendicitis may be instituted when any ileus or bowel obstruction secondary to the perforation has resolved as indicated by a flat, soft abdomen and the presence of flatulence.

Education for the patient and family should address the treatment plan, advancement of diet, pain management, antibiotic administration if indicated, incision care, signs and symptoms of infection to watch for, when to return to school or daycare, and the need for follow-up appointments.

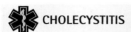 CHOLECYSTITIS

See Chapter 28, Jaundice.

Constipation and Fecal Impaction
Constipation is a common symptom with a wide variety of interpretation from patients regarding its etiology and the actual frequency of stooling; it is commonly defined as passing fewer than three stools per week. Many patients attempt to remedy their constipation with over-the-counter laxatives with modest success. For some patients, especially children, constipation and fecal impaction can become a chronic condition that requires a detailed workup to rule out functional and/or systemic disease conditions.

Symptoms
• Diffuse, crampy abdominal pain +++

Signs
• Often physical examination is unremarkable. ++++
• Physical examination may provide clues to systemic disease that contributes to constipation (e.g., hypothyroidism). ++
• Abdominal mass, potentially palpated in a child or thin adult ++

Workup
• Evaluation may include flexible sigmoidoscopy, barium enema, or colonoscopy in patients with protracted constipation that has not resolved spontaneously and in older patients for whom change in bowel habits may require further evaluation to rule out tumor or other pathology.
• Serum electrolytes, thyroid function tests, blood glucose, and serum calcium to evaluate for a metabolic disorder that may cause constipation, but this is a very uncommon cause
• Fecal occult blood testing (FOBT) as a screen for GI lesions
• Anorectal manometry may be indicated to rule out Hirschsprung's disease.
• Rectal biopsy may also be indicated in the workup of Hirschsprung's disease. Full-thickness rectal wall mucosa and muscularis must be obtained to adequately exclude the presence of myenteric ganglia.

Comments and Treatment Considerations
Symptoms may be improved by lifestyle changes, including exercise and allowing adequate time to defecate. Increase dietary fiber

through fruits, vegetables, grains, or supplemental fiber, for example. Increase fluid (water) intake. Avoid medications that may worsen symptoms (e.g., opioids, calcium channel blockers). Liberal laxative use, including mineral oil, lactulose or polyethylene glycol (PEG) may be helpful. Sometimes a vicious cycle develops: constipation is relieved by laxatives or cathartics; the patient has no urge to pass stool for several days because the bowel has been evacuated; the patient has no urge to pass stool for several days and becomes concerned; then the patient perceives constipation again and resumes laxatives. Fecal impaction may be broken manually during digital rectal examination. If this is not successful, the mass may be softened by warm water or saline lavage through a sigmoidoscope or rectal tube, or via a mineral oil enema. Rarely, surgical removal of the impaction is necessary. A combination of behavioral and medication therapy and maintenance management yields the most favorable outcomes in children with functional constipation and soiling.

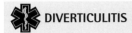 **DIVERTICULITIS**

Diverticulosis refers to the presence of diverticula, or herniations of the intestinal mucosa and submucosa, commonly present in the sigmoid colon. More than half of patients older than 50 years have incidental colonic diverticula. *Diverticulitis* is the most frequent complication of diverticulosis, occurring in up to 20% of patients, and results from a microperforation of a diverticulum by the presence of inspissated fecal material that often becomes a phlegmon, or a pericolic or intra-abdominal abscess.

Symptoms

- Most people with colonic diverticula are asymptomatic; in contrast, abdominal pain is the presenting symptom in almost all patients with diverticulitis. Other presentations are rare except in older adults and diabetic patients in whom abdominal infections may sometimes present with minimal abdominal complaints and findings. Some may complain of chronic or intermittent LLQ abdominal pain. ++++
- RLQ pain + (in some Asian populations +++)
- Infrequent bowel movements or constipation +++
- Flatulence ++
- Dyspepsia ++
- Nausea ++
- Vomiting ++
- Constipation ++
- Diarrhea ++
- Dysuria +
- Urinary frequency +
- Symptoms may overlap with irritable bowel syndrome (IBS), inflammatory bowel disease (IBD), colon cancer, ischemic colitis, bowel obstruction, and gynecologic and urologic disorders.

Signs
- LLQ tenderness +++++
- Fever ++++
- Leukocytosis ++++
- RLQ tenderness + (in some Asian populations +++)

Workup
- The American Society of Colon and Rectal Surgeons' parameters for the treatment of diverticulitis state that if a patient's clinical picture clearly suggests acute diverticulitis based on symptomatology, the diagnosis can be made on the basis of clinical criteria alone.
- The need for additional tests in a patient with suspected diverticulitis is determined by the severity of the presenting signs and symptoms and security of the diagnosis of diverticulitis.
- CT scan with oral, rectal, and intravenous (IV) contrast has become increasingly used as the initial imaging test for patients with suspected diverticulitis, particularly when moderate severity disease or abscess is anticipated. Due to the risks of extravasation of contrast from a potential colonic perforation in the patient with acute diverticulitis, barium enemas should be avoided in patients in whom perforation is a significant consideration.
- Criteria for the diagnosis of diverticulitis via water-soluble contrast enema include the presence of diverticula, mass effect, intramural mass, sinus tract, and extravasation of contrast.
- US may reveal bowel wall thickening, abscess, and rigid hyperechogenicity of the colon due to inflammation and may be helpful in female patients to exclude pelvic or gynecologic pathology.
- Criteria for the diagnosis of diverticulitis include colonic wall thickening, pericolic fat infiltration ("streaky" fat), pericolic or distant abscesses, and extraluminal air.
- CT is not sufficiently sensitive to differentiate cancer from diverticulitis and must be followed after acute treatment by contrast enema or endoscopy.
- Endoscopy is commonly avoided in the setting of acute diverticulitis because of the risk of perforating the inflamed colon, either with the instrument itself or by the insufflation of air.
- In situations in which the diagnosis of acute colonic diverticulitis is uncertain, limited flexible sigmoidoscopy with minimum insufflation of air may be performed to exclude other diagnoses.

Comments and Treatment Considerations
The decision of whether to proceed with inpatient or outpatient treatment of diverticulitis depends on the clinical judgment of the physician, the severity of the disease process, and the likelihood that the patient's condition will respond to outpatient therapy.

Patients who are able to tolerate a diet, who do not have systemic symptoms, and who do not have significant peritoneal signs may be treated on an outpatient basis with trimethoprim-sulfamethoxazole (TMP-SMX) or a fluoroquinolone plus metronidazole for 10 days. Conservative treatment results in resolution in 70% to 100% of cases.

A single dose of an IV antibiotic with coverage against gram-negative aerobes, either IV quinolone and metronidazole or oral TMP-SMX and metronidazole has been shown to be as effective as combination therapy in acute diverticulitis. A common regimen used is levofloxacin and metronidazole (Flagyl).

If the patient does not improve after several days, a colonic abscess should be suspected and diagnostic imaging should be considered.

After recovering from an initial episode of diverticulitis and when the inflammation has settled, the patient should be reevaluated. Appropriate examinations include a combination of flexible sigmoidoscopy and single- or double-contrast barium enema or colonoscopy.

Eventual resumption of a high-fiber diet is recommended after acute inflammation resolves; long-term fiber supplementation after the first episode of diverticulitis has been shown to prevent recurrence in more than 70% of patients followed up for more than 5 years.

Surgical treatment of diverticulitis, in the acute and chronic settings, has been successfully accomplished by laparoscopic and laparoscopic-assisted techniques. Primary colonic resection and anastomosis without a protective stoma has become the surgical treatment of choice for uncomplicated diverticulitis and may also be performed for patients with localized pericolic or pelvic abscesses.

Factors considered when deciding whether to proceed with resection include physiologic age of the patient; the number, severity, and interval of the attacks of diverticulitis; the rapidity and degree of response to medical therapy; and the persistence of symptoms after an acute attack of diverticulitis.

The risk of recurrent symptoms after an attack of diverticulitis ranges from 7% to 45%. With each recurrent episode, the patient is less likely to respond to medical therapy (70% chance of response to medical therapy after the first attack compared with a 6% chance after the third). Thus after two attacks of uncomplicated diverticulitis, resection is commonly recommended.

Free perforation of acute diverticulitis with fecal or purulent peritonitis is a surgical emergency that requires immediate resuscitation with IV fluids, broad-spectrum antibiotics, cardiovascular support (when indicated), and prompt operative therapy.

DYSPEPSIA

Dyspepsia (literally, "bad digestion") accounts for approximately 5% of all visits to family practitioners and is the most common reason for a referral to a gastroenterologist in the United States, comprising 20% to 40% of consultations. The lack of a standardized definition affects accurate prevalence data, given the challenge of clearly defining dyspepsia as either *functional* or *non-ulcer dyspepsia* (NUD) (approximately 60% of cases), or that caused by structural or biochemical disease (40% of cases). Regardless of cause, dyspepsia has a profoundly negative effect on patients' health-related quality of life (HRQOL) and provides a significant economic burden.

Studies examining factors that drive a primary care provider's decision to refer a patient for a gastroenterologic evaluation of dyspepsia are lacking. As a consequence, many patients with organic dyspepsia due to gastroesophageal reflux disease (GERD), peptic ulcer disease (PUD), or even malignancy are most often managed empirically in primary care. Formal management strategies of uninvestigated dyspepsia have been designed to reduce the number of endoscopic procedures, and ultimately, direct cost and inconvenience to the patient (Fig. 1-1).

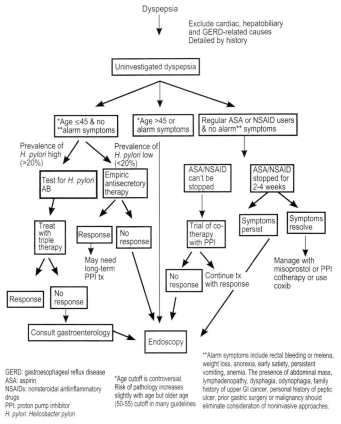

FIGURE 1-1 Evaluation of uninvestigated dyspepsia. *(Adapted from Saad R, Scheiman JM: Diagnosis and management of peptic ulcer disease, Clin Fam Pract 6:569-587, 2004.)*

Symptoms

- Episodic or recurrent epigastric "aching," "gnawing," or "hunger-like" pain or discomfort arising from the proximal GI tract on an empty stomach commonly relieved by meals ++++
- Gastric ulcer pain often occurs 5 to 15 minutes after eating and remains until the stomach empties, which may be up to several hours in duration, whereas epigastric pain is otherwise absent during times of fasting. ++++
- Pain caused by duodenal ulcers is often relieved by eating, drinking milk, or taking antacids, and may return anywhere from 90 minutes to 4 hours after eating a meal. ++++
- Both classifications of ulcers may be associated with nausea and vomiting occurring anytime shortly after eating to several hours later. ++++
- Indigestion ++++
- Heartburn +++
- Bloating +++
- Nausea commonly occurs in the setting of a gastric outlet obstruction, due to either the scarring from ulcer healing or inflammation with impaired gastric emptying. ++
- Pain may radiate to the back (suggestive of a penetrating ulcer of the posterior duodenum that erodes the pancreas). ++
- Regurgitation ++
- Early satiety ++

Signs

- Physical examination is often unreliable ++++
- Rigidity of the abdomen and absent bowel sounds suggest perforation. ++++
- Occasional upper abdominal or epigastric tenderness and guarding +++
- Weight loss ++

Workup

- FOBT
- Upper endoscopy is the preferred diagnostic modality. Some clinicians may prefer barium radiographic studies due to their availability compared to the upper endoscopy.
- Long-term cost comparisons have been shown to favor endoscopy over other diagnostic modalities, and patients have been found to actually prefer endoscopy to that of barium radiographic studies in the diagnosis of PUD.
- Upper endoscopy provides the distinct advantage of permitting biopsies and/or brushings to identify the presence of underlying pathology, namely *Helicobacter pylori* and malignancy.

Comments and Treatment Considerations—*Helicobacter pylori*

Fecal-oral infection with *H. pylori* is a major risk factor for the development of PUD. Its prevalence and association with PUD is higher in populations where the standard of living is considered to be lower than that of the United States, especially in Africa and Central

America. Approximately 90% of patients worldwide with duodenal ulcers are infected with *H. pylori*, yet in the United States, its association with PUD ranges from 30% to 60%. The strongest evidence to support the role of *H. pylori* as an etiology of PUD is the elimination of ulcer recurrence when the infection has been successfully eradicated.

Patients younger than 45 years with dyspepsia and no alarm symptoms (see Fig. 1-1) should be tested for *H. pylori* infection and then given eradication therapy if positive ("test and treat"), whereas patients older than 45 years and those with alarm symptoms should have prompt endoscopy.

H. pylori–negative patients younger than 45 years of age and without alarm symptoms should be managed empirically for functional dyspepsia.

H. pylori–positive or *H. pylori*–negative patients who do not undergo endoscopy initially should do so if their symptoms persist. The effectiveness of this approach depends on the prevalence of *H. pylori* infection in patients with ulcers in the community because in some geographic areas prevalence may be too low to make this approach effective.

H. pylori testing via nonendoscopic methods includes a quantitative assay for serum immunoglobulin G (IgG) antibodies, the radiolabeled urea breath test, and the stool antigen test. The median sensitivity and specificity for serologic IgG tests are 92% and 83%, respectively. Some patients may have persistently positive IgG antibodies for months to years after eradication therapy, yielding a false-positive result during that period if retested.

The stool antigen test has been recommended by the European *Helicobacter pylori* Study Group as the preferred initial noninvasive diagnostic test; the urea breath test is the recommended standard to determine if *H. pylori* has been successfully eradicated.

Once *H. pylori* has been identified in the setting of PUD, treatment should be initiated regardless of whether there is a history of nonsteroidal antiinflammatory drug (NSAID) use, yet treatment of *H. pylori* alone is not adequate in preventing ulcer recurrence if NSAID therapy is continued or restarted.

Although most *H. pylori*–infected patients do not develop an ulcer, as many as 95% of patients with duodenal ulcers and 80% of those with gastric ulcers are infected. Patient education regarding the need for effective eradication therapy and to encourage adherence to the drug regimen is critical.

A meta-analysis of random controlled trials (RCTs) of *H. pylori* eradication for the treatment of duodenal ulcers found that one ulcer recurrence (evidenced on endoscopy) would be prevented for every 2.8 patients successfully treated. The best evidence-based recommendation for *H. pylori* eradication is for 14-day triple therapy with the use of a proton pump inhibitor (PPI), clarithromycin, and either amoxicillin or metronidazole, yielding eradication rates from 75% to 90%.

Although no studies demonstrate any difference among the available PPIs when used in the triple therapy regimens, the chosen antibiotic has been shown to effect the eradication rates due to various antibiotic resistances. The current resistance rates of *H. pylori* in the United States are 33% for metronidazole, 11% for clarithromycin, and 0% for amoxicillin. The ideal *H. pylori* eradication regimen should reach an intention-to-treat cure rate of 80%.

Patients with documented PUD should have adequate follow-up because further diagnostic testing may be needed to ensure eradication of the *H. pylori* organism, particularly in the case of treatment failure or relapse. Because eradication therapy usually cures PUD, chronic acid suppression therapy should not be needed in most patients who have cleared the *H. pylori* infection and who are not taking NSAIDs.

Among primary care patients with a history of PUD taking chronic acid suppressive therapy, 78% of those treated for *H. pylori* were able to discontinue their therapy.

Comments and Treatment Considerations—NSAIDs
The use and overuse of these medications is the most common cause of PUD in *H. pylori*–negative patients, and up to 60% of unexplained cases of PUD are attributed to unrecognized NSAID use. Independent risk factors that augment the effect of *H. pylori* and/or NSAID-related PUD risk, and may promote ulcer complications include advancing age; a history of PUD or complicated ulcer disease with perforation, penetration, or gastric outlet obstruction; multiple NSAID use (including the concomitant use of low-dose aspirin and an NSAID); and concurrent warfarin or corticosteroid use.

Evidence suggests that smoking may augment the risk of PUD and ulcer complications by impairing gastric mucosal healing. Alcohol use may increase the risk of ulcer complications in NSAID users, but its overall effect in those patients without concomitant liver disease has not been clearly defined. There is no solid evidence to implicate dietary factors in the development of PUD.

It has been recognized that there is an increased familial incidence of PUD, most likely due to the familial clustering of *H. pylori*, and inherited genetic factors. NSAID and aspirin use is frequently associated with symptoms of dyspepsia, even in the absence of PUD. Empiric antisecretory therapy with PPIs is an attractive strategy that involves subjecting only those patients to upper endoscopy who fail to respond to a 4-week course of pharmacotherapy.

The approach to NSAID-related PUD can be divided into primary prevention, the promotion of ulcer healing, and the prevention of recurrence and its complications. The optimal management plan is the avoidance of NSAIDs in high-risk individuals (particularly in older adults), in patients with a history of PUD, and in patients taking corticosteroids and/or anticoagulants.

Management strategies for the primary prevention of NSAID-induced PUD include cotherapy with either a histamine type-2 receptor antagonist (H_2RA) or PPI, and the eradication of *H. pylori*, if present.

INFLAMMATORY BOWEL DISEASE

The incidence of ulcerative colitis (UC) and Crohn's disease is approximately 1.5 to 8 new cases per 100,000 persons per year in the United States. It is more commonly seen among whites and has no specific gender predominance, although some reviews have suggested a male predominance in Crohn's disease and a female predominance in UC. Most patients are diagnosed with IBD between the ages of 15 and 25, and there is a second peak of incidence between 55 and 65 years of age. Genetic factors have been implicated because first-degree relatives of patients with either form of IBD have been shown to have an almost 10% lifetime risk of developing disease, and they commonly present with a similar disease type and course as their affected family member. Environmental factors are also believed to be important in the pathogenesis of IBD. Although remarkably rare in Africa and Asia, the risk of IBD has been shown to increase when individuals migrate to a higher-risk region, such as the United States or Western Europe.

 ULCERATIVE COLITIS

Symptoms
- Crampy lower abdominal pain +++++
- Mild to moderate diarrhea without constitutional symptoms ++++
- The more severe the illness, the greater the number of bowel movements, and the more likely constitutional symptoms such as fever, fatigue, dehydration, and weight loss also occur. ++++
- Can be intermittent with flare-ups and remission can occur without therapy ++
- A minority of patients with UC present with severe or fulminant pancolitis, ranging from an acute abdomen to toxic megacolon. ++

Signs
- Rectal bleeding +++++
- Hematochezia +++++
- Involves the mucosal layer of the sigmoid colon and rectum in the vast majority of cases, causing proctitis and proctosigmoiditis +++++
- When there is proximal spread, it tends to be continuous and symmetric, causing intestinal mucosal inflammation with edema and friability that is visualized from the rectum proximally. +++++
- Pancolitis is caused by inflammatory exudates producing a "backwash ileitis" by way of a patent ileocecal valve, and can cause small bowel involvement. ++++
- Chronic ulcerative colitis with cycles of flares and healing can produce scarring and shortening of the colon. ++++
- Weight loss ++++
- Anemia ++++

CROHN'S DISEASE

Symptoms

- In mild cases, or when only a few inches of the terminal ileum are involved, abdominal pain may be vague, the diarrhea intermittent, and weight loss absent. ++++
- In cases with more extensive small bowel and/or colonic involvement, the presentation often consists of significant abdominal pain (often in the RLQ) and frequent diarrhea. ++++
- Rectal involvement produces more urgent and frequent small, bloody stools as a result of an inflamed, nondistensible rectum. ++++
- Mild to moderate abdominal tenderness ++++
- Postprandial crampy pain can suggest transient small bowel obstruction from inflamed or fibrotic narrowed small bowel segments. +++
- Colonic involvement with Crohn's disease may present similar to that seen in UC, with predominantly bloody diarrhea. +++
- Anorexia +++
- Pallor due to anemia of blood loss of chronic disease +++
- Low-grade fever ++
- Tachycardia secondary to dehydration and diminished blood volume +
- Malnourishment (potential) +

Signs

- Mucosal abnormalities are discontinuous ("skip lesions"), asymmetric, and patchy, which accounts for obstruction, abscesses, and perianal fistulae. Lesions to other organs and skin can also be seen in Crohn's disease. +++++
- Most commonly found in the immunologically rich terminal ileum +++++, and involves the rectum in less than 50% of cases. ++
- Weight loss ++++
- Anemia ++++
- Perianal scarring or fistulae ++++
- May involve any part of the GI tract from the mouth to the anus, including the gallbladder and biliary tree, and involves the entire thickness of the bowel wall ++++
- Endoscopic appearance of "rake marks" or "cobblestone patterns" ++++
- Recurrent disease flares and healing of the disease can result in significant muscular hypertrophy and fibrosis of the intestinal wall that lead to small bowel strictures, upstream dilation of intestine and increased fistula formation, eventual bowel obstruction and the imminent need for surgical intervention. ++++
- Abdominal distention +++
- Rebound tenderness, absence of bowel sounds, and high fever may indicate toxic megacolon. +++
- Extraintestinal manifestations of Crohn's disease:
  - Joints—Arthritis, sacroiliitis, ankylosing spondylitis +++
  - Skin—Erythema nodosum, pyoderma gangrenosum ++

- Eyes—Conjunctivitis, iritis ++
- Liver—Fatty infiltration, chronic active hepatitis, primary sclerosing cholangitis, pericholangitis, bile duct carcinoma ++
- Kidneys—Pyelonephritis, renal stones ++
- Oral—Aphthous ulcers ++
- Amyloidosis +

Workup

- Patients presenting with diarrhea containing blood and/or mucus should undergo an appropriate workup including FOBT, fecal leukocytes and lactoferrin, stool cultures, and ova and parasite smears.
- In the vast majority of cases, diarrhea is caused by infections by viral and less commonly bacterial agents. For persistent or recurrent or particularly severe complaints with abdominal findings, a diagnosis of IBD should be considered, and a prompt referral to a gastroenterologist should be arranged.
- Flexible sigmoidoscopy and colonoscopy allow for direct visualization and biopsy of colonic mucosa. Endoscopic biopsy results consistent with nonspecific inflammation are not helpful.
- Patients with explained diarrhea and hematochezia should undergo colonoscopy to rule out cancer.
- Patients with UC and Crohn's disease have an increased risk of colorectal cancer and should be followed with routine surveillance colonoscopy.
- The finding of confluent erythematous rectal inflammation is most consistent with UC and infectious colitis.
- Pseudopolyp formations indicate chronic inflammatory colitis, whereas solitary aphthous ulcers, "rakelike" lesions, strictures, and rectal sparing are consistent with Crohn's disease.
- Colonoscopic evaluation should include ileal intubation and biopsies of both normal and abnormal mucosa. Extreme caution should be taken during colonoscopy given a high risk of iatrogenic perforation.
- Anal or perianal lesions, including sinus tracts, rectovaginal fistulae, and abscesses, is consistent with Crohn's disease but not with UC. The mucosa in a patient with Crohn's disease may appear cobblestoned or nodular. Loss of haustra, distortion of normal architecture, or both may be found.
- Laboratory values usually include an elevated erythrocyte sedimentation rate (ESR) and C-reactive protein (CRP), and decreased hemoglobin and serum albumin, giving an indication of the chronicity and severity of disease.
- An elevated alkaline phosphatase in a patient who has known UC always should raise the question of coexisting primary sclerosing cholangitis.

Comments and Treatment Considerations

Pharmacologic treatment of IBD is aimed at inducing remission and maintaining a symptom-free life, and is often directed after consultation with a gastroenterologist. Treatment of active flares with systemic corticosteroids has been the mainstay of remission-induction therapy and produce remission rates of 70% in Crohn's disease versus 30% with placebo; similar results have been shown in the remission of UC.

Budesonide, a nonsystemic steroid used in an enema formulation, has been shown to be effective for the induction of remission in Crohn's disease and distal UC flares. Mild flares of UC are commonly treated with 5-aminosalicylic acid (5-ASA) derivatives such as sulfasalazine, yet RCTs have shown it is only marginally superior to placebo at controlling flares of Crohn's disease. 5-ASA and mesalamine can be used in enema or suppository formulation for patients with left-sided ulcerative colitis or proctitis; 5-ASA products are used infrequently for the induction of remission in Crohn's disease.

Azathioprine and its metabolite, 6-mercaptopurine, are slow-acting compounds proven to be effective for inducing remission in Crohn's disease. They are often added to systemic steroids to help induce and maintain remission and to ease steroid tapering. Patients using these medications should not be exposed to live vaccines and should receive high priority for annual influenza vaccines and Pneumovax.

Metronidazole and ciprofloxacin have been used for induction of remission in patients with active Crohn's disease. No evidence of benefit in induction of remission in UC has been demonstrated by using antibiotics.

Methotrexate is also effective for the induction of remission in Crohn's disease. Close monitoring of CBCs and serum transaminases is recommended, with monthly testing on initiation and with dosage changes. Pregnancy and exposure to live vaccines should be avoided.

Infliximab, an antitumor necrosis factor-α antibody, is remarkably effective in treating approximately 60% of steroid-resistant patients with Crohn's disease. It has significant side effect risks, including infusion reactions, worsening of heart failure, activation of latent tuberculosis, serum sickness, and invasive fungal infections.

In patients who are in remission and are not receiving maintenance therapy, 50% of those who have Crohn's disease will have a flare within 2 years and approximately 89% of patients who have UC will relapse within 1 year. The risk of undergoing exploratory or bowel resection surgery for complications of Crohn's disease is approximately 60% by 10 years from the diagnosis; this risk increases with an early age at diagnosis and previous surgery for Crohn's disease.

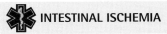 INTESTINAL ISCHEMIA

The spectrum of ischemic bowel disease is broad, and is best divided into acute and chronic mesenteric ischemia, and colonic ischemia. Management of each of these categories of ischemic injury requires its own unique strategy, largely based on descriptive studies and clinical experience summarized in the American Gastroenterological Association guidelines for intestinal ischemia because evidence based on RCTs is lacking.

Symptoms
- Acute mesenteric ischemia—Severe abdominal pain particularly in older adults and those with vascular disease whose clinical picture does not suggest another abdominal diagnosis (e.g., cholecystitis or diverticulitis) ++++
- Chronic mesenteric ischemia ("intestinal angina")—Postprandial abdominal pain and marked weight loss resulting from repeated transient episodes of inadequate intestinal blood flow provoked by the increased metabolic demands associated with digestion ("intestinal angina") ++++
- Colonic ischemia—Mild to moderate abdominal pain, diarrhea, or lower GI bleeding with minimal to moderate abdominal tenderness ++++
- Hematochezia ++++

Signs
- In acute ischemia of the bowel, pain may be severe with abdominal findings coming late at the time of bowel infarction.
- Diffuse or localized abdominal tenderness with guarding and/or rebound tenderness (a late finding) +++++
- Decreased bowel sounds ++++
- Weight loss +++
- Abdominal bruit (nondiagnostic) ++

Workup
- Acute and chronic mesenteric ischemia—Emergent surgical consultation, mesenteric angiography, CT or magnetic resonance imaging (MRI)
- Colonic ischemia—Colonoscopy or barium enema; mesenteric angiography is useful only if the ascending colon is affected

Comments and Treatment Considerations
Acute mesenteric ischemia results from either arterial or venous thrombi, or vasoconstriction secondary to decreased blood flow. Correctly diagnosing this condition prior to intestinal infarction is the single most important factor in minimizing poor outcomes, as reported mortality rates range from 59% to 93%. Patients at risk for acute mesenteric ischemia, most notably those with atherosclerotic disease or procoagulant conditions, who have severe abdominal pain should be promptly evaluated. These patients must be identified early in the clinical course of the disease and treated aggressively if survival is to be improved.

Suspected patients should undergo emergent surgical exploration or mesenteric angiography if another cause for the pain cannot be discovered via abdominal plain film radiography or CT. Vasodilators are widely used in the treatment of nonocclusive mesenteric ischemia, and are strongly suggested for occlusive disease of the superior mesenteric artery. Anticoagulants and thrombolytics have also been used, but rigorous studies comparing their outcomes to that of other modalities are lacking. In patients who develop acute ischemic colitis, expert opinion states that systemic corticosteroids should be avoided.

In patients with chronic mesenteric ischemia, mesenteric angiography commonly demonstrates partial or complete occlusion of at least two of the three major splanchnic vessels, yet these abnormalities alone are not sufficient to diagnose chronic mesenteric ischemia.

Treatment is either surgical or by percutaneous transluminal mesenteric angioplasty with or without stenting. Experience with angiographic treatment modalities is limited, and at present these modalities are best reserved for patients at a high risk for surgical revascularization. High-resolution CT and MRI have been proposed for use in diagnosing chronic mesenteric ischemia, but have not been proven sufficiently sensitive or specific to become a gold standard.

Colonic ischemia is the most common form of intestinal ischemia. Although most cases have no definable cause, it is often associated with a spectrum of disorders including transient colitis, chronic colitis, stricture, gangrene, and fulminant universal colitis. Diagnosis is made via colonoscopy or barium enema in an individual with a typical history.

Broad-spectrum antibiotics are customarily used in treatment, despite an absence of solid clinical evidence supporting their benefit. Although most cases of colonic ischemia have an excellent prognosis and resolve spontaneously, surgery may be required acutely, subacutely, or electively in chronic cases. Surgery is indicated acutely for those patients with peritoneal signs, massive GI bleeding, or fulminant colitis; subacutely for those who do not improve after 2 to 3 weeks or who develop recurrent sepsis; and electively in cases of symptomatic ischemic stricture or chronic colitis.

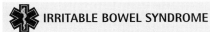 IRRITABLE BOWEL SYNDROME

IBS is one of the most common GI conditions encountered in family practices with a prevalence ranging from 14% to 24% in women and from 5% to 19% in men in the United States and England. The syndrome commonly appears in the late 20s, although it may present in teenagers and in patients as old as age 45; patients older than 45 years with suspected IBS should be evaluated for organic disease. Although the diagnosis of IBS may be a challenging one to make, it is clear that symptoms suggestive of IBS are common, and less than 25% of symptomatic patients seek medical advice for their symptoms. IBS is responsible for approximately 2.4 to 3.5 million physician visits per year in the United States, and represents 12% of primary care visits and 28% of referrals to gastroenterologists.

Studies have indicated that the HRQOL in patients in the United States with IBS is worse than that of patients suffering from clinical depression. Patients who have IBS are much more likely to exhibit health care–seeking behaviors that are related to GI and non-GI complaints. Consultations for non-GI problems are four times more common in this population compared with patients who do not have IBS.

Psychosocial stressors likely exacerbate symptoms in patients with functional GI disorders. Anxiety disorders, somatoform disorders, and a history of physical and/or sexual abuse have been identified in 42% to 61% of patients with IBS who have been referred to gastroenterologists. Patients with IBS have a hypersensitivity to bowel stimulation with stress and lumen exposures to food and bacteria as known exacerbating factors. In addition, autonomic nervous system dysfunction occurs, which has been shown to alter visceral perception and has reproducibly been shown to accelerate large bowel motility and delay gastric emptying. Overlap syndromes with fibromyalgia and interstitial cystitis have led to multidisciplinary approaches to the management of IBS with an emphasis on behavior therapies to improve HRQOL.

Symptoms
- Abdominal pain +++++
- Cramping +++++
- Bloating +++++
- Constipation or diarrhea, or both +++++
- Anxiety ++++
- Depression ++++
- Mucus in stools +++

Signs
- Physical examination is often nonspecific, and may demonstrate a normal abdominal examination, a diffusely tender abdomen, or a focally tender abdomen. ++++
- Voluntary guarding ++++

Workup
- The Rome II criteria are the most widely accepted classification for establishing a diagnosis of IBS (Table 1-1).
- Multiple diagnostic screening tests have been recommended including a CBC, ESR, serum chemistries, thyroid function tests,

Table 1-1. Rome II Criteria for Diagnosis of Irritable Bowel Syndrome

- Abdominal pain or discomfort for at least 12 weeks, although not necessarily contiguous, during the last 12 months
- At least two out of three of the following features:
  - Relief with defecation
  - Onset associated with change in form of the stool
  - Onset with change in the frequency of bowel movements
- Additional supporting features include:
  - Fewer than three bowel movements per week
  - More than three bowel movements per day
  - Hard or lumpy stool

Adapted from Cash BD, Chey WD: Irritable bowel syndrome: a systematic review, *Clin Fam Pract* 6:647-669, 2004.

stool cultures including ova and parasites, FOBT, colonoscopy, and hydrogen breath testing, specifically to rule out other causes of disease.
- Despite these recommendations, diagnostic testing should depend on the pretest probability of organic disease.
- The pretest probability of IBS depends on the presence or absence of alarm symptoms, including hematochezia, fevers, weight loss greater than 10 pounds, chronic severe diarrhea, and family history of colon cancer.
- In the absence of alarm symptoms, diagnostic testing should be limited. Studies have suggested that accurate diagnosis of IBS is imperative (although challenging), and that protracted negative workups may negatively affect symptomatology and outcomes.
- Diagnostic testing may be performed to reassure the clinician as well as the patient, yet the value of reassurance from negative diagnostic testing has never been examined.
- The differential diagnosis of IBS includes IBD, lactose intolerance, acute gastroenteritis, celiac disease, small intestinal bacterial overgrowth, colorectal cancer, and motility-altering metabolic disturbances (e.g., hypo- or hyperthyroidism).

Comments and Treatment Considerations

There is no single evidence-based consistently successful therapeutic approach for patients with IBS. Because it is largely a chronic condition, the goals of therapy should focus on patient reassurance, education about the natural course of the syndrome, and global symptomatic improvement, rather than on disease cure. This is best achieved through a well-developed patient-physician relationship with a clear delineation of realistic goals and expectations. Treatment for symptoms related to IBS is indicated when the patient and physician believe there has been a decrement in HRQOL.

Alosetron, a 5-HT3 antagonist, is indicated for women with diarrhea-predominant IBS, and has also been shown to be more effective than placebo in RCTs. Due to reports of ischemic colitis, the use of alosetron has been limited to physicians participating in the manufacturer's risk management program.

Treatment of diarrhea-predominant IBS can be achieved with the use of loperamide; however, no advantage over placebo for global IBS symptoms has been reported. To date, all other classes of medications used in the management of IBS have a more limited effect on the global symptoms of IBS. The tricyclic antidepressants, selective serotonin reuptake inhibitors (SSRIs), and peppermint oil have been shown to reduce abdominal pain.

Treatment of constipation-predominant IBS can be achieved with fiber-bulking agents. Cognitive behavioral therapy, interpersonal psychotherapy, group therapy, biofeedback, and hypnosis have been shown to improve individual aspects of diarrhea-predominant IBS. Alternative medicine techniques, including acupuncture, probiotic therapy, and Chinese herbal medicine, are becoming increasingly popular in the treatment of GI disorders, and have been shown to have some limited symptomatic improvement in selected cases of IBS.

PANCREATITIS

Mild acute pancreatitis, accounting for almost 80% of all cases, is characterized by parenchymal interstitial edema of the pancreas, and no worse than minimal distal organ dysfunction. Recovery is usually rapid (measured in days) and any distal organs affected by the acute event quickly return to their baseline function. In severe acute pancreatitis, parenchymal and fat necrosis ensues, as well as profound multisystem organ failure, infection, and life-threatening hemodynamic instability. Many patients fall somewhere between these categories.

The causes of acute pancreatitis are diverse and demonstrate changing trends over time and variation by geography. Gallstones, biliary sludge, and microlithiasis are recognized as the proximate cause in well over half of reported cases in several studies from around the world. Ethyl alcohol ingestion is the second most commonly reported cause of acute pancreatitis and accounts for up to 30% of cases. The remaining causes of acute pancreatitis account for less than 15% of total cases by most accounts, including hypertriglyceridemia, trauma, medications, endoscopic retrograde cholangiopancreatography (ERCP), neoplasms, perforated peptic ulcer disease, viral infection, and idiopathic causes. Many of the cases of idiopathic pancreatitis may be due to unrecognized microlithiasis.

Symptoms
- Gnawing epigastric abdominal pain radiating to the back that is commonly constant and can last from hours to days, but most often has been present for more than 24 hours +++++
- Substernal pain, generalized to the left upper quadrant (LUQ) or right upper quadrant (RUQ), or even the lower abdomen, worsened by food or alcohol, and may be precipitated by binge drinking ++++
- Abdominal distention ++++
- Nausea ++++
- Vomiting +++

Signs
- Decreased bowel sounds on auscultation +++
- Small bowel ileus, secondary to diffusion of inflammatory fluid around the pancreas ++
- Low-grade fever of 37.8° to 38.9° C (100° to 102° F) may be present; a temperature in excess of 38.9° C (102° F) suggests another diagnosis or complication ++
- Hypovolemia ++
- Cullen's sign, a periumbilical bluish discoloration +
- Grey Turner's sign, a bluish discoloration of the flanks +
  - *Neither of these signs are specific for pancreatitis and are rarely seen.*

Workup

- Lipase is the serum marker of choice with high sensitivity and specificity. However, lipase level does not predict the severity or course of disease.
- The sensitivity of pancreatic amylase for the diagnosis of acute pancreatitis decreases to less than 30% between the second and fourth day after the onset of the acute episode.
- Amylase levels may be elevated in a variety of nonpancreatic conditions; a small bowel obstruction is the most relevant of these when abdominal pain is of an unclear etiology.
- The clearance of pancreatic amylase is diminished with a decline in renal function, thus may cloud the clinical picture even further.
- By contrast, an elevated serum lipase level can be detected as distant as 14 days after the acute event and has a sensitivity of greater than 90% for acute pancreatitis.
- Early prognostic factors that can be measured and indicate severity of disease include Ranson's criteria and more recently the Acute Physiology and Chronic Health Evaluation II (APACHE II) score (most commonly used).
- One factor considered to be significant in the management of patients with acute pancreatitis is intravascular volume status.
- The hematocrit may be high as a secondary effect of hypovolemia secondary to third spacing of fluids. In many circumstances, patients may be as many as 6 L intravascularly depleted. Volume resuscitation during the first 24 hours is extremely important and may minimize or even prevent pancreatic necrosis.
- If the bilirubin, liver transaminases, and alkaline phosphatase rise, a common bile duct (CBD) stone may exist. Similar lab abnormalities may occur in patients with chronic pancreatitis and a bile duct stricture. This possibility could be further explored with abdominal US and possibly ERCP, which can be both diagnostic and therapeutic.
- Hypocalcemia, hypoalbuminemia, hyperglycemia, and leukocytosis in the range of 15,000 to 20,000 WBC/mL are frequently found. Leukocytosis with more than 20,000 WBC/mL suggests a more severe disease.
- Because respiratory distress syndrome may ensue, chest radiographs and arterial blood gases should be considered. In severe cases, renal failure may appear despite adequate fluid intake, thus urinary output should be closely monitored,
- Contrast-enhanced CT (CECT) is the most extensively studied modality for the confirmation of acute pancreatitis and provides the highest level of sensitivity and specificity among existing imaging technologies. Limitations include overlying gas (often seen with pancreatitis-related ileus), excessive abdominal fat, and distortions of the skin from scarring that can make visualization of the underlying organs less reliable.
- US may be added to CT scan in patients who have suspected acute pancreatitis in the uncommon situation in which the biliary system is not well visualized.

- When the pancreas is visualized in the setting of acute disease, tissue abnormalities are detected in 90% of those studied.
- MRI and magnetic resonance cholangiopancreatography (MRCP) are two newer modalities that have specific yet limited roles in diagnosing acute pancreatitis. In contrast to CT imaging, MRI is more likely to uncover mild disease but requires longer scanning times that necessitate breath-holding for often uncomfortable periods of time within cramped spaces. This modality is of particular use in patients who have allergic reactions to iodinated IV contrast, impaired renal function, or are pregnant and in patients who should not be exposed to ionizing radiation. It is superior to conventional CT imaging at detecting gallstone disease and detailing anatomic anomalies, although experience in its use in the setting of acute pancreatitis is still limited. MRI should be reserved for individuals in whom CT scanning is contraindicated and when mild acute pancreatitis is suspected.

Comments and Treatment Considerations
Medical therapy of acute pancreatitis is primarily supportive, with the major objective being hemodynamic stabilization. Nutritional status and maintenance should be considered early in the course of acute pancreatitis to minimize morbidity and mortality risk.

Most patients are kept NPO until their abdominal pain subsides and appetite returns. After several days, commencement of total parenteral nutrition (TPN) or enteral feeding through a nasojejunal tube (still somewhat controversial) in the absence of a paralytic ileus should be considered. Pain management in the hospital setting is best achieved using morphine derivatives.

CARDIOVASCULAR

 ABDOMINAL AORTIC ANEURYSM

The most common etiology of abdominal aortic aneurysm (AAA) is atherosclerosis. Additional etiologies include genetic diseases (e.g., Ehlers-Danlos syndrome), trauma, cystic medial necrosis (e.g., Marfan's syndrome), arteritis, inflammatory conditions, mycosis, and infection (e.g., syphilis). White males have the highest incidence of AAA; males are affected up to seven times more often than females. More than 75% of patients with AAA are older than age 60.

Symptoms
- Most aneurysms develop slowly over many years and are asymptomatic. ++++
- If an aneurysm expands rapidly or ruptures, or if blood dissects along the wall of the aorta, symptoms may develop suddenly and include:
  - Pulsating sensation in the abdomen ++++
  - Severe, sudden, and persistent abdominal pain that may radiate to groin, back, flank, or legs ++++
  - Abdominal rigidity ++++

- Anxiety ++++
- Nausea +++
- Vomiting +++

Signs
- In incidental cases, especially in thin individuals, a pulsatile mass may be palpated in the midline of the abdomen, yet sensitivity for detection is low when the AAA is less than 5 cm. +++
- In cases of rupture or dissection, cardiogenic shock may occur exhibited by:
  - Tachycardia +++++
  - Hypotension +++++
  - Clammy skin ++++
  - Pallor ++++
  - Venous thrombosis from iliocaval venous compression ++
  - Discoloration and pain of the feet with distal embolization of the thrombus within the aneurysm. ++

Workup
- Abdominal US is nearly 100% sensitive and specific in identifying an AAA and estimating its size. It is not very accurate in estimating the proximal extension to the renal or iliac arteries
- CT is recommended for preoperative AAA imaging and estimating size. The rate of false negatives is extremely low, and the CT scan can localize the proximal extent, detect the integrity of the wall, and rule out rupture.
- Angiography provides detailed arterial anatomy and can localize the aneurysm relative to the renal and visceral arteries.

Comments and Treatment Considerations
In patients with the clinical triad of abdominal and/or back pain, a pulsatile abdominal mass, and hypotension, immediate surgical evaluation is indicated regardless. In patients with AAAs, blood pressure and fasting serum lipid values should be monitored and controlled as recommended for patients with atherosclerotic disease. Patients with aneurysms or a family history of aneurysms should be advised to stop smoking and be offered smoking cessation interventions.

In most cases, according to Lederle (Lederle, 2003), patients with infrarenal or juxtarenal AAAs measuring 5.5 cm or larger should undergo repair to eliminate the risk of rupture. In most cases, patients with infrarenal or juxtarenal AAAs measuring 4.0 to 5.4 cm in diameter should be monitored by US or CT every 6 to 12 months to detect expansion. In patients with AAAs smaller than 4.0 cm in diameter, monitoring by US examination every 2 to 3 years is reasonable.

Surgical intervention is not recommended for asymptomatic infrarenal or juxtarenal AAAs if they measure less than 5.0 cm in diameter in men or less than 4.5 cm in diameter in women. Surgical repair can be beneficial in patients with infrarenal or juxtarenal AAAs 5.0 to 5.4 cm in diameter. Surgical repair is indicated in patients with suprarenal or type IV thoracoabdominal aortic aneurysms larger than 5.5 to 6.0 cm.

Some screening regimens suggest that men 65 years of age or older who are either the siblings or offspring of patients with AAAs should undergo physical examination and US screening for detection of AAAs, and that men who are 65 to 75 years of age who have ever smoked should undergo a physical examination and baseline US screening for detection of AAAs.

Perioperative administration of β-adrenergic blocking agents, in the absence of contraindications may reduce the risk of adverse cardiac events and mortality in patients with coronary artery disease undergoing surgical repair of atherosclerotic aortic aneurysms and their administration should be considered.

Beta-blockers should be considered to reduce the rate of aneurysm expansion in patients with aortic aneurysms. Periodic long-term surveillance imaging should be performed to monitor for an endoleak, to document shrinkage or stability of the excluded aneurysm sac, and to determine the need for further intervention in patients who have undergone endovascular repair of infrarenal aortic and/or iliac aneurysms.

Endovascular repair of infrarenal aortic and/or common iliac aneurysms is reasonable in patients at high risk of complications from open operations because of cardiopulmonary or other associated diseases. Endovascular repair of infrarenal aortic and/or common iliac aneurysms may be considered in patients at low or average surgical risk.

References

American College of Emergency Physicians (ACEP): Clinical policy: critical issues for the initial evaluation and management of patients presenting with a chief complaint of nontraumatic acute abdominal pain, *Ann Emerg Med* 36:406–415, 2000.

American Gastroenterological Association Medical Position Statement: Guidelines on intestinal ischemia. [published erratum appears in *Gastroenterology* 119:280–281, 2000]. *Gastroenterology* 118:951–953, 2000.

American Society of Colon and Rectal Surgeons: Practice parameters for the treatment of sigmoid diverticulitis. Standards Task Force, *Dis Colon Rectum* 43:289, 2000.

Avunduk C: Social impact of digestive diseases. In *Manual of gastroenterology, diagnosis and therapy*, 3rd ed, Philadelphia, 2002, Lippincott Williams & Wilkins.

Brandt LJ, Locke GR, Olden K, et al: Evidence-based position statement on the management of irritable bowel syndrome in North America, *Am J Gastroenterol* 97:S1–S5, 2002.

Cash BD, Chey WD: Irritable bowel syndrome: a systematic review, *Clin Fam Pract* 6:647–669, 2004.

Cincinnati Children's Hospital Medical Center: *Evidence based clinical practice guideline for emergency appendectomy*, Cincinnati, OH, 2002, Cincinnati Children's Hospital Medical Center.

Cutler AF, Havstad S, Ma CK, et al: Accuracy of invasive and noninvasive tests to diagnose *Helicobacter pylori* infection, *Gastroenterology* 109:136–141, 1995.

Department of Health and Human Services: *Abdominal aortic aneurysm (AAA) screening*, Available at www.medicare.gov/Health/AAA.asp (accessed February 2009).

Dickerson LM, King DE: Evaluation and management of nonulcer dyspepsia, *Am Fam Physician* 70:107–114, 2004.

European *Helicobacter pylori* Study Group (EHPSG): Current European concepts in the management of *Helicobacter pylori* infection: the Maastricht Consensus Report, *Gut* 41:8–13, 1997.

Feagan BG: Maintenance therapy for inflammatory bowel disease, *Am J Gastroenterol* 98:S6–S17, 2003.

Felt BT, Brown P, Coran A, et al: Functional constipation and soiling in children, *Clin Fam Pract* 6:709–730, 2004.

Gilbert DN, Moellering RC, Eliopoulos GM, Sande MA: *The Sanford guide to antimicrobial therapy*, 35th ed. Oregon Health Sciences University, Portland, Oregon 2005, Antimicrobial Therapy, Inc.

Halter JM, Baesl T, Nicolette L, Ratner M: Common gastrointestinal problems and emergencies in neonates and children, *Clin Fam Pract* 6:731–754, 2004.

Hernandez-Diaz S, Rodriguez LA: Association between nonsteroidal anti-inflammatory drugs and upper gastrointestinal tract bleeding/perforation: an overview of epidemiologic studies published in the 1990s, *Arch Intern Med* 160:2093–2099, 2000.

Higgins PDR, Zimmerman EM: An evidence-based approach to inflammatory bowel disease, *Clin Fam Pract* 6:671–692, 2004.

Hirsch AT, Haskal ZJ, Hertzer NR, et al: *ACC/AHA 2005 guidelines for the management of patients with peripheral arterial disease (lower extremity, renal, mesenteric, and abdominal aortic): a collaborative report* [trunc], Bethesda, MD, 2005, American College of Cardiology Foundation.

Hopkins RJ, Girardi LS, Turney EA: Relationship between *Helicobacter pylori* eradication and reduced duodenal and gastric ulcer recurrence: a review, *Gastroenterology* 110:1244–1252, 1996.

Jones MP, Lacy BE: Dyspepsia: the spectrum of the problem. In Fass R, editor: *GERD/dyspepsia: hot topics*, Philadelphia, 2004, Hanley and Belfus, pp. 285–302.

Lederle FA, Wilson SE, Johnson GR: Immediate repair compared with surveillance of small abdominal aortic aneurysms, *N Engl J Med* 346:1437–1444, 2002.

Lederle FA: Ultrasonographic screening for abdominal aortic aneurysm, *Ann Intern Med* 139:516–522, 2003.

Mayerle J, Simon P, Lerch MM: Medical treatment of acute pancreatitis, *Gastroenterol Clin North Am* 33:855–869, 2004.

Merkle EM, Gorich J: Imaging of acute pancreatitis, *Eur Radiol* 12:1979–1992, 2002.

Miller AR, North CS, Clouse RE, et al: The association of irritable bowel syndrome and somatization disorder, *Ann Clin Psychiatry* 13:25–30, 2001.

Numans M, van der Graaf Y, de Wit NJ, et al: How much ulcer is ulcer-like? Diagnostic determinates of peptic ulcer in open access gastroscopy, *Fam Pract* 11:382–388, 1994.

Orbuch M: Optimizing outcomes in acute pancreatitis, *Clin Fam Pract* 6:607–629, 2004.

Papachristou GI, Whitcomb DC: Predictors of severity and necrosis in acute pancreatitis, *Gastroenterol Clin North Am* 33:871–890, 2004.

Saad R, Scheiman JM: Diagnosis and management of peptic ulcer disease, *Clin Fam Pract* 6:569–587, 2004.

Salzman H, Lillie D: Diverticular disease: diagnosis and treatment, *Am Fam Physician* 72:1229–1234, 1241–1242, 2005.

Scottish Intercollegiate Guidelines Network (SIGN): *Dyspepsia. A national clinical guideline*, *Edinburgh (Scotland)*, Scottish Intercollegiate Guidelines Network (SIGN); 2003.

Wofford SA, Verne GN: Approach to patients with refractory constipation, *Curr Gastroenterol Rep* 2:389–394, 2000.

CHAPTER 2

Abnormal Vaginal Bleeding
Evelyn Figueroa

The problem of abnormal vaginal bleeding can be daunting, given the vast differential it may represent. When caring for patients with this complaint, it is essential to be systematic during the physical examination and workup. Keeping the focus on common problems is helpful, and risk stratifying the patient will prevent unnecessary testing and save time.

Categorizing the patients as prepubertal, premenopausal, perimenopausal, and postmenopausal is a valuable approach. For prepubertal girls, trauma, abuse and malignancy are frequent causes. In patients younger than 35 years with a normal examination anovulatory causes are responsible for most episodes of irregular vaginal bleeding. In perimenopausal patients, however, endometrial hyperplasia and carcinoma are relatively common; endometrial sampling and pelvic imaging are indicated as part of the initial investigation.

Malignancy is of primary concern when confronted with vaginal bleeding in a postmenopausal woman. Because bleeding may also occur from the lower genital tract, vulvar, vaginal, and cervical causes must be excluded.

PREPUBERTAL VAGINAL BLEEDING

Before menarche, common causes of abnormal vaginal bleeding are trauma, sexual abuse, and malignancy. A careful examination under anesthesia is preferred because more than half of these cases involve a focal lesion of the genital tract and more than 20% are malignant.

Symptoms
- Vaginal bleeding of any quantity
- Pelvic pain
- Dysuria
- Vaginal discharge
- History of blunt trauma to genitals (e.g., falling onto a bicycle bar)

Signs
- Friable cervix
- Malodorous or mucopurulent vaginal discharge
- Genital tract lesion; trauma versus infection versus malignancy
- Pelvic mass on bimanual examination

Workup

- Examination (under anesthesia if necessary) to exclude genital tract lesions and infection
- Wet mount to exclude *Trichomonas* and yeast
- Cervical cultures for *Neisseria gonorrhoeae* and *Chlamydia trachomatis*
- Pelvic ultrasound

Comments and Treatment Considerations

Minimal vaginal bleeding is frequently seen in neonates due to withdrawal from maternal estrogen in the postpartum period. Treatment of sexually transmitted infections and involvement of child welfare agencies in the event of abuse are important aspects of treatment. Evaluation by a pediatric gynecologist for lower genital tract masses should be considered for cases in which the diagnosis is uncertain.

VAGINAL BLEEDING DURING THE REPRODUCTIVE YEARS

During the reproductive years, most causes of irregular bleeding are benign. In patients younger than age 35, the most common cause is pregnancy. Once pregnancy is excluded, the lower genital tract is evaluated for infections, lesions, or trauma. An ultrasound may be performed if fullness is found to rule out fibroids or other masses.

Although anovulatory cycles and uterine leiomyomata are frequently responsible for abnormal vaginal bleeding in the perimenopausal patient, early consideration of malignancy is important as the incidence of genital tract cancers increases dramatically after age 40. Lastly, dysfunctional uterine bleeding (DUB) is a diagnosis of exclusion, only to be made after infectious, endocrine, iatrogenic, anatomic, and malignant causes have been considered.

 VAGINAL BLEEDING IN EARLY PREGNANCY

Pregnancy-related causes vary by gestational age. During the first trimester, pregnancy failure, molar pregnancy, and ectopic pregnancy are considered. In these cases, serum β-human chorionic gonadotropin (β-hCG) levels may be useful. Ultrasonography is a valuable diagnostic tool for confirming a viable pregnancy and appropriate follow-up.

Ectopic Pregnancy

An ectopic pregnancy is one that implants after fertilization in an anatomic location outside of the uterine cavity. The most common location for an ectopic pregnancy is the fallopian tube; other locations include the ovary, abdominal cavity, and uterine cervix. Risk factors for ectopic pregnancy include one or more episodes of salpingitis or pelvic inflammatory disease, surgical manipulation of the fallopian tubes, and a previous ectopic pregnancy. Although there have been reports of ectopic pregnancies reaching term and resulting in the birth of a viable infant, ectopic pregnancies can cause life-threatening hemorrhage and should be treated as a gynecologic emergency.

Symptoms
- Abnormal vaginal bleeding ++++
- Breast tenderness +++
- Amenorrhea +++
- Lower back pain
- Pelvic pain +++
- Nausea

Signs
- Blood from cervical os ++++
- Unilateral pelvic pain +++
- Tender pelvic mass
- Bluish discoloration and softening of cervical os

Workup
- Physical examination including pelvic examination
- Urine pregnancy test
- Serial serum β-hCG as indicated
- Abdominal and/or intravaginal ultrasound
- ABO and Rh determination (to detect patients at risk of maternal Rh sensitization)
- Cervical cultures to rule out infection
- CBC
- Type and crossmatch for blood transfusion if necessary
- Culdocentesis

Comments and Treatment Considerations
Patients suspected of having an ectopic pregnancy should be rapidly assessed with ultrasound, considered the gold standard for diagnosis of this condition. Patients with ectopic pregnancies who are hemodynamically stable may be considered for medical management; those with excessive bleeding or unstable vital signs should be considered for immediate surgical management.

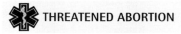 **THREATENED ABORTION**

A threatened abortion is defined as vaginal bleeding during early (<20 weeks) pregnancy, without other definitive cause. It is estimated that up to one third of all intrauterine pregnancies may end as spontaneous abortions. In patients with threatened abortions the cervical os is closed. Vaginal bleeding in pregnancy with an open cervical os may indicate an inevitable, complete, or missed abortion. Vaginal bleeding is common in intrauterine pregnancies; many cases of vaginal bleeding in early pregnancy result in delivery of term infants.

Symptoms
- Vaginal bleeding ++++
- Abdominal or pelvic pain
- Amenorrhea

Signs
- Blood from cervical os ++++
- Closed cervical os ++++
- Enlarged uterus +++
- Cervical softening and bluish discoloration

Workup
- Urine pregnancy test
- CBC
- Pelvic and/or intravaginal ultrasound
- Serum β-hCG as indicated
- ABO and Rh blood typing (to detect patients at risk for maternal Rh sensitization)

Comments and Treatment Considerations
Vaginal bleeding in early pregnancy is very common. Pelvic and/ or intravaginal ultrasound should be performed to determine fetal anatomy, fetal heart activity, and status of the cervix. If there is normal fetal anatomy, normal fetal heart activity, and no signs of excessive uterine contractions or cervical opening, the patient can be managed expectantly. Some authorities recommend avoidance of intercourse (pelvic rest) to decrease the chance of uterine stimulation. If the patient exhibits abnormal fetal anatomy, lack of fetal heart activity, or indications of significant uterine contractions or cervical dilatation, an obstetrician should be consulted.

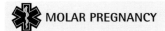 **MOLAR PREGNANCY**

A molar pregnancy occurs when an egg devoid of maternal genetic material is fertilized. In most cases, no fetus develops, and the products of conception consist of multiple intrauterine cystic structures. Less commonly, some molar pregnancies consist of some normal products of conception, along with the multiple cystic structures associated with molar pregnancies. In the United States molar pregnancies occur in approximately 1 in 1000 pregnancies. Risk factors for molar pregnancy include maternal age more than 40 years, race (some Asian and Mexican populations are at high risk, whites have a higher incidence of molar pregnancy than do African Americans), previous molar pregnancy, and a diet low in carotene.

Symptoms
- Passage of "grapelike" tissue per vagina +++
- Vaginal bleeding
- Symptoms of toxemia early in pregnancy

- Nausea +++
- Amenorrhea +++
- Lack of fetal movement +++

Signs
- Blood from cervical os
- Enlarged uterus +++
- Higher than expected levels of serum hCG +++
- Enlarged uterus +++
- Signs of toxemia early in pregnancy

Workup
- Pelvic and/or intravaginal ultrasound
- Serial serum β-hCG levels
- Pelvic examination
- CBC

Comments and Treatment Considerations
The diagnostic test of choice for molar pregnancy is pelvic and/or intravaginal ultrasound. The treatment of choice for a molar pregnancy is dilation and curettage (D&C). Following D&C, serial serum β-hCG levels must be followed until they reach normal, nonpregnant levels. Because of the possibility of the development of further trophoblastic disease, including choriocarcinoma, consultation with an obstetrician should be obtained for management of patients with molar pregnancy.

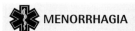 **MENORRHAGIA**

Symptoms
- Heavy menstrual bleeding, typically in excess of 7 days' duration

Signs
- Pallor
- Enlarged uterus

Workup
- Pap smear should be current
- CBC, thyroid-stimulating hormone (TSH)
- Pelvic ultrasound
- Endometrial biopsy in selected patients

Comments and Treatment Considerations
Menstrual bleeding normally lasts from 3 to 7 days, but can be as short as 1 day; regularity, however, is more important than length. Average menstrual blood loss is less than 80 mL. Consider submucosal fibroids, pregnancy, adenomyosis, endometrial hyperplasia, malignancy, and DUB.

In the perimenopausal patient, pelvic sonography and endometrial biopsy should be included in the initial evaluation. A pelvic ultrasound should also be performed to rule out uterine leiomyomata, which are present in more than half of women ages 40 or greater and 70% of women older than age 50.

In a patient younger than age 35 with a normal history and physical examination, uterine bleeding due to dysfunctional causes is most common and usually can be managed with hormonal agents, such as combined contraceptives or medroxyprogesterone. In most instances DUB is anovulatory in origin.

If the patient does not respond to initial medical treatments, pelvic sonography and endometrial biopsy should be considered. Inherited coagulopathy may present as menorrhagia in an otherwise healthy patient.

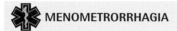 **MENOMETRORRHAGIA**

Symptoms
- Bleeding between periods at irregular intervals and flows
- Bleeding can occur at any time between menstrual cycles

Signs
- Weakness
- Fever
- Abdominal and cervical motion tenderness
- Ecchymosis and petechiae
- Tender vaginal or cervical ulcers
- Friable cervix with mucopurulent or malodorous discharge
- Cervical mass

Workup
- Cervical cultures as indicated, especially in younger patients because infectious causes are very common younger than age 25
- Wet mount demonstrating yeast vaginitis, leukorrhea, or *Trichomonas*
- Ultrasound

Comments and Treatment Considerations
Ovulatory bleeding is physiologic and can be confirmed with basal body temperatures or ovulation kits. Serious causes are endometrial polyps, endometrial hyperplasia and carcinoma, and cervical carcinoma.

Systemic diseases that may result in abnormal vaginal bleeding include many endocrine and hematologic conditions. A thorough history and physical examination usually reveal a systemic problem. Once pregnancy is excluded, the lower genital tract should be examined for infections, lesions, or trauma. Although dysplasia is rarely associated with bleeding, cervicitis may be, especially after intercourse.

Cervical and endometrial polyps are also associated with postcoital bleeding. A bimanual examination may reveal uterine enlargement (pregnancy, leiomyomata, carcinoma), tenderness (pelvic inflammatory disease), or adnexal masses (tumors, tubo-ovarian abscess).

Although iatrogenic causes are less frequent than DUB, they must be considered during the initial evaluation. Irregular menstrual bleeding can be caused by common medications such as hormonal contraceptives, corticosteroids, thyroid agents, tamoxifen, antipsychotics, SSRIs, and anticoagulants. Even herbal supplements such as soy and ginseng can contribute to abnormal uterine bleeding.

Intrauterine devices commonly cause increased and irregular vaginal bleeding.

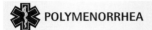 **POLYMENORRHEA**

Symptoms
• Menstrual cycles occurring more frequently than every 21 days

Signs
• Weakness
• Pallor

Workup
• CBC, TSH
• Endometrial sampling if refractory to treatment

Comments and Treatment Considerations
This pattern is usually due to a luteal phase defect. It responds well to hormonal management. Biopsy is indicated only when refractory to pharmacotherapy.

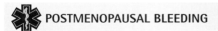 **POSTMENOPAUSAL BLEEDING**

Menopause is defined as the absence of menses for greater than 12 months and laboratory tests and/or physical findings consistent with ovarian failure.

Symptoms
• Any vaginal bleeding after menopause is reached

Signs
• Atrophic vaginal mucosa
• Firm to hard cervix
• Cervical mass or polyp
• Uterine enlargement

Workup

- Pelvic ultrasound—If the endometrial thickness is 4 to 5 mm or greater, endometrial sampling is indicated. An endometrial thickness of 4 mm or less conveys a negative predictive value of 97% for endometrial malignancy.
- Pipelle endometrial biopsy possesses a sensitivity of 85% to 90% for diagnosing endometrial abnormalities.
- D&C, once the gold standard in evaluating abnormal vaginal bleeding (AVB) in peri- and postmenopausal patients, may miss endometrial polyps and submucosal fibroids. Although Pipelle endometrial biopsy is relatively simple and usually does not involve cervical dilation, it carries a higher false-negative rate than D&C for detection of endometrial polyps and hyperplasia.
- Combined transvaginal measurement of the endometrial thickness and Pipelle endometrial biopsy, has a sensitivity of nearly 100% for detection of endometrial carcinoma.

Comments and Treatment Considerations

Aside from bleeding on initiation (first 3 months) or discontinuation of hormone replacement therapy, postmenopausal bleeding of any quantity warrants aggressive investigation. Simple endometrial hyperplasia without atypia is treated with medroxyprogesterone 10 mg daily for 3 months. The dose may be increased to 40 mg for breakthrough bleeding.

Atrophic vaginitis is best managed with topical estrogen. If topical estrogen is used in full strength (one applicator vaginally three times weekly), progestin supplementation should also be prescribed in order to prevent endometrial proliferation.

References

Albers J, Hull S, Wesley R: Abnormal uterine bleeding, *Am Fam Phys* 69(8): 1915–1926, 2004.

American College of Obstetricians and Gynecologists (ACOG): Practice Bulletin. Management of anovulatory bleeding, *Int J Gynaecol Obstet* 72:263, 2001.

American College of Obstetricians and Gynecologists (ACOG): Practice Bulletin. Management of endometrial cancer, *J Obstet Gynecol* 106: 413–425, 2005.

American College of Obstetricians and Gynecologists (ACOG): Practice Bulletin. Polycystic ovarian syndrome, *Obstet Gynecol* 114(4):936–949, 2009.

American College of Obstetricians and Gynecologists (ACOG): Practice Bulletin. Surgical alternatives to hysterectomy in the management of leiomyomas, *Obstet Gynecol* 112(2 Pt 1):387–400, 2008.

American College of Obstetricians and Gynecologists (ACOG) Technology Assessment. Saline infusion sonohysterography, *Obstet Gynecol* 102(3):659–662, 2003.

Centers for Disease Control and Prevention: STD facts. Available at www.cdc.gov/std/hiv/STDFact-STD-HIV.htm (accessed December 27, 2010).

Centers for Disease Control and Prevention: STD & pregnancy factsheet. Available at www.cdc.gov/std/pregnancy/STDFact-Pregnancy.htm (accessed December 27, 2010).

DeCherney, A, Pernoll M: *Current obstetric and gynecologic diagnosis and treatment*, 8th ed. New York, 1994, McGraw Hill, pp. 124–136, 665–669, 710–145, 938–945.

Dijkhuizen F, Bralmann H, Potters A, et al: The accuracy of transvaginal ultrasonography in the diagnosis of endometrial abnormalities, *J Obstet Gynecol* 87(3):345–359, 1996.

Dilley A, Drews C, Miller C, et al: Von Willebrand disease and other inherited bleeding disorders in women with diagnosed menorrhagia, *J Obstet Gynecol* 97:630–636, 2001.

Goldchmit R, Katz Z, Blickstein I, et al: The accuracy of endometrial pipelle sampling with and without sonographic measurement of endometrial thickness, *Obstet Gynecol* 82(5):727–730, 1993.

Hill NC, Oppenheimer LW, Morton KE: The etiology of vaginal bleeding in children. A 20-year review, *Br J Obstet Gynaecol* 96:467–470, 1989.

Hunter MH, Sterrett JJ: Polycystic ovary syndrome: it's not just infertility, *Am Fam Phys*. Published Sept. 1, 2000. http://www.aafp.org. (accessed December 27, 2010).

Janssen C, Scholten P, Heintz P: A simple visual assessment technique to discriminate between menorrhagia and normal menstrual blood loss, *Obstet Gynecol* 85(6):977–982, 1995.

National Cancer Institute: SEER Fast Stats. Available at http://seer.cancer.gov/faststats (accessed August 27, 2010).

Oriel K, Schrager S: Abnormal uterine bleeding, *Am Fam Physician*; 60:1371–1380, 1999.

Udoff L, Langenberg P, Adashi EY. Combined continuous hormone replacement therapy: a critical review, *Obstet Gynecol* 86(2):306–316, 1995.

CHAPTER 3

Amenorrhea
T. Edwin Evans

Patients with amenorrhea can be classified as "primary" (absence of menses in a 14-year-old who has failed to develop any secondary sexual characteristics, or in a 16-year-old who has had otherwise normal development) or "secondary" (lack of menses in a woman who previously menstruated and has missed either three normal cycles or has had 6 months of amenorrhea).

After evaluation for pregnancy it is helpful to categorize patients with primary or secondary amenorrhea based on sex hormone production, which may be normal, increased, or decreased. For instance, a primary amenorrhea patient with müllerian dysgenesis would have normal sex hormone levels, whereas a Turner syndrome patient would have low estrogen and progesterone with correspondingly high gonadotropins. Sex steroid levels (17-hydroxyprogesterone) are high in patients with congenital adrenal hyperplasia.

Any diagnosis that can present as secondary amenorrhea can also present as primary amenorrhea. The first step is a physical examination focused on signs of malnutrition, abnormal growth and development, an anatomically intact reproductive tract, central nervous system (CNS) disease, and galactorrhea.

PRIMARY—GENETICS/ENDOCRINE

Symptoms
- Failure of onset of menses (by age 14 in patients without development of secondary sexual characteristics; age 16 with normal development)
- Monthly abdominal pain without menstruation (suggests an imperforate hymen or transverse vaginal septum)
- Abnormal body hair distribution (virilizing)

Signs
- Galactorrhea
- Hirsutism

Workup
- Physical examination for developmental anomalies. The examiner should particularly be alert to findings consistent with an imperforate hymen, vaginal aplasia, or Turner syndrome (short

stature, webbed neck and a "shield" chest deformity [all +++++]).
Assignment of a Tanner stage should be documented.
- Pregnancy testing
- TSH and prolactin level
- Pelvic ultrasound if necessary to document presence of the uterus
- Imaging of the sella turcica if galactorrhea present by history or exam

 ## ANOVULATION: SEE SECONDARY AMENORRHEA

 ## CONGENITAL ADRENAL HYPERPLASIA

Signs
- Most cases are detected before puberty and are partial 21-hydroxylase deficiency. +++++
- Mild forms present as a short-statured individual. +
- Early epiphyseal closure demonstrated on x-rays for bone age ++++

 ## POLYCYSTIC OVARY SYNDROME (PCOS) AND ANDROGEN–SECRETING TUMORS: SEE SECONDARY AMENORRHEA

 ## PSEUDOHERMAPHRODITISM

Signs
- These individuals have 46, XY genetics but are phenotypically female due to deficient androgen production or androgen resistance at the tissue level.

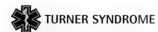 ## TURNER SYNDROME

Signs
- 45, XO genetics
- Patients appear to have Turner syndrome but have pure X,O genetics, while others are mosaics or have structural abnormalities of either an X or Y chromosome. +++
- Gonadal dysgenesis +++++

Symptoms
- Low neck hairline +++++
- Webbed neck +++++
- A high-arched palate +++++
- Aortic coarctation +++
- Hearing loss ++

SECONDARY AMENORRHEA

The traditional approach has been to localize the organ system responsible for the amenorrhea (hypothalamus, pituitary, ovary, or uterus), then zero in on the specific problem. The majority of cases have a simple solution, with only the occasional referral necessary for diagnosis or treatment.

 HYPOTHALAMIC–PITUITARY–OVARIAN AXIS

The hypothalamic-pituitary-ovarian axis is a way of referring to the combined effects of the hypothalamus, pituitary gland, and ovaries. The hypothalamic-pituitary-ovarian axis is a critical part in the development and regulation of the reproductive system.

The pathway begins with gonadotropin-releasing hormone (GnRH) secretion from the hypothalamus. GnRH acts on the anterior pituitary, causing the release of luteinizing hormone (LH) and follicle-stimulating hormone (FSH) into the bloodstream. LH and FSH both act on the ovaries causing secretion of estrogen and progesterone. Estrogen and progesterone then act on the uterus, regulating the growth and sloughing of the endometrial lining in a cyclical fashion.

Hormone release in the hypothalamic-pituitary-ovarian axis is regulated by a negative feedback mechanism. Estrogen and progesterone can provide negative feedback to the anterior pituitary and hypothalamus. Stimulation and regulation complete the pathway among hypothalamus, pituitary, and ovaries.

Symptoms
- Amenorrhea (in the absence of pregnancy)
- Galactorrhea (secretion of milky fluid from one or both breasts in a nulliparous woman or one whose last pregnancy or weaning is more than 12 months prior) +
- Hair growth in a virilizing pattern +

Signs
- Loss of menstrual function for at least 3 months (the sine qua non for diagnosis)
- Galactorrhea +
- Hirsutism +

Workup

- On physical examination, normal vaginal mucosal appearance and presence of thin, mucoid secretions is indicative of the presence of adequate estrogen.
- Pregnancy testing
- TSH
- Serum prolactin level—Hyperprolactinemia is present in the majority of patients presenting with amenorrhea and galactorrhea. ++++ Prolactin levels greater than 300 ng/mL virtually always denote a prolactinoma.
- Imaging of sella turcica, if galactorrhea present or prolactin level elevated
- If the examination, pregnancy test, TSH, prolactin and imaging of the sella turcica are normal, administer 10 mg oral medroxyprogesterone acetate (Provera, others) for 5 days. Onset of menses within a week after treatment confirms an intact genital tract and the presence of endogenous estrogen. At this point, the management of the patient centers around whether conception is desired. If not, a monthly 5-day course of progestin will suffice to eliminate the increased risk of endometrial cancer.
- The absence of withdrawal bleeding following progestin necessitates administration of estrogen for 21 days, concurrent with progestin for the final 5 days. Ensuing menstruation confirms an intact reproductive tract and an absence of endogenous estrogen. Gonadotropin levels (FSH, LH) are then indicated.

Comments and Treatment Considerations

Amenorrhea traumatica: Often referred to as Asherman syndrome, which constitutes endometrial scarring and synechiae from prior instrumentation. Scarring may also be present from prior infectious processes. These patients have normal sex hormone levels.

Anovulation: Other than pregnancy, the most common cause of secondary amenorrhea. This diagnosis has been established when a patient with normal TSH and prolactin levels has a withdrawal bleed after supplemental progesterone challenge. Women who do not currently desire conception can be treated with conventional oral contraceptive pills (OCPs) or with monthly progesterone (10 mg daily for 10 days), and should be instructed to present for reevaluation if they have return of amenorrhea. If conception is desired, evaluation for polycystic ovary syndrome (PCOS) should be considered prior to any attempt at induction of ovulation.

Emotional stress/illness: Low gonadotropins result from dysfunction of the hypothalamic/pituitary axis in patients with anorexia nervosa or excessive exercise +++++ in women at or less than 22% body fat, in addition to many endocrine diseases such as thyroid dysfunction and adrenal insufficiency.

Hyperprolactinemia: A pituitary tumor secreting prolactin will, in virtually every case, be accompanied by low gonadotropin levels. A "coned-down" view of the sella turcica is an excellent, quick, and inexpensive screening tool, whereas CT or MRI can give more definitive information. Many accept that patients with small prolactin-secreting tumors with serum prolactin levels less than 100 ng/mL may be managed conservatively with bromocriptine. Large tumors with prolactin levels greater than 300 ng/mL are unlikely to respond; with levels less than 100 ng/mL, a large tumor is probably not a prolactin-secreting mass and neurosurgical referral is indicated.

Ovarian failure: A woman who fails to have a withdrawal bleed after progesterone administration either does not have endogenous estrogen (necessary to create proliferative endometrial changes) or has a uterine defect. Simple evaluation for this scenario is described above ("workup").

Autoimmune ovarian failure is not uncommon. Initial workup (after demonstrating elevated gonadotropins) should include CBC, metabolic panel including calcium and phosphorus, thyroid studies, serum proteins, antinuclear antibody (ANA), and rheumatoid factor.

Other possible etiologies for early ovarian failure include radiation changes, chemotherapeutic agents, surgery, malignancy, infection and interruptions in vascular supply to the ovaries. Ovarian tumors producing androgens will *suppress* FSH and LH levels, resulting in amenorrhea.

A young woman diagnosed with ovarian failure (secondary amenorrhea with elevated gonadotropins) should be referred for consideration of gamete intrafallopian transfer (GIFT) or other fertility measures if desired.

The unusual scenario of low gonadotropins in the setting of secondary amenorrhea should prompt further evaluation for hypothalamic and/or pituitary failure, including CNS imaging even in the absence of an elevated prolactin level.

PCOS: Sometimes referred to as Stein-Leventhal syndrome, these patients are anovulatory +++++ and have hirsutism +++ and obesity +++. Ultrasound demonstrates enlarged, cystic ovaries. ++++ An elevated LH/FSH ratio is commonly seen. ++++. Test these patients for glucose intolerance (SORT "C").

PREGNANCY

Pregnancy and age-appropriate ovarian failure are the only normal physiologic causes of amenorrhea. Because pregnancy is the most common cause of amenorrhea and the easiest to diagnose, testing for pregnancy should be carried out as the initial evaluation in all cases of amenorrhea.

Symptoms
- Breast tenderness ++
- Nausea ++
- Sensation of fetal movement (+++ beyond 18 weeks' gestation)

Signs
- Enlargement of the abdomen (beyond first trimester)
- Cervical softening
- Bluish discoloration of vaginal mucosa (Chadwick's sign) ++++
- β-hCG detection in plasma or urine +++++
- Detection of fetal heartbeat by Doppler or ultrasound (+++++ beyond 12 weeks)
- Perception of fetal movement by examiner

Workup
- Pregnancy testing: Plasma and urinary levels are detectable prior to a missed menses, as early as 7 to 10 days after conception. Urine tests commonly available have a threshold for detecting hCG of 20 mIU/mL (plasma tests are 10 mIU/mL); by day 7 to 10 postconception, typical urine levels are 25 mIU/mL. A first-morning urine has the greatest concentrations of hCG.
- Ultrasound: In normal pregnancy a gestational sac should be visible with vaginal scanning when the hCG level is 1800 or greater (exact number varies between institutions). Ectopic pregnancy can occur at any level of β-hCG. Absence of definitive signs of pregnancy at β-hCG levels above the institutional threshold are very concerning for the possibility of ectopic pregnancy.

Comments and Treatment Considerations
Note: Any patient with a positive β-hCG who is hemodynamically unstable should have immediate surgical evaluation for ectopic pregnancy!

In addition to ectopic pregnancy, many pregnancy-related conditions may present with vaginal bleeding. The absence of amenorrhea therefore does not necessarily rule out pregnancy. A recent menstrual history, in addition to pregnancy testing, is essential to the evaluation of all patients with abnormal vaginal bleeding.

Elevated hCG levels may also be present in trophoblastic and nontrophoblastic disease; the possibility of these conditions should be considered before a diagnosis of pregnancy is given.

Establishment of a diagnosis of intrauterine pregnancy terminates the workup for amenorrhea. The hormonal manipulation described previously in the evaluation of a preexisting secondary amenorrhea is not possible (nor advised!) during pregnancy. Important areas for discussion between practitioner and patient in the setting of pregnancy include:
- Clear evidence supporting the cessation of smoking and alcohol use, and the expert consensus on cessation of recreational drug use
- Medications to avoid or discontinue during pregnancy
- Identification of providers for prenatal care and delivery, as well as for any preexisting medical conditions that complicate pregnancy (e.g., hypertension, diabetes, thyroid disease)
- Nutrition during pregnancy, including periconception folate supplementation to prevent neural tube defects

References

American College of Obstetricians and Gynecologists (ACOG): Clinical management guidelines for obstetrician-gynecologists: Practice Bulletin No. 41, December 2002, *Obstet Gynecol* 100:1389–1402, 2002.

Lumley J, Watson L, Watson M, et al: Periconceptional supplementation with folate and/or multivitamins for preventing neural tube defects, *Cochrane Database Syst Rev* 2006, CD001056.

Nordstrom ML, Cnattingius S: Smoking habits and birth weights in 2 successive births in Sweden, *Early Hum Dev* 37:195–204, 1994.

Speroff L, Fritz M: *Clinical gynecologic endocrinology and infertility*, 7th ed. Philadelphia, 1999, Lippincott Williams, and Wilkins. (This is an indispensable text for a thorough understanding of the topics discussed in this chapter.)

Yang Q, Witkiewicz BB, Loney RS, et al: A case-controlled study of maternal alcohol consumption and intrauterine growth retardation, *Ann Epidemiol* 11:497–503, 2001.

CHAPTER 4

Anemia

Rogena Johnson and Roberto Rodriguez

Anemia is a type of red blood cell disorder that has a multitude of etiologies as well as varying degrees of severity ranging from completely asymptomatic anemia to the most severe form, which can cause death in utero. It is defined by low total body RBC mass that leads to a low hemoglobin and low hematocrit. The normal hemoglobin and hematocrit vary from individual to individual depending on age, sex, menstruation status, race, altitude, and exposure to tobacco smoke. Conditions that decrease oxygen delivery to cells, at any level, may necessitate an increase in RBC mass to compensate because hemoglobin is the sole oxygen transporter for the body. Table 4-1 gives the normal hemoglobin and hematocrit levels for different populations.

The change in hemoglobin levels as children age can be attributed to changes in erythropoietin levels. A normal physiologic period of anemia is expected in all infants at 1 to 2 months. This anemia begins to resolve at about 1 to 2 years of age.

Anemias can be categorized by two main classification systems: morphologic and pathophysiologic. The pathophysiologic system of anemia classification is less commonly used, but is just as easy to understand. This system broadly separates anemias by the *cause* of low red blood cell (RBC) mass into two categories: increased destruction versus decreased production. The more commonly used classification system, however, is the morphologic system that categorizes anemias based on the size of the red cells. In order to understand this classification system it is important to remember what the various lab values within the complete blood cell (CBC) count mean. Table 4-2 defines these values.

The morphologic classification system uses the mean corpuscular volume (MCV) to categorize anemias into three major types: macrocytic, normocytic, and microcytic. Normocytic anemia is defined by an MCV of 80 to 100 fL. Macrocytic anemia includes anemias with an MCV of more than 100 fL, whereas microcytic anemia includes those with an MCV less than 80 fL. The other two values mentioned in Table 4-3 (in macrocytic anemia; megaloblastic vs nonmegaloblastic; in normocytic anemia; hemolytic vs nonhemolytic) can be used to further identify the type of anemia once the general category is determined. In this chapter we address each general morphologic category of anemia separately. Table 4-3 lists the types of anemia by morphologic categorization.

Table 4-1. Normal Laboratory Values

AGE	HEMOGLOBIN	HEMATOCRIT
Men and nonmenstruating women	13-14 g/dL	41%
Menstruating women	12 g/dL	37%
Infants at birth	16.5 g/dL	50%
First week of life	18.5 g/dL	56%
Age 1-2 months	11.5 g/dL	36%
Adolescent boy	15 g/dL	47%
Adolescent girl	14 g/dL	47%

Table 4-2. Understanding the Complete Blood Count

Hematocrit	Percent of total blood occupied by red blood cells (RBCs)
MCV	Average size of RBC; used to classify anemias; normal is 80 to 100 fL
MCHC	Amount of hemoglobin per RBC; normal is 32 to 36 g/dL
RDW	Variation in size among RBCs; normal is 12% to 15%

MCV, mean corpuscular volume; *MCHC,* mean corpuscular hemoglobin; *RDW,* red cell distribution width.

The screening recommendations per the US Preventive Services Task Force (USPSTF) are as follows: (1) all pregnant women at their first prenatal visit and all nonpregnant women beginning in adolescence and then every 5 to 10 years until menopause; and (2) screen high-risk infants with a single hemoglobin and hematocrit between 6 and 12 months of age.

MACROCYTIC ANEMIA

Macrocytic anemia is defined by an MCV of greater than 100 fL. It is further divided into megaloblastic or nonmegaloblastic. Megaloblasts are large, immature, nucleated RBCs. Megaloblastic anemia is caused by impaired deoxyribonucleic acid (DNA) synthesis, which causes dyssynchrony of cell replication and division. It is usually due to a deficiency of either cobalamin (vitamin B_{12}) or folic acid. Severe macrocytic anemia (MCV >125 fL) is almost always

Table 4-3. Morphologic Anemia Classification

MACROCYTIC (MCV >100 fL)	NORMOCYTIC (MCV 80-100 fL)	MICROCYTIC (MCV <80 fL)
MEGALOBLASTIC	**HEMOLYTIC (2 subclasses)**	Iron deficiency
B_{12} deficiency	**(1) RBC INTRINSIC**	Thalassemias
Folate deficiency	Membranopathy (i.e., HS)	Sideroblastic
Drug related, (i.e., hydroxyurea)	Hemoglobinopathy (i.e., SCD)	Anemia of chronic disease
NONMEGALOBLASTIC	Enzymopathy (i.e., G6PD deficiency)	Lead poisoning
Hypothyroidism	**(2) RBC EXTRINSIC**	Hodgkin's lymphoma
Liver disease		Castleman's disease
Alcoholism	Autoimmune mediated (SLE, drug, virus, lymphoid disorder, idiopathic)	
Myelodysplasia	Alloimmune mediated (transfusion reaction, neonatal hemolysis)	
Reticulocytosis (hemolysis, bleeding)	Microangiopathic (i.e., TTP/HUS)	
	Infection (i.e., malaria)	
	Chemical agents (i.e., venoms)	
	Splenomegaly	
	NONHEMOLYTIC	
	Acute blood loss	
	Anemia of chronic disease	
	Chronic renal insufficiency	
	Intrinsic bone marrow problem (aplastic anemia, PNH, pure red cell aplasia, etc.)	
	Extrinsic bone marrow problem (drugs, toxins, radiation, endocrine, infiltrative cancer, immune mediated, etc.)	

G6PD, Glucose-6 phosphate dehydrogenase; HS, hereditary spherocytosis; HUS, hemolytic uremic syndrome; MCV, mean corpuscular volume; PNH, paroxysmal nocturnal hemoglobinuria; RBC, red blood cell; SCD, sickle cell disease; SLE, systemic lupus erythematosus; TTP, thrombotic thrombocytopenic purpura.

megaloblastic, with a few exceptions for the myelodysplastic syndromes. Nonmegaloblastic macrocytic anemias encompass the rest of the macrocytic anemias including drugs, alcoholism, hypothyroidism, myelodysplasia, and chronic liver disease. Vitamin B_{12} and folate deficiency are discussed in this section.

 FOLIC ACID DEFICIENCY

Folic acid is tetrahydrofolate, which is needed for many reactions involving one-carbon transfers. Two of the important reactions it is required for are shown in the following text. The products are important in DNA synthesis.

Symptoms
- Fatigue
- Anorexia ++
- Weight loss
- Diarrhea ++
- Lightheadedness
- Abdominal pain

Signs
- Pallor
- Glossitis
- Jaundice
- Absent neurologic symptoms

Workup
History is the initial step in workup. Folate is found in most fruits and vegetables and daily requirements (50 to 100 mcg/day) are usually met with diet. The body stores only 2 to 3 months of folic acid, so dietary deficiency is more common than with B_{12}. At-risk patients include alcoholics, anorexic patients, older adult patients, those who avoid fruits and vegetables, and those who overcook their food, because the vitamin is labile.
- Unlike B_{12} deficiency, folate deficiency is less likely due to malabsorption because the entire GI tract absorbs folic acid. Occasionally, however, small intestine diseases such as gluten enteropathy, tropical sprue, and Crohn's disease can be a factor, so comorbid conditions should always be considered. Drugs such as trimethoprim, phenytoin, oral contraceptives, and sulfasalazine may interfere with absorption.
- During times of growth, such as pregnancy, the folic acid requirement is 5 to 10 times greater than normal. Other causes of increased demand include exfoliative skin disease, chronic hemolytic anemia, and dialysis.
- Laboratory workup reveals an anemia with an MCV more than 100 fL and normal B_{12} levels. The peripheral blood smear will look identical to one found in B_{12} deficiency. Serum homocysteine

levels will also be elevated in folate deficiency. An RBC folate level of less than 150 ng/mL is diagnostic and is a more precise indicator of chronic folate deficiency. Total serum folate is also reduced but this is influenced more by recent dietary intake.

Comments and Treatment Considerations
Treatment is with replacement of folic acid, 1 mg/day orally. This is also the recommended dose for pregnant patients. In cases of malabsorption, doses of up to 5 mg/day may be required. Parenteral folate is rarely necessary. Foods rich in folate should be encouraged. These include leafy green vegetables, citrus fruits, nuts, beans, wheat germ, and liver. There is rapid improvement as seen with B_{12} supplementation. There is an immediate sense of well-being, and reticulocytosis occurs within 5 to 7 days. Within 2 months one can expect a total correction of the anemia. Treating folic acid deficiency can allow underlying neurologic damage from B_{12} deficiency to progress, so it is important to rule out a coexisting condition.

 ## VITAMIN B_{12} DEFICIENCY

Vitamin B_{12} is a member of the cobalamin family and is essential for important enzymatic reactions in DNA synthesis. B_{12} is also required for the body to hold on to its folic acid stores. Therefore, if a patient is B_{12} deficient, he or she will likely also become folate deficient. Lack of B_{12} can lead to abnormal myelin synthesis due to inefficient methionine production. Meat contains B_{12} and an acidic stomach is necessary for the vitamin to be freed. After B_{12} is ingested it is bound to intrinsic factor (IF) in the stomach and transported to the terminal ileum, where it is absorbed. Gastric parietal cells secrete IF.

Symptoms
- Fatigue
- Weight loss
- Anorexia ++
- Diarrhea ++
- Lightheadedness
- Abdominal pain
- Peripheral paresthesias, then balance disturbance
- If severe, cerebral function may be affected, as well as vision, taste, smell
- Rarely dementia and neuropsychiatric changes precede hematologic changes.

Signs
- Glossitis
- Pallor
- Jaundice
- Decreased vibration and position sense
- Weakness
- Reflexes may be diminished or increased.

Workup

- The history is a key part of the workup. Specific attention should be given to diet. All animal products contain B_{12}, so rarely is dietary intake to blame for deficiency. Additionally, the liver stores 2 to 3 years' worth of B_{12}. Complete vegetarians, however, are at risk.
- More often, the cause of B_{12} deficiency is due to a defect in absorption and transport. The most common cause is pernicious anemia, which is caused by the absence of IF due to atrophy of the gastric mucosa or autoimmune destruction of the gastric parietal cells. It occurs most often in people around age 60, although a form of juvenile pernicious anemia is known. The incidence of pernicious anemia is increased in patients with other autoimmune diseases. Laboratory examination may reveal antiparietal cell antibodies (90%) or anti-IF antibodies (60%). The most characteristic finding is gastric atrophy sparing the antrum. Hypergastrinemia is also characteristic.
- Surgical history is also important. Total gastrectomy removes the source of IF. Partial gastrectomy may also be a cause although the exact mechanism is unclear. Ileal resection is another inciting factor.
- Ingestion of corrosive agents that damage the gastric mucosa can also remove IF.
- Many drugs can interfere with many levels of red cell production.
- Drugs that decrease gastric acid production can interfere with the release of B_{12} from food. Patients older than age 70 commonly have low gastric acid levels so are unable to absorb B_{12} from food. They are able to absorb the B_{12} found in vitamins, however.
- Chronic diarrhea can indicate malabsorption such as tropical sprue. Chronic constipation can indicate intestinal stasis due to strictures, diverticula, diabetes mellitus, scleroderma, or amyloidosis, which results in stasis in the bowel and an overgrowth of bacteria that degrade B_{12} before it can be absorbed.
- More rare causes of B_{12} deficiency are fish tapeworm infection, pancreatic insufficiency, and severe Crohn's disease.
- Laboratory examination reveals an anemia with a MCV between 110 and 140 fL. It is possible to have B_{12} deficiency with a normal MCV, however. This is sometimes explained by a concomitant thalassemia or iron deficiency. If severe, the hematocrit may be as low as 10% to 15% and one may also see thrombocytopenia and/or leukopenia. Serum B_{12} levels are less than 170 pg/mL (170 to 240 is borderline) and there is an increase in methylmalonic acid (MMA) and homocysteine levels. The peripheral smear shows anisocytosis and poikilocytosis, but the characteristic finding is the macro-ovalocyte. Reticulocyte count is reduced and lactate dehydrogenase (LDH) is elevated.

Comments and Treatment Considerations

Intramuscular B_{12} injections are historically used to treat vitamin B_{12} deficiency anemia. Injections of 100 mcg are given daily for 1 week, then weekly for 1 month, then monthly for life. Oral B_{12} can also be used with similar results. The dose currently supported in the literature is 2000 mcg/day. Patients respond with reticulocytosis within 5 to 7 days and feel a sense of wellness almost immediately. Hypokalemia and salt retention can occur during early therapy. CNS effects are generally irreversible unless they have ensued within the last 6 months. Folate supplementation may increase the likelihood of neurologic sequelae of B_{12} deficiency.

MICROCYTIC ANEMIA

Microcytic anemia is defined as a MCV less than 80 fL. Microcytic anemia may result from iron deficiency, thalassemia, anemia of chronic disease, lead toxicity, or sideroblastic anemia. Iron deficiency and thalassemia are two of the more common causes of microcytic anemia.

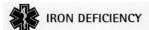 **IRON DEFICIENCY**

Iron is needed for hemoglobin synthesis among other things. If iron stores are inadequate, then anemia ensues.

Symptoms
• May be asymptomatic, especially in early stages +++
• Pallor
• Fatigue
• Orthostatic hypotension
• Exercise intolerance
• Palpitations

Signs
• Koilonychia (spoon nails)
• Atrophic glossitis
• Alopecia
• Esophageal web (Plummer-Vinson syndrome)
• Pica (a craving for nonfood items such as ice or clay)
• Tachycardia
• Blue sclera

Workup
• Perform CBC and MCV. If the MCV is less than 80 fL and the hemoglobin falls below the expected range, then the patient has microcytic anemia. The next step is to perform a serum iron panel including a ferritin, iron level, total iron-binding capacity (TIBC), and percent saturation. Refer to Table 4-4 for differential diagnosis based on laboratory results. If the diagnosis is still not clear, hemoglobin electrophoresis, peripheral blood smear, and lead levels should be obtained.
• Serum iron levels less than 60 μg/dL, ferritin levels less than 30 ng/dL, TIBC greater than 400 μg/dL, and percent transferring saturation less than 15% are indicative of iron deficiency. It is important to

Table 4-4. Iron Studies in the Evaluation of Anemia

STUDY	IRON DEFICIENCY	CHRONIC DISEASE	THALASSEMIA
Ferritin	Low	Normal or high	Normal or high
Iron	Low	Low or normal	Normal or high
TIBC	Normal or high	Normal	Normal
% Saturation	Low	Low or normal	Normal or high

TIBC, Total iron-binding capacity.

note that ferritin is an acute phase reactant and can be elevated during times of stress. On peripheral smear, iron deficient red cells appear small and hypochromic. They also demonstrate a high red-cell distribution width (RDW).
- An easy way to diagnose iron deficiency is to monitor response to treatment. This can be done by checking a reticulocyte count several days after initiating therapy.

Comments and Treatment Considerations

Iron deficiency is the most common cause of anemia, with 11% of women and 4% of men being deficient. Not all those that are deficient are anemic. Deficiency results from either excessive loss or poor intake. The most common cause of iron deficiency is chronic blood loss.

The first consideration in treating microcytic anemia caused by iron deficiency is to identify and treat the cause of the chronic blood loss. Causes may include excessive menstrual bleeding (the most common cause in young women; oral contraceptives can be useful). GI bleeding (upper GI bleeding is seen with ulcers, hiatal hernias, and varices; lower GI bleeding can be seen in Crohn's disease, celiac sprue, colon cancer, and parasitic infection), bladder cancer, prostate cancer, and urolithiasis (standard urinalysis is the first step in determining if blood is being lost in the urine). Factitious bleeding should be considered when other chronic blood loss workup is negative.

Iron supplementation is needed to replenish depleted iron stores. Oral iron is initially used as a replacement. Ferrous sulfate, ferrous gluconate, and ferrous fumarate are all oral formulations that can be used for replacement. Ferrous sulfate is the least expensive of the oral iron preparations. The 325-mg dose given three or four times daily is used for replacement. Ascorbic acid, 250 mg, can be given with the iron supplement to enhance the degree of iron absorption.

Ferrous fumarate contains 66 mg of elemental iron combined with 125 mg of ascorbic acid. The tablet is provided in 200 mg doses and is given three or four times daily. Iron should be given 2 hours before or 4 hours after ingestion of antacids, or they will not be absorbed optimally. Patients should be informed that oral iron supplements can cause constipation, so adequate water intake is essential and stool softeners may become necessary.

There are various reasons that oral formulations may not work for an individual. GI tract symptoms caused by excessive iron intake can ultimately decrease absorption or patients may simply not tolerate oral iron. Patients with chronic malabsorption or ongoing blood loss may not be able to take oral formulations. Tetracyclines, quinolones, cereals, tea, coffee, eggs, and milk can decrease the absorption of oral iron. Infection with *Helicobacter pylori* also impairs oral iron absorption. If *H. pylori* is suspected, serum *H. pylori* antibody or a urea breath test should be obtained to test for infection.

When oral iron preparations are not being tolerated or absorbed, IV and intramuscular (IM) formulations such as INFeD and DexFerrum can also be used for iron replacement. DexFerrum, 25 to 100 mg IM, can be given daily as needed. IV and IM preparations should only be used when oral preparations fail to increase serum hemoglobin. Parenteral administration of iron preparations carries a higher risk for anaphylaxis, phlebitis, fever, and muscle breakdown.

The duration of treatment is not well agreed on. Some physicians replace iron only until hemoglobin levels return to within normal limits. Other physicians replace iron 6 months after the return of a normal hemoglobin level. Some clinicians consider iron deficiency successfully treated when the serum ferritin level reaches 50 ng/mL.

A diet high in iron should be encouraged. These foods include meats such as liver and fish, whole grains, nuts, seeds, leafy green vegetables, and dried fruit.

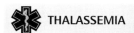 THALASSEMIA

Thalassemia results from a genetic mutation in the genes that code for the proteins that make up the alpha and beta chains of hemoglobin. This condition results in defective hemoglobin production, thus fewer red cells.

Symptoms
- Depends on the type of thalassemia
- May be asymptomatic +++
- Pallor
- Fatigue
- Irritability
- Growth restriction
- Shortness of breath
- Headache
- Dizziness

Signs
- Thalassemias may have no clinical signs evident on physical examination. +++
- Most of the signs of β-thalassemia major first become evident as fetal hemoglobin begins to convert to adult hemoglobin at 6 months of age.

- Abdominal swelling (due to hepatosplenomegaly)
- Jaundice (secondary to hemolytic anemia)
- RUQ pain (cholelithiasis, bilirubin gallstones)
- Clinical signs of congestive heart failure, severe edema
- Signs of infection

Workup

- Thalassemias are more common among patients of Mediterranean, African, and South Asian ancestry. This is partly because thalassemia confers a survival advantage to these groups should they become infected with malaria.
- Taking a careful family history is the first step because this is a genetic disease.
- Laboratory workup is the cornerstone to diagnosing thalassemia. The CBC will show microcytic anemia with an MCV less than 80 fL. The CBC may show an elevated RBC count despite decreased hemoglobin. A key difference from iron deficiency anemia is that the RDW is normal. At this point iron studies are performed that will likely rule out iron deficiency unless there is a coexisting condition. The next step therefore is hemoglobin electrophoresis. Abnormal electrophoresis results indicate thalassemia as the etiology of the microcytic anemia and differentiate the type.

Comments and Treatment Considerations

Adult hemoglobin, hemoglobin A, consists of two α- and two β-globin chains. Thalassemias result when defects are present in the production of either of these two chains via genetic defects.

β-Thalassemia major is characterized by a defect in both β-globin genes. These patients have a severe phenotype and 80% die within the first 5 years of life. They require the close care of a hematologist with frequent transfusions or splenectomy. Patients with β-thalassemia minor are heterozygous for the β-globin gene defect and therefore have varying concentrations of abnormal β-globin. Many times patients with β-thalassemia minor are clinically asymptomatic and rarely require treatment. These patients may require transfusions after vaginal delivery or surgery.

Four genes code for the α-globin subunits; therefore, the degree of severity depends on the number of genes affected. Hydrops fetalis results when all four copies of the α-globin genes are damaged. The lack of α-globin subunits causes fetal γ-globin subunits to aggregate resulting in tissue anoxia and intrauterine fetal death. This form is referred to as hemoglobin Bart's disease. Hemoglobin H disease results when three α-globin genes are defective. The diminished amount of α-globin results in aggregates of β-globins, called hemoglobin H. Hemoglobin H has a disproportionately high affinity for oxygen, thus delivering less oxygen to peripheral tissues. There are severe clinical consequences such as chronic hemolysis, frequent hospitalizations, and decreased life span. Care of these patients is similar to that of β-thalassemia major patients.

α-Thalassemia minor has two of the four α-globin genes affected, resulting in clinically minimal symptoms that do not require treatment. Again, they may require transfusion after blood loss.

The silent carrier state is present when a single α-globin gene is deleted. A patient with this condition may not know and would not require treatment. This is also called α-thalassemia minima.

In general, transfusions are used for severe microcytic anemia caused by thalassemia. Chronic blood transfusions leave a patient susceptible to iron overload. Iron chelation therapy is classically done with deferoxamine. Deferoxamine is given IM 0.5 to 1 mg daily. However, deferasirox (Exjade) can also be used and is questionably tolerated better by patients. Splenectomy and allogenic bone marrow transplantation should be considered in severe thalassemia cases.

All patients with thalassemia should be offered genetic counseling prior to family planning.

NORMOCYTIC ANEMIA

Normocytic anemias consist of a very widespread group of anemias that can be grouped into two basic categories: hemolytic or non-hemolytic. Normocytic anemias are those with an MCV that is within the normal range of 80 to 100 fL. In this section hemolysis and blood loss are discussed.

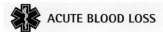 **ACUTE BLOOD LOSS**

The investigation of chronic blood loss can be found in the discussion of iron deficiency anemia within this chapter. In this section we focus on acute losses only.

Symptoms
- Relate to the amount of blood lost (>2 L is severe)
- Shortness of breath at rest or with exertion
- Restlessness
- Anxiety
- Syncope with change in position
- Confusion

Signs
- Vasovagal reaction
- Orthostatic hypotension
- Hypotension
- Tachycardia
- Shock

Workup
- Following a trauma it is usually customary to rule out massive bleeding with inspection and rapid scans. In the nontrauma

setting, ruling out bleeding is not always at the forefront. If the bleed is external, it is usually obvious that the patient is bleeding. If the bleeding is internal, it is not always that obvious. Close observation of vital signs and mental status are thus important when caring for a patient. Patients can bleed into their GI tract, abdomen, chest, or retroperitoneum from GI tract varices, broken bones, ruptured vessels or organs, or cancers. Sometimes large volumes of blood can acquire before any symptoms develop. Usually this volume is around 1 L or 20% of total blood volume. The first sign is usually tachycardia, which usually occurs prior to hypotension. Initial resuscitation generally proceeds with IV fluids; however, in trauma fluid resuscitation prior to definitive care may negatively effect outcome in some circumstances. The anemia is usually then only discovered after attempts at volume replacement to combat the hypotension.

- Screening for a bleed in the GI tract can be done via stool Hemoccult test or gastric lavage and Gastroccult for upper GI bleeds. Exact localization of the bleed may require either an esophagogastroduodenoscopy (EGD) and/or a colonoscopy. Bleeds in the GI tract not able to be seen with either of these two modalities may require a tagged red blood cell scan.

Comments and Treatment Considerations

Treatment of the cause of the bleed is critical. The endpoint for transfusions depends on patient status and comorbidities. If the anemia is not severe, no specific therapy is required because the body will compensate for the loss. The patient must have functioning kidneys in order to make erythropoietin, and functioning bone marrow for this to take place. Adequate iron is also required. Reticulocytosis will be noticed within days.

Each unit of packed RBCs raises the hematocrit by about 4%.

There are 300 mL in 1 unit of packed RBCs and 200 of them are RBCs.

Signs of major transfusion reactions are fever, chills, backache, and headache. If severe there may be dyspnea, hypotension, and vascular collapse. Stop the transfusion! Disseminated intravascular coagulation (DIC) and renal failure can occur. The patient will need aggressive hydration.

If the patient develops fever and chills within 12 hours of transfusion, it is a reaction to antigens on the white cells still present in the blood given. These reactions are usually not severe and can be treated with acetaminophen and diphenhydramine. Often patients are pretreated with these agents. If a patient requires frequent transfusions, leukopoor blood can be ordered. This blood has the white cells totally washed out.

The risk of hepatitis B virus (HBV) infection from a transfusion is 1:200,000 per unit, and of human immunodeficiency virus (HIV) 1:250,000 per unit. The most common infection risk is hepatitis C virus (HCV), with a risk of 1:3300 per unit.

✽ HEMOLYSIS

There is a wide variety of causes of hemolytic anemias, which can be characterized as intrinsic red cell defects or extrinsic red cell defects. Intrinsic red cell defect implies that there is something wrong with the red cell itself that causes it to be destroyed. Extrinsic red cell defects include things that happen outside the red cell that bring attention to the red cell, which in turn causes it to be destroyed. Extrinsic defects also include various environmental hazards red cells wander through that may end up terminating their life. Refer to Table 4-5 for a classification of hemolytic anemias.

Symptoms
• Fatigue
• Red-brown urine
• Acute pain episodes (sickle cell disease [SCD])
• Vary widely depending on the disease

Signs
• Jaundice
• Splenomegaly
• Chronic leg ulcers (hereditary spherocytosis [HS], SCD)
• Vary widely depending on the disease

Workup
• A careful history and physical examination are essential, particularly regarding medications and possible toxin exposures. Many of the anemias in this category are inherited.
• Due to the survival time of RBCs (120 days), one can expect a fall in hematocrit of up to 3% per week if the bone marrow is dysfunctional. If it declines at a faster rate, blood loss or hemolysis are to blame.
• The laboratory workup will reveal reticulocytosis as a key feature in the diagnosis of hemolysis. The exceptions to this rule are (1) reticulocytosis *does not* occur with hemolysis in the setting of a second disorder such as infection, or folate deficiency, and (2) reticulocytosis *does* occur during recovery from other nonhemolytic anemias such as B$_{12}$ or folate deficiencies and from an acute bleed. Another laboratory value that is shared among all hemolytic anemias is serum haptoglobin level. Haptoglobin is a binding protein for hemoglobin, so its levels decrease during hemolysis. Haptoglobin is not a reliable indicator alone. Urine can be examined for hemoglobin and hemosiderin if the hemolysis is intravascular. Hemoglobin and methemoglobin can also be measured in serum with severe intravascular hemolysis. Increased total and indirect bilirubin are also indicators of hemolysis because they are stored inside red cells. Total bilirubin may rise above 4 mg/dL; suspect liver dysfunction if higher. Finally, LDH levels should be included. The microangiopathic anemias will elevate LDH.

Table 4-5. Classification of Hemolytic Anemias

INTRINSIC RBC DEFECTS	EXTRINSIC RBC DEFECTS
MEMBRANE DEFECTS: • Hereditary spherocytosis • Hereditary elliptocytosis • Paroxysmal nocturnal hemoglobinuria	AUTOIMMUNE Warm antibody mediated • CLL • SLE • Idiopathic Cold antibody mediated • *Mycoplasma* • Idiopathic
ENZYME DEFICIENCIES: • Pyruvate kinase deficiency • G6PD deficiency • Methemoglobinemia • Severe hypophosphatemia	LOCAL ENVIRONMENT Microangiopathic • TTP/HUS • DIC • Valve hemolysis • Metastatic adenocarcinoma • Vasculitis Hypersplenism Burns
HEMOGLOBINOPATHIES: • Sickle cell syndromes • Unstable hemoglobins • Methemoglobinemia	RBC INFECTIONS • Malaria • *Clostridium* • *Borrelia* OTHER • Drug-induced (e.g., PCN)

CLL, Chronic lymphocytic leukemia; *DIC,* disseminated intravascular coagulation; *G6PD,* glucose-6-phosphate dehydrogenase; *HUS,* hemolytic-uremic syndrome; *PCN,* penicillin; *RBC,* red blood cell; *SLE,* systemic lupus erythematosus; *TTP,* thrombotic thrombocytopenic purpura.

- Peripheral blood smear is useful (i.e., sickled cells). RBC membrane defects are readily diagnosed here. Enzyme deficiencies can also be diagnosed via this method combined with specific enzyme assays and DNA sequencing. Hemoglobinopathies require the use of hemoglobin electophoresis in addition to peripheral smear.
- Immune-mediated hemolysis is diagnosed with the Coombs' antiglobulin test. The direct Coombs' test assays whether there are immunoglobulins or complement components attached to red cells. If immunoglobulins are present on the red cells, they will clump together when the Coombs' reagent is added. If this happens at body temperature, the patient has a "warm" antibody-mediated hemolytic anemia. If it has to be cooled to clump, then the patient has a "cold" antibody-mediated hemolytic anemia. The indirect Coombs' test may also be needed to diagnose the immune-mediated anemias. Serum complement levels, specifically C3 and C4, may be depressed during immune-mediated hemolysis.

- When RBCs are destroyed due to mechanical trauma they encounter in their environment they are fragmented and this can be seen on peripheral smear (schistocytes). The other clinical symptoms and objective signs of the microangiopathic hemolytic anemias are used to key into their diagnosis. One important form of mechanical hemolysis that may be encountered in the primary caregiver's office is runner's anemia. This is when hemolysis occurs from the repetitive pounding of the feet on the pavement during frequent running. This causes hemolysis and anemia that is easily diagnosed with a little time off from running and rechecking the CBC.
- Splenomegaly can be diagnosed by physical examination versus simple imaging.
- Diagnosing infection-induced hemolysis requires looking at the red cell for characteristic signs of infection such as those associated with *Plasmodium falciparum*. Serologic markers are used for specific infections.

Comments and Treatment Considerations

It is important to give patients with hemolytic anemia folic acid supplementation to keep up with the demand of reticulocytosis.

Following splenectomy, patients are at risk for infection with encapsulated bacteria, so immunize against *Pneumococcus* and *Meningococcus*.

Cholecystectomy is an option for bilirubin gallstone-induced cholecystitis.

Specific treatment depends on the type of hemolysis. The common forms are discussed here.

Hereditary spherocytosis is inherited in an autosomal dominant pattern. Diagnosis is via peripheral smear and the osmotic fragility test. The MCHC will be elevated on the CBC. The severity of the disease determines treatment; splenectomy is the definitive treatment. Blood transfusions are given as needed.

Glucose-6-phosphate dehydrogenase (G6PD) deficiency is transmitted in an X-linked pattern. Oxidative stress causes hemolysis and occurs when patients are exposed to things such as fava beans, sulfa drugs, moth balls, or primaquine. Infections can also incite acute events. The flares are sporadic and can be prevented with avoidance of culprit substances. During acute events patients may need hospitalization, transfusions, and hydration.

Sickle cell anemia is an autosomal recessive disease and is diagnosed via hemoglobin electrophoresis. A wide spectrum of disease exists from asymptomatic to severe. Patients that are homozygous for the disease are discovered during childhood. When attacks occur, red cells sickle and become clogged in the microvasculature. The most common presentation is the acute pain crisis with pain anywhere in the body. These episodes are treated with hydration, oxygenation, adequate pain control, transfusions as needed, and attention to any underlying infection or stress that may have precipitated the attack. Hydroxyurea may reduce sickling and is given prophylactically. "Acute chest syndrome" is the triad of chest pain, pulmonary infiltrate, and fever. This can represent pneumonia or pulmonary infarct, or sometimes both. Prompt attention is required. These patients usually autoinfarct their spleen early in life, so it is as if they have had a splenectomy. Children are given prophylactic penicillin until age 5.

Autoimmune hemolytic anemia is often treated with corticosteroids, especially the warm antibody-mediated type. Other options for long-term treatment include azathioprine, cyclosporine, and rituximab. Intravenous immune globulin (IVIg) can be used in the acute setting only for adults. Exchange transfusions are also an option. Splenectomy is used for refractory cases.

References

Choi J: Serum-soluble transferring receptor concentrations in *Helicobacter pylori*–associated iron-deficiency anemia, *Ann Hematol* 30:735–737, 2006.

Dang C: Runner's anemia, *JAMA* 286:714–771, 2001.

Gonzales R, Kutner J: Current practice guidelines in primary care 2006. Available at www.accessmedicine.com (accessed December 29, 2010).

Kasper D, Braunwald E, Fauci A, et al: *Harrison's manual of medicine*, 16th ed, New York, 2005, McGraw-Hill.

Linker C: *Current medical diagnosis and treatment 2007*, 46th ed, New York, 2006, McGraw-Hill.

McKenzie SB, *Textbook of hematology*, 2nd ed, Baltimore 1996, Lippincott, Williams & Wilkins.

Microcytic anemia, UpToDate. Nov. 11, 2006 Available at www.uptodateonline.com/utd/index.do (accessed 12/29/2010).

O'Connell C, Dickey V: *Hematology and oncology*, Singapore, 2005, Malden: Blackwell.

South-Pauly J, Matheney S, Lewis E: *Current diagnosis and treatment in family medicine*, New York, 2004, McGraw-Hill.

Vidal-Alaball J, Butler C, Cannings-John R, et al: Oral vitamin B_{12} versus intramuscular vitamin B_{12} for vitamin B_{12} deficiency, *Cochrane Database Syst Rev* 2005, CD004655.

CHAPTER 5

Anxiety
W. Scott Craig

Studies have shown that 14.6% to 15.6% of patients in primary care settings have anxiety disorders. These patients do not typically identify themselves as having "anxiety." Many of these patients initially present with nonspecific somatic complaints, and they tend to exhibit high health care use; 50% of patients with diagnosed anxiety disorders receive treatment services for these symptoms in primary care settings. Anxiety disorders can significantly impair individuals' ability to function in daily routines, so they are at risk for financial problems, interpersonal problems, poor health habits, academic decline, and work productivity problems. Anxiety disorders often elicit cardiopulmonary, GI, genitourinary, and neurologic symptoms. Anxiety disorders have even been shown to exacerbate coronary artery disease and increase cardiovascular mortality rate. It is important to recognize that certain medical conditions and chemicals can cause symptoms of anxiety (see "Secondary Causes of Anxiety"). These secondary or organic causes of anxiety should be addressed primarily.

Anxiety disorders include:
• Generalized anxiety disorder
• Panic disorder
• Agoraphobia
• Social phobias
• Specific phobias
• Obsessive-compulsive disorder
• Posttraumatic stress disorder
• Acute stress disorder
• Separation anxiety disorder
• Anxiety disorder due to a general medical condition
• Substance-induced anxiety disorder
• Anxiety disorder not otherwise specified (typically mixed anxiety-depression)

Adjustment disorder with anxiety can temporarily mimic some of these clinical anxiety disorders.

Epidemiology data (Table 5-1) for anxiety disorders show a strong familial pattern, yet it is apparent that both genetic and environmental factors play a role in anxiety disorders.

Table 5-1. Epidemiology of Common Anxiety Disorders

	LIFETIME PREVALENCE	GENDER DIFFERENCE	AGE OF ONSET	TYPICAL FAMILIAL PATTERN	GENERAL COURSE
Generalized anxiety disorder (GAD)	5%	F > M	20s	Yes	Fluctuating/chronic
Obsessive-compulsive disorder (OCD)	1% to 2.5%	F = M	Childhood to early adult	Yes	Episodic/potentially chronic
Panic disorder (PD)	1% to 3.5%	F > M	18-35	Yes	Episodic/potentially chronic
Posttraumatic stress disorder (PTSD)	8%	F = M	Any	Yes	Variable/potentially chronic
Separation anxiety disorder (SEP)	4%	F ≥ M	Childhood	Yes	Episodic/situational
Social phobia (SOP)	3% to 13%	F ≥ M	Mid-teens	Yes	Continuous/chronic
Specific phobia (SPP)	7.2% to 11.3%	F ≥ M	Childhood or mid-20s	Yes	Episodic/situational

GENERALIZED ANXIETY DISORDER

Generalized anxiety disorder (GAD) is characterized by excessive apprehension and uncontrollable worry about multiple events or activities. The focus of the worry often shifts from one area of concern to another. Children and adolescents tend to focus more on performance issues, while adults will worry more about routine life circumstances. These symptoms can be distressing, and they interfere with the patient's quality of life or daily functioning. The anxiety is not confined to the features of another psychiatric disorder, medical condition, or the physiologic effects of a substance. Although a minimum of 6 months of anxiety symptoms is necessary for diagnosis, many patients have experienced these symptoms for years prior to seeking treatment.

GAD has a high comorbidity rate with depression, panic disorder, social phobia, specific phobias, somatization disorders, substance abuse, and personality disorders. GAD also has a high co-occurrence with hyperthyroidism, chronic fatigue syndrome, fibromyalgia, diabetes, irritable bowel syndrome, peptic ulcer disease, tension headaches, hypertension, ischemic stroke, chronic obstructive pulmonary disease (COPD), and heart disease. Some electroencephalogram (EEG) abnormalities are common with GAD (e.g., alpha rhythm and evoked potentials), and EEG sleep discontinuity includes a decrease in stage 1, delta, and rapid eye movement (REM) sleep.

Symptoms
- Excessive anxiety ++++
- Uncontrollable worry ++++
- Irritability ++++
- Restlessness ++++
- Muscle tension +++
- Concentration problems +++
- Sleep problems (typically insomnia) +++
- Stomachache or nausea +++
- Shortness of breath ++
- Palpitations ++
- Headache ++
- Fatigue ++

Signs
- Cognitive vigilance +++
- Excessive sweating +++
- Diarrhea +

Workup
- Medical examination for differential diagnosis: Review medical history. Endocrine system problems, brain tumors, toxin exposure, stimulant intoxication, and withdrawal (e.g., from alcohol, benzodiazepines, sedatives) can present symptoms of GAD.

- Thyroid function tests (TSH, T$_4$) are generally recommended. A basic metabolic panel (BMP) and an ECG may also be warranted (see "Secondary Causes of Anxiety").
- Clinical interview: Include mental status examination current psychosocial stressors; family (genetic) history of substance abuse, medical, or psychiatric disorders; and patient history of psychiatric, medical, or substance abuse problems or treatment services.
- Differential diagnosis or comorbidity screening indicated for other anxiety disorders, mood disorders, adjustment disorders, somatoform disorders, personality disorders, factitious disorders, eating disorders, psychosis, and suicidal ideations
- Structured diagnostic interviews and instruments: Primary Care Evaluation of Mental Health Disorders (PRIME-MD), Mini-International Neuropsychiatric Interview (MINI), Symptom Driven Diagnostic System for Primary Care (SDDS-PC), Structured Clinical Interview for DSM-IV (SCID), and Quick PsychoDiagnostics (QPD) Panel
- Screening checklists: Generalized Anxiety Disorder Questionnaire (GADQ-IV), Generalized Anxiety Disorder-7 (GAD-7), Beck Anxiety Inventory for Primary Care (BAI-PC), Penn State Worry Questionnaire (PSWQ), and Depression Anxiety Stress Scale (DASS).

Comments and Treatment Considerations

Initiate patient education regarding GAD and discuss treatment options. Consider the high comorbidity of GAD with depression (as well as other psychiatric/ medical conditions) when developing the treatment plan and when selecting psychotropic medications.

Buspirone is effective with GAD (without the risk of dependency, withdrawal, or relapse risks common with benzodiazepines), although it is often not effective with the associated comorbidities of GAD.

Benzodiazepines are primarily useful for acute symptoms of GAD, yet antidepressants are considered to be more effective for long-term symptom management.

SSRIs (escitalopram, paroxetine, and sertraline) and serotonin-norepinephrine reuptake inhibitor (SNRIs) (venlafaxine) antidepressants are approved by the US Food and Drug Administration (FDA) for treatment of GAD. Other SSRI medications are likely to be effective as well due to class effect. Tricyclic antidepressants can be effective with GAD, yet they are not a "front-line" option due to anticholinergic side effects, overdose potential, and cardiovascular risks. The FDA has advised monitoring patients for suicidal ideations after starting antidepressant medications.

Strong evidence-based research supports the effectiveness of cognitive-behavioral therapy (CBT) for GAD. It has shown effectiveness equal to pharmacotherapy. Applied relaxation is another very effective therapeutic technique for GAD. CBT is compatible with pharmacotherapy, and CBT maintains gains beyond medication discontinuation. Collaborative care models of treatment have promise for GAD.

PANIC DISORDER

Panic disorder (PD) is characterized by having unexpected panic attacks and an intense discomfort or fear regarding the possibility of having future panic attacks. It is common for people to worry about the implications of the panic attacks because they may feel that they are having a heart attack, breathing problems, or that they are "going crazy." Panic attacks are defined as an intense and abrupt fear or discomfort with multiple somatic or cognitive symptoms. These symptoms are out of context to the setting (i.e., no emergency is actually taking place). Panic attacks typically peak within 10 minutes and often end within 20 to 60 minutes. Panic attacks tend to occur on a variable frequency rate. During a panic attack the person may fear death, loss of control, or imminent danger.

Nocturnal panic attacks can occur during stage II and stage II sleep. Situationally bound panic attacks may actually stem from a phobia instead of a panic disorder, whereas panic disorder is typically signaled by unexpected panic attacks. Panic attacks have been associated with cerebral vasoconstriction, temporal lobe involvement, and multiple neurotransmitters: norepinephrine (NE), serotonin (5-HT), gamma-aminobutyric acid (GABA), and cholecystokinin tetrapeptide (CCK-4). It is of note that cigarette smokers are up to three times more likely to have panic attacks than nonsmokers.

If patients associate the panic attack with a certain setting or situation they may attempt to avoid certain environments in a quest to prevent panic attacks. They sometimes make major life decisions (such as quitting a job or refusing a promotion that involves travel) to reduce the perceived odds of having a panic attack. They may be especially avoidant of settings and situations in which escape is difficult or help appears difficult to access (e.g., agoraphobia). Not all panic disorders include agoraphobia, and some people have agoraphobia without a history of panic disorder (this is not common). PD has a very high comorbidity with social phobia and specific phobias.

Symptoms
- Panic attacks (recurrent and unexpected) ++++
- Intense fear of having additional panic attacks ++++
- Behavioral changes +++
- Agoraphobia +++
- Nausea +++
- Dizziness +++
- Paresthesias ++
- Concentration problems +

Signs
- Palpitations or chest pain +++
- Autonomic hyperactivity +++
- Depersonalization or derealization +++
- Sweating +++
- Tachycardia +
- Dyspnea +

Workup

- Medical examination for differential diagnosis: Review medical history. Screen for endocrine disorders, cardiovascular disease, respiratory disorders, temporal lobe epilepsy, vestibular disorders, and substance abuse.
- Due to the cardiac symptoms of this disorder, an ECG is often warranted.
- Depending on the patient's presenting symptoms, the utility of a CBC, complete metabolic panel (CMP), TSH, urinalysis, and a drug screen should be considered (see "Secondary Causes of Anxiety").
- Clinical interview: Include mental status examination; current psychosocial stressors; family (genetic) history of substance abuse, medical, or psychiatric disorders; and patient history of psychiatric, medical, or substance abuse problems and treatment services.
- Differential diagnosis or comorbidity screening indicated for other anxiety disorders, mood disorders, somatoform disorders, personality disorders, factitious disorders, eating disorders, psychosis, and suicidal ideations
- Structured diagnostic interview and instruments: Primary Care Evaluation of Mental Health Disorders (PRIME-MD), Mini-International Neuropsychiatric Interview (MINI), Symptom Driven Diagnostic System for Primary Care (SDDS-PC), Structured Clinical Interview for DSM-IV (SCID), and Quick PsychoDiagnostics (QPD) Panel
- Screening checklists: Brief Panic Disorder Screen (BPDS), Panic Disorder Severity Scale (PDSS), NIMH Panic Questionnaire, Panic and Agoraphobia Scale (PAS), Albany Panic and Phobia Questionnaire (APPQ), and Beck Anxiety Inventory for Primary Care (BAI-PC)

Comments and Treatment Considerations

After a diagnosis of panic disorder, a health care provider will need to spend psychoeducational time with the patient. Because of the intensity of the distress and somatic symptoms, it is initially difficult for a patient to believe that the panic attacks stem from an anxiety disorder. Reassurance and supportiveness from a health care provider can go a long way with helping the patient gain acceptance of this diagnosis.

Consider the high comorbidity of PD with social phobia or specific phobias when developing the treatment plan.

Alprazolam can be effective for rapid symptom control, whereas SSRIs are considered to be a more conservative option for long-term symptom management. Both alprazolam and paroxetine have FDA approval for the treatment of panic disorder. Benzodiazepines must be slowly discontinued because abrupt discontinuation can elicit a recurrence of panic attacks.

Tricyclic medications (such as clomipramine and imipramine) can be effective for PD; however, they can be deadly in overdose. Monitor the risks of anticholinergic side effects, overdose potential, and cardiovascular distress. The FDA has advised monitoring patients for suicidal ideations after starting antidepressant medications.

There is strong evidence-based research supporting the effectiveness of CBT for panic disorder, and these gains appear to be long lasting. Exposure techniques, cognitive strategies, and relaxation techniques have shown effectiveness.

Collaborative care models of treatment have promise for PD because studies have shown that combining psychologic treatments with psychotropic medication improves treatment prognosis. Routine exercise has also been shown to reduce symptoms of PD. A reduction in caffeine and nicotine use is generally advisable.

 ## SECONDARY CAUSES OF ANXIETY

Secondary conditions that cause anxiety symptoms include anxiety disorder due to a general medical condition and substance-induced anxiety disorder. These anxiety disorders cause significant distress and impairment in daily functioning, and they can mimic the symptoms of other anxiety disorders. Neither diagnosis is given if the anxiety symptoms occur only during a delirium or if the anxiety is best accounted for by another psychiatric disorder.

Anxiety disorder due to a general medical condition is diagnosed when the direct physiologic effects of a medical condition have caused clinical anxiety features. Endocrine (e.g., hyperthyroidism, hypoparathyroidism, hypoglycemia, pheochromocytoma), cardiovascular (e.g., cardiac arrhythmia, cardiomyopathy, mitral valve prolapse), respiratory (e.g., asthma, COPD), metabolic (vitamin B_{12} deficiency, porphyria), and neurologic (cerebral neoplasms, encephalitis, etc.) problems can directly produce anxiety. Inflammatory disorders (e.g., lupus erythematosus, rheumatoid arthritis), pregnancy, and perimenopause are also associated with anxiety.

Substance-induced anxiety disorder is diagnosed when the physiologic consequences of a substance have directly caused anxiety symptoms. Toxin exposure, substance intoxication, and substance withdrawal can produce symptoms of various clinical anxiety disorders. Substances that often cause anxiety during intoxication and withdrawal include alcohol, cocaine, amphetamine, cannabis, hallucinogens, inhalants, hypnotics, anxiolytics, sedatives, phencyclidine, nicotine, and caffeine.

Many over-the-counter medications (i.e., decongestants and weight-loss tablets) and prescription drugs (i.e., methylphenidate, narcoleptics, corticosteroids, anticholinergics, β-adrenergic agonists, and SSRIs) have anxiety as a possible side effect. Antianxiety medications (such as benzodiazepines) can actually induce anxiety when discontinued. Toxins that can induce anxiety include mercury, phosphorus, arsenic, benzene, and carbon disulfide, for example. Dioxin and theophylline toxicity can cause anxiety symptoms.

Symptoms
- Panic attacks ++
- Obsessions and compulsions ++
- Generalized anxiety ++
- Agitation +
- Phobias (not common in general medical conditions) +
- Palpitations and chest pain +
- Nausea +
- Dizziness +
- Paresthesias +

Signs
- Cognitive impairments +
- Tachycardia +
- Dyspnea +
- Sweating +
- Autonomic hyperactivity +

Workup
- *Clinical interview:* Include mental status examination; current psychosocial stressors; family (genetic) history of substance abuse, medical, or psychiatric disorders; and patient history of psychiatric, medical, or substance abuse problems and treatment services. Screen for mood disorders, personality disorders, and malingering.
- Differential diagnosis or comorbidity screening indicated for other anxiety disorders, mood disorders, somatoform disorders, personality disorders, factitious disorders, eating disorders, psychosis, and suicidal ideations
- *History:* Etiology of the anxiety symptoms must be shown to be related to the general medical condition or substance exposure. Temporal associations (onset, exacerbation, and remission of symptoms) and atypical symptoms for clinical anxiety disorders provide clues to the secondary causes of the anxiety.
- Consider side effect profiles and interactions between current medications.
- *Structured diagnostic interviews and instruments:* Symptom Driven Diagnostic System for Primary Care (SDDS-PC)
- *Medical examination for differential diagnosis:* Screen for endocrine disorders, cardiovascular disease, respiratory disorders, temporal lobe epilepsy, vestibular disorders, toxin exposure, and substance abuse.
- A CMP, TSH, CBC, ECG, urinalysis, and a drug screen provide important information regarding secondary causes of anxiety. A CMP helps assess for diabetes, liver disease, and kidney disease. The TSH helps to screen for hyper- or hypothyroidism. A CBC can be helpful to screen for anemia, infections, and inflammation. The ECG helps to reveal cardiac problems. Urinalysis helps detect metabolic and kidney disorders. The drug screen detects substance abuse problems (which the patient may not initially disclose).

- Spirometry testing and bronchodilator reversibility testing can be useful to screen for asthma and COPD. Additional studies may necessitate an EEG or vestibular testing.

Comments and Treatment Considerations

A full substance abuse assessment is indicated when it is determined that alcohol, illicit drugs, or prescription drug abuse contributes to the patient's anxiety level. Inpatient substance abuse services, outpatient substance abuse services, Alcoholics Anonymous or Narcotics Anonymous (AA/NA) meetings, or medical detox options may be necessary.

Extended removal of the substance or toxin should result in a reduction in the anxiety level. Encourage a healthy lifestyle (e.g., routine exercise, appropriate diet, good sleep hygiene, no substance abuse). A change in medication may be necessary, if any of the patient's medications have anxiety as a side effect, interaction, or withdrawal effect.

If the patient's medical problems produce anxiety symptoms, treatment of the underlying medical condition should produce a reduction in anxiety symptoms. Further assessment or differential diagnosis is indicated if improvements are not noted with the preceding approaches.

SOCIAL PHOBIA (SOCIAL ANXIETY DISORDER)

Social phobia is characterized by having a significant fear of social or performance situations in which embarrassment or humiliation can occur. It is much more intense and distressing than simply being shy, and the exposure to certain social encounters can immediately elicit a physical anxiety response. Situational panic attacks can occur in social phobia. These patients show functional impairments, avoidant behaviors, anxious anticipation, and a diminished quality of life. Despite such impairments patients are generally reluctant to seek help for social anxiety, and this diagnosis can easily be missed by health care providers.

Adults often identify that this fear is excessive, and they often want to be "normal" socially. Children and teens can display transient social anxiety symptoms without developing social phobia. Early childhood language impairment appears to be a precursor for social phobia. For those younger than 18 years of age, the symptoms must persist for at least 6 months to qualify for the social phobia diagnosis. Many people with social phobia will only display the symptoms in certain situations (such as meeting strangers, dating, or public speaking). Social phobia has a subclassification of "generalized type," which is to be noted if fear occurs in most social interaction or performance situations. This subtype represents about one third of patients with social phobia.

Patients with social phobia are likely to exhibit anticipatory anxiety regarding certain social interactions, perfectionism, and then self-criticism regarding their performance. They may worry that others are aware of their physical symptoms of anxiety (i.e., blushing, trembling, dry mouth). The diagnosis is not given if the embarrassment is primarily about symptoms of another known medical or psychiatric disorder. Social phobia has a high comorbidity rate with GAD, dysthymic disorder, major depressive disorder, PD, specific phobias, and avoidant personality disorder. It often co-occurs with eating disorders and alcohol abuse.

Symptoms
- Excessive fear (in one or more social interaction/performance situations) +++++
- Embarrassment or humiliation concerns ++++
- Anxiety or anxious anticipation ++++
- Distress +++
- Avoidance +++
- Panic attacks (situational) +
- Palpitations +

Signs
- Impaired social relationships +++
- Blushing ++
- Situational tremors ++
- Sweating +
- Diarrhea +

Workup
- Clinical interview: Include mental status examination; current psychosocial stressors; family (genetic) history of substance abuse, medical, or psychiatric disorders; and patient history of psychiatric, medical, or substance abuse problems and treatment services.
- Differential diagnosis or comorbidity screening indicated for other anxiety disorders, mood disorders, somatoform disorders, personality disorders, factitious disorders, eating disorders, psychosis, and suicidal ideations
- Screening checklists: Liebowitz Social Anxiety Scale (LSAS), Social Phobia Inventory (SPIN), Social Interaction Anxiety Scale (SIAS), Social Phobia and Anxiety Inventory (SPAI), and Social Phobia Scale (SPS)
- Medical examination for differential diagnosis (if panic attacks are present and are not entirely situational): Screen for endocrine disorders, cardiovascular disease, respiratory disorders, temporal lobe epilepsy, vestibular disorders, and substance abuse (see "Secondary Causes of Anxiety").

Comments and Treatment Considerations
Initiate patient education regarding social phobia and discuss treatment options. SSRIs (sertraline, fluvoxamine, and paroxetine) are considered to be effective for treating social phobia. Other medications that are used for social phobia include SNRIs (venlafaxine), monoamine oxidase inhibitors (MAOIs) (phenelzine), benzodiazepines (clonazepam and alprazolam), and buspirone. The FDA has

advised monitoring patients for suicidal ideations after starting anti-depressant medications.

Although β-adrenergic receptor antagonists (atenolol and propran-olol) are sometimes effective for the associated performance anxi-ety, they are not considered to be effective for generalized social phobia. Cognitive-behavioral treatments, exposure-based treatments, applied relaxation, interpersonal psychotherapy (IPT), and social skills training have all shown some effectiveness as psychologic interventions for social phobia. CBT and exposure-based treatments appear most effective (and maintain effectiveness on posttreatment follow up studies).

References

American Psychiatric Association: *Diagnostic and Statistical Manual of Mental Disorders*, Fourth Edition, Text Revision, Washington, DC, 2000, American Psychiatric Association.

Anthony MM, Swinson RP: *Phobic disorders and panic in adults: a guide to assessment and treatment*, Washington, DC, 2000, American Psychological Association.

Anthony MM, Swinson RP: *The shyness & social anxiety workbook*. Oakland, CA, 2000, New Harbinger Publications, Inc.

Anxiety Disorders Association of America: *Improving the diagnosis & treatment of generalized anxiety disorder: a dialogue between mental health profession-als and primary care physicians*. Washington, DC, 2004, ADAA.

Barlow DH: *Anxiety and its disorders: the nature and treatment of anxiety and panic*, 2nd ed, New York, 2002, Guilford Press.

Breslav N, Klein DF: Smoking and panic attacks: an epidemiologic investiga-tion, *Arch Gen Psychiatry* 56:1141–1147, 1999.

Chessick CA, Allen MH, Thase ME, et al: Azapirones for generalized anxiety disorder, *Cochrane Database Syst Rev* 2006, CD006115.

Gale C, Oakley-Brown M: *Clinical evidence: mental health: generalized anxiety disorder*. London, 2005, BMJ Publishing Group.

Kapczinski F, Lima MS, Souza JS, et al: Antidepressants for generalized anxiety disorder, *Cochrane Database Syst Rev* 2003, CD003592.

Kumar S, Oakley-Brown M: *Clinical evidence: mental health: panic disorder*. London, 2004, BMJ Publishing Group.

Moses S: *Anxiety secondary cause*. Family Practice Notebook, LLC, 2000, Minnesota, www.fpnotebook.com. Accessed December 30, 2010.

O'Donohue WT, Byrd MR, Cummings NA, Henderson DA: *Behavioral integra-tive care: treatments that work in the primary care setting*, New York, 2005, Brunner-Routledge.

Roy-Byrne P, Craske M, Stein M, et al: A randomized effectiveness trial of cognitive-behavioral therapy and medication for primary care panic disorder, *Arch Gen Psychiatry* 6:290–298, 2005.

Rygh JL, Sanderson WC: *Treating generalized anxiety disorder: evidence-based strategies, tools, and techniques*, New York, 2004, The Guilford Press.

Sadock BJ, Sadock VA: *Kaplan & Sadock's synopsis of psychiatry*, 9th ed. Philadelphia, 2003, Lippincott Williams & Wilkins.

Shearer S, Gordon L: The patient with excessive worry, *Am Fam Physician* 73:1049–1056, 1057–1058, 2006.

Spitzer R, Kroenke K, Williams J, Lowe B: A brief measure for assessing generalized anxiety disorder: The GAD-7, *Arch Intern Med* 166:1092–1097, 2006.

Stein DJ, Ipser JC, Van Balkom AJ: Pharmacotherapy for social anxiety disor-der, *Cochrane Database Syst Rev* 2004, CD001206.

Voci S, Beitchman J, Brownlie EB, Wilson B: Social anxiety in late adolescence: the importance of early childhood language impairment, *J Anxiety Disord* 20:915–930, 2006.

Wagner R, Silove D, Marnane C, Rouen D: Delays in referral of patients with social phobia, panic disorder and generalized anxiety disorder attending a specialist anxiety clinic, *J Anxiety Disord* 20:363–371, 2006.

CHAPTER 6

Arthralgia
David McBride

According to the National Center for Health Statistics' report on health in the United States published in 2009, arthritis and musculoskeletal conditions were the most common causes of limitation of work among the working-age population. Of all symptom-based visits to physician offices, musculoskeletal complaints are the most common presenting symptom, ahead of respiratory and psychological complaints, which ranked second and third, respectively.

The cardinal signs of inflammation, *rubor* or redness, *calor* or heat, *dolor* or pain, and tumor or swelling, are used as examination findings to support the diagnosis of arthritis rather than arthralgia. Redness and heat are generally seen with inflammation rather than with joint and connective tissue disease. Limitation of passive range of motion (ROM) versus active ROM may indicate joint effusion, which is seen with intra-articular disease—traumatic, inflammatory, or degenerative. Tenderness over bony surfaces raises the concern for fracture and should generally be evaluated radiologically.

SEPTIC JOINT

Joint infection is an orthopedic emergency because untreated joint infection can lead to permanent cartilage loss and ultimate joint dysfunction. Synovial tissue has no basement membrane, so bacteria can easily enter a joint and cause infection. Acute monoarthritis has a short differential diagnosis, primarily crystal arthropathy and infection. At times patients with infectious arthritis exhibit other symptoms of infection, such as fever (64%), malaise, or a primary source of infection, so joint fluid analysis is crucial to the diagnosis of an acute monoarthritis.

Infectious arthritis has three main patterns: acute monoarthritis with common organisms such as *Staphylococcus aureus;* gonococcal arthritis, which is typically polyarticular and involves small joints; and chronic infectious, which can involve large and small joints and may be migratory (i.e., Lyme disease). The knee is the most commonly affected joint. There is a high chance of permanent loss of joint function with acute infectious monoarticular arthritis and up to a 15% mortality rate, thus appropriate diagnosis and management are crucial.

Management of a septic joint typically involves either surgery, antibiotics, or both. The surgical approach can be open or arthroscopic or can involve repeated joint aspirations to remove infected fluid as it accumulates. Most practitioners advocate an approach of "septic joint until proven otherwise" when approaching an acute monoarticular arthritis.

Symptoms
- Intense joint pain +++++ (this does not differentiate infectious from other forms of arthritis)
- New joint swelling ++++
- Sweats, rigors +
- Prosthetic joint +

Signs
- Fever (50%)
- Joint warmth, tenderness, and decreased ROM

Workup
- Joint aspiration with microscopic examination, crystal analysis, and culture. Joint fluid WBC count greater than 100,000 per cubic milliliter should be considered infectious until proven otherwise. Fluid may be turbid with decreased stringing.
- CBC with WBC greater than 10,000/μL
- Elevated ESR
- Elevated CRP
- Blood culture (positive in 50%)
- Consider testing for gonorrhea by throat culture or urine, urethral, or cervical sample.

Comments and Treatment Considerations
Immediate surgical consultation is indicated to assist in decision making when a septic joint is suspected. Antibiotic coverage for *S. aureus, Streptococcus pneumoniae,* and gram-negative bacilli is generally indicated, in the form of a third-generation cephalosporin or fluoroquinolone in the case of cephalosporin allergy. Methicillin-resistant *S. aureus* (MRSA) has become an increasingly common community-acquired organism, so vancomycin may be added if this is a concern. Antibiotics may be required for 2 to 4 weeks followed by an additional 2 to 6 weeks of oral antibiotics. Coverage may be narrowed once an organism has been identified.

Surgical approaches may include arthroscopic drainage and lavage or open drainage and lavage. Drain tubes may be placed to allow persistent accumulation of pus to be removed. Serial arthrocentesis can also allow for joint fluid to be removed, but this approach does not allow for joint lavage.

Despite hospitalization, surgery, and antibiotic use, mortality from joint sepsis may be up to 15%. Immediate treatment after a high level of suspicion may help mitigate this reality.

GOUT

Gout is classically described as an acute monoarthritis, with a propensity for the first metatarsophalangeal (MTP) joint and foot in general, the knee, and sometimes the hands, wrists, and elbows. Acute gout is clinically indistinguishable from pseudogout in which calcium pyrophosphate, rather than uric acid, is the offending crystallized solute. Gout has an intercritical form in which uric acid can have other negative systemic effects, such as nephrolithiasis. Chronic gout is a destructive joint disease potentially causing significant disability.

Gout is the result of the inflammatory effect within the joint stimulated by the presence of precipitated uric acid crystals. The influx of neutrophils, releasing nonspecific inflammatory products, is the culprit in the intense inflammation and not the "needle-like" effect of the crystals themselves. Hyperuricemia raises the likelihood of a gout attack, but elevated levels of uric acid are not necessary to make the diagnosis of gout. Men are more often affected than women. Obesity, renal insufficiency, thiazide diuretic use, cyclosporine therapy, high purine intake, excess alcohol intake, and family history are also predisposing factors.

Symptoms
- Joint pain that is intense +++++ Patients often report that the lightest touch on the joint is excruciatingly painful.
- Fairly rapid onset of joint pain ++++
- Swelling and redness +++++
- Often the classic gout joints, such as the first MTP or knee affected ++++
- Chronic gout may include ongoing joint pain because of erosions of bone and joint space caused by inflammation. +
- Tophi are usually painless, developing insidiously and without inflammation. ++

Signs
- Usually one joint affected +++++
- Redness and synovitis around the affected joint. The appearance may resemble acute cellulitis. +++++
- Severe tenderness to palpation +++++
- Limited active and passive ROM ++++
- Chronic gout may have tophi, which are firm, nontender nodules, generally over joints affected and often on extensor surfaces. ++

Workup
- Look for signs of chronic gout.
- Joint aspiration with fluid analysis should be performed if possible, at least in first occurrences, to help in distinguishing from joint infection. Joint fluid findings should include negatively birefringent crystals, greater than 2000 but less than 100,000 WBCs/mL, absence of Gram-staining organisms, and negative fluid culture. Viscosity of fluid is typically low, as is fluid "stringing." +++++
- Serum uric acid may be measured, but normal levels do not rule out gout. A serum level of 9 mg/dL is associated with a 4.9% annual incidence in healthy men, compared with 0.1% annual incidence for a level of less than 7 mg/dL.

- Evaluation for predisposing factors such as hypertension, renal insufficiency ++
- Consider evaluation for insulin resistance as a factor influencing uric acid excretion and as a risk factor for heart disease. + Hyperuricemia is a documented risk factor for cardiovascular disease as well.
- Young age at first presentation (20s or 30s) may warrant evaluation for inheritable enzyme deficiencies like hypoxanthine guanine phosphoribosyltransferase. +

Comments and Treatment Considerations

Decrease pain and inflammation with NSAIDS, noting that there is no proven advantage of any one NSAID. Ibuprofen derivatives, naproxen, sulindac, indomethacin, and cyclooxygenase-2 (COX-2) inhibitors have all shown similar efficacy (e.g., naproxen sodium 500 mg twice a day for 3 days then 250 mg twice daily until resolution).

Note that all NSAIDs (including COX-2 inhibitors) carry a black box warning about increase in acute cardiovascular risk. Hyperuricemia is a risk factor for cardiovascular disease (CVD).

Systemic (either by mouth or IM) or intra-articular corticosteroids are effective, provided that joint sepsis is not a consideration (e.g., prednisone 60 mg by mouth once daily for 3 days then taper).

Oral colchicine may be started at 0.6 mg by mouth up to three doses then dosing 0.6 mg one every other day to twice daily for prophylaxis from further attacks. Colchicine is renally excreted and must be dosed based on creatinine clearance. Patients with creatinine clearance less than 10 mL/min should not receive colchicine. Side effects of diarrhea, nausea, and vomiting are common. Colchicine is most effective if started on the first day of an attack.

For chronic and suppressive conditions, lifestyle modifications such as weight loss and decreased alcohol intake (particularly beer) are important. Diets lower in carbohydrate with proportional increase in unsaturated fat and protein have been proven effective in lowering serum uric acid levels.

Discontinuation of thiazide diuretics and consideration of discontinuation of cyclosporine, if possible.

When colchicine is used for long-term prophylaxis, patients should be monitored for muscle weakness (myopathy caused by the drug), bone marrow suppression, and renal insufficiency. Colchicine or an NSAID should be started concurrently with allopurinol or a uricosuric to prevent the precipitation of a gout episode in the first 3 to 4 weeks of therapy.

Allopurinol is effective both for underexcreters (75% to 90% of gout sufferers) and overproducers (10% to 25% of gout sufferers). Allopurinol should not be started within 3 to 4 weeks of an acute attack because sudden changes in serum uric acid levels during this period may stimulate an attack. Two percent of patients may develop an allergic reaction to allopurinol, which is generally mild, although severe allergic reaction is possible. Dosing should be started at 100 mg daily and increased until serum uric acid concentrations are normalized (30% reduction in episodes if serum uric acid is 4.6 to 6.6 mg/dL). The usual daily dose is 200 to 300 mg/day. Allopurinol should be dosed based on the creatinine clearance.

Uricosurics have shown similar efficacy to allopurinol for underexcreters of uric acid in a prospective parallel study. Uric acid excretion should be documented at less than 700 mg per 24 hours. Probenecid is started at 250 mg by mouth twice daily and is increased up to 2000 mg daily in divided doses to lower serum uric acid level to less than 6 mg/dL. Sulfinpyrazone dosing starts at 50 mg by mouth twice daily and can be increased to 400 mg daily in divided doses, again with a target serum uric acid level of less than 6 mg/dL. Creatinine clearance must be monitored and uricosuric use can precipitate urolithiasis.

Uric acid oxidase is used for gout treatment and prevention in patients undergoing chemotherapy. A case study has demonstrated efficacy of tumor necrosis factor (TNF) blockade (etanercept) in treatment of refractory tophaceous gout. A novel xanthine oxidase inhibitor, febuxostat, has been shown more effective than allopurinol in a head-to-head trial.

HIP FRACTURE

Hip fracture remains a harbinger of poor outcomes in older adult patients. A 2000 report on fall prevention in older adults, notes, "Falls are the leading cause of injury deaths and disabilities among persons aged older than 65 years," and 95% of hip fractures are caused by falls.

Risks for falling are familiar territory to family physicians in working with older adult patients and include:
• Physical inactivity leading to loss of strength and balance
• Difficulty completing activities of daily living
• The presence of dementia
• Use of medications that cause cognitive impairment
• Home hazards such as poor lighting and throw rugs
• Having more than one chronic disease
• History of stroke
• Parkinson's disease
• Neuromuscular disease
• Urinary incontinence
• Visual impairment

Many of these risk factors are modifiable through intervention in the home. Interventions that Cochrane calls "likely to be beneficial" include multidisciplinary home evaluation and intervention in patients with a defined history of falls, professionally led strengthening and balance training, professional home hazard modification, withdrawal of psychotropics, cardiac pacing when indicated, and tai chi. The benefit of other interventions is less clear.

Treatment and prevention of osteoporosis using calcium and vitamin D supplementation and weightbearing exercise earlier in life, bisphosphonates, calcitonin, and raloxifene all help to increase bone density and have proved fracture reduction. Calcium and vitamin D supplementation after menopause has been historically recommended, though this recommendation has been called into question. There is some apparent benefit of vitamin D alone in preventing falls in nursing home patients.

Symptoms
- Typically follow a fall ++++
- Pain in the area often with and without movement +++++
- It is not uncommon that patients walk on the injured leg for some time before presenting for care.

Signs
- Limitation of active and passive ROM secondary to pain +++++
- Shortening, internal rotation and abduction of the affected hip ++++

Workup
- Plain x-ray: A posteroanterior (PA) view of the pelvis and lateral view of the femur +++++
- MRI (or CT if MRI is unavailable or contraindicated) can be used if a high index of suspicion is present and the fracture is not apparent on plain x-ray.
- Hip fracture can occur at the femoral neck, between the greater and lesser trochanter (intertrochanteric), or below the lesser trochanter. The third is the least common type.

Comments and Treatment Considerations
Early surgical repair within 24 to 48 hours is optimal. If surgical risk assessment needs to be done prior to the procedure, outcomes are better if this is done in less than 72 hours. Displaced femoral neck fractures treated with primary arthroplasty result in similar mortality but better function and fewer surgery-related complications.

Most patients undergoing hip fracture repair should be treated with thromboprophylaxis with unfractionated heparin, low-molecular-weight heparin (LMWH), direct thrombin inhibitors, or warfarin. If anticoagulation is contraindicated, antithrombotic pumps are also effective in preventing deep vein thrombosis (DVT). Anticoagulation should be continued for 10 to 14 days after surgery and longer if the patient has risk factors for DVT such as inability to ambulate, obesity, malignancy, history of DVT, and older age.

Patients should be mobilized as early after fracture repair as possible. Antibiotics during surgery reduce the incidence of infection. Pain control is important in the management of any operative procedure. Addressing hospital- or surgery-associated delirium in older adult patients is important in preventing perioperative complications of repeat falling and patient distress.

KNEE AND ANKLE TRAUMA

Knee and ankle trauma are two of the most common concerns that bring patients to a family physician office. Family physicians should recognize and appropriately manage these injuries as they present to the office. The patient's story will give pertinent clues to lead to the appropriate diagnosis. Often the injury can be intuited from the mechanism of injury that the patient reports.

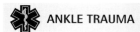 **ANKLE TRAUMA**

Common mechanisms of sports injury in the foot and ankle occur on the playing field and with extreme, sudden force or impact of the joint and its surrounding soft tissue. For the ankle a mechanism of inversion versus eversion, dorsiflexion versus plantar flexion narrows the differential. Immediate swelling and non-weightbearing status after the injury are a concern. The anterior talofibular ligament is the most commonly injured structure in an acute ankle injury.

Symptoms
- Immediate swelling is a sign of ligamentous rupture or bony trauma because both of these injuries lead to subcutaneous bleeding. +++++ Blood typically accumulates more rapidly than other edema fluid.
- Inability to bear weight is a very important symptom +++++ because it is more indicative of bony injury.
- The majority of ankle injuries involve inversion. +++++ The patient's report of the location of the pain will most often be on the lateral ankle in this case.
- Patients may report the feeling or sound of a "pop" when a ligament or tendon is ruptured. ++++ Patients often report feeling like they were "shot" in the calf when an Achilles tendon rupture occurs. ++++

Signs
- Location of swelling should be noted (Table 6-1). Most often the swelling is laterally located. +++ Swelling across the anterior flexor crease of the ankle may be an indication of an intra-articular injury, like a talar dome fracture. ++++
- Ecchymosis is most often associated with ligamentous injury. +++++ Ligaments have a rich blood supply and partial or complete tear leads to a large amount of subcutaneous bleeding.
- The anterior drawer test is used to assess the integrity of the anterior talofibular ligament. +++++ It may reveal stability compared to the opposite side and laxity with an endpoint or laxity without a clear endpoint. It is important to compare with the uninjured side in special testing because preexisting laxity can be confused for acute ligamentous injury.

Table 6-1. Common Ankle Traumatic Injuries and Specific Signs

INJURY	COMMON SIGNS
First degree	Swelling and point tenderness anterior to the distal fibula. Edema and bruising are generally mild.
Inversion sprain	Stability should be present on anterior drawer and talar tilt.
Second degree	Swelling and point tenderness as above are more severe.
Inversion sprain	There may be laxity with an endpoint on anterior drawer and talar tilt.
Third degree	This injury represents complete tear of the ATF. Swelling, tenderness and ecchymosis are severe.
Inversion sprain	Anterior drawer and talar tilt reveal laxity without a clear endpoint.
High ankle sprain	Pain with dorsiflexion and eversion over syndesmosis.
	Positive squeeze test.
Peroneal tendon injury	Tenderness posterior to the lateral malleolus. The patient may experience difficulty with plantar flexion or eversion.
	Subluxation of the peroneal tendon over the lateral malleolus may be appreciated on palpation while the patient everts the foot.
Achilles tendon rupture	Tenderness over the Achilles. Inability to plantar flex when standing on one foot. Thompson test does not reveal plantar response.
Proximal fifth metatarsal fracture/Jones fracture	Pain over proximal fifth metatarsal.
Stress fracture	Metatarsal or calcaneus tenderness and pain.

- The talar tilt test also assesses the integrity of the lateral ankle ligamentous structures. +++++ Laxity and pain with testing compared with the opposite side indicate a higher grade of injury.
- The squeeze test involves compressing the tibiofibular axis. Pain with this maneuver suggests a rupture of the tibiofibular syndesmosis. +++++
- The Thompson test of the Achilles tendon involves squeezing the relaxed calf musculature with the knee in 90 degrees of flexion (patient kneeling on a chair) and noting for the presence of plantar flexion of the foot. +++++

Workup

- Radiography is indicated in the evaluation of ankle injuries, particularly if any of the following are present:
  - Pain on the posterior edge of the lateral malleolus
  - Pain on the posterior edge of the medial malleolus
  - If patient is totally unable to bear weight after the episode or for four steps in the office
  - Pain at the base of the fifth metatarsal
  - Pain at the navicular
- Mortise view should generally be included in an ankle x-ray series. Inversion stress views can also be obtained to determine the degree of joint opening, with more joint opening associated with complete ligamentous tear. MRI can detect ligamentous injury, but data on treatment favor functional treatment regardless of the degree of sprain.
- When a stress fracture is suspected, early radiography may be negative. Family physicians have the option to wait and repeat an x-ray in 1 to 2 weeks, at which point one may see signs of callus formation. Bone scan is more sensitive and reveals changes earlier or when no plain radiographic findings are apparent.

Comments and Treatment Considerations

Table 6-2. Treatment of Ankle Injuries

INJURY	TREATMENT
First degree Inversion sprain	Rest, ice, compression, elevation. Progressive weight bearing.
Second degree Inversion sprain	Rest, ice, compression, elevation. Crutches initially for comfort with progressive weightbearing. Early weightbearing yields better results. Medial, lateral stabilizing brace is indicated for 2 weeks continuously and up to 4 weeks with exercise. Patients should be taught range of motion, proprioception and strengthening exercises at the 2-week follow-up.
Third degree Inversion sprain	Rest, ice, compression, elevation. Crutches may be required. Functional treatment with progressive weightbearing and activity seem to be favored over immobilization. There is suggestion that surgical repair of rupture yields better outcomes than immobilization.
High ankle sprain	Rest, ice, compression, elevation. Non-weightbearing and orthopedic referral. This injury is often associated with higher-grade ankle sprain and even proximal fibular fracture.
Peroneal tendon injury	Rest, ice, compression, elevation. Non-weightbearing and referral to orthopedics.

Table 6-2. Treatment of Ankle Injuries—cont'd

INJURY	TREATMENT
Achilles tendon rupture	Often requires urgent surgical repair. Rest, ice, compression, elevation. Non-weightbearing and referral to orthopedics.
Proximal fifth	Rest, ice, compression, elevation. Fracture of the distal tip of the fifth metatarsal can be treated with 2-4 weeks in a hard-bottom shoe.
Metatarsal fracture/ Jones fracture	Rest, ice, compression, elevation. Fracture of the more distal portions of the metatarsal may require controlled ankle motion (CAM) walker immobilization and possible pinning.
Stress fracture	Rest, ice, compression, elevation. Non-weightbearing for 4-6 weeks and graded return to play are necessary.

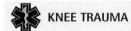

KNEE TRAUMA

Knee trauma can occur on and off the playing field. The mechanism of injury will strongly lead the family physician in the direction of a correct diagnosis (Table 6-3).

Symptoms
- Immediate swelling is a symptom of ligamentous rupture or bony trauma because both of these injuries lead to subcutaneous bleeding. Blood typically accumulates more rapidly than other edema fluid. Effusions typically occur within 24 hours of injury, but especially in the first 4 to 6 hours. +++++
- Inability to bear weight is a very important symptom because it is more indicative of bony injury. ++++
- Patients may report the feeling or sound of a "pop" when a ligament or tendon is ruptured, especially in an anterior cruciate ligament (ACL) injury. ++++
- Typical ACL injury history involves foot planting and a twist. +++++
- Posterior cruciate ligament (PCL) is generally a dashboard injury. +++++
- Medial collateral ligament (MCL) and lateral collateral ligament (LCL) injuries often involve a blow to the opposite side of the knee from the affected ligament. +++++

Signs
- With ligament tear, the swelling is centrally located and hinders both knee flexion and extension. Ligaments have a rich blood supply and partial or complete tear leads to a large amount of subcutaneous bleeding or effusion.
- The Lachman test is used to assess the integrity of the ACL. It may reveal stability compared to the opposite side, laxity with

Table 6-3. Common Knee Traumatic Injuries and Specific Symptoms and Signs

INJURY	SYMPTOM	COMMON SIGNS
ACL tear	Pop with twisting Immediate swelling	Positive Lachman Pivot shift, anterior drawer
MCL tear/sprain	Pain on medial knee Lateral blow to the knee	First degree—negative valgus stress Second degree—positive stress but firm endpoint Third degree—positive stress without an endpoint
Meniscal tear	Medial/lateral twist, stress Locking/clicking sensation	Positive McMurray test with click Joint line tenderness and pain with squatting
PCL tear	Dashboard type injury	Positive posterior drawer
LCL sprain/tear	Lateral knee pain Medial blow to knee	First degree—negative varus stress Second degree—positive stress but firm endpoint Third degree—positive stress without an endpoint
Tibial plateau fracture	Axial loading and inability to bear weight	Knee effusion, positive x-ray

ACL, Anterior cruciate ligament; *LCL*, lateral collateral ligament; *MCL*, medial collateral ligament; *PCL*, posterior cruciate ligament.

an endpoint or laxity without a clear endpoint. It is important to compare to the uninjured side because preexisting laxity or history of ipsilateral knee surgery can be confused for acute ligamentous injury. The Lachman test eliminates the stabilization of the hamstring tendons and tends to isolate the ACL to a greater degree. It has a sensitivity of 86% and specificity of 91%. ++++

- The anterior drawer test of the knee may also assess for ACL injury using the same guidelines as above. It has a sensitivity of 20% and a specificity of 88%. The low sensitivity is due to patient guarding with the hamstring tendons or a PCL injury. ++++
- The pivot shift test assesses the ACL and has a sensitivity of 48% and specificity of 99%. +++++ Examiner skill is a determinant in the sensitivity of this test.
- The posterior drawer test assesses the integrity of the PCL. Again, laxity, endpoint, and comparison to the other knee should be noted. The sensitivity is 90% and specificity is 99%. +++++
- The McMurray test assesses the integrity of the medial and lateral meniscus. This test is performed in many different fashions; however, all methods involve a valgus stress with foot inversion and a varus stress with foot eversion while flexing and extending the knee. A positive test involves a palpable pop over the joint line of the affected side. The sensitivity is 26% and specificity is 94%. +++
- The combination of medial joint line tenderness (sensitivity 76%, specificity 29%) and painful squatting have good predictive value for meniscal injury. +++
- A valgus stress should be placed on the lateral knee to test the medial collateral ligament. A lateral blow to the knee is likely to yield a medial collateral ligament tear. The MCL and medial meniscus are continuous structures and are often injured together. +++++
- A varus stress should be placed on the medial knee to test the lateral collateral ligament. A medial blow to the knee may produce an LCL tear. ++++
- A patella apprehension test should be performed on a knee in which subluxation is suspected. A positive test is pain and laxity with a lateral stress to the medial patella. ++++

Workup
- Radiography is indicated in the evaluation of knee injuries, particularly if the following are present:
  - Patient is unable to bear weight immediately or in the office
  - Patient is tender over the patella
  - Patient is tender over the proximal fibular head
  - Patient is unable to flex knee past 90 degrees
  - Patient is more than 55 years old
- Order three x-ray views: the AP, lateral, and sunrise.
- A Hughston view may be substituted for the sunrise for a more specific view of the patella.

- If ligamentous or cartilage injury is suspected, an MRI of the knee without contrast may be ordered. Of note, although MRI is often ordered in the workup of ACL tear, MRI has not been shown superior to clinical examination in making this diagnosis.
- Wait 1 week for the knee effusion to decrease prior to ordering more studies and reexamine the knee when ROM is more accessible.

Comments and Treatment Considerations

Table 6-4. Treatment of Common Knee Injuries

INJURY	TREATMENT
ACL tear	Rest, ice, analgesics. For higher-grade tears, crutches and knee immobilization are often needed for patient comfort. Physical therapy is often initiated prior to surgery to maintain strength and range of motion. Consider referral to sports medicine or orthopedics within 1-2 weeks.
MCL tear/sprain	Relative rest, ice and analgesics. First degree: physical therapy and hinged medial/lateral stabilization brace Second degree: physical therapy and hinged medial/lateral stabilization brace Third degree: referral to sports medicine or orthopedics and possible surgery
Meniscal tear	Rest, ice, analgesics. Physical therapy versus surgical debridement or repair
PCL tear	Rest, ice, analgesics. Physical therapy and consideration of surgery
LCL sprain/tear	Rest, ice, analgesics. Physical therapy Surgical consideration if complete tear
Tibial plateau fracture	Immediate orthopedic referral

ACL, Anterior cruciate ligament; *LCL,* lateral collateral ligament; *MCL,* medial collateral ligament; *PCL,* posterior cruciate ligament

OSTEOARTHRITIS

Of all joint disorders worldwide, osteoarthritis (OA) occurs with the greatest frequency. OA is defined by joint pain, functional loss, and radiologic evidence of degeneration in the absence of significant systemic inflammatory response. "Wear and tear" is blamed for osteoarthritis and a specific injury is not always identifiable. Local inflammatory mediators do lead to articular degeneration, and local cytokines and interleukins do contribute to joint damage, but the disease is not one of systemic inflammation. Articular cartilage and subchondral bone are the tissue types most affected by OA. Predisposing factors such as joint deformity, repetitive joint loading, trauma, and obesity do raise an individual patient's risk of developing OA.

Symptoms
- Joint pain +++++
- Stiffness, generally less pronounced after rest ++++
- A pattern of joint pain and/or stiffness over most days of a month ++++
- Swelling of the affected joint(s) ++++

Signs
- Patient age more than 38 to 40 years, depending on the joint affected. Younger patients tend not to have degenerative joint disease. +++
- Overweight or obese
- Angular deformity that may predispose to OA (i.e., genu valgum or varum)
- Effusion of joints where this finding is appreciable (knees).
- Bony enlargement.
  - Heberden's nodes (distal interphalangeal [DIP] joints of the fingers) +++
  - Bouchard's nodes (proximal interphalangeal [PIP] joints of the fingers) +++
- Limited active ROM secondary to stiffness or pain +++
- Limited passive ROM if effusion is present or if bony exostoses are prominent ++
- Crepitance or "crunching or grinding" feeling when joints are taken through range of motion ++
- Antalgic gait secondary to pain if knees or hips are affected

Workup
- Plain radiography may reveal typical patterns of OA. These changes may include osteophyte (bony spur) formation, joint space narrowing (often asymmetric), eburnation (increase in subchondral bone density), and subchondral cysts. The correlation of radiographic OA findings and arthroscopic disease is limited (correlation coefficient of 0.41 to 0.56 in one study of 125 patients). Additionally, bony spur formation may be present in asymptomatic individuals. Hence the need to use radiography in the context of appropriate history and physical examination. +++
- MRI is much better at detecting subtle changes in articular cartilage, but is not often needed to diagnose OA.
- Serum evaluation for inflammation using ESR typically reveals a normal value. +++++
- Joint fluid analysis typically reveals decreased viscosity and decreased fluid "stringing" and WBC count less than 2000/mL. +++++

Comments and Treatment Considerations
Lifestyle modification and nonpharmacologic interventions such as weight loss and exercise for muscle strengthening are very

important. Aerobic exercise is effective in improving gait, pain, and functional status. Ice massage may improve ROM, strength, and swelling in an osteoarthritic joint but the effect on pain is unproven. Heat does not appear to offer a benefit. Physical therapy and occupational therapy should be targeted at joint protection and strengthening of supporting muscles around the affected joint.

Pharmacologic interventions can also prove beneficial. Acetaminophen is the safest drug (in terms of GI events) used to treat OA in the absence of preexisting hepatic problems and can be used at the maximum dose of 4 g/day.

NSAIDs are more effective, though modestly, for improving pain, particularly in patients with moderate to severe disease. NSAID GI risk can be mitigated by the addition of a PPI.

COX-2 inhibitors may be considered for patients who cannot tolerate NSAIDs for renal or GI reasons. The GI risk reduction is actually greater with PPIs and NSAIDs, however, compared with COX-2 inhibitors. COX-2 inhibitors, additionally, may raise the risk of adverse cardiac events.

Tramadol and other opioid analgesics offer pain relief in OA. Tolerance, addiction, and side effects may limit the use of this class of medications.

Pain reduction can be achieved with injection of intra-articular steroid, particularly the knee. Triamcinolone appears to be superior to betamethasone. Functional improvement may not be achieved with intra-articular steroid.

Viscosupplementation gives pain relief comparable to steroid, but with a longer duration of effect. Brand-name products such as Hyalgan, Hylan G F 20, Orthovisc, and Synvisc have been studied in placebo-controlled trials and show benefit.

Joint fluid aspiration at the time of injection should generally be performed.

Semirigid bracing of joints and weight distribution change with shoe lifts are helpful for OA of the knee. Bracing of the first metacarpophalangeal (MCP) joint helps relieve pain.

Surgery for OA takes a number of forms. Arthroscopic debridement of damaged cartilage does provide relief, particularly for patients with cartilage damage that causes locking. Osteotomy repairs angular deformities that contribute to OA, but outcomes on the knee are not better than conservative therapy. Arthrodesis, or surgically decreasing joint mobility, helps with pain at the cost of ROM and is considered a salvage procedure in those who are not candidates for joint replacement.

Joint replacement relieves pain, although prosthesis failure with time is a concern. Typical life span of a prosthetic joint is 10 to 15 years.

Complementary and alternative measures including acupuncture offer relief from pain in OA, but studies are mixed in its superiority to sham acupuncture.

Certain brands (Rotta) of glucosamine are somewhat helpful for pain in OA, but can be expensive.

OVERUSE INJURIES

Chronic overuse tendon injuries are commonly mislabeled "tendinitis," whereas histologic findings demonstrate tendon degeneration without inflammation. As a result, the terms *tendinosus* or *tendinopathy* are more appropriate.

Tendons have a poor vascular supply proximal to their insertion, hence the osteotendinous junction is the most commonly affected site. However, these tendon injuries can occur at any level of the tendon.

The pathophysiology of tendinosis involves degeneration of highly arranged collagen fiber structures within the tendon. Disorientation of these fibers leads to tendon weakening and an increase of proteoglycan substance with neovascularization.

Radiographs can evaluate bony structures and joints, but films cannot be used to evaluate soft tissues. Films may demonstrate calcification at the osteotendinous junction. MRI is commonly used to evaluate soft tissues as is ultrasound, although it is highly operator dependent. MRI and ultrasound are commonly ordered for preoperative evaluation.

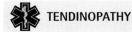 **TENDINOPATHY**

Symptoms
- May persist for up to 6 months
- Many patients respond more rapidly to nonoperative measures.

Comments and Treatment Considerations
Pain control, relative rest, ice, stretching, and eccentric strengthening are the mainstay of treatment. Analgesics such as acetaminophen or tramadol may be used. NSAIDs have a limited role because inflammation is often not present, although they may be beneficial during the acute stage.

Rest from the offending activity or sport prevents further tendon damage and may promote healing. Activities that do not cause pain symptoms may continue to be performed.

Cryotherapy has a potential benefit of analgesia, and may offer short-term relief. Prolonged application should be avoided to prevent injury to the skin. Its use should not exceed 15- to 20-minute intervals, and a moist towel should be used to avoid injury to the skin.

Stretching is widely accepted and considered beneficial.

Eccentric exercise involves lengthening of muscle fibers while the muscle is still contracting. These exercises stimulate collagen formation and aid in proper alignment of newly formed fibers.

Therapeutic ultrasound and massage are often used with varying results.

The use of corticosteroid injections is controversial. These injections aid in temporary relief of symptoms, but they can also weaken the tendon and ultimately lead to tendon rupture.

Braces are used to protect or unload the tendon during activity. Results vary, but braces are a safe treatment option.

Surgery is generally reserved for cases refractory to 6 months of nonoperative treatment. The procedure involves resection of the degenerative portion of the affected tendon.

 ## ACHILLES TENDINOPATHY

Achilles tendinopathy is often seen in adult running athletes and its incidence increases with age. Causes include improper training techniques, sudden increase in activity, anatomic lower extremity deformities, uneven training surfaces, and poor-fitting shoes. Fluoroquinolone exposure has also been implicated in tendon degeneration and even rupture.

Symptoms
- Pain at the heel proximal to the tendon insertion +++
- Increase in pain associated with increased training schedule

Signs
- Tendon thickening and tenderness 2 to 6 cm proximal to its insertion ++++
- Frequently accompanied by foot alignment abnormalities (i.e., flat feet, heel varus, or foot pronation) +++
- Tightness of the calf muscles is often seen. +++
- Thomson's squeeze test (squeezing the gastrocnemius with the patient in the prone position) should be performed to verify that the tendon has not ruptured.

Workup
- The diagnosis is based primarily on physical examination and history.

Comments and Treatment Considerations
Eccentric or decline calf raises may be particularly helpful in this overuse injury. Stretching of the gastrocnemius-soleus complex and deep friction massage are often helpful.

 ## LATERAL ELBOW TENDINOPATHY

Tendinopathy of the elbow can affect both the medial and lateral elbow. Lateral elbow tendinopathy is 10 times more common than its medial counterpart, and the patient's dominant arm is affected 75% of the time. Elbow tendinopathy more commonly occurs after age 40 +++, but may present at an earlier age.

Mechanisms causing lateral elbow tendinopathy, commonly mislabeled "lateral epicondylitis," include racquet sports ("tennis elbow") and repetitive activities that involve wrist extension or gripping.

Symptoms
- Insidious onset of dull or sharp pain in the lateral elbow +++++
- Typically affect the dominant arm +++
- Symptoms present with increased activity, and may appear at night in advanced stages.

Signs
- Tenderness at the lateral epicondyle, along the wrist extensor tendons, and the tendon insertion
- Resisted wrist extension commonly reproduces the patient's symptoms, especially with the elbow in extension.

Workup
- Lateral elbow tendinosis is a clinical diagnosis, but ultrasound and MRI are sometimes performed if treatment has failed.

Comments and Treatment Considerations
Tennis elbow brace or counterforce brace can sometimes be helpful. Equipment modification such as larger grip or vibration absorption devices may be useful. Corticosteroid injection provides short-term relief, although long-term outcomes are poorer in injection versus noninjection groups at 12 months.

 MEDIAL ELBOW TENDINOPATHY

Medial elbow tendinopathy, commonly mislabeled "medial epicondylitis," can be seen in golfing ("golfer's elbow"), throwing sports, racquet sports, or activities that require repetitive wrist flexion.

Symptoms
- Insidious onset of dull or sharp pain in the medial elbow ++++
- More common in the dominant elbow
- Grip weakness
- Can be associated with nerve irritation in an ulnar distribution

Signs
- Tenderness along the medial epicondyle and tendons of the flexor pronator mass +++++
- Pain with resisted pronation and wrist flexion ++++
- Positive Tinel's testing (tapping on the nerve) posterior to the medial epicondyle suggests ulnar nerve irritation.
- Ulnar collateral ligament tear should also be suspected in throwing athletes. This can be assessed clinically with a valgus stress test of the elbow.

Workup
- The diagnosis is based primarily on physical examination and history.
- MRI or diagnostic ultrasound should be ordered if an ulnar collateral ligament tear is suspected.

Comments and Treatment Considerations
Corticosteroid injection should be used with caution because of the
proximity of the lateral epicondyle to the ulnar groove and nerve.
Injection into the nerve can cause damage.

 ROTATOR CUFF TENDINOPATHY

Rotator cuff tendinopathy commonly presents with a history of
repetitive overhead activities ++++, and this tendinopathy affects
approximately 2% of the population. Incidence increases with age
and is more common with overhead activities (i.e., throwing athletes, volleyball, and tennis) and in labor workers.

Pathophysiology is thought to involve repeat "impingement" or
rubbing of the supraspinatus muscle with the coracoacromial arch
during shoulder abduction. Tendon hypovascularity, which occurs
approximately 2 cm from the distal supraspinatus insertion, also
plays a role in this degenerative process.

Symptoms
- Pain at the region of the deltoid, which is worse with activity
  ++++
- Difficulty sleeping while lying on the affected shoulder ++++

Signs
- Positive *empty* can test (weakness/pain with resistance, arms 70
  degrees abduction, 30 degrees forward flexion, and internal rotation with thumbs pointing down) +++
- Positive Hawkin's test (arm forward flexed 90 degrees and elbow
  flexed 90 degrees with progressive shoulder internal rotation)
  +++
- Positive Neer's test (fully pronated arm with maximum forward
  flexion) +++

Workup
- Radiographs: Radiographs may demonstrate spur formation of
  the acromion or tendon calcification.
- Ultrasonography: Diagnostic ultrasound can detect full-thickness
  rotator cuff tears, and can demonstrate chronic tendinopathy.
- MRI: Highly sensitive and specific for detection of rotator cuff
  tears and tendinopathy

Comments and Treatment Considerations
Avoidance of overhead activities in the acute phase, and patients
should not be immobilized to prevent muscle atrophy. It is crucial
to differentiate between rotator cuff tendinosis and tear. Tendinosis
improves with rest, whereas tears often do not.

The goal of physical therapy is to reestablish pain free ROM
through stretching exercises, and strengthen shoulder muscle once
the patient has recovered from the acute phase.

Subacromial corticosteroid injections have shown to have a small benefit compared with placebo up to 1 month postinjection.

Subacromial decompression surgery involves shaving of the undersurface of the acromion to better accommodate the supraspinatus.

PATELLAR PROBLEMS

Dysfunction of the patellofemoral joint is the most common cause of anterior knee pain. It can be seen in all ages and professions but is especially frequent in athletes, and most specifically runners. Thirty percent of athletes experience anterior knee pain at some point during their competitive careers. Despite being a common problem, the specific etiology is frequently difficult to establish and is often multifactorial in nature. The patient history can be very helpful in suggesting a diagnosis, especially when a single traumatic event is involved and the mechanism of injury can be elucidated. However, frequently anterior knee pain is not associated with a specific traumatic event, but rather is insidious in onset. In these cases, a careful examination and appropriate use of diagnostic imaging tests are essential in establishing a diagnosis.

 PATELLAR DISLOCATION

Acute, first-time patella dislocations are common in sports, and frequently occur in individuals younger than age 20. Studies have shown that the highest incidence occurs in women, ages 10 to 17 years. The mechanism can be a direct blow causing a valgus force across the knee, a direct medial blow to the patella, or with a twisting force associated with strong quadriceps contraction. Redislocation rates can be very high, approaching 60% in some studies.

Symptoms
- Sensation of the knee "popping" out of place +++++
- Anterior knee pain +++++
- Swelling +++++
- Medial bruising +++
- Instability or weakness +++
- Reluctance to bear weight

Signs
- If seen acutely the knee will typically be held in a flexed position with the patella prominent along the anterolateral side of the knee. +++++
- Large effusion/hemarthrosis +++++
- Tenderness along the medial retinaculum, often with ecchymosis in this area ++++
- May be marked hypermobility of the patella ++
- Apprehension when the patella is displaced laterally +++++

Workup

- Thorough knee examination looking for other associated injuries such as disruption of the ACL, MCL, or menisci.
- All suspected patella dislocation should have a radiograph to evaluate for associated osteochondral injury.
- Evaluation of possible predisposing anatomic factors:
  - Increased Q angle
  - Trochlear dysplasia
  - High-hiding patella
  - Vastus medialis obliquus (VMO) weakness or atrophy
  - Increased femoral anteversion
  - External tibial torsion
  - Pes planus or foot hyperpronation
  - Genu valgum

Comments and Treatment Considerations

If seen in the acute setting, the patella can often be easily relocated by extending the knee with gentle lateral to medial pressure on the patella. The examiner may hear or feel a "clunk" as the patella is reduced.

If a large hemarthrosis is present, aspiration under sterile techniques can often provide some symptomatic relief and allow improved ROM. Presence of fat globules in the aspirated blood can indicate an associated fracture.

Apply ice to minimize swelling. NSAIDs provide pain reduction.

It is generally accepted that a short period (2 to 3 weeks) of immobilization with the knee in extension may allow disrupted structures to heal and minimize redislocation rates. Early physical therapy will also help.

Return to sports when full ROM and strength are regained, without symptoms of instability. This may take 6 to 12 weeks. Consider surgery for recurrent dislocations.

 ## PATELLAR TENDINOSIS (TENDINITIS)

Tendinopathy of the patella tendon is an overuse condition resulting from repetitive loading of the knee extensor mechanism. This loading typically occurs with jumping, and therefore the condition has been termed "jumper's knee." It is believed that repetitive stresses cause microdamage, and tendon fiber failure, without allowing adequate time for tendon healing.

Symptoms

- Well-localized pain typically at the inferior pole of the patella ++++
- Pain begins gradually and may only be present during intense physical activity or after activity. As symptoms persist, the pain becomes present during normal daily activities and even at rest. +++++
- Pain may be intensified with rising from squatting position, prolonged sitting with bent knees, and the use of stairs. ++++

Signs
- Tenderness at the inferior pole of the patella, and upper portion of the patella tendon when the knee is in full extension ++++
- Pain may be elicited with repetitive squats. +++
- Palpable thickening of the tendon compared with the contralateral side ++
- Atrophy of the quadriceps musculature ++

Workup
- History and clinical examination should be used to differentiate patella tendinosis from patellofemoral pain.
- Careful questioning as to potential aggravating activities
- The only anatomic factor shown prospectively to be predisposing is tight musculature, particularly the quadriceps muscles.
- X-rays may be helpful to differentiate patella tendinosis from other conditions such as patellofemoral OA.

Comments and Treatment Considerations
Relative rest and avoiding all potentially aggravating activities are the key features of treatment. Despite this being a relatively non-inflammatory condition there is still debate as to whether inflammatory mediators such as COX play a role in its pathogenesis, so NSAIDs may still have a role in a treatment regimen.

Ice can be used as an analgesic. It may also reduce the neovascularization that histologically has been shown to occur, and may play a role in the pathogenesis.

Eccentric exercise is most helpful for tendinopathy.

Deep tissue massage has shown some promise in animal studies.

The length of time to recover is generally related to the severity of the disease progression. It is not unusual for full recovery to take 4 to 6 months. Conservative treatment has been shown to be equal to surgical treatment in terms of length of time to recovery, and outcomes. However, cases not responding to a prolonged, intensive course of conservative treatment may be considered possible candidates for surgery.

 PREPATELLA BURSITIS

The prepatella bursa is a fluid-filled sac lying between the patella and the skin. The main function of the bursa is to provide cushioning against external pressure over the patella, such as occurs with kneeling. Inflammation of the bursa can occur from a single traumatic event, from repetitive pressure on the patella, or rarely from an infection. This condition is frequently seen in professions that involve kneeling such as carpet layers, tilers, gardeners, and roofers.

Symptoms
- Anterior knee swelling +++++
- Anterior knee pain especially when pressure is placed over the patella such as with kneeling ++++
- Occasionally may have some surrounding skin erythema ++

Signs
- Enlarged, boggy bursa on palpation ++++
- Bursa may be tender to the touch. +++
- May lack full flexion due to skin tension around the inflamed bursa ++
- May be palpable crepitance ++
- Occasional surrounding skin erythema, warmth, or cellulitis ++

Workup
- Aspiration of the bursa can be performed under sterile conditions if the bursa is very tense and limiting full joint motion, or if infection is suspected.
- X-rays should be performed in cases that occur from single traumatic fall or blow to the patella to rule out a fracture.

Comments and Treatment Considerations
Ice and NSAIDs: If a bursa aspiration is performed, a compression wrap should then be applied, followed by a short period (1 to 2 days) of immobilization. Aspiration in chronic bursitis is usually not helpful.

In chronic bursitis the goal is to avoid inciting activities or use protective knee pads. If a septic bursa is suspected the bursa should be aspirated, and fluid sent for analysis. Mild cases may be treated with oral antibiotics, but more severe cases may need IV antibiotics, bursal lavage, or incision and drainage. The typical bacterial causes are *S. aureus* and group A β-hemolytic *Streptococcus*.

Surgery to remove the bursa is elective, and is typically performed if there is an excessively large, chronically inflamed bursa that extends beyond the margins of the patella.

 PATELLOFEMORAL PAIN SYNDROME

Patellofemoral pain syndrome is a term used to describe anterior knee pain that seems to lack a clear-cut anatomic or pathologic cause. Usually this diagnosis is considered when other conditions have been ruled out by history, examination, and radiographic evaluation. The exact origin of the pain in patellofemoral pain syndrome is unclear. It is theorized that the pain may originate from the subchondral bone, or surrounding soft tissue structures and the cause is likely multifactorial, hence the wide variety of treatment options that have been recommended.

Symptoms
- Dull, achy anterior knee pain that can be described in a diffuse area centered around the patella, or localized very specifically to the patella ++++
- Insidious in onset +++++

- Knee may be described as "stiff," or the pain intensified after prolonged sitting with the knee in a flexed position ++++
- Occasional sense of instability when the pain is intense ++

Signs
- Absence of effusion and stable ligament examination ++++
- May have a positive patella grind test in which compression of the patella with the knee in extension reproduces pain +++
- May have tenderness along the medial and lateral facets of the patella +++

Workup
- X-rays to rule out other causes such as advanced patellofemoral OA and to assess the bony anatomy of the patellofemoral joint
- Complete evaluation of the lower extremity mechanics including the hip, ankle, foot, and general analysis of gait
- Consider an MRI if the diagnosis is in doubt, or if the patient fails to respond to appropriate treatment. An MRI is useful in visualizing the articular cartilage and surrounding structures.

Comments and Treatment Considerations
NSAIDs may have a benefit in short-term pain relief. Conservative treatment is favored over surgical treatment unless there is correctable pathology identified, or severe alignment issues.

Treatment should be tailored toward the individual patient, emphasizing correction of any potential correctable anatomic contributors. Physical therapy has been shown in several studies to be beneficial in reducing pain in patellofemoral pain syndrome, but not necessarily in improving function. The type of therapy likely does not matter because both open and closed kinetic chain exercises have shown equal benefit. There are no data to suggest that any exercises are able to isolate and strengthen the VMO, which is essential in dynamic medial stabilization of the patella, so a generalized program aimed at lower extremity flexibility, and strengthening is adequate.

Patella taping or McConnell taping, which attempts to medially shift the patella more central into the trochlea, has been used in the treatment of patellofemoral pain syndrome. In uncontrolled trials, taping has demonstrated some benefit.

Bracing has shown no benefit.

Foot orthoses may be beneficial especially in those individuals with abnormal foot mechanics, but very few studies exist to prove efficacy.

Acupuncture has shown some benefit in reducing pain, but no placebo-controlled trials exist.

Other treatment modalities which have not shown benefit include ultrasound, chiropractic manipulation, electromyelogram (EMG) biofeedback, and low-level laser treatment. Body weight plays a significant role in stresses across the patella, so weight loss is beneficial in any patient who is overweight and has patellofemoral pain syndrome.

POLYMYALGIA RHEUMATICA

Polymyalgia rheumatica (PMR) and giant cell arteritis (GCA), or temporal arteritis, are closely related conditions. The pathogenesis of these diseases is poorly understood but a "multihit" phenomenon has been proposed with possible link to infectious agents. PMR is quite common (1/133) among certain studied populations (Olmstead County, Minnesota) to an incidence of 50/100,000 in more generalized populations in the United States. GCA incidence is between 17 and 50/100,000. Comparatively, OA affects between 42 and 296/1000 people, depending on age and sex. Fifteen percent of PMR cases are associated with GCA.

Symptoms
- Bilateral aching and stiffness for 1 month or more and involving two of the following areas: neck or torso, shoulders or proximal regions of the arms, and hips or proximal aspects of the thighs +++++
- Some patients recount difficulty initiating movement after rest known as "gelling phenomenon."
- Shoulder pain (in 75% to 90% of patients) radiating toward the elbows ++++
- Hip and neck pain are present in 50% to 70% of patients, with hip pain radiating toward the knees. +++
- Distal asymmetric join pain is present in half of patients. +++

Signs
- Patient older than 50 years +++++
- Objective physical examination findings are often out of proportion to the patient's report of pain. It is uncommon to find swelling or tenderness on joint examination. ++++
- Patients report pain with both active and passive ROM. ++++
- Asymmetric knee, hand/wrist, and dorsal foot pitting edema in some of those who have distal arthritis

Workup
- Plain radiographic imaging may be used to rule out other diagnoses such as occult fracture, calcific tendinitis, and primary or metastatic neoplasm, though it is not needed.
- MRI or ultrasonography of the shoulders can be used to detect subacromial or subdeltoid bursitis, which can be present in PMR.
- Nonspecific rheumatologic screening tests (rheumatoid factor ANA) are not useful except in ruling out other polyarthritides. Evaluation for hypothyroidism with TSH and CBC to assess for hematologic causes of weakness and fatigue helps rule out other diagnoses.
- ESR is elevated greater than 40 mm/hr. +++++
- To make the diagnosis or PMR by established criteria, all of the following must be present: patient older than 50, the joint pain

and stiffness mentioned previously, ESR greater than 40 mm/hr, and exclusion of other diseases. One diagnostic criterion set also includes response to low-dose prednisone as necessary.

• ESR measurement can be used to monitor the activity of the disease, but symptoms should guide dosing of steroids.

Comments and Treatment Considerations

NSAIDs, ice, heat, massage, and physical therapy are not useful in relieving symptoms of PMR.

The primary treatment of PMR is administration of low-dose steroids (equivalent to 10 to 20 mg of prednisone by mouth daily). Steroid should be continued for 2 to 4 weeks and then withdrawn slowly to prevent relapse. Fifty percent of patients do have spontaneous relapse of symptoms.

A randomized, double-blind controlled trial has demonstrated that the addition of methotrexate to prednisone results in steroid sparing and shorter courses of steroids. This regimen might be administered in cooperation with a consulting rheumatologist.

Complications of steroids must be attended to. In particular, patients on longer-term steroids should be treated with calcium and vitamin D and monitored for the development of osteoporosis.

RHEUMATOID ARTHRITIS

Rheumatoid arthritis (RA) is the most common inflammatory arthritis. It is an appendicular arthritis, meaning that it preferentially affects the peripheral joints and skeleton as opposed to the central skeleton. The primary target of the inflammation is the synovium and joint cartilage. The erosion and destruction of cartilage and bone can rapidly lead to joint deformities, functional impairment, and disability. Worldwide prevalence of RA is approximately 1%. Women are affected two to three times more frequently than men and incidence peaks between the fourth and sixth decades of life.

Symptoms

• Onset is insidious (over weeks to months) in 55% to 70% of patients +++; subacute (over days to weeks) in 15% to 20%, ++ or acute (over a few days) in 8% to 15%. ++

• Joint pain is polyarticular in two thirds of patients. ++++ Symmetry is an important diagnostic feature. ++++ Pain is most often in the small joints of the hands and feet, in particular the wrists and PIP, MCP, and MTP joints.

• The presence and duration of morning stiffness are useful in diagnosis and in following the clinical course of the disease. Morning stiffness lasting greater than 60 minutes strongly suggests inflammatory arthritis. ++++

• Systemic symptoms may include fatigue, malaise, weakness, low-grade fever, and weight loss. ++

Signs

- Characteristic involvement of small joints of hands and feet ++++
- RA often affects larger joints such as the elbows, knees, shoulders, and cervical spine.
- DIP joints, sacroiliac joints, and the spine are rarely affected.
- The key physical finding is synovitis, warmth, bogginess, and tenderness around the joints affected. ++++ Joints may be red. ++++ The swelling is a result of both effusion within the joint and synovial proliferation.
- Limitation of active and passive ROM ++++
- Weakness may be out of proportion to pain.
- Late findings:
    - Joint deformity such as radial deviation of the wrists and ulnar deviation at the MCP joints.
    - Swan-neck deformity (extension at PIP, flexion at DIP) and boutonniere deformity (flexion at PIP, extension at DIP) result from tendon rupture and subluxation.
    - Joint instability
    - Rheumatoid nodules are present in 15% to 25% and occur over extensor surfaces and areas under pressure. Nodules may develop abruptly or gradually. ++

Workup

There is no single test to diagnose RA—its diagnosis is primarily clinical. The disease needs to present for at least several weeks to make a diagnosis. The American College of Rheumatology (ACR) criteria require four out of a possible seven criteria that provides a sensitivity and specificity of 90%.

- Morning stiffness that lasts longer than 1 hour (present for >6 weeks).
- Arthritis of three or more joint areas (>6 weeks)
- Arthritis of hand joints (wrist, MCP, PIP) (>6 weeks)
- Symmetric arthritis (present for >6 weeks)
- Rheumatoid nodules
- Serum rheumatoid factor positive
- Radiographic changes (erosions or periarticular osteopenia)

Careful observation of disease activity over time can also help to establish the diagnosis.

The differential diagnosis includes systemic lupus erythematosus, psoriatic arthritis, arthritis associated with viruses such as parvovirus, hepatitis B and C, and seronegative spondyloarthropathies.

Baseline lab studies recommended by the ACR subcommittee of RA include:

- Complete blood count (CBC) may reveal anemia in 80% ++++ of patients, which is usually normochromic, normocytic with thrombocytosis (platelets are an acute phase reactant and typically increase with systemic inflammation).
- Rheumatoid factor is present in 70% to 85% of patients. ++++ High titers correlate with more severe disease, the presence of

rheumatoid nodules, and extra-articular manifestations of RA. The titer does not have prognostic value in individual patients and serial titers are not useful. False positives are seen in numerous conditions including viral illnesses such as mononucleosis, bacterial infections such as spontaneous bacterial endocarditis, and other chronic inflammatory conditions such as sarcoidosis.

- ESR or CRP is elevated in 90%. ++++ These tests can correlate with the degree of synovial inflammation but it varies greatly from patient to patient. The tests can be a useful objective measure to follow clinical response.
- Baseline renal and hepatic function can be useful to establish a baseline before starting medications with potential renal or hepatic toxicity.
  Other tests:
- ANA is positive in 30% of RA patients. ++ Positive results are not specific to RA and the presence of ANA does not rule rheumatoid arthritis in or out.
- Anti-citrullinated peptide (CCP) antibodies are present in about 80% of RA patients. ++++ The anti-CCP2 test has equal sensitivity to rheumatoid factor (RF) test, but far better specificity (90% to 98%).
- Synovial fluid reveals 2000 to 20,000 leukocytes per mL, with 50% to 80% being neutrophils.
- X-ray reveals joint space narrowing that is symmetric, bony erosions, osteopenia, resorption of ulnar styloid, C1-2 subluxation, and instability. Radiographic evidence of erosions becomes apparent after the disease has been present for at least several months.

Comments and Treatment Considerations

Complications of rheumatoid arthritis can affect almost every body system:

- Hematologic: Includes anemia, +++ increased rate of lympho-proliferative diseases including Hodgkin's and non-Hodgkin's lymphoma, multiple myeloma, and leukemia
- Cardiac: Pericarditis (rare clinically but 50% at autopsy, +++), myocarditis, increased rates of coronary artery disease
- Pulmonary: Interstitial fibrosis, rheumatoid nodules
- Ophthalmologic: Keratoconjunctivitis, sicca syndrome, ++ episcleritis and scleritis
- Vascular: Vasculitis
- Neurologic: Myelopathy from cervical spine instability, peripheral nerve impingement
- Renal: Drug toxicity can lead to renal impairment.
- Felty syndrome: Triad of RA, splenomegaly, and neutropenia. These patients are at increased risk of serious bacterial infections of the lungs, skin, and perianal areas.
- RA is treated with a "reverse pyramid" approach in which disease modifying antirheumatic drugs (DMARDs) are begun early. This is done because joint destruction begins within weeks of symptom onset and DMARDs have significant benefits when used early. It is

therefore of critical importance to recognize and diagnose RA so that treatment can begin as rapidly as possible.

The goals of therapy are to relieve pain, reduce inflammation, improve function, prevent complications, and resolve the pathogenic process. There is no evidence that any medical therapy can heal erosions, reverse joint deformity, or cure RA.

The categories of current pharmacologic treatment are:

- NSAIDs/COX-2 inhibitors: Relieve symptoms of pain and swelling but do not alter disease course. There is no one consistently superior NSAID for RA.
- Glucocorticoids: Highly effective at relieving symptoms and can slow joint damage. Side effects of this class of medications are severe, so glucocorticoids are most often used as a bridge therapy until DMARDs take effect.
- DMARDs: Include sulfasalazine, hydroxychloroquine, methotrexate, and leflunomide. This class includes immunosuppressives such as azathioprine and cyclosporine.
- Biologic response modifiers: Infliximab, adalimumab, rituximab, etanercept, abatacept, anakinra.

Generally speaking, early referral to rheumatology is advisable to speed access to disease-modifying drugs. There is increasing evidence that combinations of DMARDs may be more effective than single-drug regimens. There is no clear evidence for dietary interventions such as supplemental fatty acids and vegetarian diets.

References

Akuthota V, Chou L, Drake D, et al: Achilles tendinopathy, *J Bone Joint Surg* 84-A:2062–2076, 2002.

Arden N, Nevitt M: Osteoarthritis: epidemiology, *Best Pract Res Clin Rheumatol* 20:3–25, 2006.

Arendt EA, Fithian DC, Cohen E: Current concepts of lateral patella dislocation, *Clin Sports Med* 21:499, 2002.

Arroll B, Ellis-Pegler E, Edwards A, et al: Patellofemoral pain syndrome. A critical review of the clinical trials on nonoperative therapy, *Am J Sports Med* 25:207, 1997.

Atkin DM, Fithian DC, Marangi KS, et al: Characteristic of patients with primary acute lateral patella dislocation and their recovery within the first 6 months of injury, *Am J Sports Med* 28:472, 2000.

Becker M, Schumacher HR Jr., Wortmann RL, et al: Febuxostat compared with allopurinol in patients with hyperuricemia and gout, *N Engl J Med* 353:2450–2461, 2005.

Bellamy N, Campbell J, Welch V, et al: Intraarticular corticosteroid for treatment of osteoarthritis of the knee, *Cochrane Database Syst Rev*, 2006, CD005328.

Bhatti J: Posterior cruciate ligament injury, *eMedicine* Topic 102.

Bischoff-Ferrari HA, Dawson-Hughes B, Willett WC, et al: Effects of vitamin D on falls: a meta-analysis, *JAMA* 291:1999–2006, 2004.

Bisset L, Beller E, Jull G, et al: Mobilisation with movement and exercise, corticosteroid injection, or wait and see for tennis elbow: randomised trial, *BMJ* 333:939, 2006.

Bizzini M, Childs JD, Piva SR, et al: Systematic review of the quality of randomized controlled trials for patellofemoral pain syndrome, *J Orthop Sports Phys Ther* 33:4, 2003.

British Society of Rheumatology: Current concepts in the management of tendon disorders, *Rheumatology* (Oxford, England) 45:508–521, 2006.

Brosseau L, Casimiro L, Robinson V, et al: Therapeutic ultrasound for treating patellofemoral pain syndrome, *Cochrane Database Syst Rev,* 2001, CD003375. In 2008 Number 4. Oxford: Update Software Ltd. Available at www.update-software.com. (Translated, 2008 Issue 3. Chichester, UK: John Wiley & Sons, Ltd.).

Brosseau L, MacLeay L, Robinson VA, et al: Intensity of exercise for the treatment of osteoarthritis, *Cochrane Database Syst Rev*, 2003, CD004259.

Brosseau L, Yonge KA, Robinson V, et al: Thermotherapy for treatment of osteoarthritis, *Cochrane Database Syst Rev*, 2003, CD004522.

Brouwer RW, Jakma TSC, Verhagen AP, et al: Braces and orthoses for treating osteoarthritis of the knee, *Cochrane Database Syst Rev*, 2005, CD004020.

Buchner M, Baudendistel B, Sabo D, et al: Acute traumatic primary patella dislocation: long-term results comparing conservative and surgical treatment, *Clin J Sports Med* 15:62, 2005.

Burroughs K: Lisfranc injury of the foot: a commonly missed diagnosis, *Am Fam Physician* 58:118–120, 1998.

Caporali R, Cimmino MA, Ferraccioli G, et al: Prednisone plus methotrexate for polymyalgia rheumatica: a randomized, double-blind, placebo-controlled trial, *Ann Intern Med* 141:493–500, 2004.

Cosgarea AJ, Browne JA, Kim TK, et al: Evaluation and management of the unstable patella, *Phys Sports Med* 30:2002 Oct.

Cox JS, Blanda JB: Peripatella pathologies. In: Delee JC, Drez D, editors: *Orthopaedic sports medicine*, Philadelphia, 1994, Saunders.

Crossley K, Bennell K, Green S, et al: A systematic review of physical interventions for patellofemoral pain syndrome, *Clin J Sports Med* 11:103, 2001.

D'hondt NE, Struijs PA, Kerkhoffs GM, et al: Orthotic devices for treating patellofemoral pain syndrome, *Cochrane Database Syst Rev*, 2002, CD002267.

Duri ZA, Aichroth PM, Wilkins R, et al: Patella tendonitis and anterior knee pain, *Am J Knee Surg* 12:99, 1999.

Durson N, Durson E, Kilic Z: Electromyographic biofeedback-controlled exercise versus conservative care for patellofemoral pain syndrome, *Arch Phys Med Rehabil* 82:1692, 2001.

Eakin CL: Arthrometric evaluation of posterior cruciate ligament injuries, *Am J Sports Med* 26:96–102, 1998.

Eriksson E: Pain in the patella tendon, knee surgery, sports traumatology, *Arthroscopy* 14:107, 2006.

Eriksson E: Patella dislocation, knee surgery, sports traumatology, *Arthroscopy* 13:509, 2005.

Felson D: Osteoarthritis of the knee, *N Engl J Med* 354:841–848, 2006.

Fithian DC, Paxton EW, Stone ML, et al: Epidemiology and natural history of acute patellar dislocation, *Am J Sports Med* 32:1114, 2004.

Galanty HL: Anterior knee pain. In Puffer JC, editor: *20 Common problems in sports medicine*, New York, 2002, McGraw-Hill.

Geary M, Schepsis A: Management of first time patellar dislocations, *Orthopedics* 27:1058, 2004.

Cameron ID, Murray GR, Gillespie LD, et al: Interventions for preventing falls in older people in nursing care facilities and hospitals, *Cochrane Database Syst Rev*, 2010, CD005465.

Gupta MN, Sturrock RD, Field M, et al: A prospective 2-year study of 75 patients with adult-onset septic arthritis, *Rheumatology* 40:24–30, 2001.

Hart LE: Long-term prognosis for jumper's knee, *Clin J Sports Med* 13:196, 2003.

Hay E, Paterson S, Lewis M, et al: Pragmatic randomised controlled trial of local corticosteroid injection and naproxen for treatment of lateral epicondylitis of elbow in primary care, *BMJ* 319:964–968, 1999.

Heintjes E, Berger MY, Bierma-Zeinstra SM, et al: Exercise therapy for patellofemoral pain syndrome, *Cochrane Database of Syst Rev*, 2003, CD003472.

Heintjes E, Berger MY, Bierma-Zeinstra SM, et al: Pharmacotherapy for patellofemoral pain syndrome, *Cochrane Database Syst Rev,* 2004, CD003470.

Hing E, Cherry D, Woodwell D: National ambulatory medical care survey, 2004
summary, *Adv Data Vital Health Stat* 374:3, 2006.

Hong QN, Durand M-J, Loisel P: Treatment of lateral epicondylitis: where is the
evidence? *J Bone Spine* 71:369–373, 2004.

Jackson RD, LaCroix A, Gass M, et al: Calcium plus vitamin D supplementation
and the risk of fractures, *N Engl J Med* 354:669–683, 2006.

Jonsson P, Alfredson H: Superior results with eccentric compared to concen-
tric quadriceps training in patients with jumper's knee: a prospective randomized study, *Br J Sports Med* 39:847, 2005.

Kannus P, Natri A, Paakkala T, et al: An outcome study of chronic patellofemoral pain syndrome. Seven-year follow-up of patients in a randomized, controlled trial, *J Bone Joint Surg* 81:355, 1999.

Lawrence R, Helmick C, Arnett F, et al: Estimates of the prevalence of arthritis
and selected musculoskeletal disorders in the United States, *Arthritis Rheum*
41:778–799, 1998.

Matheny JM, Brinker MR, Elliott MN, et al: Confidence of graduating family
practice residents in their management of musculoskeletal conditions, *Am
J Orthop* 29:945–952, 2000.

Mehallo C, Drezner J, Bytomski J: Practical management: nonsteroidal antiinflammatory drug (NSAID) use in athletic injuries, *Clin J Sports Med* 16:170–
174, 2006.

Mysnyk MC, Wroble RR, Foster DT, et al: Prepatella bursitis in wrestlers, *Am J
Sports Med* 14:46, 1986.

Naradzy J: Ankle fractures. *eMedicine* Topic 188.

Nomura E, Inoue M: Injured medial patellofemoral ligament in acute patellar
dislocation, *J Knee Surg* 17:40, 2004.

Pijnenburg A, van Dijk C, Bossuyt P, et al: Treatment of ruptures of the lateral
ankle ligaments: a meta-analysis, *J Bone Joint Surg* 82:761–773, 2000.

Post WR, Teitge R, Amis A: Patellofemoral malalignment: looking beyond the
viewbox, *Clin Sports Med* 21:521, 2002.

Rao S: Management of hip fracture: the family physician's role, *Am Fam
Physician* 73:12, 2006.

Reilly JP, Nicholas JA: The chronically inflamed bursa, *Clin J Sports Med* 6:345,
1987.

Rogmark C, Johnell O: Primary arthroplasty is better than internal fixation of
displaced femoral neck fractures: a meta-analysis of 14 randomized studies
with 2,289 patients, *Acta Orthop* 77:3–367, 2006 359.

Salvarani C, Cantini F, Boiardi L, et al: Polymyalgia rheumatica and giant-cell
arteritis, *N Engl J Med* 347:261–271, 2002.

Sharma P, Maffulli N: Tendon injury and tendinopathy: healing and repair,
J Bone Joint Surg 87:187-202, 2005.

Sorosky B, Press J Plastaras C, Rittenberg J: The practical management of
Achilles tendinopathy, *Clin J Sports Med* 14(1):40–44, 2004.

Spiegel BM, Farid M, Dulai GS, et al: Comparing rates of dyspepsia with coxibs
vs NSAID+PPI: a meta-analysis, *Am J Med* 119:448.e27–e36, 2006.

Stein BE, Ahmad CS: Patellofemoral disorders. In Schepsis AA, Busconi BD,
editors: *Sports medicine*, Philadelphia, 2006, Lippincott Williams & Wilkins.

Stevens J, Olson S: Reducing falls and resulting hip fractures among older
women, *MMWR* 49(RR02):1–12, 2000.

Stiell IG: Implementation of the Ottawa ankle rules, *JAMA* 274:827–832, 1994.

Stratford PW: A review of the McMurray test: definition, interpretation, and
clinical usefulness, *J Orthop Sports Phys Ther* 22:116–120, 1995.

Suresh E: Diagnosis and management of gout: a rational approach, *Postgrad Med J* 81:572–579, 2005.

Tandeter H: Acute knee injuries: use of decision rules for selective radiograph ordering, *Am Fam Physician* 60:2599–2604, 1999.

Tausche AK, Inokuchi T, Moriwaki Y, et al: Severe gouty arthritis refractory to anti-inflammatory drugs: treatment with anti-tumour necrosis factor alpha as a new therapeutic option, *Ann Rheum Dis* 63:1351–1352, 2004.

Terkeltaub R: Clinical practice—gout, *N Engl J Med* 349:1647–1655, 2003.

Timm KE: Randomized controlled trial of protonic on patellar pain, position, and function, *Med Sci Sports Exercise* 30:665, 1998.

Towheed T, Maxwell L, Judd M, et al: Acetaminophen for osteoarthritis, *Cochrane Database Syst Rev*, 2006, CD004257.

Visnes H, Hoksrud A, Cook J, et al: No effect of eccentric training on jumper's knee in volleyball players during the competitive season: a randomized clinical trial, *Clin J Sports Med* 15:227, 2005.

Visser S, Tupper J: Septic until proven otherwise: approach to and treatment of the septic joint in adult patients, *Can Fam Physician* 55:374–375, 2009.

Warden SJ, Brukner P: Patellar tendinopathy, *Clin Sports Med* 22:743, 2003.

Wilson J, Best T: Common overuse tendon problems: a review and recommendations for treatment, *Am Fam Physician* 72:811–818, 2005.

Witvrouw E, Lysens R, Bellemans J, et al: Open versus closed kinetic chain exercises for patellofemoral pain. A prospective, randomized study, *Am J Sports Med* 28:687, 2000.

Zigang G, Yang H, Boom C, et al: Osteoarthritis and therapy, *Arthritis Rheum* 55:493–500, 2006.

CHAPTER 7

Back Pain
Deepak Patel, Pritesh Patel, Vanathi Anan Siddaiah,
Sunita Kalra, and Amanpreet Singh

Low back pain (LBP) is one of the most common complaints seen in the family medicine practice. It is estimated that 70% to 80% of the population will suffer from this at some point in their lifetime. A detailed history and examination are essential to ascertain the etiology and diagnosis. Although we are able to determine some potential etiologies of back pain, often the actual causes of pain-producing components are unknown. Complicating this situation, multiple factors and triggers may exist in an anatomically normal back that may create pain. Conversely, anatomic abnormalities, such as the presence of herniated disks have been demonstrated in asymptomatic individuals.

In some cases, back pain can represent a life-threatening emergency. A history of bony point tenderness raises the concern for infection or fracture. Associated abdominal pain or unexplained pain in older patients could represent an aortic aneurysm. It remains critical for the family physician to recognize situations requiring a more detailed workup and treatment. The most common etiology, mechanical (myofascial) back pain, can typically be treated conservatively without imaging, hospitalization, surgery, or strict activity restrictions.

Aortic aneurysm: Abdominal aortic aneurysms can present as back pain (see Chapter 1).

Osteomyelitis of the lumbosacral spine can present as back pain. This condition typically presents with local signs of inflammation and infection. Osteomyelitis of the lumbosacral spine often occurs because an infected skin wound or superficial infection in the area of the lumbosacral spine extends deeper and involves the bones of the spinal cord.

Epidural abscess can present as back pain. An epidural abscess in the area of the lumbosacral spine typically presents with systemic findings such as fever and malaise in addition to the back pain. In cases of epidural abscess there are usually predisposing factors, such as immune deficiency, or instrumentation of the epidural space, either for diagnostic or therapeutic reasons.

HERNIATED LUMBAR DISK

A herniated lumbar disk (sometimes called a ruptured disk) is different from a bulging disk or protrusion. It occurs when the gel-like center of a disk actually ruptures out through a tear in the tough

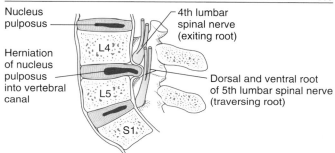

FIGURE 7-1 Herniated lumbar intervertebral disk. Herniation occurs posterolaterally and affects traversing root, not exiting root, i.e., herniation at L4-L5 affects L5 root, whereas herniation at L5-S1 affects S1 root. *(From Moore NA, Roy WA:* Rapid review gross and developmental anatomy, *3rd ed, Philadelphia, 2011, Elsevier.)*

disk wall (annulus) (Fig. 7-1). The gel material is irritating to the spinal nerves, causing something like a chemical irritation. The pain is believed to be a result of spinal nerve inflammation and swelling caused by pressure of the herniated disk. Usually, disks herniate because of injury or improper lifting, but aging also contributes. Herniated disks are most common in people in their 30s and 40s.

Each disk has two parts, the nucleus pulposus (the inner, central, soft part of the intervertebral disk) and the annulus fibrosis (the thick, outer part). As the nucleus pulposus loses its turgor and the elasticity of the annulus diminishes, the disk bulges outward beyond the vertebral body margins. A herniated nucleus pulposus (HNP) through an annular defect causes focal protrusion of the disk material beyond the margins of the adjacent vertebral endplate, resulting in disk herniation.

Trauma is the single most common cause of rupture of the nucleus pulposus through the annulus fibrosis resulting in protrusion or extrusion of the disk material into the vertebral canal. This outcome can be due to a single event or repeated trauma. The injury most often occurs on the posterior or posterolateral aspect of the disk (Table 7-1). Other potentiating factors include age, apoptosis, abnormalities in collagen, vascular ingrowth, loads placed on the disk, abnormal proteoglycan, obesity, sedentary lifestyle, and poor physical fitness. Although a commonly suspected cause of LBP, herniated disks represent only 4% of cases of LBP.

Symptoms
- Sciatica (pain radiating below the knee) +++++
- Sharp, burning, or stabbing pain that radiates from the lower back area, down one or both legs ++++
- Pain like an electrical shock that is severe with standing, walking, or sitting ++++

Table 7-1. Location of Pain and Motor Deficit in Association with Nerve Root Involvement

DISK LEVEL	LOCATION OF PAIN	MOTOR DEFICIT
T12–L1	Pain in the inguinal region and medial thigh	None
L1–L2	Pain in anterior and medial aspect of upper thigh	Slight weakness in quadriceps; slight diminished suprapatellar reflex
L2–L3	Pain in anterolateral thigh	Weakened quadriceps; diminished patellar or suprapatellar reflex
L3–L4	Pain in posterolateral thigh and anterolateral tibial area	Weakened quadriceps; diminished patellar reflex
L4–L5	Pain in dorsum of foot	Extensor weakness of big toe and foot
L5–S1	Pain in lateral aspect of foot	Diminished or absent Achilles reflex

- Activity such as bending, lifting, twisting, and stooping increases the pain +++
- Lying supine may be the only relief ++
- Muscle spasms in the back or leg ++
- Cauda equina syndrome produces symptoms requiring immediate referral to a specialist to prevent permanent damage.
  - Leg muscle weakness +++
  - Knee or ankle reflex loss +++
  - Footdrop +++
  - Loss of bowel and bladder function ++

Signs
- Straight-leg test is positive in patients with herniated lumbar disks ++++
- When in doubt of authenticity of symptoms, the distracted (seated) straight-leg test should be performed.
- Crossed straight-leg raise (reproduction of pain on the affected side, while raising the contralateral leg) (most specific test) +++
- Weak ankle dorsiflexion or ankle reflex +++
- Leg sensory abnormality ++

Workup
- Emergent MRI of the spine (lumbosacral, thoracic, or cervical images) in severe cases in which cauda equina or cord impingement is of concern
- MRI may be considered after failure of 6-week trial of conservative treatment or for severe or progressive neurologic deficits (the

high rate of disk abnormalities in asymptomatic patients require appropriate selection and clinical correlation of MRI findings.
- X-ray in person older than age 50 with or without history of mechanical cause to rule out metastatic disease or compression fracture as cause of symptoms
- EMG may help to correlate the disk herniation to the nerve affected, but is rarely done.
- Bone scan is an option to evaluate for bony abnormality but has been largely replaced in most cases by MRI.
- CT scan of the spine (lumbosacral, thoracic, or cervical images) if concern for fracture
- Myelography with CT scanning is indicated when MRI is not possible (i.e., hardware in patient such as pacemaker) or when surgery is contemplated in cases of:
  - Spinal stenosis
  - Lateral recess stenosis
  - Multiple abnormal disks
  - Spondylolisthesis
  - Possible neoplasm
  - After severe trauma

Comments and Treatment Considerations

In the absence of red flags, patients should be treated conservatively. Approximately 90% of cases improve within 6 weeks and progress to symptom resolution within 12 weeks. Recommending bed rest shows no benefit and may actually delay recovery.

Aerobic exercise and physical therapy strengthening of abdominal and back muscles can relieve symptoms of radicular pain, but have limited supporting evidence. Exercise and massage techniques are easily taught to patients and family members. Extension and isometric exercises are performed first and after sufficient strength and pain relief, flexion exercises are allowed. Exercise may be beneficial for prevention of recurrence. Ultrasound, transcutaneous electrical nerve stimulation (TENS), and acupuncture/massage are of limited value for pain control only.

 MEDICATIONS—NSAIDS, ANALGESICS, STEROIDS

In patients with nonspecific LBP, NSAIDs, acetaminophen and muscle relaxers may be effective based on systematic reviews and RCTs, but lack specific studies for lumbar disk herniation. NSAIDs reduce inflammation and alleviate pain, but clinical evidence shows NSAIDs to be no different than placebo based on one systematic review in treating sciatica pain associated with herniated lumbar disk. Tramadol and opioid analgesics are effective for moderate to severe pain, but have not been studied specifically for disk herniation. Nortriptyline and amitriptyline are often recommended for neuropathic pain, but lack specific evidence in disk herniation. Systemic steroids are no better than placebo for the treatment of lumbar disk herniation pain studied using consistent RCTs.

Trigger point injections—1 to 2 mL of 1% lidocaine without epinephrine—can be administered to provide extended relief for localized pain sources (trigger points). Epidural steroid injections are often considered. One systematic review demonstrated limited evidence that epidural corticosteroid injections increased global improvement compared with placebo. RCTs following this initial study showed no significant difference between epidural corticosteroid injections plus conservative treatment and conservative treatment alone. It may modestly improve pain in the short term but has no effect on the long-term outcomes.

Spinal manipulation is controversial, but may warrant consideration as a recent study demonstrated pain improvement (see "Mechanical Back Pain").

Surgical intervention has been controversial. Studies have had limitations in study design. Patients who have microdiskectomies have faster improvements than patients receiving conservative treatment, but long-term improvement rates in both groups are similar.

Surgical indications include:
• Cauda equina syndrome
• Progressive neurologic deficit
• Profound neurologic deficit
• Severe and disabling pain refractory to 4 to 6 weeks of conservative treatment

In the absence of these "red flags," systematic reviews show conservative management is appropriate for up to 6 weeks prior to obtaining imaging or considering surgical approaches.

MECHANICAL BACK PAIN

Back pain is the second most common presenting complaint in the United States. Mechanical back pain is most commonly attributed to acute trauma or injury from overuse. The mechanism of injury is frequently twisting of the back while lifting a heavy object. Injury may also result from motor vehicle accidents, prolonged sitting, or falls. Mechanical back pain often results from lumbar strain or sprain, disk herniation, spinal stenosis, degeneration (osteoarthritis), or fractures either due to trauma or compression. Muscle spasms are the result of protective muscle splinting following joint or soft tissue disease or injury, and may be another source for LBP. Acute trauma or repetitive microtrauma may lead to the formation of trigger points and can also cause LBP.

Although the precise etiology for back pain is often difficult to establish, it is widely assumed that nonradiating LBP is secondary to musculoligamentous injury, degenerative changes in the spine, or both. Tenderness of the bony spine itself should raise concern for non–soft tissue (and potentially emergent) diagnoses. The etiology of LBP is mechanical in 97% of cases.

RISK FACTORS FOR MECHANICAL BACK PAIN

- Heavy physical work, heavy lifting, twisting, vibration, and posture ++
- Increasing age +
- Work dissatisfaction and monotonous work +
- Depression +
- Smoking, drug use +
- Obesity +
- Severe scoliosis ++
- Extremes of physical fitness ++

Symptoms
- History of trauma or injury ++++
- Pain at the site of injury or occasional radiation of pain to the legs ++++
- Stiffness +++
- Numbness, weakness, tingling at the site of pain or of extremity +++
- Position of pain reproduction (for nonradicular pain) may suggest etiology:
  - Flexion: interspinous ligament (sitting) +++
  - Extension: facet related (standing) +++
- Muscle spasm ++

Signs
- Swelling +
- Tenderness, warmth over musculature +
- Palpable mass, spasm ++
- Trigger points are focal, hyperirritable nodules located in a taut band of skeletal muscle that produce pain locally and in a referred pattern with palpation. +++
- Limited ROM due to pain +++
- Manual medicine clinicians commonly use the PART (Pain and Tenderness; Asymmetry; Range of motion abnormality; Tone, Texture, and Temperature abnormality) acronym to identify the categories of joint dysfunction. +++
- Motion between adjacent vertebrae to detect hypomobility with tenderness and pain +++
- Decreased sensation over site of injury ++
- Sciatic nerve and piriformis muscle tenderness may indicate piriformis syndrome. +++
- Supraspinous or interspinous ligament tenderness, due to injury or spondylolisthesis +++
- Stork test may indicate spondylolysis ++
- Gait: Antalgic to the ipsilateral side of spasm ++
- Patrick or flexion abduction external rotation (FABER) test to differentiate hip versus sacroiliac (SI) joint etiology of pain ++

Workup

- Consider nonmechanical conditions as a source of back pain such as malignancy, infection, and inflammatory conditions and aortic vascular disease (<5% of cases).
- Diagnosis is based mainly on history and physical examination, although testing is sometimes required to rule out emergent conditions.
- Mechanical LBP is difficult to diagnose due to the absence of any screening or confirmatory tests. As mentioned earlier, urinalysis, x-ray, CT, ultrasound, and MRI may occasionally be required to rule out more ominous causes of pain. A recent guideline advises against routine imaging for nonspecific LBP.
- MRI is indicated for severe or progressive neurologic deficits (should be ordered cautiously due to the high rate of disk abnormalities in asymptomatic patients).
- Patients with loss of bowel or bladder sphincter tone or progressive neurologic deficit from LBP should be appropriately referred for immediate aggressive treatment.
- Long-term management of patients with chronic back pain may be aided by MRI, though many patients without pain have findings and those with pain may have limited findings.

Comments and Treatment Recommendations

Approximately 90% of LBP cases improve within 4 to 6 weeks and spontaneously recover usually within 3 months. If pain persists or symptoms worsen, further workup may be necessary to evaluate for other causes. Follow-up examinations are recommended to provide education and psychologic support to patients. Because treating and reversing the causes of chronic pain can be challenging at best, treatment is directed to prevent transition from acute to chronic. Chronic pain treatment goals involve maximizing functional ability and limiting pain because these patients may never be completely pain free.

It is important to return to activities of daily living as soon as possible, and bed rest should be limited to 2 to 3 days even in severe cases. There is strong evidence to support limited best rest.

Ice is recommended for the first 24 to 48 hours along with pain medication. Heat can be applied after 48 hours to increase blood flow locally and decrease stiffness and spasms. The effectiveness of heat has been supported by recent literature. There is also some evidence to support the use of topical counterirritants for acute injury.

NSAIDs maybe useful for pain control and mobility. Acetaminophen may also be recommended for pain control because evidence for superiority for NSAIDs over acetaminophen is lacking. Short-term opiate analgesics should be considered if necessary in severe cases. Muscle relaxants can also be used to reduce spasms or for more severe pain, but their use may be limited by the drowsiness side effect.

Braces may offer support to the back and relieve pain. No strong evidence to support their use and concerns for potential muscle weakening should limit this as a treatment option.

Physical therapy has proven benefits. Therapists are able to provide further education, treatment modalities and address additional underlying physical confounders. Although preferred by many patients, strong evidence to support massage treatments is lacking.

Studies on manipulation have demonstrated some short-term benefit. Because an increasing number of patients and providers are using manipulation, a brief description is included in the following text. Manipulation is a high-velocity procedure that moves a joint past its passive range and into the end barrier. The ROM is increased and, unlike mobilization, the patient does not have control in cases with severe spasm. The provider instead has control over the joint and the patient. Therefore, only those skilled in manipulation should perform this procedure. The negative pressure created within the joint commonly produces a cracking sound, which allows for greater passive range of motion and gapping of the zygapophyseal/facet joint. Spinal manipulation has shown to be beneficial for acute and chronic pain. Patients treated with manipulation for LBP have been shown to use fewer overall number of treatments when compared with physical therapy alone. Other forms of manipulation use more traction forces in order to decrease diskal pressure or increase foraminal dimensions.

 CONTRAINDICATIONS TO SPINAL MANIPULATION

- Cancer or other destructive lesions
- Severe osteopenia
- Active spondyloarthropathies
- Cauda equina symptoms

METASTATIC DISEASE TO THE SPINE

Metastatic spinal disease is 25 times more common than primary tumors. The most common tumors to metastasize to the spine include lymphoma, melanoma, and tumors of the breast, lung, prostate, kidney, and GI tract. Blood flows through the Batson plexus in the epidural space, which communicates with blood spaces in the vertebral marrow. Lung and breast metastases mostly affect the thoracic spine, whereas renal metastasis affects the lumbosacral spine. Although metastasis may compromise the vascular supply causing edema or ischemia, nerve tracts are vulnerable to compression. This includes the corticospinal and spinocerebellar tracts and the posterior spinal columns.

Symptoms
- Back pain is the presenting symptom in 90% of patients who have spinal metastasis; it tends to be worse when patients are supine and may awaken them during the night. ++++
- Fever, chills ++
- Weight loss +++

- Weakness in 75% of patients ++++
- Autonomic or sensory symptoms in 50% of patients +++
- More than 50% of patients have bowel and bladder dysfunction. +++

Signs

- Red flags: History of cancer, age less than 20 or more than 50 years, weight loss, or radiculopathy +++
- Spinal instability because the pain is mechanical in origin ++++
- In early diagnosis, patients are more likely to show flaccidity and hyporeflexia. ++
- In later diagnosis, spasticity and hyperreflexia are more common. +++

Workup

- Frequently, early metastasis is not visualized on plain radiographs.
- Positive findings when present can be osteoblastic or osteolytic or mixed changes on x-ray.
- The advantage of CT is its good anatomic resolution, soft-tissue contrast, and detailed morphology. Both cortical and trabecular bone components are well defined. The sensitivity of CT for detecting bone metastasis ranges between 71% and 100%. Because cortical destruction is required for visualization of a metastasis by CT, the sensitivity of this modality in detecting early malignant bone involvement is relatively low.
- Bone scans are positive in 85% of patients who have spinal metastasis.
- Technetium bone scan shows increased uptake. By injecting radioactive dye, the dye has a propensity to accumulate in damaged or cancerous bone areas that are detected by a scan. The bone scan is most helpful to rule out metastatic spread to bone, especially if new bone pain is noted and surgery is contemplated.
- Published sensitivity rates of bone scan in detecting bone metastases vary between 62% and 100% with a specificity of 78% to 100%.
- Repeat bone scans may be needed to help confirm if an area seen is actually cancer, or just an old area of trauma. A baseline bone scan, as is done with breast cancer, may be reasonable for reference to follow up bone scans.
- MRI is the most sensitive and specific modality for imaging spinal metastases.
- Paraspinal tumors that enter the epidural space through the neuroforamen result in back pain, and progressive neurologic symptoms are often unseen on bone scan but are typically detectable on MRI.
- MRI may identify spinal metastasis in patients who have normal radiographs and bone scans. MRI has a sensitivity ranging from 83% to 100%.
- MRI is mainly reserved for regional assessment of a bone lesion suggested by bone scan or CT.

Comments and Treatment Considerations

Treatment focuses on two aspects: treatment of the primary disease and symptomatic pain control. Symptomatic pain control is typically conducted with opioids, chemotherapy, and radiotherapy. Radiotherapy remains the standard for spinal metastases due to myeloma, lymphoma, and many types of adenocarcinoma. Myelopathy, which occurs secondary to compression, can be pretreated with high-dose corticosteroids to decrease cord edema and alleviate pain. Radiation therapy is the standard approach for treatment.

Surgery is indicated for certain biopsies, treating mechanical instability, and decompressing the spinal cord in cases of bony impingement, failed radiotherapy, or tumors resistant to radiotherapy. Spinal cord compression (also discussed in this chapter) is also a serious complication.

VERTEBRAL COMPRESSION FRACTURE

Vertebral compression fracture is the most common complication of osteoporosis and the most common type of osteopathic fracture. There are about 500,000 new cases of vertebral fractures yearly in the United States and it is estimated to occur in 26% of women older than age 50 years. The prevalence of this condition increases with advancing age, reaching 40% in women 80 years of age. Acute fractures occur when the weight of the upper body exceeds the ability of the bone within the vertebral body to support the load. The risk factors are categorized as modifiable and nonmodifiable. Nonmodifiable factors include advanced age, female gender, white race, and presence of dementia. Modifiable factors are alcohol use, tobacco use, presence of osteoporosis, and estrogen deficiency.

Symptoms
- LBP, which can also occur in the upper back, abdomen, and thigh +++++
- Paresthesias +++
- Bowel and bladder incontinence ++
- Kyphosis, lumbar lordosis +++
- Early satiety secondary to compressed abdominal organs +
- Weight loss ++

Workup
- Physical examination: Typically has tenderness directly over the area of the acute fracture, and commonly increased kyphosis is noted. In an uncomplicated fracture straight-leg raise is negative and the neurologic examination is normal.
- Plain radiographs: The recommended initial imaging study obtained, which may show the classic wedge-shaped vertebral body
- CT and MRI are used for evaluating the posterior vertebral wall integrity and for ruling out alternative causes of the back pain. MRI is also recommended when patients have suspected spinal cord compression or other neurologic symptoms.
- A nuclear medicine bone scan: Indicated when symptoms are atypical. It is also helpful in diagnosing sacral insufficiency fractures.

Comments and Treatment Considerations

Traditional treatments are nonoperative and conservative. Most patients can fully recover or show improvement from the fracture in about 6 to 12 weeks. Bed rest is indicated. Prolonged inactivity should be avoided.

Analgesics and NSAIDs offer pain relief. Use caution in older adults because of the risk of GI bleeding. Calcitonin-salmon nasal spray has also shown to be beneficial for pain. Prescribe a muscle relaxant for symptomatic relief of associated muscle spasms.

In addition to treating osteoporosis and thereby reducing the risk of fracture, bisphosphonates may be beneficial in treatment of fracture. In one study, alendronate was shown to reduce the number of days of bed disability and days of limited activity caused by back pain in postmenopausal women with preexisting vertebral fracture.

Physical therapy helps stabilize the spine and improves posture.

External back braces are uncomfortable and typically unnecessary for fractures with minimal compression.

Patients who do not respond to conservative treatment or continue to have severe pain are good candidates for percutaneous kyphoplasty or vertebroplasty. An ongoing multicenter randomized controlled trial is examining the outcomes from vertebroplasty versus kyphoplasty.

Preventive measures are the best way to avoid these fractures. These include a well-balanced diet, regular exercise, smoking cessation, appropriate calcium and vitamin D, and bisphosphonates (for osteopenia and osteoporosis).

References

Aaron JE, Gallagher JC, Anderson J, et al: Frequency of osteomalacia and osteoporosis in fractures in the proximal femur, *Lancet* 1:229, 1974.

Alvarez DJ, Rockwell PG: Trigger points: diagnosis and management, *Am Fam Physician* 65:653–660, 2002.

Arce D, Sass P, Abul-Khoudoud H: Recognizing spinal cord emergencies, *Am Fam Physician* 64:631–638, 2001.

Aslan S, Karcioglu O, Katirci Y, et al: Speed bump-induced spinal column injury, *Am J Emerg Med* 23:563, 2005.

Bartynski WS, Heller MT, Grahovac SZ, et al: Severe thoracic kyphosis in the older patient in the absence of vertebral fracture: association of extreme curve with age, *AJNR Am J Neuroradiol* 26:2077, 2005.

Bigos S. Bowyer O. Braen G., et al: Acute low back problems in adults. AHCPR publication no.

Bilsky M, Lis E, Raizer J, et al: The diagnosis and treatment of metastatic spinal tumor, *Oncologist* 4:459–469, 1999. 95-0642. Rockville, MD, 1994, Agency for Health Care Policy and Research.

Black DM, Arden NK, Palermo L, et al: Prevalent vertebral deformities predict hip fractures and new vertebral deformities but not wrist fractures. Study of Osteoporotic Fractures Research Group, *J Bone Miner Res* 1999; 14:821.

Cambron J, Gudavalli MR, McGregor J, et al: Amount of health care and self-care following a randomized clinical trial comparing flexion-distraction with exercise program for chronic low back pain, *Chiropr Osteopat* 14:19, 2006.

Campbell SE, Phillips CD, Dubovsky E, et al: The value of CT in determining potential instability of simple wedge-compression fractures of the lumbar spine, *AJNR Am J Neuroradiol* 16:1385, 1995.

Carek PJ, Dickerson LM, Sack JL: Diagnosis and management of osteomyelitis, *Am Fam Physician* 63:2413–2420, 2001.

Chao D, Nanda A: Spinal epidural abscess: a diagnostic challenge, *Am Fam Physician* 65:1341–1346, 2002.

Chapman-Smith DA: In *The chiropractic profession: its education, practice, research, and future directions*, West Des Moines, IA, 2000, NCMIC Group Inc.

Chou R, Qaseem A, Snow V, et al: Diagnosis and treatment of low back pain: a joint clinical practice guideline from the American College of Physicians and the American Pain Society, *Ann Intern Med* 147:I45, 2007.

Cooper C, Atkinson EJ, O'Fallon WM, Melton LJ, 3rd: Incidence of clinically diagnosed vertebral fractures: a population-based study in Rochester, Minnesota, 1985–1989, *J Bone Miner Res* 7:221, 1992.

Cox JL: Low back pain: mechanism, diagnosis, treatment, 6th ed, Philadelphia, 1999, Lippincott Williams & Wilkins.

Cramer GD, Gregerson DM, Knudsen JT, et al: the effects of side-posture positioning and spinal adjusting on the lumbar Z joints, *Spine* 27:2459–2466, 2002.

Cramer GD, Tuck NR, Knudsen JT, et al: Effects of side-posture positioning and side-posture adjusting on the lumbar zygapophyseal joints as evaluated by magnetic resonance imaging: a before and after study with randomization, *J Manipulative Physiol Ther* 23:380–394, 2000.

De Smet AA, Robinson RG, Johnson BE, Lukert BP: Spinal compression fractures in osteoporotic women: patterns and relationship to hyperkyphosis, *Radiology* 166:497, 1988.

Devereaux M: Low back pain: primary care clinical office practice, *Occup Med* 26:443, 2004.

Dublin AB, Hartman J, Latchaw RE, et al: The vertebral body fracture in osteoporosis: restoration of height using percutaneous vertebroplasty, *AJNR Am J Neuroradiol* 26:489, 2005.

Even-Sapir E: Imaging of malignant bone involvement by morphologic, scintigraphic, and hybrid modalities, *J Nucl Med* 46:1356–1367, 2005.

Genant HK, Cooper C, Poor G, et al: Interim report and recommendations of the World Health Organization Task-Force for Osteoporosis, *Osteoporos Int* 10:259, 1999.

Genant HK, Wu CY, van Kuijk C, Nevitt MC: Vertebral fracture assessment using a semiquantitative technique, *J Bone Miner Res* 8:1137, 1993.

Gilbert JR, Taylor DW, Hildebrand A, Evans C: Clinical trial of common treatments for low back pain in family practice, *BMJ* 291:791–794, 1985.

Giles LGF, Singer KP: *The clinical anatomy and management of back pain series. Volume 1: clinical anatomy and management of low back pain*, Oxford, UK, 1997, Butterworth-Heinemann.

Gold RI, Seeger LL, Bassett LW, Steckel RJ: An integrated approach to the evaluation of metastatic bone disease, *Radiol Clin North Am* 28:471–483, 1990.

Green AD, Colon-Emeric CS, Bastian L, et al: Does this woman have osteoporosis? *JAMA* 292:2890, 2004.

Greendale GA, DeAmicis TA, Bucur A, et al: A prospective study of the effect of fracture on measured physical performance: results from the MacArthur study—MAC, *J Am Geriatr Soc* 48:546, 2000.

Gregory DS, Seto CK, Wortley GC, Shugart CM: Acute lumbar disk pain: navigating evaluation and treatment choices, *Am Fam Physician* 78:835–842, 2008.

Gudavalli MR, Cambron J, Jedlicka J, et al: A randomized clinical trial and subgroup analysis to compare flexion-distraction with active exercise for chronic low back pain, *Eur Spine J* 31(5):376–380, 2005.

Haas M, Goldberg B, Aickin M, et al: A practice-based study of patients with acute and chronic low back pain attending primary care and chiropractic physicians: two-week to 48-month follow-up, *J Manipulative Physiol Ther* 27:160–169, 2004.

Hamaoka T, Madewell JE, Podoloff DA, et al: Bone imaging in metastatic breast cancer, *J Clin Oncol* 22:2942–2953, 2004.

Hart LG, Deyo RA, Cherkin DC: Physician office visits for low back pain. Frequency, clinical evaluation, and treatment patterns from a U.S. national survey, *Spine* 20:11–19, 1995.

Harwood MI, Smith BJ: Low back pain: a primary care approach, *Fam Pract Clin* 7(2):279–303, 2005.

Hills D: *Mechanical low back pain*. Available at www.aafp.org (accessed June 2006).

Horton WC, Daftari TK: Which disc as visualized by magnetic resonance imaging is actually a source of pain? A correlation between magnetic resonance imaging and discography, *Spine* 17:S164–S171, 1992.

Huang C, Ross PD, Wasnich R: Vertebral fracture and other predictors of physical impairment and health care utilization, *Arch Intern Med* 156:2469, 1996.

Huff SJ: *Neoplasms, spinal cord*. 2001. eMedicine [serial online]. Available at www.emedicine.com/emerg/topic337.htm (accessed January, 2011).

Kandel ER, Schwartz JH, Jessell TM: *Principles of neural science*, 3rd ed, Norwalk, CT, 1991, Appleton & Lange.

Kaufmann TJ, Jensen ME, Schweickert PA, et al: Age of fracture and clinical outcomes of percutaneous vertebroplasty, *AJNR Am J Neuroradiol* 22:1860, 2001.

Khairi MR, Johnston CC: What we know—and don't know—about bone loss in the elderly, *Geriatrics* 33:67, 1978.

Kinkade S: Evaluation and treatment of acute low back pain, *Am Fam Physician* 75:1190–1192, 2007.

Klotzbuecher CM, Ross PD, Landsman PB, et al: Patients with prior fractures have an increased risk of future fractures: a summary of the literature and statistical synthesis, *J Bone Miner Res* 15:721, 2000.

Koes BW, van Tulder MW, Thoma S: Diagnosis and treatment of low back pain, *BMJ* 332:1430–1434, 2006.

Laptoiu D: *Back pain*. Available at www.sportsmed-forum.com/index-1/st_pag_patients-home/sm_pag_backpain.htm (accessed January, 2011).

Ledlie JT, Renfro MB: Kyphoplasty treatment of vertebral fractures: 2-year outcomes show sustained benefits, *Spine* 31:57, 2006.

Lewis G: Percutaneous vertebroplasty and kyphoplasty for the stand-alone augmentation of osteoporosis-induced vertebral compression fractures: present status and future directions, *J Biomed Mater Res B Appl Biomater* 27:217–223, 2006.

Lindsay R, Silverman SL, Cooper C, et al: Risk of new vertebral fracture in the year following a fracture, *JAMA* 285:320, 2001.

Malmivaara A, Hakkinen U, Aro T, et al: The treatment of acute low back pain—bed rest, exercises, or ordinary activity? *N Engl J Med* 332:351–355, 1995.

Malmros B, Mortensen L, Jensen MB, Charles P: Positive effects of physiotherapy on chronic pain and performance in osteoporosis, *Osteoporos Int* 8:215, 1998.

Nevitt MC, Ettinger B, Black DM, et al: The association of radiographically detected vertebral fractures with back pain and function: a prospective study, *Ann Intern Med* 128:793, 1998.

Peterson DH, Bergmann TF: *Chiropractic technique: principles and procedures*, 2nd ed, St. Louis, 2002, Mosby.

Peul WC, van Houwelingen HC, van den Hout WB, et al, for the Leiden-The Hague Spine Intervention Prognostic Study Group: Surgery versus prolonged conservative treatment for sciatica, *N Engl J Med* 356:2245–2256, 2007.

Raisz LG: Clinical strategy in osteopenia, *Hosp Pract* 13:11, 1978.

Rapado A: General management of vertebral fractures, *Bone* 18:191S, 1996.

Schlaich C, Minne HW, Bruckner T, et al: Reduced pulmonary function in patients with spinal osteoporotic fractures, *Osteoporos Int* 8:261, 1998.

Schliesser JS, Kruse R, Fallon LF: Cervical radiculopathy treated with chiropractic flexion distraction manipulation: a retrospective study in a private practice setting, *J Manipulative Physiol Ther* 26:160–169, 2003.

Sheon RP, Moskowitz RW, Goldberg VM: *Soft tissue rheumatic pain: recognition, management, prevention*, 3rd ed, Baltimore, 1996, Williams & Wilkins.

Sinaki M, Mikkelsen BA: Postmenopausal spinal osteoporosis: flexion versus extension exercises, *Arch Phys Med Rehabil* 65:593, 1984.

Theodorou DJ, Theodorou SJ, Duncan TD, et al: Percutaneous balloon kyphoplasty for the correction of spinal deformity in painful vertebral body compression fractures, *Clin Imaging* 26:1, 2002.

Vogt TM, Ross PD, Palermo L, et al: Vertebral fracture prevalence among women screened for the Fracture Intervention Trial and a simple clinical tool to screen for undiagnosed vertebral fractures. Fracture Intervention Trial Research Group, *Mayo Clin Proc* 75:888, 2000.

Weinstein JN, Tosteson TD, Lurie JD, et al: Surgical vs nonoperative treatment for lumbar disc herniation: the Spine Patient Outcomes Research Trial (SPORT): a randomized trial, *JAMA* 296:2441–2450, 2006.

Winters M, Klutz P, Zilberstein J: Back pain emergencies, *Med Clin North Am* 90:505–523, 2006.

Wynne AT, Nelson MA, Nordin BEC: Costoiliac impingement syndrome, *J Bone Joint Surg* 67B:124, 1985.

CHAPTER 8

Behavior Problems in Children
Arwa Nasir

The primary care physician's office is often the point of first contact for families who have children with disruptive behavior. Parents seek help for a range of problems in different age groups. Sleeping problems and excessive crying or infantile colic are the two common problems in infancy. School refusal and hyperactive behavior are observed in the early elementary school years. Learning disabilities become evident at the middle to late elementary school years. In the adolescent years, behavioral problems in the form of aggressive behavior and substance abuse are often seen. The observed increase in the incidence of autistic spectrum disorders (ASDs) in recent years and the availability of effective management of this condition makes it important for the primary care physician to have the knowledge and skills to evaluate and refer a child presenting with an ASD.

Although children with behavioral problems often arrive prelabeled, the physician should always be ready to consider alternate diagnoses if the situation warrants it. The physician should also be aware that frequently more than one behavioral problem coexists in the same individual.

A large proportion of behavioral problems is the result of maladaptive interactional patterns within the family. These maladaptive interactional patterns also maintain the problem behavior. Literature indicates strong associations between family attributes, including maternal mental health, parental discord, and parenting behavior, and the diagnosis of many behavioral disorders in children including attention-deficit/hyperactivity disorder (ADHD), oppositional defiant disorder (ODD), and conduct disorder.

The role of the physician in this situation is to clarify the problematic dynamic in a nonjudgmental fashion, and provide advice or referral for the parent and/or child.

ANXIETY DISORDERS

Anxiety disorders are the most common psychiatric disorders diagnosed in children and adolescence with a prevalence of 7% to 13%. Anxiety disorders can be classified into four different categories: generalized, separation anxiety, social anxiety disorder or social phobia, or obsessive-compulsive disorder.

Symptoms
- Excessive uncontrollable worry that is developmentally inappropriate
- Anxious anticipation
- Causes subjective distress *or* affects social or academic performance
- School refusal
- Somatic symptoms such as abdominal pain

Signs
- Tachycardia
- Diaphoresis
- Pallor or flushing
- Tremor

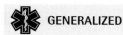 **GENERALIZED**

Signs
- Children in this category worry about all manner of upcoming events including school performance, punctuality, and crime and natural disasters.
- They tend to be perfectionists and require excessive reassurance.

 OBSESSIVE-COMPULSIVE DISORDER

Symptoms
- Recurrent, time-consuming obsessive or compulsive behaviors that cause distress and/or impairment
- Obsessions are repetitive, intrusive thoughts and impulses.
- The compulsions can be physical behaviors such as handwashing or ritualistic cleaning, or cognitive, such as counting and praying.

Comments and Treatment Considerations
Because fears and worries are common in the pediatric age group, the diagnosis should focus on demonstrating high and developmentally inappropriate intensity and pervasiveness of worry, and disruption of function. Anxiety should be included in the differential diagnosis of children who present with recurrent abdominal pain, headaches, or other somatic symptoms. Medical conditions that produce sympathetic hyperactivity may mimic anxiety symptoms and include hypoglycemic episodes, hyperthyroidism, cardiac arrhythmias, caffeine toxicity, pheochromocytoma, or medication side effects.

Pharmacologic treatment with SSRIs is effective for generalized anxiety disorder, social phobia, and obsessive-compulsive disorder. Cognitive-behavioral therapy and desensitization therapy are probably efficacious for most forms of anxiety.

SEPARATION ANXIETY

Symptoms
- Refusal to sleep alone
- Excessive distress or physical symptoms when separated such as dizziness or palpitations
- Older children and adolescents may present with somatic symptoms such as abdominal pain or headaches.

Signs
- Excessive worry about separation from an attachment figure or place
- Separation anxiety is developmentally appropriate in children younger than 5 to 6 years of age.
- School refusal is the most common presentation of separation anxiety.

 SOCIAL ANXIETY DISORDER

Symptoms
- Sweating
- Palpitations
- Tremor
- Flushing or pallor

Signs
- Children have a persistent fear of being humiliated or embarrassed in social situations.
- More common in girls than boys

Workup
- The prognosis for remission depends on the severity and pervasiveness of symptoms and on life events that may reassure the individual or validate and reinforce his or her fears.

ATTENTION–DEFICIT/HYPERACTIVITY DISORDER

ADHD is a behavioral syndrome defined as the presence of symptoms of inattention, impulsivity, or hyperactivity that are maladaptive and inconsistent with developmental stage. There must be evidence that symptoms compromise social, academic, or occupational function in more than one setting. Evidence of some of the behaviors needs to have been observed before age 7 years and persisted for more than 6 months (*Diagnostic and Statistical Manual of Mental Disorders, Fourth Edition* [DSM-IV]). The DSM-IV lists nine behaviors in each of the categories of inattention and hyperactivity. Diagnosis is considered if the child meets six of the criteria in one or both categories. A child may have a predominantly inattentive or predominantly hyperactive or a combined type ADHD. Symptoms of inattention or hyperactivity that do not cause impairments in learning or social functioning do not meet the criteria for ADHD.

Symptoms
- Inattention and/or impulsivity
- Impairments in learning or occupational function
- Comorbid neuron-developmental conditions such as learning disabilities, ODD, anxiety disorders +++

Signs
- Beginning prior to 7 years of age ++++
- Persisting more than 6 months ++++
- Symptoms occur in more than one setting (e.g., home and school) +++++

Workup
- Impaired social (peer relations) or occupational (school) functioning
- Demonstrated impairment in more than one setting. Frequently obtain input from parents and teachers.
- Several assessment tools that are based on the DSM-IV criteria are available for evaluating children with ADHD. The two most commonly used are the National Initiative for Children's Healthcare Quality (NICHQ) Vanderbilt Assessment and the Conner's Rating Scale Revised. Both include screening questions for comorbid conditions commonly associated with ADHD such as ODD (both) and depression (Vanderbilt).

Comments and Treatment Considerations
Most children who are diagnosed with ADHD are diagnosed during the early elementary school years, when their inattention or hyperactivity interferes with their learning or ability to comply with standards of behavior in the classroom.

The American Academy of Pediatrics (AAP) has published treatment guidelines based on comprehensive evidence-based review of the literature. The AAP guidelines stress the importance of accurate diagnosis and close follow-up and monitoring in addition to the pharmacologic and nonpharmacologic components of the management of the child with ADHD.

The nonpharmacologic component of management includes:
- Educating the family and the child about the nature of the problem and management options. Parent training in behavior management and structuring the environment of the child are helpful.
- Educational management: Identifying possible coexistent learning disabilities, and identifying academic issues that may improve classroom performance, including preferential seating, and one-on-one tutoring.
- Cognitive-behavioral therapy

Pharmacotherapy with stimulant medications has been shown to be effective in decreasing undesired behavior and improving function in the majority of children with ADHD. Monitoring of efficacy and side effects of stimulant medications is imperative. The reader is referred to other sources for a more detailed discussion of the pharmacologic management of ADHD.

AUTISM

Autism is a neurodevelopmental disorder characterized by impairments in three domains:
- Reciprocal social interaction
- Verbal and nonverbal communication
- Range of activities and interests

Autism is a spectrum disorder, which means that it affects children differently. Autistic behaviors can range from mild to severe. The child may be recognized as unusual at birth, or symptoms may first be noted during the first 1 to 2 years of life.

Autism presents as delay in reaching developmental milestones, especially speech. Autistic children also lack normal social interaction with others, including parents, and seem to be "in a world of their own." They also display unusual behaviors including self-stimulation behaviors, limited interest, and repetitive behaviors.

Symptoms
- A child who does not babble, point, or make meaningful gestures by 1 year of age
- A child who does not speak one word by 18 months
- A child who does not combine two words by 2 years
- A child who does not respond to his/her name
- A child who does not seem to know how to play with toys
- Preoccupation with order of things: lines up toys or other objects
- A child who at times seems to be hearing impaired
- Difficulty with emotional regulation: tend to lose control, difficult to console

Signs
- Poor eye contact
- Lack of smile
- Self-stimulating behaviors
- Repetitive behaviors

Workup
- Several screening tools are available to assist the clinician to quickly gather information about the child's social and communicative development, such as the Checklist of Autism in Toddlers (CHAT).
- Once a child is suspected to have autistic features, a comprehensive evaluation by a multidisciplinary team is indicated.

Comments and Treatment Considerations

Several problems are frequently associated with autism: mental retardation, hearing impairment, seizure disorder, and associations noted with some genetic syndromes including fragile X and tuberous sclerosis.

Autistic spectrum disorders are treatable. A wide variety of treatment options can be very helpful. Left untreated, most autistic children do not develop effective social skills and may not learn to talk or behave appropriately.

OPPOSITIONAL DEFIANT DISORDER

The essential feature of ODD is a recurrent pattern of developmentally inappropriate negativistic, defiant, disobedient, and hostile behavior toward authority figures (DSM-IV). These behaviors tend to be more evident with the people the child knows well.

ODD tends to be more prevalent in families in whom parenting is harsh, inconsistent, or neglectful. Current conceptualizations of the disorder focus on maladaptive parent-child interactional patterns. ODD is considered to be the developmental antecedent of conduct disorder, which includes all the criteria of ODD, in addition to more severe violence in the form of physical aggression, destruction of property, deceitfulness, and serious violations of rules.

Symptoms
- Begins around ages 8 to 13 years +++
- Short temper +++
- Stubbornness +++
- Arguing (with adults) +++
- Defying rules and resistance to direction
- Anger and resentment
- Spitefulness and vindictiveness
- Unwillingness to compromise, negotiate, or give in
- Unwillingness to accept responsibility or blame for misdeeds, blaming others
- Verbal aggression

Signs
- Manifests in the preteen to early teen years ++++
- Characteristic behaviors appear in the home setting before extending to other settings.

Comments and Treatment Considerations

Parent training is effective in treating oppositional and defiant behaviors. Parent training programs consist of standardized, short-term interventions to teach parents specific parenting strategies including reinforcement strategies and other behavior modification techniques, in addition to positive parenting and ignoring unwanted behavior. Parent participation is critical to the success of any treatment strategy.

References

American Psychiatric Association: *Diagnostic and statistical manual of mental disorders, fourth edition*, Washington, DC, 2000, APA.

Farley SE, Adams JS, Lutton ME, et al: Clinical inquiries. What are effective treatments for oppositional and defiant behaviors in preadolescents? *J Fam Pract* 54:162,164–165, 2005.

Goldson E: Autism spectrum disorders: an overview, *Adv Pediatr* 51:63–109, 2004.

Greene RW, Doyle AE: Toward a transactional conceptualization of oppositional defiant disorder: implications for assessment and treatment, *Clin Child Fam Psychol Rev* 2:129–148, 1999.

Parker S, Zuckerman B, Augustyn M: *Developmental behavioral pediatrics: a handbook for primary care*, 2nd ed, Philadelphia, 2005, Lippincott Williams & Wilkins.

Reiff MI, Stein MT: Attention-deficit/hyperactivity disorder: diagnosis and treatment, *Adv Pediatr* 51:289–327, 2004.

Yusin AS: American Academy of Pediatrics practice parameter on attention-deficit/hyperactivity disorder, *Pediatrics* 113:428–429, 2004.

CHAPTER 9

Bleeding and Bruising
Ivan Abdouch

Normal hemostasis is dependent on a complex and balanced process of clot formation and clot lysis. A number of congenital and acquired conditions can produce disruption of this process, resulting in spontaneous, excessive, or delayed bleeding and bruising.

Determining whether a pathologic or even clinically significant process is present can be obscured by the wide variation that exists among patients in their perceptions about bleeding or bruising. Because no standardized measure of bleeding severity exists, the clinician must rely on historical clues relative to the patient's bleeding history (e.g., bleeding after tooth extraction or other surgical procedures, menstrual history, anemia), dietary habits, and medication use.

ABNORMAL PLATELET FUNCTION

Abnormal platelet function can be caused by medications and/or disruption at any of the several levels of the normal process of primary hemostasis including: (1) endothelial injury; (2) platelet adhesion as platelets interact with von Willebrand factor (vWf) in the endothelium; (3) platelet aggregation, which is mediated by platelet glycoprotein IIb/IIIa; (4) platelet activation, which involves release of alpha and dense granules; the alpha granules contain hemostatic proteins like fibrinogen, and vWf, whereas the dense granules contain proaggregatory factors like adenosine diphosphate (ADP); and (5) formation of thromboxane A_2.

Signs
- Often present in early childhood with moderate to severe bruising or bleeding, usually recognized at the time of trauma or surgery but occasionally there is spontaneous bleeding
- Females may have menorrhagia that worsens with use of nonsteroidals.

Workup
- In vitro bleeding time
- Flow cytometry
- Platelet aggregation

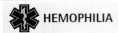 **HEMOPHILIA**

Hemophilia is a congenital sex-linked recessive disorder occurring in approximately 1 in 10,000 births. Individuals with hemophilia have limited levels of specific clotting factors resulting in prolonged bleeding. The genetic transmission of hemophilia results in males with the disorder and females as carriers. The most common forms of hemophilia include factor VIII (most prevalent) and factor IX.

Symptoms
- Bleeding or bruising +++

Signs
- Family history of bleeding disorders particularly in the male members
- Prolonged bleeding
- Hemarthrosis, joint or muscle pain
- Swollen, warm, or stiff joints
- Multiple or large contusions
- Hematomas
- Trauma-induced or postoperative uncontrolled bleeding (including circumcision)
- Altered mental status post-head injury

Workup
- Screening tests
  - Bleeding time
  - Closure time
  - Platelet count
  - Activated partial thromboplastin time (aPTT)
- Studies to rule out other causes of bleeding such as:
  - Cancer
  - Liver disease
  - Bone marrow dysfunction
  - Medications
  - Immune system–related diseases
  - DIC (often associated with childbearing, cancer, or infection)
  - Eclampsia
  - Organ transplant rejection
  - Antibodies that destroy clotting factors
  - Exposure to snake venom
- Check factor VIII and IX specific assays if any abnormal screening test results (Table 9-1).
- aPTT—Elevated in moderate to severe hemophilia; may be normal in mild hemophilia (Table 9-2)
- Females—Check factor levels before any major surgery if:
  - Father, son, and/or brother have hemophilia (may have decreased factor levels)
  - Experience hemophilia-type symptoms (some women can be symptomatic carriers; severe menstrual bleeding is the most common symptom for women with lower factor levels)

Table 9-1. Differential Diagnoses Based on Findings

POSSIBLE CONDITION	PT	aPTT	BLEEDING TIME	PLATELET COUNT
Normal	+	+	+	+
vWf	+	+ or ⇑	+ or ⇑	+ or ⇓
Hemophilia A and B	+	⇑	+	+
Platelet defect	+	+	+ or ⇑	+ or ⇓

aPTT, Activated partial thromboplastin time; +, normal; ⇑, prolonged;
PT, prothrombin; ⇓, reduced; *vWf,* von Willebrand factor.

Table 9-2. Categorization of Hemophilia by Factor Level

FACTOR LEVELS	SEVERITY OF DISEASE	COMPLICATIONS
>1 %	Severe	Spontaneous bleeds
1%-5%	Moderate	Occasional spontaneous bleeds; severe bleeds—surgery or trauma
5%-40%	Mild	Usually only bleeds with surgery or trauma

Comments and Treatment Considerations

Reduce complications by administering factor concentrate on arrival to the health care facility before any lab, intake paperwork, vitals, or ancillary services are obtained. Clotting factor replacement is very effective, but is extremely expensive; the financial stress on the family should be considered and addressed. Reaching an insurance lifetime maximum is common.

Desmopressin (DDAVP) can be used for non–life-threatening bleeds instead of factor concentrate for individuals with mild to moderate factor VIII deficiency and von Willebrand disease (Table 9-3). This medication can raise the factor two to eight times the baseline level.

Be aware of the possibility of the emergence of inhibitors—a severe complication for some individuals who use factor concentrate. This may be found when a person who normally responds to the factor concentrate continues to bleed. When this occurs the factor levels and the presence of inhibitors should be checked. A hematologist should be consulted and a second-line agent chosen.

Antifibrinolytic drugs can also be used for mouth bleeds. With all individuals with bleeding disorders, medicines that affect platelet function should not be used (e.g., aspirin and NSAIDs). Acetaminophen is a good alternative.

During testing and diagnosis, support the family by providing accurate information about the disease and educate them over

Table 9-3. Types of von Willebrand Disease

TYPE	CHARACTERISTIC	INHERITANCE	TREATMENT
1	vWf is reduced, usually do not bleed spontaneously, most common	Dominant: one parent	DDAVP by intravenous or intranasal Severe bleeds/ surgery may require factor VIII with vWf
2	vWf is abnormal (smaller and breaks down too easily or factor sticks to platelets too well)	Dominant: one parent	Factor VIII with vWf
3	Severe bleeding problems and has very low vWf and factor VIII	Recessive: both parents	Factor VIII with vWf
Pseudo	Similar to type 2 but the defects are in the platelets	Dominant: one parent	Platelet transfusion

DDAVP, Desmopressin; *vWf,* von Willebrand factor.

time. A follow-up visit should occur soon after the initial diagnosis to provide support, information, and clarification for the families. Caregiving and coping with a chronic disease should be addressed with the family in each encounter. Because many individuals with hemophilia are treated at home, establishment of a collaborative and supportive relationship is imperative.

Due to the large volume of factor concentrates and other treatment modalities a hematologist should be part of the treatment team and should be consulted when a new diagnosis occurs and when significant injury or surgeries occur.

If the individual has a history of hemophilia and there is doubt about the possibility of a bleed occurring, err on the side of caution and treat. Because hemophilia is an uncommon disorder and families have knowledge of past treatment successes, the family should be encouraged to provide guidance to the treatment team.

Life-threatening bleeds include severe trauma, or trauma to the GI, CNS, neck, and throat. Serious bleeds involve joints, muscle, urinary tract, mouth, gums, and nose—these can cause serious secondary damage (e.g., arthritis, nerve damage, urinary tract damage). Joint bleeds are the most common complication in hemophilia.

Treatment options include:
• Daily prophylactic treatment for individuals with severe disease with frequent spontaneous bleeding (due to the difficulty with daily IV administration of factor, many young children will have a Port-A-Cath placed and parents will be trained to administer the factor at home)

- Periodic treatment when injury, surgery, or spontaneous bleed occurs
- Adjunctive therapy should be used in conjunction with factor replacement to aid in healing, decrease swelling, and aid in pain reduction.
  - RICE: Rest, Ice (20 minutes every 4 hours until swelling and pain decreases), Compression, and Elevation
  - May also need splinting, crutches, or wheelchair

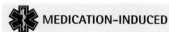 **MEDICATION-INDUCED**

Acquired platelet dysfunction has been described as being second only to thrombocytopenia as the major cause of clinical bleeding disorders. The most common of drug induced bleeding disorders arise from the ingestion of aspirin and other NSAIDs that inhibit platelet production of thromboxane A_2. These drugs inhibit COX. The other agents are competitive and reversible inhibitors with more transient effects. Table 9-4 illustrates common drugs associated with platelet dysfunction.

Signs
- Clinical evidence of bleeding, but a normal platelet count and coagulation studies
- Easy bruising and bleeding confined to skin
- Occasionally patients will have prolonged oozing after surgery, particularly with procedures involving mucous membranes.

Workup
- Ask explicit questions to identify all prescribed drugs, over-the-counter medications, and any herbal preparations.
- Prolonged Ivy bleeding time; platelet aggregometry

Comments and Treatment Considerations
- Discontinue the culprit drug.
- Platelet transfusion in the setting of clinically significant bleeding
- Patients who have taken aspirin should be treated as if they have a mild hemostatic defect for the next 5 to 7 days.

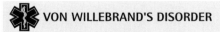 **VON WILLEBRAND'S DISORDER**

von Willebrand's disease (vWD) is an autosomal disorder with three specific types. Type 1 is an autosomal dominant disorder and types 2 and 3 are recessive disorders. vWD is the most common form of bleeding disorders, with a prevalence of approximately 1% to 2% of the population. vWf works in conjunction with platelets to stick to the damaged part of the body. It is also used to transport factor VIII to the site of the injury. Individuals with vWD have problems with one or both of these issues.

Table 9-4. Common Drugs Causing Platelet Dysfunction

INTERFERES WITH PLATELET MEMBRANE	INHIBITION OF PROSTAGLANDIN SYNTHESIS	INHIBITION OF PLATELET PHOSPHODIESTERASE	UNKNOWN MECHANISM OF ACTION
Amitriptyline	Aspirin	Caffeine	Acetazolamide
Imipramine	NSAIDs	Dipyridamole	Ethacrynic acid
Chlorpromazine	Furosemide	Aminophylline	Hydroxychloroquine
Cocaine	Verapamil	Theophylline	Nitroprusside
Lidocaine	Hydralazine	Vinblastine	Cyproheptadine
Isoproterenol	Cyclosporine A	Vincristine	Nitroglycerin
Propranolol	Hydrocortisone	Colchicine	Famotidine
Penicillin		Papaverine	Cimetidine
Ampicillin		Clopidogrel	
Cephalothin		Ticlopidine	
Promethazine			
Diphenhydramine			
Carbenicillin			

Signs
- Family history of bleeding disorders
- Prolonged bleeding
- Hemarthrosis
- Joint or muscle pain
- Swollen, warm, or stiff joints
- Multiple or large contusions
- Hematomas
- Trauma-induced or postoperative uncontrolled bleeding (including circumcision)
- Altered mental status post-head injury
- Abnormal menstrual bleeding

Workup
- Screening tests
  - Bleeding time
  - Closure time
  - Platelet count
  - aPTT
- If results are abnormal, vWf and factor VIII specific assay tests should be conducted (see Table 9-1).
- Studies to rule out other causes of bleeding such as cancer, liver disease, bone marrow dysfunction, medications, immune system–related diseases, DIC (often associated with childbearing, cancer, or infection), eclampsia, organ transplant rejection, antibodies that destroy clotting factors, and exposure to snake venom
- Check vWf assay if any abnormal screening test results (see Table 9-1).

Comments and Treatment Considerations
Reduce complications by administering factor concentrate on arrival to the health care facility before any lab, intake paperwork, vitals or ancillary services are obtained. Clotting factor replacement is very effective, but is extremely expensive; the financial stress on the family should be considered and addressed. Reaching an insurance lifetime maximum is common.

DDAVP can be used for non–life-threatening bleeds instead of factor concentrate for individuals with mild to moderate factor VIII deficiency and vWD. This medication can raise factor two to eight times the baseline level.

Be aware of the possibility of the emergence of inhibitors—a severe complication for some individuals who use factor concentrate. This may be found when a person who normally responds to the factor concentrate continues to bleed. When this occurs the factor levels and the presence of inhibitors should be checked. A hematologist should be consulted and a second-line agent chosen.

Antifibrinolytic drugs can also be used for mouth bleeds. With all individuals with bleeding disorders, medicines that affect platelet function should not be used (e.g., aspirin and NSAIDs). Acetaminophen is a good alternative.

During the testing and diagnosis, support the family by providing accurate information about the disease, and educate them over time. A follow-up visit should occur soon after the initial diagnosis to provide support, information and a clarification for the families. Caregiving and coping with a chronic disease should be addressed with the family in each encounter. Because many individuals with hemophilia are treated at home, establishment of a collaborative and supportive relationship is imperative.

Due to the large volume of factor concentrates and other treatment modalities a hematologist should be part of the treatment team and should be consulted when a new diagnosis occurs and when significant injury or surgeries occur.

Disease should be categorized so that treatment can be specific to disease type (see Table 9-3).

THROMBOCYTOPENIA

Symptoms
• Bleeding or bruising +++

Signs
• Platelet count less than 150,000 ++++
• Less than 50,000: petechiae appear +++
• Less than 20,000: bleeding from gums, nose, GI tract, or brain may occur ++
• Splenomegaly and systemic symptoms (e.g., fever) suggest that thrombocytopenia is secondary to another condition.
• Hemarthrosis occurs with coagulation disorders but not with platelet dysfunction.

Workup
• May be due to medications, decreased platelet production, increased destruction, or sequestration.
• Medication history—explicit questions to identify all prescribed drugs, over-the-counter medications, and any herbal preparations; medication-induced thrombocytopenia is often am empirical diagnosis, supported only by resolution of thrombocytopenia after discontinuation of therapy with the suspected drug (Table 9-5).
• CBC and platelet count
• Bone marrow analysis if needed (decreased megakaryocytes signal decreased platelet production; increased megakaryocytes signal increased platelet destruction)
• Other studies as dictated by specific circumstances as outlined in the following text. May need radiologic confirmation of splenomegaly.

Comments and Treatment Considerations
Treat the underlying disorder if feasible. In the case of medications, remove the offending agent and maintain symptomatic treatment of the patient (give oral prednisone 1 mg/kg once daily if platelet count <10,000/mm^3); platelet counts should recover within 5 to 7 days.

Table 9-5. Drugs Associated with Thrombocytopenia, with Level I Evidence (Definite) or Level II Evidence (Probable)

Abciximab	Clozapine	Gold salts	Olanzapine	Simvastatin
Acetaminophen	Cyclosporine	Haloperidol	Ondansetron	Sulfadiazine
Acetazolamide	Desmopressin	Hydantoin	Penicillin	Sulfathiozole
Acyclovir	Diazepam	HCTZ	Phenytoin	Suramin
Ampicillin	Diazoxide	Hydroxyurea	Piroxicam	Teicoplanin
Atorvastatin	Diclofenac	Hepatitis B vaccine/interferon	Plicamycin	Terbinafine
Benztropine	Diltiazem	Levamisole	Prednisone	Ticlopidine
Bleomycin	Doxepin	L-Tryptophan	Procainamide	Trimethoprim
Carbamazepine	Enalapril	Measles vaccine	Prochlorperazine	Valproate
Cephalosporins	Famotidine	Mesalamine	Pyrimethamine	Vancomycin
Chlorpromazine	Fluphenazine	Methylphenidate	Quinidine	
Cimetidine	Furosemide	Moxalactam	Ranitidine	
Ciprofloxacin	Ganciclovir	Naproxen	Rifampin	
Clopidogrel	Gentamicin	Octreotide	Rituximab	

If major bleeding is present, platelet transfusions, IVIg, and high doses of parenteral glucocorticoids (comparable to treatment of idiopathic thrombocytopenia [ITP]) are appropriate.

Medication-induced thrombocytopenia typically presents as isolated thrombocytopenia in a patient who is taking several medications. The main issue is to distinguish between drug-induced thrombocytopenia and ITP. Medications begun within the last month are more likely the cause of thrombocytopenia than are medications taken regularly for many years. Mechanisms include hapten-type immune reaction, innocent bystander–type immune reaction, direct toxicity, and heparin-induced reaction.

Direct Toxicity
- Causes suppressed thrombopoiesis
- Cancer chemotherapy agents, pesticides, and organic solvents have been implicated in this type of thrombocytopenia.

 HAPTEN–TYPE IMMUNE REACTIONS

Symptoms
- Most common type of thrombocytopenia
- Usually appears at least 7 days after the start of a new medication
- Can occur sooner in cases of reexposure to a drug that was previously taken

 HEPARIN–INDUCED THROMBOCYTOPENIA I (HIT I)

- Occurs within the first 2 days after heparin initiation
- Often returns to normal with continued heparin administration
- More common than HIT II
- Is of no clinical consequence

 HEPARIN–INDUCED THROMBOCYTOPENIA (HIT II)

HIT II, the more serious form, is an immune-mediated disorder characterized by the formation of antibodies against the heparin-platelet factor IV complex.

Symptoms
- Bleeding and bruising +++

Signs
Early:
- Increased bruising +
- Petechiae +

- Ecchymoses +
- Epistaxis +
- Necrotic skin lesions +

Later:
- Bleeding ++
- Severe purpura
- Platelet count that has fallen 50% or more from a prior value +
- Heparin therapy within the preceding 5 to 10 days, or in a patient receiving prolonged treatment with LMWH
- Thrombosis associated with thrombocytopenia +++

Workup
- Diagnosis of HIT is made on clinical grounds; assays with the highest sensitivity and specificity may not be readily available and have a slow turnaround time.
- Most specific diagnostic tests: Serotonin release assays, heparin-induced platelet aggregation assays, and solid phase immunoassays.
- Patients with HIT II also have elevated platelet-associated IgG levels, but this is a nonspecific finding.
- 14C-Serotonin release assay: Gold standard among the diagnostic tests for HIT II
- Heparin-induced platelet aggregation: More than 90% specific, but lacks sensitivity.
- Solid phase enzyme-linked immunosorbent assay (ELISA) immunoassay: Best used along with one of the functional assays rather than as a single test

Comments and Treatment Considerations
Immediately stop exposure to heparin, including heparin-bonded catheters and heparin flushes. Avoid LMWH.
- Lepirudin (Refludan): Recombinant hirudin, FDA-approved treatment of HIT complicated by thrombosis.
  - Initial dose of 0.4 mg/kg (up to 44 mg) IV bolus followed by an infusion of 0.15 mg/kg/hr (up to 16.5 mg/hr) for 2 to 10 days
  - Adjust infusion rate according to aPTT ratio
- Warfarin: Initiate while the patient has been stably anticoagulated with a thrombin-specific inhibitor, and when the platelet count has increased to $100,000/\mu L$ or higher. The use of warfarin in the absence of other anticoagulants should be avoided. Dose is patient specific.
- Bivalirudin: Hemodialyzable direct thrombin inhibitor and hirudin analog; FDA approved for patients with or at risk of HIT who are undergoing percutaneous coronary intervention.
- Argatroban: Another direct thrombin inhibitor; monitor its effect with aPTT
  - In patients with normal hepatic function, the starting dose is 2 mcg/kg/min by continuous IV infusion.
  - Adjust rate to maintain the aPTT at 1.5 to 3 times baseline

Decreased platelet production can be due to:
- Infections (including HIV)
- Chemotherapy or radiation therapy
- Deficiency of folate or vitamin B_{12} (especially seen with ethanol abuse)
- Marrow infiltration by tumor or storage diseases
- Marrow failure due to aplastic anemia
- Leukemia
- Myelodysplastic syndrome

 INCREASED PLATELET DESTRUCTION

Alloimmune Thrombocytopenia
- Posttransfusion purpura: Up to 3% of the population is homozygous human platelet antigen (HPA)-1b due to amino acid substitution in the platelet glycoprotein IIb/IIIa antigen. When exposed to blood products from a person who is HPA-1a, antibodies develop that become clinically apparent 10 days posttransfusion. The resulting thrombocytopenia may last for weeks but will respond to IVIg.
- Neonatal alloimmune thrombocytopenia: Occurs in 1/200 pregnancies but is clinically significant in 1/1500. Most cases involve a mother who is HPA-1b and a baby who is HPA-1a. Thrombocytopenia occurs during the first pregnancy in half of cases.

Immune Thrombocytopenic Purpura
- Variety of immune conditions that result in problems with primary hemostasis (formation of the initial hemostatic plug)
  - Acute ITP: Self-limited form that usually occurs after a viral illness. Predominantly in children with peak age from 3 to 5 years. Incidence 5/100,000.
  - Chronic ITP: Platelet count low for more than 6 months. Peak age 20 to 40 years old. More common in females (1.7:1). Incidence 3 to 5/100,000.
  - Secondary ITP: Can occur with systemic lupus erythematosus, antiphospholipid antibody syndrome, IgA deficiency, hepatitis C, lymphomas and chronic lymphocytic leukemia, HIV, heparin, and quinidine.

 THROMBOTIC THROMBOCYTOPENIC PURPURA

Thrombocytopenic purpura is characterized by the presence of increased vWf precursors in the endothelial cells due to abnormal function of the enzyme ADAMTS13. Ultralarge multimers induce platelet aggregation, resulting in platelet consumption and occlusion of the small blood vessels. They are especially dangerous in brain and kidney.
- Sporadic form: Due to antibodies or toxins that inhibit ADAMTS13. These include cancer, chemotherapy, medications such as ticlopidine, cyclosporine A, tacrolimus, and quinine. Presents with

petechiae and neurologic symptoms ranging from headache and confusion to seizures and coma. May occur about 3 weeks after a flulike illness.
• Chronic, recurrent form (childhood thrombotic thrombocy-topenic purpura [TTP]): Probably due to congenital deficiency of ADAMTS13. May be treated with transfusions of platelet-poor fresh-frozen plasma every 3 weeks.

Innocent Bystander–Type Immune Reaction
• Most often associated with quinidine

Sequestration of Platelets
• Platelets are sequestered in spleen or liver due to liver disease or malignancy.
• Presents with mild to moderate thrombocytopenia
• Presents with mild decrease in neutrophils and hemoglobin in the peripheral blood
• Presents with normal bone marrow
• May need radiologic confirmation of splenomegaly

THROMBOCYTOSIS

The most common condition is essential thrombocythemia—a myelo-proliferative disorder (along with polycythemia vera and idiopathic myelofibrosis). Consider this diagnosis if there are no other causes of increased platelets such as arthritis, iron deficiency anemia, splenectomy, or chronic myelogenous leukemia.

Signs
• Mildly enlarged spleen
• Abnormal clotting in the brain or heart can be deadly.
• In pregnancy, fetal growth restriction, spontaneous abortion, and placental abruption

Workup
• Platelet count greater than 600,000; may be as high as 2 million
• Increased megakaryocytes in the bone marrow
• Abnormal clonal stem cell

References
Aster RH: Drug-induced immune thrombocytopenia: an overview of pathogenesis, *Semin Hematol* 36:2, 1999.
Baz R, Mekhail T: *Platelet disorders*, The Cleveland Clinic Disease Management Project. Available at www.clevelandclinicmeded.com (accessed December 1, 2003).
Bick RL: Acquired platelet function defects, *Hematol Oncol Clin North Am* 6:1203–1226, 1992.
Enayat M, Guilliatt A, Lester W, et al: Distinguishing between type 2B and pseudo-von Willebrand disease and its clinical importance, *Br J Haematol* 133:664–666, 2006.
Favaloro EJ: 2B or not 2B? Differential identification of type 2B, versus pseudo-von Willebrand disease, *Br J Haematol* 135:141–142, 2006.

Geil J: *Von Willebrand disease*. Available at www.emedicine.com/ped/topic2419 .htm (accessed May 2006).

George JN, Raskob GE, Shah SR, et al: Drug-induced thrombocytopenia: a systematic review of published case reports, *Ann Intern Med* 129:886, 1998.

Goldenberg NA, Jacobson L, Manco-Johnson MJ: Brief communication: duration of platelet dysfunction after a 7-day course of ibuprofen, *Ann Intern Med* 142:506, 2005.

Greinacher A, Eichler P, Lubenow N, et al: Heparin-induced thrombocytopenia with thromboembolic complications: meta-analysis of 2 prospective trials to assess the value of parenteral treatment with lepirudin and its therapeutic aPTT range, *Blood* 96:846, 2000.

Guidelines for the management of hemophilia. http://www.ehc.eu/fileadmin/ dokumente/Gudelines_Mng_Hemophilia.pdf.

Johns TE, Harbilas JW: Drug-induced hematologic disorders. In DiPiro JT, Talbert RL, Yee GC, et al, editors: *Pharmacotherapy: a pathophysiologic approach*, Stamford, CT, 1999, Appleton & Lange.

Kappers-Klunne MC, Boon DMS, Hop WCJ, et al: Heparin-induced thrombocytopenia and thrombosis: a prospective analysis of the incidence in patients with heart and cerebrovascular diseases, *Br J Haematol* 96:442, 1997.

Kaufman DW, Kelly JP, Johannes CB, et al: Acute thrombocytopenic purpura in relation to the use of drugs, *Blood* 82:2714, 1993.

Khair K, Liesner R: Bruising and bleeding in infants and children: a practical approach, *Br J Haematol* 133:221–231, 2006.

Lee CA, Berntorp EE, Hoots WK, editors: *Textbook of hemophilia*, Malden, MA, 2005, Blackwell Publishing.

Li X, Hunt L, Vesely SK: Drug-induced thrombocytopenia: an updated systematic review, *Ann Intern Med* 142:474, 2005.

Madan M, Berkowitz SD, Christie DJ, et al: Rapid assessment of glycoprotein IIb/IIIa blockade with the platelet function analyzer (PFA-100) during percutaneous coronary intervention, *Am Heart J* 141:226, 2001.

Marshall PW, Williams AJ, Dixon RM, et al: A comparison of the effects of aspirin on bleeding time measured using the Simplate method and closure time measured using the PFA-100, in healthy volunteers, *Br J Clin Pharmacol* 44:151, 1997.

National Hemophilia Foundation: www.hemophilia.org.

Newman P, Chong B: Heparin-induced thrombocytopenia: new evidence for the dynamic binding of purified anti-PF4-heparin antibodies to platelets and the resultant platelet activation, *Blood* 96:182, 2000.

Pedersen-Bjergaard U, Andersen M, Hansen, PB: Drug-induced thrombocytopenia: clinical data on 309 cases and the effect of corticosteroid therapy, *Eur J Clin Pharmacol* 52:183, 1997.

Rice L, Attisha WK, Drexler A, Francis JL: Delayed-onset heparin-induced thrombocytopenia, *Ann Intern Med* 136:210, 2002.

Rizvi MA, Kojouri K, George JN: Drug-induced thrombocytopenia: an updated systematic review, *Ann Intern Med* 134:346, 2001.

Warkentin TE: Clinical presentation of heparin-induced thrombocytopenia, *Semin Hematol* 35:9, 1998.

Warkentin TE: Current agents for the treatment of patients with heparin-induced thrombocytopenia, *Curr Opin Pulmon Med* 8:405–441, 2002.

Warkentin TE, Greinacher A: Heparin-induced thrombocytopenia: recognition, treatment, and prevention: the Seventh ACCP Conference on Antithrombotic and Thrombolytic Therapy, *Chest* 126:311S, 2004.

White J: Golgi complexes in hypogranular platelet syndromes, *Platelets* 16:51–60, 2005.

CHAPTER 10

Blood in Stool
Richard B. English

GI bleeding can arise from any area of the alimentary tract, and presentation can vary greatly. Bleeding can be insidious with minimal signs or symptoms as with occult blood loss, or dramatic with shock and hematemesis from esophageal varices. Common symptoms include hematemesis (vomiting of blood), the vomiting of "coffee grounds"–appearing emesis, hematochezia (red blood in the stool), and melena (dark black, tarry, foul-smelling stool).

For this discussion we consider only GI sources of bleeding as the cause of blood in the stool, and consider bleeding above the ligament of Treitz as upper gastrointestinal bleeding (UGIB) and below it as lower gastrointestinal bleeding (LGIB). Due to significant variations in presentation, UGIB can be further divided into variceal and nonvariceal bleeding sources. UGIB has an incidence of 40 to 150 episodes per 100,000 population per year, with mortality ranging between 6% and 10%. LGIB accounts for 20 to 27 hospitalizations per 100,000 population per year with mortality rates between 4% and 10%. Additionally, there is a 200-fold increase in the rate of bleeding with advancing age from the third to the ninth decades of life.

Patients with acute, severe, GI bleeding can deteriorate rapidly and immediate and appropriate interventions must be initiated during the primary assessment of the patient. The ABCs—airway, breathing, circulation—of acute resuscitation must be borne in mind at all times.

In addition to bleeding from esophageal varices, nonvariceal bleeding sites including peptic ulcer disease, gastric erosions, Mallory-Weiss tears, and Dieulafoy lesions are discussed. The discussion of LGIB includes diverticulosis, ischemic bowel sources, angiodysplasia, inflammatory bowel disease (IBD), polyps and neoplasia, and anorectal sources.

DIEULAFOY LESION

The characteristic feature is a large-caliber artery in the submucosa, which bleeds on erosion of the overlying mucosa. The lesion can be difficult to locate endoscopically unless actively bleeding. They are usually solitary lesions often in the proximal stomach.

Symptoms
- Dyspepsia ++
- Abdominal or epigastric pain +++
- Hematemesis +++
- "Coffee grounds" emesis +++
- Hematochezia +++
- Melena ++++

Signs
- Hematemesis or "coffee grounds" emesis +++
- Hematochezia +++
- Melena ++++
- Tachycardia and hypotension
- Positive nasogastric aspirate for blood or "coffee grounds" material ++++
- Positive stool testing for blood ++++
- Anemia

Workup
- Evaluate hemodynamic stability immediately. Orthostatic testing: Positive orthostatic testing is variably defined, but usually a drop of at least 20 mm Hg of systolic blood pressure (BP) is considered positive. A report from the American Society of Gastrointestinal Endoscopy (ASGE) showed an improvement in survival if postural changes were not present on initial examination.
- Lab: Hemoglobin, hematocrit, blood urea nitrogen (BUN), creatinine liver function tests, amylase, lipase, and coagulation studies
- In the absence of overt hematemesis, placement of a nasogastric (NG) tube for confirmation of bleeding and assessment of prognosis is generally recommended. NG aspiration has a low false-positive rate, yet may be negative in up to 25% of UGIB.
- Type and crossmatch for 2 to 4 units of packed red blood cells, more if clinically indicated.
- GI consultation for endoscopic evaluation and treatment of the acute bleeding site is recommended. Although most bleeding stops spontaneously, endoscopy provides an accurate diagnosis and the ability to directly coagulate the bleeding site. Various methods of hemostasis are used, but none has been found to be superior to the others.
- Selective visceral angiography should be considered if endoscopy fails to identify a bleeding source. Bleeding must be at rates exceeding 0.5 to 1 mL/min for examination to be optimal and have high yield.
- Radionuclide technetium-99m-labeled red cell scan may also be considered for continued bleeding because it can detect bleeding at rates that exceed 0.1 mL/min. However, pooled blood may sometimes be mistaken for active bleeding.

Comments and Treatment Considerations
Obtain IV access with two large-bore catheters and begin immediate fluid resuscitation with crystalloid solutions as needed. Efforts

to assess the patient's rate and severity of bleeding, and to gather essential historical information to elucidate the possible source of bleeding should occur simultaneously with the evaluation and stabilization of the hemodynamic status.

Assessment is important because a direct correlation has been shown to exist between the number of disease categories present and mortality rates. Risk factors include the use of tobacco, NSAIDs, selective SSRIs, and alcohol, as well as prior *Helicobacter pylori* infection.

In patients awaiting endoscopy, empirical therapy with a high dose PPI should be considered. Omeprazole 8 mg/hr IV for 72 hours is one therapeutic regimen. Long-term acid-suppression therapy with PPIs is recommended along with eradication of *H. pylori* infection using one of the standard treatment protocols.

In certain cases of major bleeding, selective arterial embolization may be attempted, or intra-arterial vasopressin for 24 hours for selective vasoconstriction may be used. This latter therapy has a 70% rate of bleeding control but an 18% rebleeding rate. Indications for surgery include uncontrolled hemorrhage, rebleeding despite endoscopic therapy, large ulceration (>2 cm) or bleeding vessel (>2 mm), continuous posterior duodenal wall bleeding, or transfusion requirement of more than 4 units of blood per 24 hours.

ANGIODYSPLASIA

Angiodysplasia is a submucosal arteriovenous (AV) malformation occurring predominantly in patients between 60 and 80 years old. Their pathogenesis is unknown. They are most commonly found in the proximal colon but can occur anywhere along the GI tract. Bleeding occurs in less than 10% of patients and usually resolves spontaneously, but rebleeding is common.

Symptoms
- Fatigue or weakness +++
- Brisk intermittent rectal bleeding +++
- Syncopal episode

Signs
- Hypotension or tachycardia
- Positive tilt test
- Heme-positive stool +++

Workup
- CBC
- Coagulation studies
- Colonoscopy: 1.5- to 2-mm red patches in the mucosa are seen
- Angiography

Comments and Treatment Considerations
Volume Replacement
Localize bleeding site and stop bleeding with local injection, contact thermal methods, or endoscopic laser therapy. Correct coagulopathy; 80% to 90% of patients will stop bleeding with the preceding measures.

ANORECTAL DISORDERS

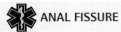 **ANAL FISSURE**

An anal fissure is a tear in the anal mucosa from constipation or trauma. Pain and a small amount of bleeding may occur with bowel movements.

Symptoms
- Anal pain that intensifies during defecation ++++
- Blood on stool surface or on toilet tissue ++

Signs
- Tenderness on digital rectal examination and palpation of fissure (most commonly posterior) +++++
- Visible externally when patient bears down +++

Workup
- Diagnosis is made by the patient's history and gentle physical examination
- Anoscopy may be needed if the fissure is not visualized easily.

Comments and Treatment Considerations
Spontaneous recovery occurs in 60% to 80% of anal fissures. Patients should avoid constipation with a high-fiber diet or the use of a bulking agent such as psyllium. They should take frequent sitz baths and apply topical anesthetic ointment if needed.

A fissure lasting more than 2 months is considered chronic. Nitroglycerin gel (0.2%) daily will heal 50% of chronic fissures. Botulinum toxin injections are an alternative treatment. If medical therapy fails, lateral internal sphincterectomy is the procedure of choice.

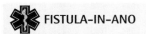 **FISTULA–IN–ANO**

A fistula-in-ano is a tunnel that connects an internal opening, usually at an anal crypt, with an external opening on the perianal skin. Half of patients who undergo incision and drainage of an anorectal abscess will develop a fistula-in-ano.

Symptoms
- Perianal itching ++
- Anal discharge
- Pain

Signs
- Drainage of pus, blood, and sometimes stool from the external opening ++++

Workup
- Anoscopy may reveal the internal opening of the fistula.

Comments and Treatment Considerations
Surgery, fistulotomy, or unroofing of the tunnel are the treatments of choice. Care must be taken to avoid division of the anal sphincter, which could result in fecal incontinence.

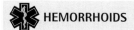 **HEMORRHOIDS**

Hemorrhoids are the most common anorectal source of lower GI bleeding. Other sources to consider include anal fissure and fistula-in-ano.

Internal hemorrhoids are located above the dentate line, are covered by mucosa, and more commonly present with bright red bleeding after defecation. Internal hemorrhoids are described by degree of prolapse with grade 1 having no prolapse to grade 4 with a persistent prolapse.

External hemorrhoids are located below the dentate line, are covered with squamous epithelium, have sensory innervation, and when thrombosed present with pain.

Symptoms
- Bright red rectal bleeding on toilet tissue after bowel movement ++++
- Rectal pain usually with bowel movement ++++

Signs
- External hemorrhoids appear as a swollen bluish mass +++++
- Tenderness on rectal examination ++++
- Prolapsed internal hemorrhoids may be visible on examination +++

Workup
- CBC
- Anoscopy can be done without bowel prep in office
- Hemorrhoids are common but other sources of GI bleeding should be investigated with sigmoidoscopy or colonoscopy (especially in patients >50 years).

Comments and Treatment Considerations
Thrombosed external hemorrhoids can be excised within 72 hours of onset. Topical local anesthetics can be used to relieve pain and itching. High-fiber diet and adequate hydration can be used to prevent constipation. Psyllium or docusate can be used to create softer stools. Rubber band ligation of internal hemorrhoids is performed when pharmacologic methods fail. Surgical excision is usually reserved for grade 4 internal hemorrhoids.

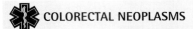 **COLORECTAL NEOPLASMS**

In the United States only lung cancer causes more cancer-related deaths than cancer of the colon and rectum. It is recognized that more than 95% of colorectal cancers develop from benign, neoplastic adenomatous polyps (adenomas). Therefore, it is important to identify and remove adenomatous polyps and early-stage cancers to lower the mortality rate for colorectal cancer. This can be achieved with fecal occult blood testing.

Symptoms
- Abdominal pain (left-sided colon cancer) +++
- Fatigue or weakness (right-sided colon cancer) +++
- Change in bowel pattern or stool caliber/tenesmus (left-sided colon cancer) +++
- Weight loss +++

Signs
- Heme-positive stool ++++
- Mass on rectal examination
- Tenderness on abdominal palpation

Workup
- CBC
- Coagulation studies
- Liver function tests
- Colonoscopy with biopsy
- Computed axial tomography (CAT) scan of the abdomen and pelvis

Comments and Treatment Considerations
All patients with colorectal cancer should be staged because prognosis is closely associated with depth of tumor penetration, presence of regional lymph nodes and distant metastasis. The most frequently used staging system is the Dukes classification.

Resection offers the greatest potential for cure in patients with invasive colorectal cancer. Before surgery, a carcinogenic embryonic antigen (CEA) titer should be determined and colonoscopy performed. CEA assay is not useful as a screening test because elevations usually occur with cancers of at least stage B2.

DIVERTICULAR DISEASE OF THE COLON

Colonic diverticuli are herniations of colonic mucosa and submucosa through the muscularis propia. Most diverticular disease in Western countries occurs in the left colon, although 50% of diverticular bleeding originates from a diverticulum proximal to the splenic flexure. Diverticulitis results from inflammation and/or perforation of a diverticulum. Diverticulosis is more common in women and whites and generally presents with pain and not GI bleeding. Only 10% to 25% of patients with diverticulosis will develop diverticulitis.

Symptoms
- Abdominal pain especially in the left lower quadrant ++++
- Change in bowel habit ++
- Nausea or vomiting ++
- Orthostatic symptoms if acute blood loss or chronic over a long period of time +

Signs
- Elevated temperature (usually <38.5° C but may be higher) ++++
- Tenderness and/or mass palpated in the left lower quadrant ++++
- Heme-positive stool++
- Tachycardia or hypotension (occurring with complications such as abscess, fistula, or perforation)

Workup
- CBC
- ESR or CRP
- Coagulation studies
- Type and crossmatch if hemodynamically unstable.
- Helical CT of the abdomen with oral water-soluble contrast
- Bleeding scan with technetium helps localize the site of bleeding when rate is greater than 0.5 mL/min
- Angiography

Comments and Treatment Considerations
A stable patient who can maintain oral fluids and has mild diverticulitis may be managed as an outpatient with a liquid diet and oral antibiotics to cover gram-negative and anaerobic bacteria. Patients with moderate to severe diverticular disease should be managed as an inpatient. Management includes keeping the patient NPO, volume replacement with IV fluids and /or blood products, Foley catheter to monitor output, NG tube insertion, and pain management.

Surgical intervention may be needed for perforation, abscess/fistula formation, stricture or obstruction. Long-term medical management for patients with diverticular disease includes high-fiber diet and avoidance of food with seeds, nuts, and kernels.

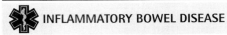

INFLAMMATORY BOWEL DISEASE

Ulcerative colitis and Crohn's disease are the two most common inflammatory bowel disorders although their etiologies still remain unknown. These diseases are most common in the second and third decades of life, affecting males and females equally. A genetic predisposition exists and cigarette smoking may affect the disease.

Symptoms
- Blood in stool (gross or hematochezia) ++++
- Crampy abdominal pain ++++
- Diarrhea (more often bloody in ulcerative colitis) ++++
- Urgency to have a bowel movement ++++

Signs
- Elevated temperature ++++
- Weight loss ++++
- Heme-positive stools (ulcerative colitis) +++
- Hypotension/tachycardia
- Diffuse abdominal tenderness that may have associated rebound, guarding, or rigidity

Workup
- CBC
- Electrolytes
- ESR or CRP
- Serum albumin
- Stool studies such as WBC, ova, and parasites
- Colonoscopy with biopsy
- CT of abdomen with oral contrast

Comments and Treatment Considerations
Medical
- Aminosalicylates
- Steroids
- 6-Mercaptopurine
- Antirheumatic drugs such as azathioprine, methotrexate, and infliximab

Surgery
Indications for surgery include failure to respond to medication, cancerous or precancerous changes, fistula, abscess, or stricture.

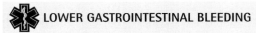

LOWER GASTROINTESTINAL BLEEDING

Lower GI bleeding when acute causes frequent hospital admissions and affects morbidity and mortality. Most series indicate the average age of patients with lower GI bleeding is 60 years old. The most common causes of lower GI bleeding are diverticular disease of the colon, IBD, anorectal disorders, neoplasms, and angiodysplasias.

MALLORY-WEISS TEAR

A Mallory-Weiss tear is a longitudinal laceration of the mucosa usually near the gastroesophageal junction caused by forceful retching or vomiting.

Symptoms
- Forceful retching or vomiting precedes hematemesis +++
- Small volume of blood in vomitus ++++

Signs
- Hematemesis +++
- Hematochezia and/or melena
- Tachycardia and hypotension
- Positive nasogastric aspirate for blood +++
- Positive stool testing for blood
- Anemia

Workup
- See workup for PUD or gastric erosions.

Comments and Treatment Considerations
The history of antecedent forceful retching is key to making this diagnosis. Bleeding is usually minimal and self-limited. Treatment should focus on symptom control and treatment of nausea or the underlying cause of the vomiting. If there are symptoms of GERD, PPI therapy should be initiated. For continuing bleeding or hemodynamic instability, treatment is as noted under "Peptic Ulcer Disease/Gastric Erosions."

PEPTIC ULCER DISEASE/GASTRIC EROSIONS

PUD, gastric erosions, a Mallory-Weiss tear, and the Dieulafoy lesions are all examples of nonvariceal bleeding, and represent more than two thirds of the sources of major UGIB. PUD and gastric erosions have similar risk factors, and are often associated with heavy alcohol use and the use of NSAIDs.

Scoring systems have been developed in an attempt to identify patients at high risk for continued bleeding or rebleeding. However, the difficulty in using these systems is that an important question remains unanswered: whether endoscopy is essential or whether some population of patients can be detected clinically who do not require endoscopy.

Assessment for comorbid conditions is important because the presence of a higher number of comorbid conditions is associated with poorer prognosis. Other factors that increase the risk of morbidity and mortality are advancing age, hemodynamic instability, and increased bleeding intensity.

A peptic ulcer is a localized process resulting from the erosion of the gastric mucosa exposing the submucosa. Gastric erosion (gastritis) is a more generalized process encompassing a larger surface area of the gastric mucosa and is accompanied by diffuse inflammatory changes. Bleeding is the result of erosion extending to the underlying blood vessel, and the rate and severity of bleeding are determined by the size of the vessel(s) involved.

Symptoms
- Dyspepsia ++
- Abdominal or epigastric pain +++
- Hematemesis +++
- "Coffee grounds" emesis +++
- Hematochezia +++
- Melena ++++

Signs
- Hematemesis or "coffee grounds" emesis +++
- Hematochezia +++
- Melena ++++
- Tachycardia and hypotension
- Positive nasogastric aspirate for blood or "coffee grounds" material ++++
- Positive stool testing for blood ++++
- Anemia

Workup
- Evaluate hemodynamic stability immediately. Orthostatic testing: Positive orthostatic testing is variably defined, but usually a drop of at least 20 mm Hg of systolic BP is considered positive. A report from the ASGE showed an improvement in survival if postural changes were not present on initial examination.
- Lab: Hemoglobin, hematocrit, BUN, creatinine (BUN:creatinine ratio of >36:1 in patients without renal failure is suggestive of UGIB), liver function tests, amylase, lipase, and coagulation studies
- In the absence of overt hematemesis, placement of an NG tube for confirmation of bleeding and assessment of prognosis should occur. NG aspiration has a low false-positive rate yet may be negative in up to 25% of UGIB.
- Type and crossmatch for 2 to 4 units of packed red blood cells, more if clinically indicated.
- GI consultation for endoscopic evaluation and treatment of the acute bleeding site is recommended. Although most bleeding stops spontaneously, endoscopy provides an accurate diagnosis and the ability to directly coagulate the bleeding site. Various methods of hemostasis are used, but none has been found to be superior to the others.
- Selective visceral angiography should be considered if endoscopy fails to identify a bleeding source. Bleeding must be at rates exceeding 0.5 to 1 mL/min for examination to be optimal and have high yield.
- Radionuclide technetium-99m-labeled red cell scan may also be considered for continued bleeding because it can detect bleeding at rates that exceed 0.1 mL/min. However, pooled blood may sometimes be mistaken for active bleeding.

Comments and Treatment Considerations

Obtain IV access with two large-bore catheters and begin immediate fluid resuscitation with crystalloid solutions as needed. Efforts to assess the patient's rate and severity of bleeding, and to gather essential historical information to elucidate the possible source of bleeding should occur simultaneously with the evaluation and stabilization of the hemodynamic status.

Assessment regarding prior UGIB and the presence of comorbid conditions are important because a direct correlation has been shown between the number of disease categories present and mortality rates. Risk factors include the use of tobacco, NSAIDs, SSRIs, and alcohol, as well as prior *H. pylori* infection.

In patients awaiting endoscopy, empirical therapy with a high-dose PPI should be considered. Omeprazole 8 mg/hr IV for 72 hours is one therapeutic regimen. Long-term acid-suppression therapy with PPIs is recommended for PUD, along with eradication of *H. pylori* infection using one of the standard treatment protocols.

In certain cases of major bleeding from PUD and gastritis, selective arterial embolization may be attempted, or intra-arterial vasopressin for 24 hours for selective vasoconstriction may be used. This latter therapy has a 70% rate of bleeding control but an 18% rebleeding rate. Indications for surgery include uncontrolled hemorrhage, rebleeding despite endoscopic therapy, large ulceration (>2 cm) or bleeding vessel (>2 mm), continuous posterior duodenal wall bleeding, or transfusion requirement of more than 4 units of blood per 24 hours.

Although EGD is the gold standard for evaluation of UGIB, exactly when it should occur in the hemodynamically stable patient is not established. Most studies refer to EGD within 24 hours of admission.

UPPER GASTROINTESTINAL BLEEDING

UGIB is five times more common than LGIB, and often presents with hematemesis or "coffee grounds" emesis, but can also present with hematochezia or melena. The initial assessment for UGIB should begin with a rapid assessment of the patient's hemodynamic stability. Rapid transfer to an inpatient setting is appropriate when any hemodynamic instability is found.

VARICEAL BLEEDING

Esophageal varices are abnormally dilated veins found predominantly in the distal esophagus, are often associated with cirrhosis, and are the result of increased portal pressure. They are the most common single cause of "severe and persistent" UGIB (33% of cases), are significantly more likely to present with bright red hematemesis (76% versus 49% for ulcers), and have a mortality rate of about 30% or greater (Table 10-1).

Table 10-1. Causes of Major Upper Gastrointestinal Bleeding

DISEASE STATE	% OF BLEEDING
Peptic ulcer disease	60%
Variceal bleeding	10%-30%
Gastric erosions	6%-30%
No diagnosis	7.6%-22%
Mallory-Weiss tear	5%-11%
Dieulafoy lesion	5%

Symptoms
• Sudden onset of vomiting a large volume of bright red blood with or without clots ++++

Signs
• Tachycardia
• Positive orthostatic testing
• Hemodynamic instability
• Anemia
• Hematochezia

Workup
• Initial evaluation of hemodynamic stability. Orthostatic testing: Positive orthostatic testing is variably defined, but usually a drop of at least 20 mm Hg of systolic BP is considered positive. One report showed an improvement in survival if postural changes were not present on initial examination.
• Lab: hemoglobin, hematocrit, BUN, creatinine (BUN:creatinine ratio of >36:1 in patients without renal failure is suggestive of UGIB), liver function tests, amylase, lipase, and clotting studies
• Type and crossmatch for 2 to 4 units of packed red blood cells
• Depending on age, ECG and cardiac monitoring may be appropriate.
• Emergent GI consult and endoscopy are required for endoscopic treatment with sclerotherapy or band ligation.

Comments and Treatment Considerations
Obtain IV access with two large-bore catheters and begin immediate fluid resuscitation with crystalloid solutions as needed. Assess the vital signs quickly and repeatedly for hypotension or postural hypotension. Intensive care unit (ICU) admission is indicated for hemodynamically unstable patients.

Consider octreotide 25 to 50 mcg/hr IV infusion for 5 days in combination with endoscopic therapy (works better than either therapy alone). Consider vasopressin drip at 0.2 to 0.4 unit/min IV (max is 0.9 unit/min), taper after 12 hours. Give with nitroglycerin (NTG) IV; this regimen has a 50% success rate, and a high rebleeding rate. For continued bleeding despite therapy, consider intubation and insertion of a Sengstaken-Blakemore tube pending surgical/radiologic evaluation.

If bleeding persists, consider the insertion of a transjugular intra-hepatic portosystemic shunt (TIPS) by an interventional radiologist. Although TIPS has many contraindications, it is also reported to control bleeding in 90% of patients. However, this procedure has a high rate of complications and a mortality of 1% to 2%. Surgery is considered when other measures have been ineffective. Procedures include portosystemic venous shunting and esophageal devascularization.

References

Achkar J-P: Inflammatory bowel disease. The American College of Gastroenterology. Available at http://gi.org/patients/gihealth/ibd.asp (accessed Oct 24, 2006).

Arnell T, Saver D: *Hemorrhoids*. Available at www.firstconsult.com/fc_home/members/?urn=com.firstconsult/1/101/1014780 (accessed Oct 21, 2006).

Arnell T, Scherger J, Murray J: *Anal fissure*. Available at www.firstconsult.com/fc_home/members/?urn=com.firstconsult/1/101/6030201 (accessed Oct 21, 2006).

Barkun A, Bardou M, Marshall J: Consensus recommendations for managing patients with nonvariceal upper gastrointestinal bleeding, *Ann Intern Med* 10:843–859, 2003.

Bond J: Polyp guideline: diagnosis, treatment, and surveillance for patients with colorectal polyps, *Am J Gastroenterol* 11:3053–3063, 2000.

Calkins B: A meta-analysis of the role of smoking in inflammatory bowel disease, *Dig Dis Sci* 12:1841–1854, 1989. Available at www.springerlink.com/content (accessed Apr 23, 2005).

Feldman M, Scharschmidt B, Fordtran J: *Sleisenger & Fordtran's gastrointestinal and liver disease*, 7th ed., New York, 2002, Saunders.

Kunnamo I, editor: *Diverticulitis and diverticulosis; evidence-based medicine guidelines*, West Sussex, England, 2005, Duodecim Medical Publications, Ltd.

Peter M, David J, Dougherty J: Evaluation of the patient with gastrointestinal bleeding: an evidence based approach, *Emerg Med Clin North Am* 17.1:239–261, 1999.

Pfenninger J, Zainea G: Common anorectal conditions: part 1—symptoms and complaints, *Am Fam Physician* 12:2391–2398, 2001.

Pfenninger J, Zainea G: Common anorectal conditions: part II—lesions, *Am Fam Physician* 64.1:77–88, 2001.

Read T, Kodner I: Colorectal cancer: risk factors and recommendations for early detection, *Am Fam Physician* 11:3083–3096, 1999.

Rockey M, Don C: Gastrointestinal bleeding, *Gastroenterol Clin North Am* 34:581, 2005.

Strate L: Lower GI bleeding: epidemiology and diagnosis, *Gastroenterol Clin North Am* 34:643–664, 2005.

CHAPTER 11

Breast Masses and Nipple Discharge
Gretchen Dickson, Crystal L. Jones, and George D. Harris

Breast symptoms are a common problem initiating a woman's visit to a physician's office. The most common symptoms include breast pain (mastalgia), nipple discharge, or a breast mass. Each of these complaints deserves evaluation by a physician. A thorough clinical examination should be performed as part of a complete breast assessment along with specific imaging studies.

Breast pain (mastalgia) is the most frequent breast complaint but only about half of women with breast pain seek medical evaluation. It occurs with multiple conditions but does not have a known etiology. Mastalgia occurs more often during menses and more frequently in premenopausal than in postmenopausal women. Neither hormonal fluctuations nor fluid retention has been shown to cause mastalgia. Hormonal fluctuations related to menstruation or pregnancy are often responsible for breast tenderness. They may also occur during puberty (in females and males), during breastfeeding, or as a woman approaches menopause. The occurrence of breast pain or tenderness in a teenage boy is referred to as gynecomastia and is a normal part of development. Other causes of breast pain include fibrocystic breast disease, mastitis, premenstrual syndrome, alcoholism with liver damage, and local injury or trauma to the breast.

NIPPLE DISCHARGE

Nipple discharge is the third most common breast complaint. The incidence of symptomatic nipple discharge in patients referred to a breast clinic is between 4.8% and 7.4%. It is not unusual for a woman to express either spontaneously or with external pressure, a physiologic discharge from her breast in the form of a few drops of sticky, gray, green, or black viscous fluid (nonpuerperal galactorrhea). However, any abnormal nipple discharge is a symptom of pathology within the breast and requires further evaluation.

Symptoms
- Unilateral or bilateral nipple discharge ++++
- May or may not have associated breast mass +++
- Spontaneous or provoked
- Mastalgia

Signs
- Visible or expressed nipple discharge: The secretion can be bloody, serous, serosanguineous, or watery. ++++
- May or may not have associated breast mass +++
- Spontaneous or provoked
- Breast tenderness may be present if there is an abscess or infection.

Workup
- A comprehensive, detailed medical history and a physical examination are imperative in the evaluation of a nipple discharge.
- The patient's age, the type and duration of the discharge, pregnancy history, the presence of a mass, history of breast cancer, trauma or other breast conditions, unilateral or bilateral discharge, family history of nipple discharge, and whether the discharge is spontaneous or provoked are important.
- Medication history is also important because various hormones (estrogen, oral contraceptives, thyrotropin-releasing hormone [TRH]), psychotropic medications (risperidone, SSRIs, tricyclic antidepressants), antihypertensives (methyldopa, verapamil), antiemetics (metoclopramide), and H_2-receptor blockers (cimetidine) can cause increased prolactin levels and galactorrhea.
- A mammogram is indicated in all women with unilateral spontaneous nipple discharge.
- An ultrasound may be the initial modality to evaluate breast abnormality in women younger than age 35.
- Cytology and occasionally biopsy of a nipple discharge and any breast mass, respectively, may be indicated.
- One should perform cytologic examination on all guaiac-positive nipple discharges to evaluate the fluid for breast carcinoma. This procedure is done by placing a glass slide at the ductal opening, expressing the discharge onto the slide, and immediately spraying the slide with a fixative. Up to four slides should be prepared.
  - If the slides test negative for occult blood, the patient should have a prolactin level and TSH performed.
  - If the test is positive for occult blood, then surgical consultation is needed.

Comments and Treatment Considerations
In nonpregnant or nonlactating women, the more likely diagnosis of nipple discharge includes intraductal papilloma, ductal ectasia, pituitary adenoma, breast abscess or infection, and breast carcinoma.

A mammogram is indicated in all women with unilateral spontaneous nipple discharge. An ultrasound may be the initial modality to evaluate the breast abnormality in women younger than age 35.

A pathologic nipple discharge is usually spontaneous, unilateral, and from a single duct opening on the nipple. The secretion can be bloody, serous, serosanguineous, or watery.

The most common cause of pathologic nipple discharge is a benign intraductal papilloma followed by ductal ectasia. Carcinoma is the least likely cause and occurs in about 10% to 15% of cases.

BREAST MASS

A breast mass is the most common presenting symptom or complaint in most breast clinics. In these situations a clinical breast examination reveals a palpable dominant breast mass in about half of the possible breast mass cases. However, breast masses are often detected by the patient and are associated with localized swelling, thickening, tenderness, or pain. Breast masses are a common occurrence throughout the life span of a woman.

Even though most breast masses are benign, their diagnostic evaluation should proceed as expeditiously as possible to allow optimal clinical benefit and to alleviate patient fears because for her, this can be one of the most traumatic experiences of her life. A thorough clinical examination should be performed as part of a complete breast assessment along with specific imaging studies. Ultrasonography and mammography are two basic imaging techniques for routine diagnostic imaging of breast diseases. Screening mammography is typically conducted among asymptomatic women and a diagnostic mammogram is usually the first imaging study performed for women older than the age of 35 with a palpable or suspected breast mass.

If a mass is present, ultrasound is also ordered to determine whether the mass is a simple cyst, a complex mass, or a solid mass. It is not clear how much the presence of symptoms increases the risk of breast cancer at screening exams, but studies have shown that the specificity of screening and diagnostic exams may be lower for women with breast symptoms compared with women without symptoms.

Because a breast mass is the most common symptom associated with breast cancer, all masses deserve clinical evaluation. The presence of a breast mass on palpation requires a mammogram, fine-needle aspiration (FNA), and surgical evaluation for excisional biopsy. This approach is necessary because the majority (55% to 68%) of breast cancer cases continue to present with palpable masses, despite the widespread use of screening mammography. The breast mass may be cystic or solid. An ultrasound can be used to distinguish between a solid and cystic lesion.

If the mass is cystic it needs to be confirmed by FNA. If the aspirated fluid is clear and the mass disappears following the aspiration, then the mass is classified as a simple cyst. This site needs to be reevaluated in 4 to 6 weeks for recurrence. Recurrence of the cyst suggests further evaluation with a biopsy or excision of the mass. If the aspirated fluid is grossly positive or positive for occult blood or it does not disappear with FNA, the mass needs cytologic evaluation. The presence of a solid mass requires mammography and a surgical biopsy. The presence of a nonpalpable breast lesion on mammography or ultrasound deserves stereotactic localization and biopsy.

Any persistent palpable breast mass must be diagnosed by FNA and cytology or with histology obtained by tissue core-needle biopsy or open surgical biopsy. Approximately 9% to 11% of breast masses result in the diagnosis of breast cancer.

Breast cancer prevalence among women presenting with a breast mass increases with age (1% for women age 40 or younger, 9% for women between ages 41 and 55, and 37% for women 55 or older). Because diagnosis and treatment options evolve quickly, early referral to a breast surgeon may be indicated. Although the prevalence of breast cancer diagnoses among women with symptoms is low, failure to diagnose breast cancer is one of the most common causes of malpractice claims and results in some of the highest liability awards and payments in medical malpractice.

 FIBROCYSTIC BREAST DISEASE

Fibrocystic breast disease is perhaps one of the most common benign conditions of the breast. Studies suggest that more than 60% of women are affected by this condition at some point in their lives with the most common ages affected being 30 to 50. Because of the associated hormonal influences, it is a much more rare condition after menopause and incidence is lower in women taking oral contraceptive pills.

Symptoms
- Irregular, dense pebble-like consistency of breast tissue ++++
- Intermittent breast fullness or discomfort
- Dull, heavy pain that occurs in association with menstrual cycles
- Nipple discomfort or itching

Signs
- Mobile, rubbery mass ++++
- Outer upper quadrant predominance
- Round mass with smooth borders

Workup
- Breast self-examination
- Clinical breast examination +++
  - Can detect up to 44% of abnormalities alone with up to 29% of those having been missed on mammogram alone
- Ultrasound ++++
  - Under appropriate criteria, sensitivity is 89% with specificity for lesions at 78%
- Mammogram
  - May be difficult to interpret in young women who are generally affected
  - Increased density of breast tissue in disease may further hinder interpretation.
- Biopsy
  - May be needed to rule out other disorders if lesions are large, painful, or persistent
  - Fibrocystic change is often present in histologic studies, although women may be asymptomatic.

- Ultrasound
- Breast self-examination
- Clinical breast examination

Comments and Treatment Considerations

A placebo effect is common and may account for as much as 20% of improvement.

A well-fitting brassiere may offer support and symptomatic relief and should be worn 24 hours a day for adequate relief.

Dietary modification should include limiting dietary fat intake to 25% of total calories. This will affect the intermediate marker of disease, but still has an unknown effect on symptoms. Eliminate caffeine. There is insufficient evidence to use vitamin E, vitamin B_6, or evening primrose dietary supplement for relief; however, much anecdotal evidence exists about effect. Typically 400 IU of vitamin E is used, but much variation exists in dosing and preparation of all of these compounds.

Oral contraceptives may limit hormonal effects thought to mediate disease process. Danazol was previously used for severe pain; however, it is being phased out because it has many androgenic side effects. Tamoxifen is noted to reduce fibrocystic breast disease, but only as a side effect when used for reduction of cancer risk.

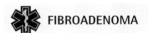 FIBROADENOMA

Fibroadenoma is the most common benign breast mass and contains both connective tissue and epithelial elements. Prevalence ranges from 2% to 23% of women and accounts for about half of all breast biopsies occurring most frequently in young women within 20 years of puberty. It has a biphasic incidence with peaks at 25 and 48 years of age. In African American women this is earlier with peaks at 16 and 25 years of age. Younger women tend to have rapid growth of the mass. Multiple lesions may present in 10% to 15% of women. Older women characteristically have a single, slower-growing lesion that frequently calcifies, and may involute after menopause. The etiology is unknown. The diagnosis of fibroadenoma is based on clinical, radiologic, and pathologic examination or a "triple test." It is not considered cancerous or premalignant and risk factors include a patient who is a postpubescent female or a postmenopausal female exposed to estrogen.

Symptoms
- Painless, smooth, breast mass ++

Signs
- Small, well-circumscribed, round or ovoid, rubbery, freely mobile, nontender mass ++
- Usually 1 to 5 cm
- Usually in the upper quadrant

Workup
- Breast self-examination
- History: Include questions related to nature and pattern of symptoms, relationship to menstrual cycle, timing of onset and course, nipple discharge, hormone use, and any prior treatments
- Clinical breast and axillary examination
- Ultrasound for localization and characterization
  - Most appropriate for women younger than the age of 35 due to breast density
- Mammogram in women older than 35 years for localization and characterization
  - Not appropriate for younger women due to dense breast tissue
- FNA or excisional biopsy +++
  - Diagnostic and definitive treatment

Comments and Treatment Considerations
Providers must consider fibrocystic condition of the breast and carcinoma in women 30 years of age or older. Triple test: Clinical breast exam, ultrasound, FNA, or core-needle biopsy is used to evaluate fibroadenomas.

No treatment is necessary and the lesion may be observed if benign triple test unless one of the three components is discordant or the lesion enlarges. Conservative management with serial ultrasounds every 6 months is acceptable for stable lesions. Benign fibroadenomas can change size. A change in 20% in any one of the three dimensions over a 6-month interval was not associated with malignancy. Fibroadenomas may increase significantly in size during pregnancy. If the change in size is more significant, the lesion may be associated with malignancy or phylloides tumor. Fibroadenomas may also regress or become smaller. This is more likely in very young women, new-onset lesions, small masses, and those that occur during pregnancy.

If diagnosis is uncertain, excision or vacuum-assisted core needle removal with cytologic examination is recommended. Complex fibroadenomas include epithelial calcification, apocrine metaplasia, sclerosing adenosis, and size larger than 3 mm.

Epithelial hyperplasia with atypia occurs in 0.3% and does not correlate with an additional increased long-term risk of breast carcinoma.

Fibroadenomas may increase the long-term risk of developing breast cancer. There is a 2.17 to 3.1 relative risk in those with a family history of breast cancer and complex fibroadenomas.

Cryoablation and ultrasound-guided vacuum-assisted biopsy are being studied as an alternative to excision. MRI is being studied as a noninvasive and reliable alternative to tissue diagnosis.

 BREAST ABSCESS AND INFECTION

The diagnosis of a breast abscess is characterized by breast pain, redness, tenderness, flulike symptoms, and a fluctuant mass. Breast abscesses are most commonly associated with lactation and occur within the first month postpartum or at weaning, but may be fistulous tracts from squamous epithelial neoplasm or duct occlusion. Prevalence of breast abscess in breastfeeding women is 0.1%. A breast abscess develops in 5% to 11% of women with mastitis.

Risk factors are maternal age more than 30 years, primiparity, gestational age 41 weeks' or more, mastitis, diabetes, RA, steroids, silicone or paraffin implants, lumpectomy with radiation, heavy cigarette smoking, nipple retraction, history of a bite, or penetrating trauma.

Symptoms
- Mastalgia +++
- Erythema
- Myalgia
- Malaise
- Fever ++
- Chills ++

Signs
- Breast tenderness ++++
- Localized swelling or pitting edema
- Localized warmth
- Fluctuant mass
- Usually unilateral +++
- Purulent exudates
- Proximal (axillary) lymphadenopathy

Workup
- CBC: Helps quantify infection and monitor response to therapy
- Ultrasound: Helps differentiate between mastitis and abscess in addition to localizing the lesion for definitive treatment
- Aspiration: Helps in obtaining culture sample and is also for definitive treatment
- Culture and sensitivity: Help identify the pathogen and sensitivity or resistance to antibiotic therapy
- ESR may be used in monitoring the inflammatory response.

Comments and Treatment Considerations
Cold Compresses
Continue expression of milk, if lactating, by pumping on the affected side. Initiate empiric antibiotic therapy with appropriate drugs early. Common etiologic agents include *Staphylococcus aureus, Streptococcus,* and *Escherichia coli.* Nonlactational abscesses are associated with anaerobic bacteria. Drugs of choice include first-generation cephalosporin, erythromycin, Augmentin, and clindamycin.

Drainage of the localized abscess can usually be performed by needle aspiration, with or without ultrasound guidance. If needle aspiration is not effective, incision and drainage are needed with the removal of loculations and opening of all fistulous tracts. If the incision does not interfere with latch-on, breastfeeding may continue on both breasts. If the incision interferes with nursing on the affected breast, a pump should be used to remove milk regularly for 3 to 4 days until the wound is sufficiently healed to allow nursing. Nursing should continue on the unaffected breast. Antiinfective properties of the milk that drains from the abscess may bathe the wound and accelerate healing.

Biopsy should be performed on all nonlactating abscesses to rule out inflammatory carcinoma. NSAIDs should be used for pain relief and to decrease the local inflammatory response.

Treat mastitis early with cold compresses and milk expression if lactating. Follow patient until resolution to exclude carcinoma. Complete healing should be within 8 to 10 days. Relapse occurs in up to 38% of women within an 8-year period and is more associated with those who are not lactating.

Consider mammography and biopsy after infection has cleared.

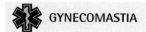 **GYNECOMASTIA**

Gynecomastia results in the most common cause of male breast evaluation throughout the male life cycle with increased prevalence in teenage (10% to 48%) and older adult men (57% of men greater than age 50). Although breast cancer is less common in men, it should be considered if a focal abnormality is present.

Symptoms
- Enlargement of one or both breasts ++++
- Typically a global enlargement as a mass or lump requires evaluation for other etiologies.
- Breast pain, nipple discharge, or change in nipple size more concerning

Signs
- Enlargement of breast ++++
  - Can be quite significant
  - Classified into lesions that are less than 5 cm and greater than 5 cm because this correlates with expected resolution and response to treatment

Workup
- Physiologic gynecomastia does not require workup, however, must ensure that enlargement is physiologic
- Thorough history is critical
- Examine for symptoms related to decreased testosterone production or other diseases.
- Kallmann's syndrome
  - Embryonic absences of GnRH-secreting neurons leading to lack of hypothalamic GnRH
- Klinefelter's syndrome
- Genotype of XXY

- Increased risk of breast cancer from 10% to 20% ++
  - Testicular tumors
  - 5-α reductase deficiency
  - Androgen insensitivity
- Age of onset of gynecomastia
  - Physiologic in newborns, adolescents, and older adult males
- History of mumps or testicular trauma
  - Rule out testicular torsion and viral orchitis
- Use of alcohol or medications
  - Heroin
  - Marijuana
  - Digitalis
  - Phytoestrogens
  - Gonadotropins
  - Clomiphene
  - Phenytoin
  - Ketoconazole
  - Metronidazole
  - Methyldopa
  - Busulfan
  - Tricyclic antidepressants (TCAs)
  - Calcium channel blockers
  - Angiotensin-converting enzyme (ACE) inhibitors
  - Cisplatin
  - Spironolactone
  - Cimetidine
  - Flutamide
  - Finasteride
  - Etomidate
  - Atorvastatin
- Family history of similar changes ++++
- Infertility or sexual dysfunction
- Thorough physical examination
  - For stigmata of liver, thyroid, or renal disease
  - Look for other signs of feminization such as abnormal body hair or voice tone.
  - Testicular examination
    - Rule out masses or asymmetry
    - Obtain ultrasound if concern exists for neoplasm
- Breast examination
  - Examine size of breasts and consistency of tissue.
    - Gynecomastia is enlargement of glandular tissue and can be treated.
    - Pseudogynecomastia is enlargement of adipose tissue typically noted in those that are obese.
      - This does not warrant treatment other than ongoing encouragement for weight loss.
  - Nipple discharge
  - Axillary lymphadenopathy
  - Obtain a mammogram if a concern exists for male breast cancer.

- Workup then does not significantly differ from that typically followed for females with mass for concerning cancer
- BMP to rule out chronic liver or renal disease
- TSH to rule out hyperthyroidism
- If other features of feminization exist, consider:
  - Total testosterone
    - If elevated check testicular ultrasound
  - Luteinizing hormone (LH)
  - Estradiol
  - Dehyroepiandrosterone sulfate levels
- If no features of feminization exist, instead consider:
  - Total testosterone
    - If elevated check testicular ultrasound
  - LH
  - FSH
  - Prolactin
  - β-hCG and estradiol levels
    - If elevated, check chest x-ray and CT of chest, abdomen and pelvis to find primary secreting tumor.

Comments and Treatment Considerations

Physiologic gynecomastia does not require treatment; 90% of adolescent gynecomastia resolves within weeks to 3 years. If breasts are larger than 4 cm, full regression is less likely.

Treat underlying diseases if gynecomastia is not physiologic. Remove offending medications. Consider replacing testosterone through parenteral or transdermal systems if androgen is low.

Idiopathic or residual gynecomastia can be pharmacologically treated with clomiphene (50 to 100 mg/day for up to 6 months with 50% of patients having reduction in breast size and 20% of patients having full resolution), tamoxifen (10 to 20 mg twice daily with 80% reporting resolution within 3 months), danazol (inhibits LH and FSH to decrease estrogen synthesis, 200 mg twice daily, with complete resolution noted in 23% of cases), or testolactone (150 mg three times daily for 6 months; can cause significant side effects with less than 40% of patients having decrease in breast size).

Reduction mammoplasty can be considered if medical therapy has failed. This option is also considered for cosmetic reasons. Liposuction may be sufficient if pseudogynecomastia is suspected.

 INTRADUCTAL PAPILLOMA

Symptoms
- Nipple discharge
  - Often bloody +++
  - Unilateral +++
- Breast mass
  - Typically small, hard nodule ++++
  - Found behind nipple most commonly

- Breast pain +++
- Breast enlargement
  - Unilateral difference in breasts that is of new onset

Signs
- Bloody or serous nipple discharge +++
  - May be expressed on examination
  - Can be spontaneous
- Breast lump
  - May or may not be palpable by examiner
  - Found behind nipple most commonly

Workup
- Mammogram
  - Typically not useful because women may be younger with denser breasts
  - Papillomas often not appreciated on mammogram
- Ultrasound
  - Most useful modality
  - Diagnostic features
    - Dense, coarse calcifications
    - Highly vascular
      - Propensity to bleed spontaneously
      - Vascular pedicle may be found
- Ductogram
  - May be useful because contrast can outline papilloma
- Breast biopsy with pathology ++++
  - Cytokeratin stains of biopsy can be useful for differentiating this from other breast lesions.
  - Cell clumping and nuclear change may help differentiate benign and malignant disease.

Comments and Treatment Considerations
Surgical excision is required to aid in symptom control and remove papilloma. Typically local area excision of affected duct can be undertaken. Wide surgical excision is not typically needed.

 IN SITU LOBULAR OR DUCTAL CARCINOMA

Ductal carcinoma in situ (DCIS) is a noninvasive premalignant breast disease that is diagnosed by pathologic examination of tissue specimens. DCIS is considered a precursor to invasive ductal carcinoma (IDC), the most common histologic type of invasive breast cancer. DCIS carries a 2- to 8.6-fold increased risk of invasive breast cancer. DCIS is diagnosed in up to 20% of breast cancer patients.

Lobular carcinoma in situ (LCIS) is noninvasive and now also considered a premalignant breast disease based on pathologic exam of tissue specimens. LCIS is considered a precursor to invasive lobular carcinoma (ILC) and carries a 3- to 4.2-fold increased risk of invasive breast cancer.

There is difficulty in classification alone due to the fact that histologic criteria differentiating ductal carcinoma in situ from atypical ductal hyperplasia and similarly lobular carcinoma in situ from atypical lobular hyperplasia are not strongly established. DCIS is further differentiated by comedo or non-comedo classifications.

Non-comedo is the most common histologic type of DCIS and thought to be the precursor to comedo or poorly differentiated or high-grade DCIS. Despite the problem with correct classification of each lesion, the incidences of both have been increasing. The yearly incidence of DCIS is 4.5 to 5.4/1000 and has increased 7.2-fold, with the highest rates of increase in women 50 years of age and older and non-comedo classifications increasing while comedo DCIS is decreasing. IDC rates have remained constant. The yearly incidence of LCIS is 5.2 to 7.3/1000 and has increased 2.6-fold, primarily among older women. In addition, ILC rates have also increased (65%) and similarly vary with age. This may be a factor of screening practices, skills, technology, and the increased use of mammography.

Risk factors are similar in both instances and are similar to the risk factors for invasive carcinomas: family history of breast cancer, previous breast biopsy, nulliparity, fewer full-term pregnancies, older at first full-term pregnancy, older at menopause, and ethnicity (African American and Hispanic).

Symptoms
- Ductal—With or without palpable breast mass or nipple changes +++
  - May complain of itching or burning of the nipple
  - Previously presented with palpable breast mass and/or nipple discharge
- Lobular—With or without palpable breast mass

Signs
- Ductal—With or without palpable breast mass
  - May have superficial erosion or ulceration of the nipple
- Lobular—With or without palpable breast mass

Workup
- Breast self-examination
- Family history
- Clinical breast examination
- Routine screening mammography (picks up majority of the diagnosed cases, most of which are nonpalpable breast masses) +++
- Ultrasound for localization and characterization of any abnormalities found on mammography
- Large-core needle biopsy, especially in lesions with associated microcalcifications
- Excisional biopsy ++++

Comments and Treatment Considerations
Those with a family history of breast cancer have a two- to three-fold associated risk, especially if multiple first-degree relatives have

been diagnosed with breast or ovarian cancer and at younger ages. These families have a high correlation to the *BRCA1* and *BRCA2* alleles but there have not been any studies investigating the prevalence of these gene mutations with in situ breast carcinomas.

LCIS lacks any clinical signs and is almost always an incidental finding in breast biopsies that have been done for other reasons. Thought not to have any specific findings, it is associated with calcifications on mammography (21% to 67%).

It is hypothesized that postmenopausal hormones are a risk factor for LCIS based on studies showing an associated increased risk for ILC and molecular similarities between ILC and LCIS.

E-cadherin, a cell adhesion molecule, is not expressed in almost all ILCs and is used to distinguish lobular from ductal carcinomas. Loss of expression seems to occur early in the development in ILCs. LCIS has been shown to have complete loss of e-cadherin expression.

There remains no good way to differentiate those who will go on to develop invasive breast cancer from those who will not. DCIS patients are currently recommended for total mastectomy or lumpectomy with radiation. Axillary dissection is not routinely indicated.

Local recurrence rates are higher in those treated with lumpectomy alone and lumpectomy with radiation. This is still controversial given that the majority of DCIS patients will not develop invasive breast cancer.

LCIS is considered a nonsurgical disease and appropriate treatment remains controversial. Options include observation, lumpectomy, chemoprevention with a selective estrogen receptor modulator, or prophylactic mastectomy.

Studies have shown that LCIS patients have the same likelihood to develop invasive tumors in the ipsilateral breast as they do in the contralateral breast, making bilateral mastectomy the best treatment option, which would be unnecessary in up to 80% of patients.

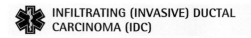 INFILTRATING (INVASIVE) DUCTAL CARCINOMA (IDC)

Invasive breast cancer accounts for approximately 75% to 85% of breast malignancies with the majority (85%) being IDC. It starts in the duct of the breast and spreads to the fatty tissue of the breast. It may metastasize through the lymphatic system or bloodstream. IDC is an invasive adenocarcinoma that demonstrates differentiation characteristics of breast ductal cells. Histologic diagnostic criteria includes: (1) irregular infiltration of stroma, (2) variable ductal formation by infiltrating cells, (3) a wide range of cytologic atypia and mitotic rates, and (4) the absence of myoepithelial cells in the invasive areas.

Infiltrating carcinoma should be separated from ductal carcinoma in situ by the minimal stromal invasion (microinvasion).

Symptoms
- A mass that has changed in size +++
- Painless palpable mass
- Breast pain or deformity
- Nipple discharge +++
- Breast erythema
- Breast skin ulceration
- Bone pain, dyspnea, or meningitic syndrome may suggest distant metastases requiring a more extensive workup.

Signs
- A malignant mass that is firm and hard, usually painless (8% to 90%), irregular, and fixed to the skin or chest wall ++++
- Skin dimpling (the result of shortening or retraction of the Cooper ligaments induced by the tumor; does not have prognostic value)
- Nipple changes or retraction
- Bloody nipple discharge
- Peau d'orange (reflects the invasion of the subdermal lymphatic plexus and lends to a shortened survival)

Workup
- These lesions should undergo the triple test—a combination of careful, clinical examination, breast imaging, and needle biopsy (pathologic evaluation).
- Noncystic breast masses in women younger than 40 years of age are common and most often benign.
- No matter what her age, malignancy must be considered in any woman presenting with a dominant breast mass.
- If imaging studies reveal no suspect findings for a patient with an equivocal result on clinical breast examination, repeat breast examination should be scheduled in 6 to 8 weeks.
- Diagnostic mammography should be obtained before biopsy if clinical concern of malignancy is high.
- Negative imaging studies do not eliminate the need for further evaluation of a suspect mass.
- After breast imaging, a needle biopsy—either a core or FNA—should be performed.
- Ultrasound can be used to determine if the mass is solid or cystic along with the use of FNA biopsy. ++++
- Fine-needle aspiration biopsy (FNAB) of the breast is a well-established method for the diagnosis of breast carcinoma. +++++
- The presence of nonbloody fluid and complete resolution of the cyst can confirm its benign nature. However, if the fluid is bloody or the cyst does not resolve after aspiration or has a complex appearance on the ultrasound image, a biopsy is indicated.
- Mammography can provide signs suggestive of cancer that include architectural distortions, microcalcifications, or masses. These changes require further evaluation using diagnostic mammograms with or without ultrasound. Biopsies are indicated if these changes are confirmed.

Comments and Treatment Considerations

Invasive ductal carcinomas have the poorest prognosis of all invasive breast cancers. The patient and physician must discuss the benefits and risks of mastectomy compared with those of breast conservation therapy (BCT) in each individual case.

Women whose breasts are preserved have more positive attitudes about their body image and experience fewer changes in their frequency of breast stimulation and feelings of sexual desirability. Patients can be offered BCT followed by local irradiation, modified-radical mastectomy alone, or modified-radical mastectomy with immediate reconstruction.

Women with two or more primary tumors in separate quadrants of the breast or with diffuse, malignant-appearing microcalcifications are not considered candidates for BCT. Persistent positive margins after reasonable surgical attempts absolutely contraindicate BCT with radiation.

A history of therapeutic irradiation to the breast region that, combined with the proposed treatment, would result in an excessively high total radiation dosage to a significant volume is an absolute contraindication. Adjuvant systemic therapy should be considered for most women with invasive breast cancer.

Adjuvant tamoxifen citrate similarly substantially reduces the rate of local recurrence in patients treated with breast conservation surgery and local irradiation, but does not seem to reduce greatly the rate of local recurrence after breast conservation surgery alone.

 INVASIVE LOBULAR CARCINOMA

ILC constitutes the second most frequent type of invasive breast cancer accounting for approximately 5% to 10% of invasive breast carcinomas. Invasive lobular carcinomas are characterized by multifocality in the ipsilateral breast and appear to be bilateral more often than other types of invasive breast cancer. Invasive lobular carcinomas show distinctive cytologic features and patterns of tumor cell infiltration of the stroma. In their classic form there are relatively uniform neoplastic cells that invade the stroma singly, resulting in the formation of linear strands that encircle mammary ducts in a target-like manner.

There are variant forms of ILC (solid, alveolar, and tubulolobular), which differ from the classic form with regard to architectural or cytologic features. In the variant forms, the cells comprising the lesion have features characteristic of the classic form, but differ with regard to the growth pattern of the tumor cells. Classical invasive lobular carcinomas typically show expression of estrogen and progesterone receptors.

Symptoms
- A mass that has changed in size
- Painless palpable mass +++

- Breast pain or deformity
- Tender, thickened area over the breast

Signs
- Discrete, firm mass on palpation
- Spiculated mass on mammogram
- Only a vague area of thickening or induration, without definable margins
- Abdominal pain

Workup
- A breast mass should undergo the triple test—A combination of careful, clinical examination, breast imaging, and needle biopsy (pathologic evaluation).
- If imaging studies reveal no suspect findings for a patient with an equivocal result on clinical breast examination, repeat breast examination should be scheduled in 6 to 8 weeks.
- Ultrasound can be used to determine if the mass is solid or cystic along with the use of FNAB. +++
- Diagnostic mammography should be obtained before biopsy if clinical concern of malignancy is high. ++++
- After breast imaging, a needle biopsy—either a core or FNA—should be performed. +++++

Comments and Treatment Considerations
Metastases to the lungs, liver, and brain parenchyma appear to be less common in patients with lobular than ductal cancers. Lobular carcinomas have a greater propensity to metastasize to the leptomeninges, peritoneal surfaces, retroperitoneum, GI tract, and reproductive organs than do ductal cancers.

The patient and physician must discuss the benefits and risks of mastectomy compared with those of BCT in each case. Patients can be offered BCT followed by local irradiation, modified-radical mastectomy alone, or modified-radical mastectomy with immediate reconstruction.

Women whose breasts are preserved have more positive attitudes about their body image and experience fewer changes in their frequency of breast stimulation and feelings of sexual desirability.

Women with two or more primary tumors in separate quadrants of the breast or with diffuse, malignant appearing microcalcifications are not considered candidates for BCT. Persistent positive margins after reasonable surgical attempts absolutely contraindicate BCT with radiation.

A history of therapeutic irradiation to the breast region that, combined with the proposed treatment, would result in an excessively high total radiation dosage to a significant volume is an absolute contraindication. Adjuvant systemic therapy should be considered for most women with invasive breast cancer. Adjuvant tamoxifen citrate similarly substantially reduces the rate of local recurrence in patients treated with breast conservation surgery and local irradiation, but does not seem to reduce greatly the rate of local recurrence after breast conservation surgery alone.

INFLAMMATORY CARCINOMA

Inflammatory carcinoma is an aggressive but fortunately rare disease, accounting for 1% to 5% of breast cancers. It has a sudden onset and a rapidly progressive course. It is a distinct form of breast cancer that warrants special clinical considerations. It must be diagnosed promptly to avert progression and death. Because of its aggressive and rapid course, it carries a higher morbidity and mortality than the invasive cancers. It has distinct clinicopathologic features characterized by an early age at diagnosis, poor nuclear grade, negative hormone receptor status, and an overall poor survival outcome.

Inflammatory carcinoma occurs mainly in premenopausal women and is associated with a 95% risk of distant metastases. It is characterized clinically by redness and erythema involving more than half the breast and pathologically by tumor involving the dermal lymphatics of the breast.

Inflammatory breast carcinoma must be distinguished from a common lactational mastitis or abscess. This is usually accomplished by sampling the skin by tissue biopsy at the time the area is incised and drained.

In contrast to inflammatory breast cancer, mastitis often presents with fever, leukocytosis, and systemic malaise. In addition, antibiotics tend to be of immediate benefit in mastitis and breast abscess, but not with inflammatory breast cancer.

Symptoms
- Discoloration (red to purple) of the skin affecting at least one third of the breast with rapid onset (weeks to months) ++++
- Thickening and/or fine dimpling (peau d'orange) of the skin with rapid onset (weeks to months) ++++
- Warmth and a palpable ridge present at the margin of induration
- Erythematous, nonblanchable nodules over the chest
- Mastalgia (breast pain) +++
- Ecchymosis
- Bone pain

Signs
- Nipple inversion or retraction +++
- Diffuse erythema
- Breast edema
- Skin ridging (peau d'orange) ++++
- May not be an underlying palpable mass
- Fine dimpling of the skin
- Warmth over the skin
- Palpable or matted axillary lymph nodes
- No distinct mass (occurs in 50% of cases) +++

Workup
- Biopsy of the affected skin
- Diagnostic mammogram

- Breast ultrasound
- Assess for metastatic disease for patients who are asymptomatic outside the breast. These studies include a bone scan and CT scan of the chest and abdomen.
- The diagnostic workup must include marking the original tumor bed for future radiotherapy planning and other evaluations.

Comments and Treatment Considerations

The patient and physician must discuss the benefits and risks of mastectomy compared with those of BCT in each case. Chemotherapy with a modified radical mastectomy plus radiotherapy may be an alternative to a radical mastectomy.

Metastases are the major determinant of survival in patients with inflammatory breast cancer. Urgent and aggressive treatment with neoadjuvant anthracycline–based chemotherapy is the current standard for initial treatment.

The neoadjuvant chemotherapy is followed by multimodality locoregional therapy.

References

Arisio R, Cuccorese C, Accinelli G, et al: Role of fine-needle aspiration biopsy in breast lesions: analysis of a series of 4,110 cases, *Diagn Cytopathol* 18:462–467, 1998.

Arpino G, Allred DC, Mohsin SK, et al: Lobular neoplasia on core-needle biopsy-clinical significance, *Cancer* 101:242, 2004.

Berens PD: Prenatal, intrapartum, and postpartum support of the lactating mother, *Pediatr Clin North Am* 48:365, 2001.

Boni R: Tumescent power liposuction in the treatment of the enlarged male breast, *Dermatology* 213:140–143, 2006.

Bradley, SJ, Weaver, DW, Bouwman, DL: Alternatives in the surgical management of in situ breast cancer. A meta-analysis of outcomes, *Am Surg* 56:428, 1990.

Braunstein GD, Glassman HA: Gynecomastia, *Curr Ther Endocrinol Metab* 6:401–404, 1997.

Carter BA, Page DL, Schuyler P, et al: No elevation in long-term breast carcinoma risk for women with fibroadenomas that contain atypical hyperplasia, *Cancer* 92(1):30–66, 2001.

Choi YD, Gong GY, Kim MJ, et al: Clinical and cytologic features of papillary neoplasms of the breast, *Acta Cytol* 50:35–40, 2006.

Claus, EB, Stowe, M, Carter D: Breast carcinoma in situ: risk factors and screening patterns, *J Natl Cancer Inst* 93:1811, 2001.

Dener C, Inan A: Breast abscesses in lactating women, *World J Surg* 27:130, 2003.

Dupont WD, Page DL, Parl FF, et al: Long-term risk of breast cancer in women with fibroadenoma, *N Engl J Med* 331:10, 1994.

Fisher B, Bryant J, Dignam J, et al: Tamoxifen, radiation therapy, or both for prevention of ipsilateral breast tumor recurrence after lumpectomy in women with invasive breast cancers of one centimeter or less, *J Clin Oncol* 20:4141, 2002.

Fitzgibbons PL, Henson DE, Hutter RV: Benign breast changes and the risk for subsequent breast cancer: an update of the 1985 consensus statement. Cancer Committee of the College of American Pathologists, *Arch Pathol Lab Med* 122:1053, 1998.

Foster, MC, Helvie, MA, Gregory, NE, et al: Lobular carcinoma in situ or atypical lobular hyperplasia at core-needle biopsy: is excisional biopsy necessary, *Radiology* 231:813, 2004.

Frykberg, ER, Bland, KI: Management of in situ and minimally invasive breast carcinoma, *World J Surg* 18:45, 1994.

Ganesan S, Karthik G, Joshi M, et al: Ultrasound spectrum in intraductal papillary neoplasms of breast, *Br J Radiol* 79, 843–849, 2006.

Glass AR: Gynecomastia, *Endocrinol Metab Clin North Am* 23:825–837, 1994.

Gordon PB, Gagnon FA, Lanzkowsky L: Solid breast masses diagnosed as fibroadenoma at fine-needle aspiration biopsy: acceptable rates of growth at long-term follow-up, *Radiology* 229:233, 2003.

Greenberg R, Skornick Y, Kaplan O: Management of fibroadenoma, *J Gen Inter Med* 13:640, 1998.

Hammons KB, Edwards RF, Rice WY: Golf-inhibiting gynecomastia associated with atorvastatin therapy, *Pharmacotherapy* 26:1165–1168, 2006.

Hance KW, Anderson WF, Devesa SS, et al: Trends in inflammatory breast carcinoma incidence and survival: the surveillance, epidemiology, and end results program at the National Cancer Institute. *J Natl Cancer Inst* 97:966–975, 2005.

Harris J, Lippman M, Morrow M, Osborne C: *Diseases of the breast*, 3rd ed. Philadelphia, 2004, Lippincott Williams & Wilkins.

Harris GD, White RD, Carlson B, Sisodia T: *Common breast problems*. Monograph, Edition No. 259, Home study self-assessment program. Leawood, KS, 2000, American Academy of Family Physicians.

Hussain AN, Policarpio C, Vincent MT: Evaluating nipple discharge, *Obstet Gynecol Surv* 61:278–282, 2006.

Jacobs TW, Connolly JL, Schnitt SJ: Nonmalignant lesions in breast cancer core needle biopsies: to excise or not to excise, *Am J Surg Pathol* 26:1095, 2002.

Jones DJ, Holt SD, Surtees P, et al: A comparison of danazol and placebo in the treatment of adult idiopathic gynecomastia: results of a prospective study in 55 patients, *Ann R Coll Surg Engl* 72:296–298, 1990.

Karstrup S, Solvig J, Nolsøe CP, Nilsson P, et al: Acute puerperal breast abscesses: US-guided drainage, *Radiology* 188:807, 1993.

King TA, Carter KM, Bolton JS, Fuhrman GM: A simple approach to nipple discharge, *Am Surg* 10:960–965, 2000.

Kuijper A, Mommers EC, Van der Wall E, et al: Histopathology of fibroadenoma of the breast, *Am J Clin Pathol* 115:736, 2001.

Kvist LJ, Rydhstroem H: Factors related to breast abscess after delivery: a population-based study, *BJOG* 112:1070, 2005.

Li CI, Daling JR, Malone KE: Age-specific incidence rates of in situ breast carcinomas by histologic type, 1980 to 2001, *Cancer Epidemiol Biomarkers Prev* 14:1008, 2005.

Li CI, Malone KE, Saltzman BS, et al: Risk of invasive breast carcinoma among women diagnosed with ductal carcinoma in situ and lobular carcinoma in situ, 1988-2001, *Cancer* 106:2104, 2006.

Mahoney CP: Adolescent gynecomastia. Differential diagnosis and management, *Pediatr Clin North Am* 37:1389–1404, 1990.

Moriya T, Kasajima A, Ishida K, et al: New trends of immunohistochemistry for making differential diagnosis of breast lesions, *Med Molec Morphol* 39:8–13, 2006.

Morrow M: Evaluation of common breast problems, *Am Fam Physician* 61:2371–2378, 2000.

Morrow M, Wong S, Venta L: The evaluation of breast masses in women younger than forty years of age, *Surgery* 124:634–641, 1998.

Neuman JF: Evaluation and treatment of gynecomastia, *Am Fam Physician* 55:1835–1844, 1849–1850, 1997.

O'Hara RJ, Dexter SP, Fox JN: Conservative management of infective mastitis and breast abscesses after ultrasonographic assessment, *Br J Surg* 83:1413, 1996.

Plourde PV, Kulin HE, Santner SJ: Clomiphene in the treatment of adolescent gynecomastia. Clinical and endocrine studies, *Am J Dis Child* 137:1080–1082, 1983.

Schwarz RJ, Shrestha R: Needle aspiration of breast abscesses, *Am J Surg* 182:117, 2001.

Sperber F, Blank A, Metser U, et al: Diagnosis and treatment of breast fibroadenomas by ultrasound-guided vacuum-assisted biopsy, *Arch Surg* 138:796, 2003.

Thompson DF, Carter JR: Drug-induced gynecomastia, *Pharmacotherapy* 13:37–45, 1993.

Ulitzsch D, Nyman MKG, Carlson RA: Breast abscess in lactating women: US-guided treatment, *Radiology* 232:904, 2004.

Varey AHR, Shere MH, Cawthorn SJ: Treatment of loculated lactational breast abscess with a vacuum biopsy system, *Br J Surg* 92:1225, 2005.

Weinstein D, Strano S, Cohen P, et al: Breast fibroadenoma: mapping of pathophysiologic features with three-time-point, contrast-enhanced MR imaging-pilot study, *Radiology* 210:233, 1999.

Wilkinson S, Anderson TJ, Rifkind E, et al: Fibroadenoma of the breast: a follow-up of conservative management, *Br J Surg* 76:390, 1989.

CHAPTER 12

Chest Pain

Daniel S. Clark, Stephanus Philip, Joseph S. Esherick,
Mark Lepore, and Bryan Wong

Chest pain is one of the cardinal symptoms in medicine. Chest pain is the chief complaint responsible for more than 5.3 million emergency room (ER) visits per year; it accounts for 5% of all ER visits. The challenge to the primary care physician is to differentiate patients who have chest pain as a result of a life-threatening cause from those presenting with chest pain from a benign cause. A thorough history and physical examination are critical in the evaluation of all cases of acute chest pain.

The life-threatening causes of chest pain include acute coronary syndromes, aortic dissection, pulmonary embolus, pneumothorax, and pericarditis with tamponade. Despite our best efforts, up to 8% of patients with chest pain from a life-threatening cause will be incorrectly diagnosed and inappropriately sent home. This chapter focuses on the more common causes of chest pain: acute coronary syndrome, stable angina, aortic dissection, pulmonary embolism, pericarditis, pneumonia, pneumothorax, gastroesophageal reflux, musculoskeletal chest wall pain, and herpes zoster.

ACUTE CORONARY SYNDROME

Acute coronary syndrome (ACS) is the most common life-threatening cause of chest pain. More than 1.4 million patients are admitted annually for ACS.

More than 1 million myocardial infarctions occur each year. ACS includes three distinct conditions: ST-segment elevation syndrome (STEMI), unstable angina (UA), and non–ST-segment elevation myocardial infarction (NSTEMI).

The three acute coronary syndromes are usually the result of the sudden rupture of a *soft* cholesterol-rich coronary artery plaque. This event occurs commonly between 6 AM and noon. The three syndromes are distinguished by the electrocardiographic findings, and cardiac biomarker levels.

Risk factors for ACS include hypertension (blood pressures >140/90 mm Hg), dyslipidemia, diabetes mellitus, smoking, obesity, physical inactivity, family history for premature coronary artery disease (CAD), and metabolic syndrome.

Symptoms
- ACS presents with chest pain *qualitatively* similar to typical angina; however, *quantitatively* it is more frequent, intense, or prolonged than typical angina.
- New onset anginal pain
- Anginal pain at rest or at low effort
- Anginal pain occurring at a decreased effort
- Anginal pain occurring with increased duration (>20 minutes) or intensity despite rest or NTG
- Anginal pain occurring post acute myocardial infarction (MI)
- Atypical anginal pain presenting in a sudden onset or crescendo pattern

Signs
- Few signs with ACS unless there is a sudden decrease in systolic or diastolic left ventricular (LV) function
- Transient hypotension during chest pain +
- Transient cardiac gallops (S_3 or S_4) at the cardiac apex during chest pain ++
- Transient mitral insufficiency secondary to papillary muscle dysfunction during chest pain, associated with a soft S_1 at the left lower sternal border ++

Workup
- ECG
  - Should be measured as soon as possible after presentation with acute chest pain
  - May be normal in up to 20% of patients with ACS and 10% with acute MI ++
  - If ECG is normal, but high clinical suspicion of ischemia is present, ECG should be repeated.
    - Determine *location* of ECG change—Related to coronary anatomy
      - II, III, aVF inferior wall—Right coronary artery (RCA)
      - V1-3 anteroseptal wall—Left anterior descending coronary
      - I, aVL, V4-6 anterolateral wall—Circumflex coronary
      - I, aVL, V1-6 anterior wall—Left main coronary
      - V1-2 reciprocal changes—Posterior wall, proximal RCA
    - Determine the type of ECG change
      - ST-segment depression—UA or NSTEMI (or "reciprocal" change of infarction in another location)
      - ST-segment elevation—STEMI or spasm (Prinzmetal's angina)
  - In an inferior wall MI (proximal RCA obstruction), check for a right ventricular infarction
    - An ECG with reversed V leads (right-sided ECG) demonstrates ST-segment changes in the right-sided V3-4.
  - In ACS the number of leads in which ST segment and T wave abnormalities are noted correlates with increased cardiac risk

- Sinus bradycardia, Wenckebach (Mobitz I) second-degree atrio-ventricular (AV) block, slow ventricular tachycardia (ventricular rate <100 bpm) suggests RCA involvement.
- Sustained rapid junctional tachycardia or Mobitz II second-degree AV block suggests left anterior descending (LAD) coronary artery involvement.
- Underlying conditions that interfere with the ECG diagnosis of ACS by obscuring the typical ST and T wave changes are:
  - Left bundle branch block (LBBB), ventricular pacemaker rhythm, preexcitation syndrome, myopericarditis, left ventricular hypertrophy with strain pattern and marked hyperkalemia
- Chest x-ray—portable technique
  - Chest x-ray is often totally normal with ACS.
  - May help exclude other causes for chest pain (pneumothorax, pulmonary embolus, aortic dissection, and pneumonia)
  - Cardiomegaly and heart failure point to intrinsic heart disease and increase the pretest likelihood of CAD.
- Cardiac biomarkers
  - Troponin T or I is a marker of choice.
    - Troponin elevates in 6 to 8 hours and may remain elevated up to 10 days.
    - Troponin T and I are equally sensitive and specific (90% sensitive and 95% specific), and both have enhanced prognostic value compared with creatinine kinase-MB fraction (CK-MB).
    - Serial troponin levels every 4 to 6 hours increase diagnostic capability for MI
    - Troponin levels are abnormal in STEMI and NSTEMI.
      - The World Health Organization's criterion for MI is a troponin level more than 99th percentile of normal (usually ≥0.6 ng/mL).
      - Troponins remain normal in UA (<0.6 ng/mL).
    - Normal troponin levels obtained less than 6 to 8 hours after the onset of pain cannot exclude acute myocardial damage.
    - Normal troponin levels obtained after 6 to 8 hours from the onset of pain may exclude MI but not unstable angina.
      - Of note, cell death often does not correspond with the onset of chest pain.
    - A single normal troponin level in a patient with suspected ACS should not generally be used as reassurance that discharge is safe.
    - The peak troponin elevation is directly related to the amount of myocardial damage.
  - CK-MB elevates in 6 hours but usually returns to normal within 3 days.
  - CK-MB is a better marker than troponins to diagnose reinfarction, if recurrent ischemic chest pain occurs post MI.
  - Troponin and CK-MB elevation may be noted in nonischemic cardiac disease (myopericarditis, cardiac contusion) and in noncardiac conditions (hypothyroidism, pulmonary embolus, sepsis, and renal failure on dialysis).

- Routine laboratory workup
  - Obtain a CBC, basic metabolic panel, and renal and liver panels.
  - Check for risk factors with a fasting lipid panel and fasting glucose levels.
  - Recommend checking resting oximetry and consider a TSH level.

 RISK STRATIFICATION

- Echocardiogram
  - If ECG is nondiagnostic, and the patient is particularly ill, a transthoracic echo may demonstrate new segmental LV contraction abnormalities suggestive of ischemic heart disease.
  - Can help exclude other cardiac causes of chest pain (aortic stenosis, hypertrophic cardiomyopathy, or aortic dissection)
- Noninvasive stress or myocardial perfusion testing
  - Exercise treadmill or echocardiogram and pharmacologically assisted testing (adenosine/persantine, or dobutamine) is contraindicated in high-risk UA, acute NSTEMI, or STEMI.
- American College of Cardiology/American Heart Association (ACC/AHA) high-risk ACS criteria
  - New or presumed new ST-segment elevation
  - New or presumed new ST-segment depression
  - Recurrent ischemia despite intensive therapy
  - Recurrent ischemia with heart failure
  - Sustained ventricular tachycardia
  - Hemodynamic instability
  - Decreased systolic function
  - Elevated troponin level (>0.1 ng/mL)
  - High-risk finding on noninvasive stress or myocardial perfusion test
  - History of percutaneous coronary intervention (PCI) within 6 months
  - History of prior coronary artery bypass surgery

 MEDICAL THERAPY

- Aspirin (ASA) 160 to 325 mg chewed stat; give additional dose even if on daily ASA, clopidogrel, or warfarin. Hold only if ASA allergy exists
  - Indicated for UA, NSTEMI, or STEMI
  - Continue at 75 to 81 mg PO daily
  - Decreases mortality after acute MI for at least 4 years
  - Decreases the risk of recurrent MI
  - Reduces incidence of nonfatal stroke after an MI

- Clopidogrel (Plavix) 300-mg loading dose then 75 mg PO daily
  - Use if ASA allergy
  - Consider with cardiologist/surgeon when a coronary artery bypass graft (CABG) will occur as clopidogrel may be held prior to an operation to prevent perioperative bleeding.
  - Use with ASA in high-risk UA, NSTEMI, STEMI and continue up to 12 months
  - Use post PCI with stent placement.
    - Continue for 1 month if bare metal stent used and *no* associated MI.
    - Continue for at least 3 to 6 months if drug eluting stent (DES) used and *no* associated MI. Because of recent concerns about late-onset thrombosis in DES, consider indefinite use of combined ASA plus clopidogrel until issue fully clarified.
  - Stop 5 to 7 days before elective surgery (CABG).
  - Monitor CBC for infrequent occurrence of TTP or neutropenia.
  - Reduces composite outcome of cardiovascular death, nonfatal MI, and stroke after acute MI
- Glycoprotein IIb/IIIa agents
  - Indicated for high-risk UA, NSTEMI with persistent or recurrent ischemia and urgent invasive therapy not readily available
    - Use eptifibatide or tirofiban
  - Used as adjunctive therapy with invasive PCI therapy
    - Use abciximab after PCI
  - Reduces death and nonfatal MI in high-risk ACS patients
- Nitrates
  - Sublingual (0.4 mg every 5 minutes times three doses), transcutaneous paste 0.5 to 2 inches every 6 hours, transcutaneous patch 0.2 to 4 mg/hr patch/day; IV start with bolus 12.5 to 25 μg, then drip of 5 to 10 μg/min; increase by 5 to 10 μg/min every 5 minutes (range 5 to 200 μg/min); oral isosorbide 20 to 40 mg every 12 hours
  - Used for symptomatic control of angina
  - If a phosphodiesterase-5 inhibitor (commonly used for erectile dysfunction) has been used in the last 24 hours (sildenafil, vardenafil) or 36 hours (tadalafil), nitroglycerin is contraindicated.
  - Caution with nitroglycerin use in older adults, in patients with diastolic dysfunction, or with a right ventricular infarction because these conditions are very volume-dependent states
- Morphine
  - Pain and anxiety relief
  - Dosage 2 to 5 mg IV and may be repeated under careful observation. Watch for hypotension.
- Unfractionated heparin (UFH) and LMWH
  - Frequently used for high-risk UA, NSTEMI, and STEMI
  - UFH may reduce in-hospital mortality in acute MI
  - LMWH (enoxaparin) appears to have a lower risk of recurrent MI, UA, need for revascularization, and heparin-induced thrombocytopenia.

- Enoxaparin should be dose adjusted with moderate renal impairment and withheld with advanced renal disease or if urgent surgery is contemplated.
- Beta-blockers
  - Metoprolol 5 mg IV every 2 to 5 minutes for three doses if chest pain is ongoing and heart rate tolerates, then continue maintenance dosage 25 to 50 mg PO every 6 hours. Oral metoprolol should be started if chest pain has resolved.
  - Acutely, beta-blockers relieve chest pain and reduce infarct size and risk of sudden death.
  - Post MI, beta-blockers reduce risk of reinfarction and mortality.
  - Attempt to titrate beta-blockers to achieve a resting heart rate of 55 to 65 bpm
  - Avoid in decompensated HF, heart block, hypotension, severe bronchospasm, or sinus node disease.
  - May mask signs of hypoglycemia
- Calcium channel blockers (CCBs)
  - If beta-blockers are contraindicated, consider use for rhythm control or recurrent ischemia.
  - Indicated for coronary spasm (Prinzmetal's angina)
  - Long-acting diltiazem and verapamil are the drugs of choice.
  - Avoid nifedipine post MI.
  - No mortality benefit (and possible adverse outcome) noted with CCB therapy
- Thrombolysis
  - Only indicated for STEMI within 12 hours of symptom onset when access to the coronary catheterization lab will be delayed
    - ST-segment elevation greater than 0.1 mV in contiguous leads or new LBBB with ischemic chest pain
  - Alternative therapy to early invasive therapy with PCI if PCI is not available
  - Fibrin-specific agents—Reteplase, alteplase, tenecteplase
  - Non-fibrin specific—Streptokinase
  - Reduces mortality in STEMI
    - Benefit greater in anterior wall versus inferior wall STEMI
    - Benefit greater with earlier therapy
  - Restores normal (thrombolysis in myocardial infarction [TIMI] 3) blood flow in 60% of patients
  - Increases risk of intracranial hemorrhage by 1.5% to 3% +
- ACE inhibitors
  - Indicated for high-risk UA, NSTEMI or STEMI patients
  - Starting oral doses: Ramipril (2.5 mg bid), captopril (6.25 mg tid), enalapril (2.5 mg bid) and lisinopril (5 mg daily)
  - Usually started 24 hours after an MI, but may be started earlier if persistent hypertension (HTN) despite therapy with beta-blockers and nitrates
  - Major benefit if LV systolic dysfunction, clinical heart failure (HF) and in patients with diabetes mellitus
    - Reduces mortality post MI at 24 months
    - In patients with LV dysfunction post MI, reduces rate of death, recurrent nonfatal MI, and hospitalization for HF

- Long-term protective effect in high-risk patients with CAD by reduction in death, MI, and stroke even without systolic dysfunction or HF
- Angiotensin II receptor antagonists
  - Alternative agents if ACE inhibitors cannot be used
  - Suggest starting losartan 25 mg PO daily or valsartan 80 mg PO twice daily
- Aldosterone blockers—Selective
  - Indicated post MI in patients with either LV systolic dysfunction or clinical HF
  - Eplerenone 25 to 50 mg PO daily started day 3 post MI
  - Watch for hyperkalemia.
    - Use agent with caution if creatinine clearance less than 50 mL/min
  - Reduces mortality and morbidity if used in patients post MI
- Warfarin
  - Indicated for ACS with atrial fibrillation, DVT, or endocardial thrombus
  - Reduces long-term mortality and venous and arterial thromboembolism
- HMG-CoA reductase inhibitors (statins)
  - Statins reduce cardiovascular death and provide primary and secondary prevention for stroke and MI.
  - Recommend early, aggressive statin therapy for their pleiotropic benefit
    - Atorvastatin 80 mg PO daily is the only proven agent for acute ACS treatment.
    - Evidence suggests that early aggressive statin therapy in ACS reduces symptomatic ischemia and recurrent hospitalizations.
  - Statins cause plaque stabilization, improve endothelial function, increase spontaneous thrombolysis and fibrinolysis, lower low-density lipoprotein (LDL) cholesterol, and decrease inflammation.
  - Cholesterol lowering begins within 2 weeks with maximal benefit at 6 weeks.

EARLY INVASIVE PERCUTANEOUS CORONARY INTERVENTION

- PCI is the preferred alternative to thrombolysis in high-risk UA, high-risk NSTEMI, and all STEMI and patients with cardiogenic shock.
- Goal is rapid primary PCI performed within 90 minutes of presentation to medical attention at a site with proven expertise (large volume centers with low mortality and morbidity).
- Hospital-to-hospital transfer for primary PCI is beneficial if procedure is performed within 2 hours of presentation.
- PCI after failed thrombolysis (salvage PCI) should be considered if persistent chest pain is present.

- Restores normal (TIMI 3) coronary blood flow in more than 90% of patients
- PCI reduces death, reinfarction, and stroke rate in ACS.

 EARLY CORONARY BYPASS SURGERY (CABG)

- UA, NSTEMI, and STEMI patients with persistent or recurrent ischemia with unsuitable coronary anatomy for PCI
- Consider in patients with a critical left main coronary stenosis
- More frequently considered as a delayed form of complete revascularization in diabetic patients with multivessel disease, or in patients who otherwise require heart surgery (e.g., severe valve disease or rupture of mitral valve or intraventricular septum)

ACUTE PERICARDITIS

Acute pericarditis involves the acute inflammation of the pericardial sac. Ninety percent of cases are either of idiopathic or viral etiology. Most cases of acute pericarditis are self-limited, but recurrent pericarditis develops in 15% to 32% of cases. Other causes of pericarditis include neoplasm, infections (tuberculous [Tb], bacterial, fungal, rickettsial or parasitic), sarcoidosis, Dressler's syndrome (post MI), post irradiation, chest trauma, uremia, hypothyroidism, post pericardiotomy, connective tissue diseases (systemic lupus erythematosus, scleroderma, and RA) and medications (hydralazine, methyldopa, isoniazid, phenytoin, and procainamide).

Symptoms
- Constant, sharp, or stabbing retrosternal chest pain
- Exacerbating factors: Deep inspiration and lying down, +/- with swallowing
- Alleviating factors: Improved with leaning forward
- Radiation pattern: Neck, shoulders, arms, trapezius ridges, or epigastrium
- Malaise, myalgias, dry cough, and dyspnea are common.

Signs
- Pericardial rub heard ++++
- Harsh, high-pitched, scratchy sound best heard at end expiration, leaning forward
- Classic rub with three components best heard at the cardiac apex: Ventricular systole, early diastole, and atrial contraction
- Triphasic +++
- Biphasic and monophasic rubs ++
- Signs of cardiac tamponade: Hypotension, tachycardia, jugular venous distension and pulsus paradoxus (fall in systolic BP >10 mm Hg with inspiration) and muffled heart sounds if associated with a large pericardial effusion.
- Temperature greater than 38° C uncommon + except in purulent pericarditis

ELECTROCARDIOGRAPHIC CHANGES

- Stage 1: Diffuse, concave ST-segment elevations and diffuse PR segment depressions (mainly in leads I, II, aVL, aVF and V3-6); however, lead aVR will demonstrate ST-segment depression and PR segment elevation.
- Stage 2: ST and PR segments normalize and T waves progressively flatten.
- Stage 3: Diffuse T wave inversions
- Stage 4: Normalization of the T waves
- ECG changes can be seen. ++++
- No Q wave formation or loss of precordial R wave progression in acute pericarditis
- Electrical alternans may be seen if a large pericardial effusion exists.
- The ratio of ST-segment elevation (in millimeters) to T wave amplitude (in millimeters) greater than 0.24 in lead V6 is highly specific for acute pericarditis.
- Diffuse T wave inversions and concave ST elevation with PR depression suggests myopericarditis

 INDICATIONS FOR HOSPITALIZATION

- Fever more than 38° C, subacute onset over weeks, immunocompromised, history of trauma, anticoagulant therapy, myocarditis, elevated troponin I, evidence of cardiac tamponade or a large pericardial effusion (echo-free space >2 cm)

Workup
- Routine labs: CBC, renal panel, ESR, and troponins
- Troponin I: Mild elevations in up to 70% of patients ++++ with pericarditis and marked elevations consistent with myopericarditis
- Potential labs: Antinuclear antibody, rheumatoid factor and a tuberculous skin test
- Pericardial fluid analysis: Glucose, protein, lactic dehydrogenase, cell count, culture, and Gram stain. If Tb or neoplasm is suspected, send fluid for cytology, *Mycobacterium tuberculosis* ribonucleic acid (RNA) by PCR assay and adenosine deaminase activity (>30 units/L suggests Tb pericarditis)
- Chest radiograph
- Echocardiogram indications: All patients with acute pericarditis should have a transthoracic echocardiogram. This is especially important for prolonged symptoms, any evidence of cardiac

tamponade, or any suspicion of purulent or neoplastic pericarditis or myocardial involvement.
- Global or regional wall motion abnormalities suggest myopericarditis.

Treatment
- Treatment of symptomatic pericarditis related to viral, idiopathic, autoimmune, or connective tissue etiologies
- Oral indomethacin 75 to 225 mg/day or ibuprofen 1600 to 3200 mg/day
- Oral colchicine 1 to 2 mg/day on day 1 then 0.5 to 1 mg/day for 6 months can be added if symptoms persist for more than 2 weeks or for recurrent pericarditis.
- Prednisone 1 to 1.5 mg/kg/day orally for at least 1 month then taper over several months if severe, recurrent pericarditis or if connective tissue disease etiology.
- Idiopathic and viral pericarditis will spontaneously resolve in 2 to 6 weeks.
- Acute pericarditis from bacterial, Tb or neoplastic causes requires treatment of underlying condition and often requires creation of a pericardial window.
- Most common bacteria found in purulent pericarditis are *Staphylococcus, Streptococcus,* and *Haemophilus.* Empiric antibiotics typically include an antistaphylococcal antibiotic and an aminoglycoside antibiotic. Obtain an early cardiothoracic surgery consultation.
- Start isoniazid, ethambutol, rifampin, and pyrazinamide for Tb pericarditis.
- Pericardiectomy is indicated only in highly symptomatic, recurrent pericarditis refractory to medical management.
- Indications for pericardiocentesis: Therapeutic for clinical evidence of tamponade or diagnostic for possible purulent, Tb, or neoplastic pericarditis

AORTIC DISSECTION

No chest pain diagnosis is more dependent on the evaluator's index of suspicion than thoracic aortic dissection. Studies show that physicians correctly suspect aortic dissection in as few as 15% to 43% of patients on initial presentation—in a condition with a 48-hour mortality rate approaching 40% to 68% in untreated patients. Failure to correctly and expediently diagnose aortic dissection may lead to disastrous results, particularly if anticoagulation and/or thrombolysis is used for presumed cardiac ischemia.

Symptoms
- Sudden onset, severe, "tearing" chest pain radiating to the back, neck, or abdomen caused by the extension of a tear between the

intima and adventitia layers of the thoracic aorta, thereby creating a "false lumen" in the arterial wall ++++
- Often has a migrating quality to the chest pain +++
- May present as syncope or sudden collapse ++

Signs
- Reduced or asymmetric pulses (carotid, femoral, and radial) or blood pressures +++
- Diastolic murmur (aortic regurgitation from extension to the aortic valve) with radiation to the right or left sternal border +++
- Neurologic deficits such as stroke or paraplegia from carotid or spinal artery involvement ++
- Acute limb ischemia (look for the six "P's") ++
  - Affected limb with pain, pallor, paralysis, paresthesia, pulseless, poikilothermia
- Acute inferior wall MI (right coronary artery occlusion) +
- Cardiogenic shock from dissection into the pericardium causing tamponade ++
- Acute renal failure by involvement of the renal arteries (decreased urine output) ++

Workup
- Chest x-ray often shows a widened mediastinum (44% to 80%) or abnormal aortic contour (56% to 84%).
- Chest CT with IV contrast (preferably helical), transesophageal echocardiogram (TEE), or MRI of the chest with gadolinium
- ECG, cardiac enzymes, and D-dimer are all nonspecific.

Comments and Treatment Considerations
Risk factors include age greater than 50 years; hypertension; coarctation of the aorta; bicuspid aortic valve; trauma; Marfan, Ehlers-Danlos, and Turner syndromes; giant-cell arteritis; syphilitic aortitis; third-trimester pregnancy; family history of aortic dissection or rupture; cocaine abuse; intra-aortic catheterization; and history of cardiac surgery.

Classification systems for aortic dissection include Stanford classification and Debakey classification. Stanford classification has two kinds of classifications. Type A involves ascending aorta, regardless of the site of origin. Type B involves descending aorta with origin distal to the left subclavian artery.

Debakey classification has four types. Type I involves ascending the aorta, aortic arch, and possibly descending aorta. Type II involves the ascending aorta only. Type III A involves the descending aorta only, with proximal and distal extension. Type III B involves the descending aorta with distal extension into abdominal aorta.

Patients need excellent blood pressure and heart rate control in acute aortic dissection. Using labetalol IV to keep systolic blood pressure less than or equal to120 mm Hg is first-line therapy. Alternative agents include IV nitroprusside, esmolol, or diltiazem.

Ascending aorta dissections usually require urgent surgical repair and management. Descending aorta dissections may be medically managed.

CHRONIC STABLE ANGINA

In the medical office of a primary care physician, the majority of chest pain is noncardiac in origin (90%), +++++ whereas in the ER the likelihood may exceed 50%. +++ The probability that CAD is present is based on the characterization of the patient's chest pain, gender (men > female,) and advancing age.

 CLASSIC ANGINA

Symptoms
- Typically, chest pressure or squeezing sensation
- Pain radiates to the shoulders, neck, jaw, epigastrium or left arm
- Pain similar to prior angina or MI
- Pain associated with nausea, vomiting, or diaphoresis
- Precipitated by physical (upper > lower extremity) or emotional stress
- Lasts up to 15 minutes
- Resolves with rest or nitrate therapy within 5 to 15 minutes
- May resolve more slowly if related to emotional stress
- Stable angina is chest pain with a reproducible onset after a predictable level of exertion or stress and of a predictable duration.

 ATYPICAL ANGINA

- One or at most two of the above classic characteristics
- Pain localized to a small discrete area of the chest wall
- Pain starting at maximal intensity, or constant pain lasting for hours to days
- Atypical pain is more commonly noted in women, older adult patients, diabetic patients, and patients with renal disease.
- May present as dyspnea, sudden fatigue, or nausea

 TRADITIONAL CHARACTERIZATION OF "NONCARDIAC PAIN"

- Up to 25% of MIs may be "silent," so clinical criteria are not completely reliable.
- None or at most one of the classic characteristics ++++
- Pain that is not exacerbated by effort ++++

- Pain lasting only seconds ++++
- Pain exacerbated with swallowing, deep breathing, coughing, palpation, or position changes ++++

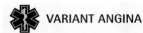 **VARIANT ANGINA**

- Has typical angina characteristics but occurs only at rest
- It is not initiated by physical effort

Signs
- Not common with stable angina
- Are related to sudden decrease in systolic or diastolic LV function
- Transient hypotension during chest pain +
- Transient cardiac gallops (S_3 or S_4) during chest pain +
- Transient mitral insufficiency (papillary muscle dysfunction) during pain +

 ELECTROCARDIOGRAM

Workup
- May be normal in 50% of patients with CAD, even if obtained during pain
- Location: ECG leads related to coronary anatomy
  - II, III, aVF—Inferior wall, RCA
  - V1-V3—Anteroseptal wall, left anterior descending coronary
  - I, aVL, V4-6—Anterolateral wall, circumflex coronary
  - I, aVL, V1-6—Anterior wall, left main coronary
  - V1-2 reciprocal changes—True posterior wall, proximal RCA
- Type of ECG change
  - ST-segment depression—Cardiac ischemia (typical angina)
  - ST-segment elevation—Cardiac injury or spasm (Prinzmetal's angina)
- Treadmill
  - Can diagnose angina and risk-stratify patient
  - The severity of the pain does not correlate with the quantity of myocardium at risk.
  - If baseline ECG is normal or only mildly abnormal (<1 mm ST depression or right bundle branch block [RBBB]), and patient can exercise, order routine treadmill (sensitivity 68%/specificity 77%).
  - If baseline ECG is abnormal, and patient can exercise, order exercise echocardiogram (sensitivity 76%/specificity 88%) or exercise myocardial perfusion imaging (MPI) study (sensitivity 88%/specificity 77%).

- If patient cannot exercise, adenosine/persantine (sensitivity 90%/specificity 75%) or dobutamine MPI (sensitivity 82%/specificity 75%)
  - Thallium isotope if weight less than 250 pounds and Cardiolite if more than 250 pounds
- Consider using Duke Treadmill Score for risk stratification.

 ## ECHOCARDIOGRAM

- CAD is associated with segmental LV contraction abnormalities.
- Can help exclude other cardiac causes of chest pain (aortic stenosis, hypertrophic cardiomyopathy, mitral valve prolapse, or aortic dissection)

 ## ROUTINE LABORATORY WORKUP

- Obtain a CBC, basic metabolic panel, renal, liver panels, and a TSH level.
- Check for risk factors with a fasting lipid panel and fasting glucose levels.

 ## MEDICAL THERAPY

- Reduces symptoms, prevents myocardial infarction, and improves survival
- Nitrates (sublingual, spray, oral, or transdermal)
  - Reduces symptoms by decreasing cardiac preload and by coronary dilation
  - Sublingual tablet or spray every 5 minutes for three doses or until pain resolves
  - Long-acting nitrates as effective as long-acting CCBs and cause less BP lowering
  - Can be used with either beta-blocker or CCB
  - Need a 14-hour nitrate-free interval to prevent drug tolerance

 ## ASPIRIN

- Dosage: 75 to 325 mg PO daily
- Recommended in acute or chronic disease with or without symptoms

Clopidogrel
- 300-mg loading dose then 75 mg PO daily
- Use if ASA allergy

- Should stop 5 to 7 days before elective major surgery (e.g., CABG) (use with caution if going to catheterization for STEMI and possibility of early CABG)
- Monitor CBC for rare occurrences of TTP or neutropenia.
- Less GI bleeding and GI upset compared with ASA

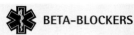

BETA-BLOCKERS

- Improve survival in patients with prior MI
- Reduce symptoms by decreasing cardiac demand
- Titrate beta-blockers to achieve a resting heart rate 55 to 65 bpm.
- Avoid in patients with sinus or AV nodal disease, severe reactive airway disease, or decompensated heart failure.

CALCIUM CHANNEL BLOCKERS

- Improve symptoms by coronary dilation, and by decreasing cardiac demand and systemic afterload
- Long-acting CCBs are indicated when beta-blockers are contraindicated, not effective, or cause unacceptable side effects.
- They relieve angina, increase exercise time to ischemia, and decrease the need for sublingual nitrates.
- They should be combined with beta-blockers or long-acting nitrates whenever possible.
- Long-acting CCBs offer no mortality benefit and possibly confer an increased risk of cardiovascular events when used as a solo agent.
- Short-acting CCBs should be avoided due to increased risk of adverse cardiac events.
- Long-acting non-dihydropyridine CCBs (diltiazem, verapamil) decrease angina, slow sinus and AV nodal function, and are negatively inotropic
  - Avoid use with beta-blockers.
  - Use with long-acting nitrates is beneficial.
- Long-acting dihydropyridine CCBs decrease angina by coronary dilation and by decreasing afterload
  - May be used with beta-blockers
  - Use with long-acting nitrates may cause excessive hypotension.

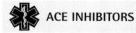

ACE INHIBITORS

- Not indicated for angina relief
- Improve survival if CAD is associated with LV dysfunction, diabetes mellitus, HTN, or prior MI

- Beneficial with chronic proteinuria by delaying progression of renal disease
- May be beneficial in all high-risk patients with CAD (HOPE trial)

 INVASIVE THERAPY

- PCI indications
  - High-risk angina
  - High-risk treadmill (large area of ischemia or ischemia at low workload)
  - Resistant angina despite optimal medical therapy
  - Two- or three-vessel CAD in nondiabetic patients
- Coronary artery bypass surgery (CABG)
  - Improves survival with left main coronary disease, triple vessel disease with decreased ejection fraction, double vessel disease with proximal left anterior descending artery stenosis
  - Significant coronary artery disease associated with need for open heart surgery for other reasons
  - Significant coronary artery disease not amenable to PCI
  - Symptomatic angina with triple vessel disease in diabetic patients

Comments and Treatment Considerations

Angina pectoris is a symptom of imbalance between oxygen *supply* via the coronary arteries and cardiac *demand* based on elevated heart rate, blood pressure, contractility, or wall stress (related to ventricular volume and mass). This imbalance occurs most commonly by decreasing supply due to plaque formation ($\geq$70% obstruction), plaque rupture, or ulceration. Decreased supply may also be due to hypotension, coronary spasm, or embolism.

Increasing cardiac demand may be related to sustained systemic hypertension, increased physical activity, emotional stress, or the presence of cardiac hypertrophy or cardiac enlargement. Because coronary perfusion occurs predominantly during diastole, prolonged tachycardia adversely affects both cardiac supply and demand.

Risk factors for stable angina are identical to those for ACS.

GERD-RELATED CHEST PAIN

See Chapter 26.

HERPES ZOSTER

Included in every differential diagnosis of chest pain should be a consideration of herpes zoster infection or "shingles." Most clinicians assume that a diagnosis of herpes zoster would be self-evident by a simple visual inspection of a patient's chest and trunk. Classically, herpes zoster reactivation manifests as a painful, itchy, erythematous vesicular eruption that follows a unilateral dermatome. However, the key is that pain with shingles may precede any semblance of rash by several days.

Varicella-zoster virus, which causes chickenpox, remains in a dormant stage in the dorsal root ganglia. On reactivation the virus travels through the sensory nerve fibers, manifesting as a rash in specific dermatomal distributions. Zoster is most commonly seen in older adults and in chronically immunosuppressed patients, particularly HIV/acquired immunodeficiency syndrome (AIDS) patients, and those receiving chemotherapy, corticosteroids, and other immunosuppressive medications.

Symptoms
- Prodrome of headache, ++ malaise, ++ dysesthesias, ++ and rarely fever +
- Pain of variable severity and typically "burning" in quality ++++
- History of chickenpox +++++

Signs
- Erythematous, pruritic, painful eruption with fluid-filled vesicles that follow a specific dermatome and does not cross midline ++++
- Vesicles and rash usually evolve over days to form ulcerations and crust.
- Resolution phase occurs over weeks and may be complicated by scarring, variation in pigmentation, and postherpetic neuralgia (PHN).
- Contiguous dermatomes may be involved in 20% of cases, but are nonadjacent. ++
- Bilateral dermatomal involvement is exceedingly rare except in immunocompromised patients in whom disseminated zoster can occur. +
- Thoracic and lumbar dermatomes are involved most commonly. ++++

Workup
- Herpes zoster is usually a clinical diagnosis based on historical and physical examination findings.
- If the presentation is atypical, particularly in immunocompromised patients, there are several methods to confirm the diagnosis:
  - Viral cultures of vesicular fluid for herpes zoster
    - Long turn-around time and false-negative results are common if inadequate specimen obtained
  - Tzanck smear
    - Floor of the vesicle scraped onto slide and then stained with Wright's or Giemsa stain
    - Will have result fast, but does not distinguish from herpes simplex infection
  - Direct antigen staining
    - Similar to Tzanck smear except material on slide sent to laboratory for direct antigen staining for herpes zoster antigen

- Advantages include quick turn-around time and test is highly sensitive and specific.
- In otherwise healthy, young patients without apparent risk factors for zoster, consider checking HIV status.
- In patients with evidence of involvement of the first branch of the trigeminal nerve (vesicles on the forehead, tip or side of the nose, swelling of the eyelid, or conjunctivitis) consider emergent consultation with ophthalmologist because of the risk of herpes zoster ophthalmicus, which may threaten vision.
- Patients with involvement of the pinna or external auditory canal may develop facial nerve palsy, often with ipsilateral hearing impairment (Ramsay-Hunt syndrome).

Comments and Treatment Considerations

The goals of treatment are to reduce symptoms of zoster and to prevent complications. Zoster is usually a self-limited illness in immunocompetent patients. The main complication in these patients is the development of PHN, which is defined as pain that persists beyond 30 days from the onset of rash and may last up to months or years. There is a direct correlation between a patient's age and duration of PHN.

In immunosuppressed patients, diligent observation must be undertaken for the development of disseminated zoster infection.

The mainstay of treatment for zoster are antiviral medications. Initiate antivirals if rash started in the last 72 hours and treat for 7 to 10 days with acyclovir (800 mg five times a day), valacyclovir (1000 mg every 8 hours), and famciclovir (500 mg every 8 hours). Studies have shown benefit compared with placebo administration in halting new lesion formation, shortening the duration of viral shedding and zoster-associated pain, but no conclusive evidence for the prevention of PHN. Antivirals are more beneficial the sooner they are started after symptom onset. Adjust antiviral dosages in patients with renal impairment.

Adjunctive corticosteroids therapy: Evidence suggests that steroids lead to an acceleration in cutaneous healing and an earlier resolution of acute pain. Steroid therapy has no clear effect on PHN. Symptomatic treatment may include narcotics when pain is not relieved with oral analgesics. Care should also be taken to keep lesions clean and dry to prevent bacterial superinfection.

Patients infected with zoster remain infectious up to the point when the last lesion crusts over. Care should be taken for contagious patients to avoid contact with anyone who does not have a history of varicella infection; the most vulnerable individuals are pregnant women and immunocompromised hosts. Zostavax is a new vaccine that has been FDA approved for the prevention of herpes zoster in persons 60 years and older who have a history of chickenpox.

MUSCULOSKELETAL CHEST WALL PAIN

Musculoskeletal chest wall pain is the established cause of chest pain in up to one third of cases seen in an outpatient setting. +++ It also must be entertained as a diagnosis in the ER despite the lower prevalence there (approximately 7%). ++ It is difficult to make this diagnosis within the ER because a sizable percentage of patients who ultimately are shown to have chest pain of cardiac etiology will have "reproducibility" of pain through palpation or movement. Establishing a musculoskeletal cause of chest pain can not only alleviate anxiety around the concern of a life-threatening cause of pain, but also obviate the need for expensive testing.

A diverse array of anatomic structures in and around the thorax (e.g., muscles, fascia, bone, cartilage, and nerves) may be responsible for musculoskeletal chest pain. Chest pain of musculoskeletal origin is a diagnosis of exclusion; more serious disorders involving the cardiovascular, pulmonary, and gastrointestinal systems must be excluded.

Symptoms
- Pain is often localized, nagging, and insidious in onset.
- Pain may be acute, stabbing, and often radiates to other locations.
- Pain is often exacerbated by movement.
- Pain is usually relieved by analgesics and local application of heat.

Signs
- Biceps tendinitis, pectoral myofasciitis, intercostal muscle spasm, or inflammation
  - Localized pain at the respective anatomic site worsened by direct palpation or movement of those muscle groups ++++
- Costochondritis
  - Tenderness at the costochondral junction ++++
  - "Tietze's syndrome" if localized swelling also present
- Sternoclavicular arthritis, manubriosternal arthritis, xiphoid process pain
  - Localized tenderness at these articulations ++++
  - Often present with systemic arthritides
- Cervical or thoracic spine arthritis or disk disease
  - Tenderness often elicited on spinous process palpation +++
  - Dermatomal distribution of pain is elicited by careful examination of the chest wall.
  - High index of suspicion is needed if pain is the only symptom
  - Distal neurologic findings may be found with progression of the lesion.
- Rib or intercostal muscle trauma
  - Tenderness at the site of trauma ++++
  - Often exacerbated by truncal movement and breathing +++
- Bony pain from metastases
  - Palpable tender mass may be appreciated at the site of metastasis.
- Shoulder pain
  - Provocative testing of passive and active ROM of the shoulders will elicit pain with radiation to the chest wall.

- Fibromyalgia
  - Tenderness elicited at 11 or more of a possible 18 tender points ++++
  - Trigger point image available at www.triggerpoints.net

Workup
- ECG is generally indicated even if suspicion of musculoskeletal etiology is high.
- Chest radiography may be indicated to rule out pneumothorax, pneumonia, or rib fractures among other etiologies.

Comments and Treatment Considerations
Replication of the patient's chest pain by palpation of the chest wall is 87% specific for the diagnosis of musculoskeletal chest wall pain. Nevertheless, 7% of chest pain reproduced by palpation may be associated with cardiac ischemia or pulmonary emboli.

Musculoskeletal chest pain may occur in isolation, or may be present concurrently with other causes of chest pain. Analgesics, including acetaminophen, NSAIDs, and/or opiate analgesics along with local measures such as heat application may be indicated for symptomatic relief of musculoskeletal chest pain. Physical therapy may be beneficial for musculoskeletal chest pain unresponsive to these measures. Complete resolution of the chest pain after local injection of lidocaine into the affected region can both diagnose musculoskeletal chest pain and provide therapeutic relief.

PNEUMONIA

See Chapter 16.

PNEUMOTHORAX

See Chapter 38.

PULMONARY EMBOLUS

Approximately 600,000 cases of pulmonary embolus (PE) are diagnosed in the United States annually. PE accounts for 10% of all hospital deaths, and the attributable mortality from a PE is 15% to 30%. Making a firm diagnosis of a PE can be challenging because the diagnosis of a PE must take into account the clinical pretest probability (by the modified Wells clinical prediction tool [Fig. 12-1]), results of a high sensitivity D-dimer test, and results of noninvasive imaging studies. The clinical pretest probability for a PE is a critical determinant for the interpretation of noninvasive imaging studies during a PE workup.

PE falls under three different classifications: uncomplicated, submassive, and massive. An uncomplicated PE has no hemodynamic

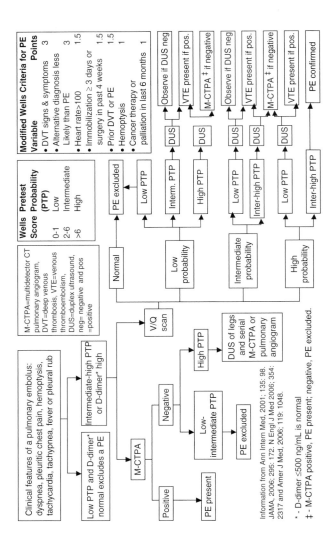

FIGURE 12-1 Diagnosis of pulmonary embolus.

Clinical features of a pulmonary embolus: dyspnea, pleuritic chest pain, hemoptysis, tachycardia, tachypnea, fever or pleural rub

M-CTPA=multidetector CT pulmonary angiogram, DVT=deep venous thrombosis, VTE=venous thromboembolism, DUS=duplex ultrasound, neg= negative and pos =positive

Modified Wells Criteria for PE	
Variable	**Points**
• DVT signs & symptoms	3
• Alternative diagnosis less Likely than PE	3
• Heart rate>100	1.5
• Immobilization ≥ 3 days or surgery in past 4 weeks	1.5
• Prior DVT or PE	1.5
• Hemoptysis	1
• Cancer therapy or palliation in last 6 months	1

Wells Score	Pretest Probability (PTP)
0-1	Low
2-6	Intermediate
>6	High

Information from Ann Intern Med, 2001; 135: 98. JAMA, 2006; 295: 172. N Engl J Med 2006; 354: 2317 and Amer J Med, 2006; 119: 1048.

* - D-dimer ≤500 ng/mL is normal
‡ - M-CTPA positive, PE present; negative, PE excluded.

compromise or ventilatory dysfunction. A submassive PE causes secondary pulmonary hypertension and right heart strain, but there are no signs of shock. A massive PE is usually the result of a "saddle embolus," which obstructs blood flow to the pulmonary arteries causing obstructive shock.

Symptoms
- Dyspnea ++++
- Pleuritic chest pain +++
- Cough +++
- Leg pain ++
- Hemoptysis ++
- Palpitations ++

Signs
- Tachypnea: Respiratory rate greater than 20 ++++
- Rales +++
- Leg swelling +++
- Tachycardia: Heart rate more than 100 bpm +++
- Wheezes ++
- Diaphoresis ++
- Fever: Temperature more than or equal to $38.5°$ C ++
- Pleural rub +

Workup
- Investigate for any risk factors for a venous thromboembolism (VTE).
- All patients should have a thorough history and examination because 10% to 20% of patients with an idiopathic VTE have an underlying malignancy.
- Investigate for any family history of clotting problems or cancer.
- The chest radiograph may be normal or show either atelectasis or a pleural-based density.
- An ECG typically shows only sinus tachycardia.
- In one third of patients with a submassive or massive PE, the ECG shows signs of acute right heart strain, often with an S1Q3T3 pattern.
- CBC, BMP, and high-sensitivity D-dimer test
- Recommend using a quantitative, rapid ELISA D-dimer test (sensitivity 95%)
- Pulse oximetry is usually adequate.
- An arterial blood gas is generally not helpful in making the diagnosis of PE because there is a normal alveolar-arterial oxygen gradient in up to 20% of patients with a PE. It can provide information about ventilation (assess $PaCO_2$).

RISK STRATIFICATION OF PE

Troponin I

- Troponin I is increased in 16% to 39% of patients with a documented acute PE.
- Troponin I is thought to be a surrogate marker for right ventricular dysfunction.
- The mortality rate approaches 33% when troponin I levels exceed 2 ng/mL.

Echocardiogram

- Right ventricular dysfunction/strain exists if any of the following are present:
  - RV diameter/LV diameter greater than 0.9
  - RV enlargement and loss of inspiratory collapse of the inferior vena cava
  - Evidence of marked pulmonary hypertension

 NONINVASIVE IMAGING TESTS FOR PE

Ventilation–perfusion (V/Q) Scans

- Diagnostic algorithm using V/Q scans
- Most V/Q scans will be indeterminate (73% of scans in the original Prospective Investigation of Pulmonary Embolism Diagnosis [PIOPED] study).

 MULTIDETECTOR CT PULMONARY ANGIOGRAMS (MCTPAS)

- The sensitivity of MCTPA alone is 83% and the specificity is 96%.
- In low-risk populations a negative MCTPA has a negative likelihood ratio of 0.07 and a negative predictive value (NPV) of 99.1% against having a significant venous thromboembolic event within 3 months. The predictive value of an MCTPA depends on the pretest probability as shown in Table 12-1. The NPV of a normal MCTPA is identical to that of a negative catheter pulmonary angiogram.
  - Additional benefits: MCTPAs can identify an alternative diagnosis two thirds of the time when a PE is not present; and the scan can assess for right ventricular enlargement, which can be a marker of right ventricular strain in a submassive PE.
  - MCTPA limitations: They are often not interpretable if there is motion artifact or in very obese patients with a body mass index (BMI) greater than 35; they have poor sensitivity for detecting subsegmental pulmonary emboli; and they require the administration of IV contrast.

Table 12-1. Predictive Value of Diagnostic Tests Based on Clinical Pretest Probability (PTP) in Patients with an Elevated D-Dimer Level

TESTING	LOW PTP	INTERMEDIATE PTP	HIGH PTP
MCTPA	NPV = 96% PPV = 58%	NPV = 89% PPV = 92%	NPV = 60% PPV = 96%
MCTPA-CTV	NPV = 97% PPV = 57%	NPV = 92% PPV = 90%	NPV = 82% PPV = 96%

MCTPA-CTV, Multidetector computed tomography pulmonary angiogram-computed tomography venogram; *NPV,* negative predictive value; *PPV,* positive predictive value.

Adapted from PIOPED II data in Stein PD, Woodard PK, Weg J, et al: Diagnostic pathways in acute pulmonary embolism, *Am J Med* 119:1048-1055, 2006.

 DUPLEX ULTRASOUND OF LOWER EXTREMITIES

- A lower extremity duplex ultrasound is indicated when the V/Q scan results are indeterminate. In this case, a duplex ultrasound documenting a DVT obviates the need for an MCTPA.

 CT VENOGRAM (CTV)

- Can be performed simultaneously with an MCTPA and increases sensitivity of VTE detection from 83% to 90%. Specificity is 95%.

 A HYPERCOAGULABLE WORKUP

- Candidates for a hypercoagulable workup
  - High likelihood of a thrombophilia: Idiopathic PE less than 45; recurrent PE; first-degree relative with PE less than 50; cerebral or visceral vein thrombosis; any pregnancy-, postpartum- or estrogen-related VTE; or any history of a stillbirth or three or more unexplained spontaneous abortions in less than 10 weeks
- What to order: Check activated protein C (APC) resistance, prothrombin gene mutation, anticardiolipin antibody, lupus anticoagulant, and levels of plasma homocysteine, antithrombin III, protein C, factor VIII activity, and protein S
- When to order it: Check all lab tests after completing anticoagulation and the patient has been off of warfarin for at least 2 weeks.

DIAGNOSIS OR EXCLUSION OF PE (See Fig. 12–1)

- PE is excluded if:
  - A normal high-sensitivity D-dimer and a low pretest probability.
    - Normal high-sensitivity D-dimer and intermediate pretest probability exclude most cases of PE (NPV is 95%).
  - A normal MCTPA and low-intermediate pretest probability
  - Normal serial MCTPA and high pretest probability
  - Normal catheter pulmonary angiogram
  - A normal V/Q scan
  - A low-probability V/Q scan and a low clinical pretest probability
- Diagnosis of PE if:
  - PE visualized on an MCTPA
  - A high-probability V/Q scan and intermediate to high pretest probability

Comments and Treatment Considerations

The vast majority of patients with an acute PE will be treated in the hospital with acute heparinization and transitioned to long-term warfarin therapy. Exceptions include a submassive/massive PE for whom thrombolysis should be considered and those with a contraindication to anticoagulation who need placement of an inferior vena cava (IVC) filter. Patients with active cancer who have had an acute PE should receive LMWH for 3 to 6 months prior to transitioning to warfarin therapy.

In patients without absolute contraindications, start either heparin or LMWH and warfarin simultaneously and overlap at least 5 days and until international normalized ratio (INR) is greater than or equal to 2 for 24 hours. Give 80 units/kg IV bolus of heparin, then begin a drip at 18 units/kg/hr and titrate to maintain aPTT 1.5 times the upper limit of normal. LMWH: enoxaparin 1 mg/kg subcutaneously q12h or tinzaparin 175 units/kg subcutaneously daily. Warfarin: Typical starting dose is 5 mg PO daily in most adults.

Duration of anticoagulation:
- 3 months: DVT with transient risk factors
- 6 to 12 months: Idiopathic PE
- Until 6 weeks postpartum: PE during pregnancy
- Indefinite: Idiopathic life-threatening PE, PE with permanent thrombophilic state (e.g., cancer or high-risk hypercoagulable state)

 THROMBOLYSIS

- The American College of Chest Physicians suggests that patients who are hemodynamically unstable from a massive PE are candidates for systemic thrombolysis with tPA 100 mg infused over 2 hours (grade 2B).
- Thrombolysis for submassive PE resulted in a decreased need for vasopressor use, but no statistically significant mortality benefit.
- IV tPA has a 2% to 3% risk of intracranial hemorrhage and a 0.5% risk of death.

References

Abrams J: Chronic stable angina, *N Engl J Med* 352:2524–2533, 2005.

ACC/AHA Task Force: ACC/AHA guidelines for the management of patients with ST segment elevation MI—executive summary, *J Am Coll Cardiol* 44:671–719, 2004.

ACC/AHA Task Force: ACC/AHA guidelines for the management of patients with unstable angina and non-ST segment elevation MI, *J Am Coll Cardiol* 40:1366–1374, 2002.

AHA/ACC guidelines for secondary prevention for patients with coronary and other atherosclerotic vascular disease: 2006 update, *J Am Coll Cardiol* 47:2130–2139, 2006.

AHA Scientific Statement: Practical implementation of the guidelines for unstable angina/non ST segment elevation MI in the emergency department, *Ann Emerg Med* 46:185–197, 2005.

Cayley W: Diagnosing the cause of chest pain, *Am Fam Physician* 72:2012–2021, 2005.

Cheitlin MD, Armstrong WF, Aurigemma GP, et al: ACC/AHA/ASE 2003 Guideline Update *Circulation* 108:1146–1162, 2003.

Chinthamuneedi M: Diseases of the aorta in the critically ill, *Crit Care Resusc* 2:117–124, 2000.

Clark AM, Hartking L, Vandermeer B, et al: Meta-analysis: secondary prevention programs for patients with CAD, *Ann Intern Med* 143:659, 2005.

Constant J: The clinical diagnosis of nonanginal chest pain: the differentiation of angina from nonanginal chest pain by history, *Clin Cardiol* 6:11–16, 1983.

Fam AG, Smythe HA: Musculoskeletal chest wall pain, *Can Med Assoc J* 133:379–389, 1985.

Gnann JW, Whitley RJ: Herpes zoster, *N Engl J Med* 347:340–346, 2002.

Hagan PE, Nienaber CA, Isselbacher EM, et al: The international registry of acute aortic dissection (IRAD), new insights into an old disease, *JAMA* 283:897–903, 2000.

Harvey WP: Cardiac Pearls. Laennec Publishing MCMXCIII. ACC/AHA Writing Committee. Pocket Guidelines on the Management of Patients with Chronic Stable Angina, *J Am Coll Cardiol* 41:159–168, 2003.

Imazio M, Bobbio M, Cecchi E, et al: Colchicine as first-choice therapy for acute pericarditis, *Arch Intern Med* 165:1987–1991, 2005.

Isselbacher E: Thoracic and abdominal aortic aneurysms, *Circulation* 111:816–828, 2005.

Klompas M: Does this patient have an acute aortic dissection? *JAMA* 287:2262–2272, 2002.

Sarasin FP, Louis-Simonet M, Gaspoz J-M, et al. Detecting acute thoracic aortic dissection in the emergency department: time constraints and choice of the optimal diagnostic test, *Ann Emerg Med* 28:278–288, 1996.

Schmader K: Herpes zoster in older adults, *Aging Infect Dis* 32:1481–1486, 2001.

Shiga T, Wajima Z, Apfel C, et al: Diagnostic accuracy of transesophageal echocardiography, helical computed tomography, and magnetic resonance imaging for suspected thoracic aortic dissection, *Arch Intern Med* 166:1350–1356, 2006.

Swap CJ, Nagurney JT: Value and limitations of chest pain history in the evaluation of patients with suspected ACS, *JAMA* 294:2623–2629, 2005.

Troughton RW, Asher CR, Klein AL: Pericarditis, *Lancet* 363:717–727, 2004.

Whitley RJ, Weiss H, Gnann JW, et al: Acyclovir with and without prednisone for the treatment of herpes zoster: a randomized, placebo-controlled trial, *Ann Intern Med* 125:376–383, 1996.

Wood MJ, Johnson RW, McKendrick MW, et al: A randomized trial of acyclovir for 7 days and 21 days with and without prednisolone for treatment of acute herpes zoster, *N Engl J Med* 330:896–900, 1994.

CHAPTER 13

Child Abuse
Arwa Nasir

There are four recognizable forms of child maltreatment: child neglect, physical abuse, sexual abuse, and emotional abuse. Physical and sexual abuse tend to present acutely. Physicians should maintain a high index of suspicion for injuries among children particularly in younger age groups. Suspicion of any form of maltreatment, including neglect or emotional abuse, should prompt careful assessment and management following the principles outlined below.

PHYSICAL ABUSE

Estimates of numbers of abused children exceed reported statistics. Also, not all child maltreatment results in injuries. However, injuries resulting from intentional trauma tend to be more severe than accidental injuries.

Several factors haves been associated with an increased risk for physical abuse, including children living in households with unrelated adults (50-fold increased risk), children suffering from developmental disabilities (2.1 times higher risk), poverty (3 to 5 times higher risk in households with income less than $15,000), and adult-partner violence (4.9 times higher risk). The presence of risk factors should not be used as indicators of child abuse but rather to provide guidance for prevention and management.

Child abuse causes significant long-term medical and psychologic morbidity. Research indicates that brain development can be physiologically altered by prolonged, severe, and unpredictable stress, as frequently seen in child abuse. This alteration can negatively affect a child's physical, cognitive, emotional, and social development.

Symptoms and Signs
Child abuse should be suspected when a child presents with an injury inconsistent with the history given by the caretakers. In addition, certain injuries in children are unlikely to happen accidentally, and nonaccidental causes should be suspected whenever these injuries are encountered. For instance, long bone fractures are very uncommon in the preambulatory child and should be investigated. Skull fractures and intracranial bleeding are also unlikely to be the result of minor household accidents and should arouse suspicion.

- Injury not compatible with the history ++++
- Different stories from different caretakers ++++
- Major elements of the history change ++++
- History of previous nonaccidental trauma ++++
- History of abuse in siblings +++
- Long bone fractures in infants or toddlers ++++
- Skull fractures in infants or young children ++++
- Multiple bruises on torso +++
- Internal abdominal injuries in the absence of history of severe accidental trauma ++++
- Hollow viscus injury ++++
- Unexplained head injury in infants or young children ++++
- Retinal hemorrhages ++++
- Immersion burns +++
- Adult bite marks ++++
- Genital injuries ++++
- Sexually transmitted diseases ++++

SEXUAL ABUSE

Presentations of sexual abuse vary. However, the principles of evaluation and documentation are similar to that of physical abuse. The first priority should be given to medical evaluation and stabilization of the child. At a minimum, a superficial genital examination should be done; however, strong consideration should be given to referring the child to a physician experienced in evaluation of child abuse for a more detailed examination. This referral should be carried out expeditiously in all cases, and emergently in cases of acute sexual assault.

PRINCIPLES OF ASSESSMENT OF NONACCIDENTAL INJURIES

As in all cases of injuries and illness, the first priority for the physician treating a child with possible nonaccidental injury is to assess and provide medical care and stabilization of the child as needed. Depending on the severity of the injury, stabilization may involve activating the emergency trauma response system. This may include surgical and critical care specialists. Once stabilization has occurred, obtaining a careful history is the most critical next step.

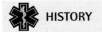 **HISTORY**

Information should be sought from all adults who witnessed the injury, and other adults who provide care for the child. History should be obtained from caretakers in a nonaccusatory manner. Important information to be elicited includes:

- Detailed history of events surrounding the injury
- Medical history including any chronic illnesses and previous injuries
- Developmental history including temperament and behavior
- Family history especially of metabolic, bone, and bleeding disorders
- Social history including household occupants, their employment, history of substance abuse, and domestic violence

The child can be interviewed if he or she is developmentally and emotionally able to answer questions. Care must be taken to ask open-ended, nonleading questions and reassure the child that the situation is not his or her fault. The child's responses, both verbal and nonverbal, should be accurately documented. The child should never be pressured to answer questions because he or she may be apprehensive about retribution for "telling." Sometimes victims of child abuse feel a sense of protectiveness toward the perpetrator.

 PHYSICAL EXAMINATION

- Complete and comprehensive physical examination to assess for other injuries that are not part of the chief complaint. This is essential in case other injuries are present that require prompt attention, such as CNS or orthopedic injury.
- Complete neurologic exam of the child. Funduscopic examination should be attempted; however, it is not recommended to dilate the eyes until the child has been stabilized so as not to interfere with the diagnostic value of the pupillary reflexes.
- Skin should be fully inspected for bruises, burns, and bites. Special attention should be paid to the face, head and neck, buttocks, upper arms, hands, and trunk. These areas are less prone to accidental trauma.
- Careful abdominal examination to detect any abdominal injuries
- Observation of the demeanor and emotional and mental status of the child and caretakers

 DOCUMENTATION

Documentation is especially important in cases of suspected nonaccidental injury or child maltreatment. This documentation should be done promptly and accurately and include all important details. Caretaker and child statements should be recorded verbatim if possible. Physical findings should be documented carefully, bruises and lacerations measured (not approximated), and photographs taken if possible. In addition, any treatments, consultations, referral, or reporting of the case should be documented, as well as plans for follow-up.

WORKUP

Laboratory workup is of limited value in the diagnosis of child abuse, except possibly for ruling out medical conditions that may mimic the presentation of nonaccidental injuries. A platelet count and coagulation profile may be needed if bruising is a major finding.

Imaging studies to document skeletal or CNS injuries play a major role in diagnosing abuse. Appropriate CNS imaging should be obtained if CNS injury is suspected. Skeletal surveys are recommended in suspected maltreatment of infants and young children.

Other laboratory and radiologic investigations may be indicated to assess the medical condition of the child and should be done accordingly.

 DIFFERENTIAL DIAGNOSIS

Rare metabolic disorders such as aminoaciduria can present with acute encephalopathy in the newborn period that may be difficult to differentiate from traumatic head injury in the acute phase before all the diagnostic tests are available. Also, some rare bone diseases such as osteogenesis imperfecta can produce fractures with little or no trauma. Children with bleeding diatheses may bruise easily and might have multiple bruises that can be confused with trauma. Occasionally skin conditions such as bullous impetigo and some chemical burns may mimic inflicted thermal burns.

It should also be kept in mind that trauma is very common in children. Most injuries in children are accidental and not inflicted. Injury patterns are seldom specific for abuse; rather it is the inconsistency of the injury with the explanation provided that should raise suspicion.

MANAGEMENT

Management of suspected physical or sexual abuse should incorporate the following major principles:
- Stabilization and treatment of the child as necessary, including activation of the emergency response system if needed, and referral for appropriate evaluation and diagnosis of injuries
- Protection from further harm
- Reporting to child protective services
- Evaluation of the family where the abuse occurred for treatment and rehabilitation or accountability

Accurate identification of possible nonaccidental injuries in children is critical in order to initiate appropriate evaluation, referral, and investigation.

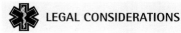

LEGAL CONSIDERATIONS

All 50 states and most countries in the world have laws that require physicians to report child abuse and neglect. Information on specific state laws are provided by the US Children's Bureau, the Administration for Children and Families, and the US Department of Health and Human Services.

PREVENTION OF CHILD ABUSE

The primary care physician is in an excellent position to prevent child maltreatment through:
• Providing anticipatory guidance in discipline and behavior management
• Awareness and screening for high-risk conditions such as domestic violence
• Early identification of signs of stress or unhealthy discipline behaviors
• Referral of parents or family to social services or mental health care as indicated
• Early identification and proper reporting and management of suspected abuse

References

Cairns AM, Mok JY, Welbury RR: Injuries to the head, face, mouth and neck in physically abused children in a community setting, *Int J Paediatr Dent* 15:310–318, 2005.

Child Welfare Information Gateway—resources from the US Department of Health and Human Services, includes information on child abuse and neglect. Available at www.childwelfare.gov/index.cfm (accessed January, 2011).

Kellogg N: The evaluation of sexual abuse in children, *Pediatrics* 116:506–512, 2005.

Kellogg ND: Evaluation of suspected child physical abuse, *Pediatrics* 119:1232–1241, 2007.

National Clearinghouse on Child Abuse and Neglect. Understanding the effects of maltreatment on early brain development. Available at http://nccanch.acf.hhs.gov (accessed January, 2011).

CHAPTER 14

Confusion
Alan Fischler and Mary Corrigan

Confusion, the impairment of higher thought processes, can be caused by a variety of illnesses, trauma, or medications. Confusion is one of the most common complaints encountered by family physicians, especially among their older adult patients. A symptomatic approach involving history, examination, and judicious use of laboratory and imaging will allow the clinician to provide optimal care for patients presenting with confusion.

DEMENTIA

Dementia is the syndrome of chronic and progressive impairment of memory and at least one other cognitive domain, resulting in decreased functional skills and impairments in social or occupational function, which does not occur only during delirium (delirium is acute with a specific "organic" cause requiring specific treatment). The vast majority of dementia is not reversible, but all treatment goals in dementia are to maintain independence, relieve patient suffering, and decrease caregiver burden, for as long as possible.

The DSM-IV-TR diagnostic criteria for Alzheimer's disease (AD) are presented in Table 14-1. AD is the most common form of dementia, followed by mixed-cause dementia (AD and vascular), vascular dementia, dementia with Lewy bodies, and Parkinson's disease with dementia (Table 14-2). "Reversible dementias," are better described as "potentially reversible," due to the low proportion who fully regain cognitive function.

Symptoms vary widely among individuals, disease stage, and type of dementia. It is important to corroborate patient history with another source. Symptoms can be classified as cognitive or behavioral.

Symptoms
- Difficulty forming new memories +++++
- Trouble recalling recent events, conversations, or objects +++++
- Difficulty recalling names of familiar people or objects
- Frequent use of imprecise terms in place of object names (calling a broom a "stick" or "a thing to sweep with")
- Map reading
- Difficulty discerning visual boundaries in the environment
- Managing financial affairs

- Planning meals, organizing shopping or excursions
- Driving
- Aggression, verbal or physical
- Repetitive vocalization or verbalization
- Delusions, often with paranoid content
- Hallucinations (seen early in dementia with Lewy bodies)
- Wandering or pacing
- Apathy and depressed affect
- Sleep cycle disturbances

Table 14-1. Alzheimer's Disease Diagnosis by DSM–IV–TR

1. Multiple cognitive impairments in both:
   - Memory impairment (difficulty learning new information or recall of previously learned information)
   - One or more of the following: aphasia, apraxia, agnosia, impaired executive functioning (planning, organizing, sequencing, and abstracting)
2. These disturbances result in significant occupational and/or social impairment and are a significant decline from prior function.
3. Gradual onset and progressive cognitive decline
4. Not due to other central nervous system, systemic, or substance-induced diseases known to cause dementia (cardiovascular disease; Parkinson's disease; Huntington's disease; subdural hematoma; normal pressure hydrocephalus; brain tumor; hypothyroidism; B_{12}, folic acid, or niacin deficiency; hypercalcemia; human immunodeficiency virus; or neurosyphilis)
5. Impairments do not occur exclusively during delirium.
6. Impairments not better accounted for by psychiatric disorders such as major depression or schizophrenia

Table 14-2. Dementias Types

DEMENTIA	SIGNS AND SYMPTOMS
Alzheimer's disease	Progressive course, prominent memory loss, language, executive functioning with symmetric neurologic examination
Vascular dementia	Asymmetric neurologic examination, risk factors or history of stroke (overlaps with Alzheimer's disease because both are common)
Dementia with Lewy bodies	Dementia with two out of three of the following: parkinsonism, fluctuating cognition, well-formed visual hallucinations. 50% have severe neuroleptic sensitivity. Some have rapid eye movement sleep behavior disorder.
Parkinson's disease with dementia	Parkinson's disease diagnosis precedes dementia by at least 1 year.
Frontotemporal dementia	Disinhibition, social inappropriateness, apathy and/or language problems worse than memory or visuospatial impairment. Onset usually before age 65.

Signs
- Neurologic examination
  - Physical examination findings depend on the stage and type of dementia.
  - In early AD the peripheral and cranial nerve examination is normal. Abnormal neurologic examination findings should prompt evaluation for conditions other than AD.
  - Parkinsonism is present in both Lewy body dementia and Parkinson's disease with dementia.
  - Myoclonus and seizures may be seen in advanced dementia.
  - Gait difficulties and urinary incontinence exist commonly in an older adult, but if newly associated with an early dementia, should raise suspicion of normal pressure hydrocephalus.
- Cognitive testing
  - The Mini-Mental State Examination (MMSE) identifies cognitive impairment in multiple domains on a 30-point scale, is used to screen for disease as well as follow disease progress over time, and takes about 10 minutes to perform. Scores less than 24 suggest cognitive impairment, but scores of 24 or more do not exclude impairment. It is relatively insensitive in early AD and shows little change with disease progression in severe AD. Educational level affects results.
  - The Mini-Cog is a 3-minute test that identifies people who need further evaluation and is relatively unbiased by education and literacy. It consists of asking the patient to register three unrelated words, followed by the Clock Drawing Test (correct placement of numbers, then hands, indicating "11:10"), then testing for uncued recall of the three words. Each word recalled yields 1 point. A normal clock drawing yields 2 points, and an abnormal clock yields 0 points. Mini-Cog scores of 0 to 2 suggest possible dementia; scores of 3 to 5 suggest no dementia.

Workup
- Blood tests to screen for comorbid conditions common in patients with suspected dementia and possible reversible causes. Syphilis and/or HIV serologic testing if high pretest probability, otherwise evidence does not strongly support routine testing
  - Complete blood cell count (CBC)
  - Electrolytes
  - Glucose
  - Folate
  - Vitamin B_{12}
  - Thyroid function
- Imaging
  - Structural neuroimaging
    - Noncontrast head CT to identify brain tumors, subdural hematoma, and normal pressure hydrocephalus (NPH) (rare)
    - Consider MRI, depending on availability, and if physical examination or risk factors suggest cerebrovascular disease.

- Functional neuroimaging
  - Single photon emission tomography (SPECT) and positron emission tomography (PET) imaging may add predictive value to the clinical diagnosis of AD, distinguishing AD from minimal cognitive impairment (MCI), and other dementias, but its routine use is not recommended at present.
- Consultation or referral considerations
  - Onset before 65 years of age
  - Behavior symptoms early or severe behavioral problems
  - Rapid course of disease (weeks to months rather than years)
  - Concerns about driving safety or independent living
  - Questions about functional neuroimaging (SPECT and PET), genetic testing, neuropsychologic testing, or genetic testing
  - Distinguishing dementia from MCI, depression, and uncommon secondary causes
- Staging
  - Use the MMSE score as follows:
    - Mild dementia: 18 to 23
    - Moderate dementia: 11 to 17
    - Severe dementia: 10 or less
    - MMSE scores decline on average about 3 points per year in AD, with a range of 0 to 6 points per year.
  - The Functional Assessment Staging Test (FAST)
    - 16-item scale reflecting the progressive functional losses of AD (Table 14-3)
    - FAST is easily understood by patients and caregivers.
    - Helps plan for future needs

Comments and Treatment Considerations

Avoid alcohol and smoking, control vascular risk factors, and encourage regular physical and mental activity. Identify drugs with anticholinergic properties and discontinue whenever possible. Vitamin E shows conflicting evidence for outcomes in AD, and is associated with increased cardiovascular mortality, so is not recommended routinely. Ginkgo biloba is not available in standardized formulations, so is not routinely recommended.

Some patients with mild to moderate AD show modest improvement in measures of cognition and function using the acetylcholinesterase inhibitors (donepezil, rivastigmine, and galantamine; Table 14-4). There is no conclusive evidence of efficacy for behavioral and neuropsychiatric symptoms in AD.

As a class these drugs commonly cause GI cholinergic side effects, such as nausea, anorexia, vomiting, and diarrhea, which may lead to weight loss. Tolerance often develops to the GI side effects. Some patients tolerate one acetylcholinesterase inhibitor better than another.

Cognition, behavior, and function (activities of daily living [ADL] and instrumental activities of daily living [IADL]) should be monitored at regular intervals (every 3 to 6 months). Continuation of the drug should be questioned if there is significant decline in MMSE and ADL 6 months after initiation of therapy, or when the patient reaches severe stage dementia (MMSE less than 10 and full ADL dependency).

Table 14-3. Functional Assessment Staging Test

FAST STAGE	FUNCTIONAL ASSESSMENT
1	No difficulties, either subjectively or objectively
2	Complains of forgetting location of objects; subjective work difficulties
3	Decreased job functioning evident to coworkers; difficulty in traveling to new locations
4	Decreased ability to perform complex tasks (e.g., planning dinner for guests; handling finances; marketing)
5	Requires assistance in choosing proper clothing
6a	Difficulty putting clothing on properly.
6b	Unable to bathe properly; may develop fear of bathing
6c	Inability to handle mechanics of toileting (i.e., forgets to flush; doesn't wipe properly)
6d	Urinary incontinence
6e	Fecal incontinence
7a	Ability to speak limited (1-5 words a day)
7b	All intelligible vocabulary lost
7c	Nonambulatory
7d	Unable to sit up independently
7e	Unable to smile
7f	Unable to hold head up

The functional staging score is highest ordinal value. Ignore item if assessed as being due to other causes apart from dementia.

Memantine has FDA approval for moderate dementia in AD. Memantine may be used alone, or in combination for patients already taking an acetylcholinesterase inhibitor. Side effects include dizziness, and less commonly confusion and hallucinations.

Caregivers should be monitored for stress and encouraged to gain support and education through their local Alzheimer's Association (1-800-272-3900 or www.alz.org). Adult daycare, respite care, and nursing home options should be discussed at the appropriate disease stages.

Patients should address choice of durable power of attorney for health care and other matters, as well as advance directives for end-of-life care while decision-making capacity is preserved.

Home safety is tied to availability of skilled caregivers and physical design of the home space. Use of the stove and other dangerous appliances and tools, cigarettes, and fireplace should be assessed at regular intervals. People with dementia who are at risk

Table 14-4. Medications for Alzheimer Disease

DRUG	CLASS	DOSE RANGE (MINIMUM THERAPEUTIC TO TARGET DOSE)	TITRATION SCHEDULE
Donepezil	Acetylcholine-sterase inhibitor	5-10 mg daily	5 mg at bedtime daily; increase to 10 mg daily after 6 weeks
Rivastigmine	Acetylcholin-esterase inhibitor	3-6 mg twice daily	1.5 mg twice daily, every 2 weeks; increase individual dose by 1.5 mg
Galantamine	Acetylcholin-esterase inhibitor	8-12 mg twice daily	4 mg twice daily; every 4 weeks increase individual dose by 4 mg
Memantine	NMDA receptor antagonist	10 mg twice daily	5 mg daily for >1 week; then increase total daily dose by 5 mg daily (divide dose twice daily), to 10 mg twice daily

for elopement should have an identification bracelet or necklace (such as Alzheimer's Association Safe Return Program) in addition to the appropriate level of supervision.

Plan for alternative transportation from the time of dementia diagnosis. Practice guideline recommendations for driving with mild dementia range from giving advice about impairment and increased risks to advising that all people with mild dementia must stop driving. Physicians should know local legal reporting requirements for dementia and options for older driver evaluation as described in the AMA/National Highway Traffic Safety Administration (NHTSA) guide.

Most people with dementia experience behavioral and neuropsychiatric symptoms. Disturbing delusions, hallucinations, and aggression symptoms increase caregiver burden and patient suffering. An organized approach is recommended, which is individualized, based on behavior type and severity, the type of underlying dementia, and patient-caregiver dynamics as follows:

• Step 1: Identify the nature of the behavior, provocatory factors, and effect of the behavior on patient and caregiver.
• Step 2: Review medication list and eliminate nonessential drugs and those with anticholinergic properties.
• Step 3: Evaluate and treat any pain symptoms and delirium (search for medication side effects, infection, systemic illness, superimposed CNS disease, bowel impaction, urinary retention).

- Step 4: Evaluate and treat any depression and anxiety (consider that pacing and repeated vocalizations may be mood symptoms, especially in dementia patients with language problems).
- Step 5: Conduct an environmental assessment, implement interventions, and provide caregiver education and support.
- Step 6: Consider starting a cholinesterase inhibitor in patients with mild to moderate AD.
- Step 7: Start an antipsychotic drug if the above interventions are ineffective, and the symptom is judged sufficiently threatening to safety and well-being of the patient or caregiver. Identify a target behavior symptom (e.g., physical aggression), goal for treatment, and time frame to attain improvement, then obtain informed consent regarding risks. Use the lowest dose of an atypical antipsychotic drug and monitor for side effects (especially sedation and extrapyramidal signs). Antipsychotic drug dose reduction should be attempted at least every 6 months. Atypical antipsychotic drugs have variable and modest effects on neuropsychiatric symptoms. The FDA has determined that atypical antipsychotic drugs are associated with increased mortality in the treatment of behavioral disturbances in older adults with dementia. Patients with Parkinson's disease and dementia can develop worsened movement disorder from typical or first-generation antipsychotic drugs (better tolerance is noted with atypical drugs, such as quetiapine). In Lewy body dementia, 50% of patients show severe neuroleptic sensitivity (worsened extrapyramidal symptoms, orthostasis, decreased level of consciousness), and first-generation antipsychotic drugs should be avoided.

Medicare guidelines for hospice referral require physician certification that life expectancy is 6 months or less, often interpreted as FAST stage 7a or higher, plus a major comorbid illness in the past 12 months.

The USPSTF states there is insufficient evidence for or against routine screening for dementia when it is not suspected by clinical presentation. Advocates of dementia screening emphasize the value of early diagnosis for planning future needs for support services.

Serum apolipoprotein E and cerebrospinal fluid (CSF) tau markers are not recommended for routine use. The results are often complex to interpret and have ethical/insurability issues requiring informed consent.

MEMORY LOSS WITHOUT DEMENTIA

People with MCI have memory problems but are not demented and are living independently. They may be experiencing memory loss without dementia. MCI is a heterogeneous group of people whose memory problems are stable, reversible, or in transition to dementia. About 6% to 25% of 65- to 89-year-olds with MCI will develop dementia per year, compared with 1% to 4% per year for similar-aged patients without MCI.

Symptoms
- Similar to early dementia memory complaints
- Do not affect ADL performance
- Subjective memory complaints, ideally confirmed by an informant ++++
- Fully independent in all ADL ++++

Signs
- Abnormal objective cognitive testing ++++
- Normal cognitive function in other domains besides memory ++++
- MMSE scores less than 24 ++++
- MMSE scores greater than or equal to 24, with further evaluation such as serial cognitive screening tests, or referral for neuropsychologic testing to confirm no physical examination abnormalities ++++
- Do not meet diagnostic criteria for dementia ++++

Workup
- Depression and sleep apnea can cause reversible memory problems. Referral for neuropsychologic testing can be useful in distinguishing normal memory from MCI and depression.
- Laboratory and imaging tests are not useful to distinguish MCI from normal or dementia, but may be applied to patients with MCI to detect underlying conditions that might cause mild cognitive problems, depending on clinical circumstances.

Comments and Treatment Considerations
Patients with MCI should be followed for development of dementia. There is no evidence to support use of vitamin E, cholinesterase inhibitors, or memantine in patients with MCI to prevent development of dementia.

DELIRIUM

Patients with delirium present acutely (hours to days) with a fluctuating course of disturbed cognition, attention, perception, and/or reduced awareness of their environment. Delirium is a syndrome associated with medical illness; therefore, its recognition should prompt a search for an underlying cause. Conditions requiring rapid diagnosis and treatment, such as hypoxia, hypoglycemia, encephalitis, and other infections should be considered.

Delirium is common, associated with high morbidity and mortality, and contributes to prolonged hospital length of stay. Poor rehabilitation and complications such as pneumonia and decubiti are often the result.

Delirium is classified as hyperactive, hypoactive, and mixed types. Psychomotor agitation is the hallmark of the hyperactive type, whereas the hypoactive type presents with lethargy or apathy. The mixed type has both hyperactive and hypoactive features. The gold standard diagnostic criteria for delirium are defined by DSM-IV-TR (Table 14-5). The Confusion Assessment Method (CAM) is a validated bedside tool (Table 14-6) that can be completed in 5 minutes and accurately diagnoses delirium.

Table 14-5. DSM-IV-TR Criteria for Delirium

- Disturbance of consciousness (i.e., reduced clarity of awareness about the environment) with reduced ability to focus, sustain, or shift attention
- A change in cognition (e.g., memory deficit, disorientation, language disturbance) or development of a perceptual disturbance that is not better accounted for by a preexisting, established, or evolving dementia
- The disturbance develops over a short period of time (usually hours to days) and tends to fluctuate during the course of a day.
- Evidence from the history, physical examination, or laboratory findings indicates that the disturbance is caused by a direct physiologic consequences of a general medical condition.

From *Diagnostic and Statistical Manual of Mental Disorders,* Fourth Edition, Washington, DC, 2000, American Psychiatric Association.

Table 14-6. Confusion Assessment Method (CAM) for Delirium Diagnosis

The diagnosis of delirium requires the presence or abnormal rating for the features (1) and (2), and either (3) or (4).

FEATURE	DELIRIUM DIAGNOSIS	CONFUSION ASSESSMENT METHOD
1	Acute onset and fluctuating course	Is there evidence of an acute change in mental status from the patient's baseline? Did this behavior fluctuate during the past day, i.e., tend to come and go or increase and decrease in severity?
2	Inattention	Does the patient have difficulty focusing attention, e.g., being easily distractible or having difficulty keeping track of what was being said?
3	Disorganized thinking	Is the patient's speech disorganized or incoherent, such as rambling or irrelevant conversation, unclear or illogical flow of ideas, or unpredictable switching from subject to subject?
4	Altered level of consciousness	This feature is shown by any answer other than "alert" to the following question: Overall, how would you rate this patient's level of consciousness?

Alert (normal), vigilant (hyperalert), lethargic (drowsy), stuporous (difficult to arouse), or comatose (unarousable)

From Inouye SK, van Dyck CH, Alessi C, et al: Clarifying confusion: the confusion assessment method, *Ann Intern Med* 113:941-948, 1990.

Symptoms
- High individual variability within a single episode
- Clouding of consciousness
- Decreased awareness of the environment
- Sleep cycle disturbances range from mild insomnia or excessive daytime sleepiness to severe nocturnal agitation and confusion
- Perceptual disturbances (illusions and hallucinations) are usually visual
- Delusions with paranoid features
- Difficulty following the direction of conversations
- Impaired orientation
- Difficulty with multistep commands

Signs
- Reverse spelling of words or sequences, such as spelling one's name or a familiar word backward
- Repeating in reverse order the days of the week or months of the year
- Counting backward from 20
- The Serial Seven Subtraction Test
- Digit-span testing
- Tests of cognition such as the Mini-Cog or MMSE are usually abnormal.
- Because delirium can complicate a preexisting dementia (diagnosed or not), subsequent serial testing to document cognition resolution or baseline is valuable.
- Focal neurologic examination findings may or may not be present. Any abnormality, if present, should provoke an evaluation for underlying neurologic disease; likewise, abnormalities in vital signs and general physical examination, if present, should prompt evaluation.

Workup
- Check oxygen saturation and blood glucose.
- Obtain a complete medical history.
- Interview secondary sources about prior level of cognition and function, recent illness, ingestions, trauma, and review the medication list, with close attention to new medications and those with anticholinergic properties.
- Perform a complete physical and neurologic examination.
- Cognitive testing: Mini-Cog or MMSE, tests of attentional ability such as reverse order word sequences or digit span
- Basic laboratory tests are urinalysis, electrolytes, glucose, liver function tests, CBCD, TSH, ECG, chest x-ray, pulse oximetry, or arterial blood gas.
- Additional laboratory tests: Depending on individual presentation, history, and physical examination signs, consider serum and urine toxicology, rapid plasma reagin (RPR) or Venereal Disease Research Laboratory (VDRL), heavy metal screen, vitamin B_{12} and folate, ANA, urine porphyrins, ammonia, HIV; drug levels (digoxin, lithium, theophylline, phenobarbital, cyclosporine).
- CT or MRI of the head, or EEG if concern for seizures
- Lumbar puncture when there is concern for CNS infection

Comments and Treatment Considerations

There are two primary goals of treatment for delirium. First, identify and treat the underlying cause. Review the medication list for adverse drug effects, anticholinergic drugs, and drug interactions. Eliminate any offending agents. Seek early diagnosis of serious, underlying medical illness, which include:

- Infections (urinary tract, pneumonia, CNS)
- Electrolyte imbalance (dehydration, hyper- and hypoglycemia)
- Acute coronary syndromes
- Acute stroke (rare cause)
- Hypoxia
- Hyper- or hypothermia
- Noninfectious encephalopathy: hypertensive/Wernicke's, liver failure, other
- Ethyl alcohol (ETOH) or drug intoxications and withdrawal syndromes

Second, relieve distress and ensure safety of both patient and caregiver from the cognitive and behavioral effects of the delirium. Delirium can impair cognition and perceptions to a degree that patients are unable to safely care for themselves and may pose a danger to themselves and others. Decisional capacity is variably affected. It may be preserved partially, intermittently, or globally impaired. Physicians should be familiar with the patient's advanced directives and local law as it relates to emergency treatment and surrogate decision making.

Patients need to be assessed for suicide risk, falls, and elopement. Medically nonessential lines should be removed. Physical restraints can increase agitation and risk for entrapment or asphyxia injuries. Continuous presence of a professional sitter is the preferred means for dealing with agitation. If physical restraints are used, documentation of indication and periodic reassessment of need is required.

Orient to time and place with wall clocks, calendars, and gentle reminders by staff; familiar pictures or objects may help reduce anxiety. Reduce noise and excess stimuli as much as possible. Windows and natural light sequences may help lessen disorientation; individuals whose symptoms worsen at night may benefit from improved lighting. Ensure use of hearing aids and eyeglasses. Engage the patient in physical activity as early as possible with therapies and nursing.

Antipsychotic medications may be required to improve patient safety and reduce distress until the underlying cause is fully treated. Of the antipsychotic medications, haloperidol has the most extensive record of use. The general dictum is to start with low doses, maintain an effective dose for several days (typically 2 to 3 days), then taper down the dose and discontinue. In older adults, haloperidol doses as low as 0.25 to 0.5 mg twice daily, and every 4 hours as needed, may be effective. In younger adults, haloperidol doses of 1 to 2 mg twice daily and every 2 to 4 hours as needed are used. Higher doses are used in more agitated patients. Benzodiazepine use is not recommended except for alcohol or benzodiazepine withdrawal.

POINTS OF INTEREST

- Vulnerable state and precipitating event: the more vulnerable the brain, the less of a precipitating event is needed to cause delirium.
- Pathophysiology of the vulnerable brain is believed related to cholinergic deficiency state, and therefore those individuals with dementia are more vulnerable to developing delirium.
- Duration of delirium and associated cognitive impairment may last weeks to months from the time of a precipitating event and some feel there is never a complete return to baseline, pointing to the need for primary prevention.
- Hospitalization and surgery, particularly hip surgery, portends a greater risk for development of delirium.

References

American Medical Association. *Physician's guide to assessing and counseling older drivers* Available at www.ama-assn.org/ama/pub/category/10791/html (accessed March 30, 2011).

American Psychiatric Association: Practice guideline for the treatment of patients with delirium, *Am J Psychiatry* 156:1–20, 1999.

American Psychiatric Association: *Diagnostic and Statistical Manual of Mental Disorders*, Fourth Edition, Washington, DC, 1994.

Borson S, Scanlan J, Brush M, et al: The Mini-Cog: a cognitive "vital signs" measure for dementia screening in multi-lingual elderly, *Int J Geriatr Psychiatry* 15:1021–1027, 2000.

Clarfield AM: The decreasing prevalence of reversible dementias: an updated meta-analysis, *Arch Intern Med* 163:2219–2229, 2003.

Crum RM, Anthony JC, Bassett SS, Folstein MF: Population-based norms for the Mini-Mental State Examination by age and educational level, *JAMA* 269:2386–2391, 1993.

Delagarza V: Pharmacologic treatment of Alzheimer's disease: an update, *Am Fam Physician* 68:1365–1372, 2003.

Dubinsky RM, Stein AC, Lyons K: Practice parameter: risk of driving and Alzheimer's disease (an evidence-based review): Report of the Quality Standards Subcommittee of the American Academy of Neurology, *Neurology* 54:2205–2211, 2000.

Folstein MF, Folstein SE, McHugh PR: Mini-mental state. A practical method for grading the cognitive state of patients for the clinician, *J Psychiatr Res* 12:189–198, 1975.

Inouye SK, van Dyck CH, Alessi C, et al: Clarifying confusion: the confusion assessment method, *Ann Intern Med* 113:941–948, 1990.

Knopman DS et al: Practice parameter: diagnosis of dementia (an evidence-based review): Report of the Quality Standards Subcommittee of the American Academy of Neurology, *Neurology* 56:1143–1153, 2001. Available at www.neurology.org/cgi/content/full/56/9/1143 (accessed Oct 17, 2006).

McKeith IG, Dickson DW, Lowe J, et al: Diagnosis and management of dementia with Lewy bodies: third report of the DLB consortium, *Neurology* 65:1863–1872, 2005.

Modi S: Which late-stage Alzheimer's patients should be referred for hospice care? *J Fam Pract* 54:984–986, 2005.

Petersen RC, Stevens JC, Ganguli M, et al: Practice parameter: early detection of dementia: mild cognitive impairment (an evidence-based review). Report of the Quality Standards Subcommittee of the American Academy of Neurology, *Neurology* 56:1133–1142, 2001.

Practice guideline for treatment of patients with Alzheimer's disease and other dementias of late life. American Psychiatric Association, *Am J Psychiatry* 154:1–39, 1997.

Reisberg B: Functional assessment staging test (FAST), *Psychopharmacol Bull* 24:653–659, 1988.

Sink KM, Holden KF, Yaffe K: Pharmacological treatment of neuropsychiatric symptoms of dementia: a review of the evidence, *JAMA* 293:596–608, 2005.

U.S. Food and Drug Administration: *FDA public health advisory: deaths with antipsychotics in elderly patients with behavioral disturbances.* Available at www.fda.gov/cder/drug/advisory/antipsychotics.htm (accessed February 17, 2011).

U.S. Preventive Services Task Force: *Screening for dementia: recommendations and rationale*, Agency for Healthcare Research and Quality, Rockville, MD. Available at www.ahrq.gov/clinic/3rduspstf/dementia/dementrr.htm (accessed February 17, 2011).

CHAPTER 15

Congestion
Ted C. Schaffer, Mary Parks Lamb, Jackie Weaver-Agostoni,
and Steven R. Wolfe

The most prevalent upper airway complaint is rhinitis—an inflammation of the nasal lining involving the cavernous tissues in the turbinates. Although nasal congestion is rarely a life-threatening problem, its patient effect in terms of frequency and cost is huge. In a given year the average adult averages two viral upper respiratory infection (URI) episodes whose major symptom is nasal congestion, whereas infants and young children experience six to eight episodes per year. An estimated 20% of the population suffers to some extent from seasonal or perennial allergic rhinitis, while an equivalent number experience nonallergic rhinitis symptoms. The pharmaceutical market for cold medicines and remedies is estimated at $5 billion, and an additional $10 billion is spent on associated disorders including allergic and nonallergic rhinitis, sinusitis, and sequelae such as otitis media and bronchitis. The four basic causes of nasal congestion include acute viral infection (rhinosinusitis), acute and chronic sinusitis, allergic rhinitis, and nonallergic rhinitis.

ACUTE RHINITIS

Acute rhinitis is overwhelmingly viral in nature, and is actually better termed acute rhinosinusitis because both sinus and nasal passages are involved. Causative agents include rhinoviruses, adenoviruses, respiratory synovial viruses, parainfluenza viruses, and enteroviruses. The greatest challenge in the care of viral rhinosinusitis is to distinguish between the acute symptoms, which are viral, and the sequelae (sinusitis, otitis media), which may have a bacterial component.

Symptoms
- Nasal congestion ++++
- Rhinorrhea: The nose may produce up to 1 L/day of discharge ++++
- May have other sequelae such as cough, sore throat, or myalgias ++

Signs
- Swollen nasal turbinates ++++
- Nasal discharge: May vary in quality +++

Workup
- Contrary to popular belief, the quality of the coryza (thin versus thick) and color (clear versus yellow or green) does not help distinguish between viral and bacterial etiology.
- The greatest differentiation is time—Symptoms less than 7 to 10 days' duration are rarely bacterial
- Viral symptoms can last 10 to 14 days—The clinical key is that the patient is improving, with the worst day usually being the second day of illness.

Comments and Treatment Considerations
Treatment is aimed at symptomatic relief. Fortunately patient expectations of antibiotic prescribing has declined. Antibiotics should be used only if symptoms have not resolved by 10 days or if there is worsening after 5 to 7 days.

Although there is some evidence to suggest that antibiotic therapy may be appropriate after 5 to 7 days of purulent drainage, most clinicians advise delaying antibiotics until there are other sequelae.

Decongestants are the first-line treatment for acute upper respiratory infections. Topical decongestants produce vasoconstriction by stimulating the lamina propria of local vessels. Sympathomimetic amines (phenylephrine and ephedrine) are less toxic to nasal cilia. Imidazoline (naphazoline, oxymetazoline, tetrahydrozoline, xylometazoline) have less myocardial and bronchiolar effect. The biggest risk for topical agents is tachyphylaxis leading to rhinitis medicamentosa in as little as 3 days. Therefore, most clinicians avoid their use.

Oral decongestants produce systemic α-adrenoceptor agonist activity. Three major products—ephedrine, pseudoephedrine, and phenylephrine—diminish nasal obstruction, but have no effect on nasal secretion. Because they produce generalized peripheral vasoconstriction, they must be used cautiously in patients with cardiovascular disease or other systemic diseases.

Antihistamines have not been proven to provide symptomatic relief in clinical trials. Topical (nasal) antihistamines are also unproven for acute viral URIs. Menthol may improve the subjective sensation of nasal congestion even though it does not actually change nasal airflow.

Unproven treatments include a number of remedies that have *not* been demonstrated to relieve common cold symptoms when subjected to clinical trials such as echinacea (studies affected by variable compounding), vitamin C (role in prophylaxis remains controversial), zinc lozenges, antiviral agents, antibiotics, humidified air, and increased fluid intake.

ACUTE AND CHRONIC SINUSITIS

Sinusitis is an infection or inflammation of the nasal mucosal passages and one or more of the paranasal sinuses. The most common sequence of events leading to sinusitis involves a viral rhinosinusitis that persists longer than 10 days to 2 weeks and becomes a secondary bacterial infection within the sinus cavity. Unilateral symptoms and double worsening of symptoms (initial improvement followed by worsening) suggest bacterial infection. *Streptococcus pneumoniae, Haemophilus influenzae,* or *Moraxella catarrhalis* are the resident bacteria most commonly involved in acute sinusitis. Acute sinusitis lasts up to 4 weeks.

Subacute sinusitis, a continuation of acute sinusitis, lasts 4 to 12 weeks. Chronic sinusitis persists at least 12 consecutive weeks. With either acute or chronic sinusitis, the osteomeatal complex (OMC), the structure through which the sinuses drain, obstructs in the face of inflammation, and leads to mucus impaction, bacterial proliferation, and pressure increases. Thus an abscess forms within the sinus cavity. Because the presentations of viral upper respiratory illness and acute bacterial sinusitis are similar, accurate clinical diagnosis is challenging. Key points in management include eliciting the time frame of symptoms and using appropriate antibiotics.

Symptoms
- Nasal congestion ++++
- Purulent rhinorrhea ++++
- Facial pain (especially unilateral) +++
- Double worsening (worse at day 2, then better, then worse a few days later) +++
- Dental pain ++
- Headache ++
- Postnasal drip ++
- Nighttime cough ++
- Hyposmia ++
- Fever ++
- Fatigue ++
- Malaise ++
- Body aches ++

Signs
- Purulent nasal drainage ++++
- Mucosal edema ++++
- Sinus tenderness, especially unilateral +++
- Fever ++
- Halitosis ++

Workup
- For acute sinusitis, the diagnosis is primarily clinical, and thus most testing is not contributory.
- Transillumination, once popular, is not now recommended.
- Radiographs of the sinuses are more readily available but are not as accurate. The presence of an air fluid level is more suggestive of sinusitis than is just mucosal thickening.
- CT imaging, though not recommended in the routine diagnosis of acute sinusitis, can play an important role in the evaluation of chronic or recurrent sinusitis.

- Sinus aspirate culture, though the gold standard for diagnosis, realistically is not performed unless the patient is very ill or immunocompromised.
- Rhinoscopy may be useful in the evaluation of chronic sinusitis, especially to rule anatomic obstruction at the OMC.
- For chronic sinusitis that fails to respond to antibiotics, other etiologies should be considered including underlying allergies, anatomic defects, or immunologic deficits.

Comments and Treatment Considerations

In the vast majority of cases, antibiotic therapy is not indicated. Reassurance, symptomatic treatment, and follow-up are recommended.

If antibiotics are used, narrow-spectrum first-line agents (amoxicillin, TMP-SMX [Bactrim], doxycycline, erythromycin) may be considered for acute sinusitis. A 10-day course is recommended. Some newer drugs have 3- to 5-day courses.

If there is no improvement after 48 to 72 hours or if sinusitis is recurrent or chronic, use second-line agents (amoxicillin-clavulanate, second- or third-generation cephalosporins, expanded spectrum macrolides, or fluoroquinolones). A 3-week course is recommended for initial treatment of chronic sinusitis.

For refractory symptoms, change to a fluoroquinolone and consider treatment for up to 6 weeks. Intranasal steroids are recommended for decreasing mucosal inflammation and swelling and for opening the OMC, especially for those with known allergic disease. Hydration may be helpful. Saline irrigation, humidification, and mechanical cleansing of the sinuses can be beneficial for chronic sinusitis. Topical decongestants may be considered but only if use is limited to 3 days or less. Systemic decongestants may provide relief, but there is little evidence to support this.

Analgesics may be useful for headache or referred dental pain. Mucolytic agents (guaifenesin) may be beneficial to thin secretions and promote sinus drainage. Surgical management should be considered for those with abnormalities of the sinuses or OMC by CT or rhinoscopy, and for those who require three or more courses of antibiotics in 12 months.

ALLERGIC RHINITIS

Allergic rhinitis (AR) ranks as the sixth most prevalent chronic disease in the United States. Affecting an estimated 40 million people, AR is also the most common chronic disease affecting children, and contributes to poor school performance and absenteeism.

AR is classified as seasonal, perennial, or occupational based on timing of symptoms. Seasonal AR produces symptoms predictably during certain times of the year and is generally triggered by outdoor allergens, including pollens and fungi. In contrast, perennial AR causes daily symptoms that last more than 2 hours for more than 9 months of the year. Perennial AR is triggered by indoor allergens, such as dust mites, cockroaches, animal dander, and mold. Occupational AR symptoms are triggered by exposure to workplace irritants.

Symptoms
- Nasal congestion or obstruction +++++
- Watery rhinorrhea ++++
- Sneezing ++++
- Pruritic nose, eyes, palate, ears +++
- Constitutional symptoms: Fatigue, malaise, weakness, headache +++
- Postnasal drip (less than nonallergic rhinitis) ++
- Sinus pressure or pain ++
- Decreased sense of smell (hyposmia/anosmia) ++
- Snoring ++
- Conjunctivitis ++
- Cough ++
- Nasal pain +

Signs
- Swollen nasal turbinates (boggy, bluish or pale, purplish red, or hyperemic) +++++
- Rhinorrhea (clear, cloudy, or colored) ++++
- Transverse nasal crease or "salute" +++
- Palatal click (results from scratching palate with tongue) ++
- High arched palate (especially in children) ++
- Mouth breathing (especially in children) +++
- Air fluid levels behind tympanic membranes +++
- Allergic "shiners" (dark circles under the eyes) +++
- Dennie-Morgan fold (accentuated lower eyelid creases) +++
- Allergic conjunctivitis may be present, with or without associated periorbital edema ++
- Pharyngeal "cobblestoning" may or may not be present ++
- Nasal polyps sometimes present ++

Workup
- Diagnostic testing should be reserved for when the diagnosis of AR is unclear, symptoms are severe or poorly controlled, there is coexisting disease (e.g., persistent asthma, recurrent sinusitis, or otitis media), or the patient is a candidate for immunotherapy.
- Percutaneous skin testing is the most common diagnostic test performed because it is quick, relatively safe, and more cost effective than alternative testing options. It is more sensitive than allergen-specific IgE antibody testing (see the following text).
- Allergen-specific IgE antibody testing (e.g., radioallergosorbent test [RAST]) high specificity, but lower sensitivity than percutaneous skin testing. Useful for identifying reactions to common allergens, but less so for food, venom, or drug allergies. Consider if percutaneous skin testing is unavailable, impractical, or patient is on medications that interfere with percutaneous test (e.g., tricyclic antidepressants or antihistamines).

- Intradermal skin testing is more sensitive but less specific than percutaneous testing. It is generally avoided because of safety concerns for anaphylaxis.
- Rhinoscopy: Especially if the predominant symptoms are nasal obstruction or congestion
- Nasal smears or cytology: Limited by its inability to differentiate allergic from nonallergic rhinitis. The presence of eosinophilia does predict a good response to treatment with topical nasal corticosteroids.
- Nasal challenge test: Typically performed when there is a discrepancy between history and diagnostic test results; can be helpful for diagnosing occupational AR

Comments and Treatment Considerations

Management for the various causes of rhinitis differs, making it essential to correctly identify the diagnosis prior to initiating treatment. Although diagnostic tests are available, AR can usually be differentiated from other causes of rhinitis based on a thorough history and physical examination. AR tends to begin in childhood, and there is commonly a family history of allergies or atopic disease. Identifying specific symptom triggers and timing also helps make the diagnosis of AR. Empiric treatment can be initiated if there is a classic presentation of AR.

The primary goal of AR treatment is to decrease nasal mucosa inflammation. IgE-mediated mast cell granulation releases histamine, which causes many of the associated symptoms of AR. The histamine release attracts eosinophils, which in turn cause much of the mucosal inflammation. Various treatments are available, and should be chosen based on the patient's predominant symptoms and complaints. If at all possible, offending agents should be avoided to halt symptom exacerbation. However, allergen avoidance can be inconvenient and costly, and may not always be an option. After starting either pharmacologic or nonpharmacologic treatment, symptom control should be reevaluated in 2 to 4 weeks, and adjustments in management made if necessary.

Primary Treatments

Intranasal corticosteroids are considered first-line treatment for moderate to severe symptoms. Their action is to attack the underlying eosinophilia. Topical corticosteroids have been shown to be the most effective monotherapy, and a meta-analysis concluded that they can be considered first-line for all classifications of AR. They are better than antihistamines at treating nasal congestion, itch and discharge, sneezing, and postnasal drip. Maximum therapeutic effect is achieved in 3 to 7 days. The various available agents appear to have similar efficacies.

Oral antihistamines generally are considered first-line treatment for mild to moderate disease. They act by negating histamine release from mast cells and are effective at quickly relieving pruritus, sneezing, rhinorrhea, and conjunctivitis but ineffective for nasal congestion. First- and second-generation antihistamines are equally efficacious, but the newer second-generation medications have fewer side effects (e.g., less sedating). There is no evidence that tolerance develops to these medications.

Alternative Treatment Options

Intranasal antihistamines treat nasal congestion and can be used as first-line medications for mild to moderate AR; they also can be combined with intranasal corticosteroids or oral antihistamines.

Ophthalmic antihistamines only treat allergic conjunctivitis. Dosing four times a day makes this impractical.

A mast cell stabilizer (intranasal cromolyn) is useful for episodic disease when started 30 minutes prior to allergen exposure. It's better at treating symptoms than placebo, but less effective than nasal corticosteroids or oral antihistamines. Dosing four times a day makes this impractical.

Oral decongestants relieve nasal congestion and improve symptoms of rhinorrhea, sneezing, and pruritus over baseline.

An intranasal decongestant can be used for the short-term treatment of nasal congestion. The patient should limit use to 2 to 3 days to avoid rebound congestion. Intranasal decongestants should be used just prior to intranasal corticosteroids.

Intranasal anticholinergics (ipratropium) are effective at decreasing rhinorrhea. They can be used in combination with nasal corticosteroids or oral antihistamines.

Consider an anti-leukotriene (montelukast) if a patient presents with coexisting asthma, but it is not as effective as intranasal steroids. Some studies have shown it to be comparable in efficacy to second-generation antihistamines, though others conclude that it is less effective than oral antihistamines; montelukast plus an oral antihistamine appears to be no better than the antihistamine alone at treating rhinitis or conjunctivitis. It is less effective than oral decongestants at treating nasal congestion but improves symptoms of rhinorrhea, sneezing, and pruritus over baseline.

Oral steroids are rarely needed. They are reserved for refractory or severe cases. Consider using them if nasal polyps are present. When prescribed, long-acting steroids should be used for a short burst of 5 to 7 days.

Combination therapies can include intranasal corticosteroids and oral antihistamines, or an oral antihistamine and decongestant. Intranasal corticosteroids and oral antihistamines are more effective at treating nasal symptoms than an antihistamine alone, but show no improvement over monotherapy with a topical corticosteroid. An oral antihistamine and decongestant combination is more effective at treating symptoms than either class alone.

Immunotherapy is generally used for severe disease when symptoms are failing to respond to avoidance or pharmacotherapy. It can be particularly useful for severe perennial AR, or when there are other associated conditions (e.g., asthma). An adequate trial generally takes 2 years.

Nasal douching with alkaline or sterile seawater solutions improves symptoms of rhinitis.

NONALLERGIC RHINITIS

The classification of rhinitis is separated into three categories: AR, nonallergic rhinitis (NAR), or mixed AR and NAR. More than 40 million Americans are estimated to have either NAR or mixed rhinitis, with a similar number having AR.

Diagnosing NAR can be confusing because the primary symptoms—nasal congestion, rhinorrhea, and postnasal drip—may be indistinguishable from AR. The primary symptoms of NAR often exist in cases of sinusitis, which can further confuse the diagnosis. Therefore, the diagnosis of NAR can be made through careful history taking and clinically distinguishing NAR from AR (Table 15-1).

Symptoms
- Congestion ++++
- Rhinorrhea +++
- Postnasal drip +++
- Pruritus +
- Sneezing +
- Anosmia +
- Headache +
- Chronic cough ++
- Throat clearing ++

Comments and Treatment Considerations
After reviewing the patient's history and presenting symptoms, a normal head, ears, eyes, nose, and throat (HEENT) examination and skin allergy testing (or RAST) can help further delineate AR versus NAR. A normal examination and negative skin test result help rule out allergic causes. However, a positive skin test does not rule out mixed rhinitis, which includes both allergic and nonallergic causes.

The most common cause of acute NAR is viral (addressed earlier). The major causes of noninfectious NAR include:
- Vasomotor rhinitis +++
- Hormonal rhinitis
- Drug-induced rhinitis
- Occupational rhinitis
- Rhinitis medicamentosa
- Eosinophilic disease
  - Nonallergic rhinitis with eosinophilia syndrome (NARES)
  - Blood eosinophilia nonallergic rhinitis syndrome (BENARS)

Table 15-1. Differential Diagnosis of Allergic Rhinitis, Nonallergic Rhinitis, and Mixed Rhinitis

MANIFESTATIONS	ALLERGIC RHINITIS	NONALLERGIC RHINITIS	MIXED
Prevalence	≈43%	≈23%	≈34%
Onset	Usually childhood	Adult	AR as a child with subsequent development of NAR as an adult*
Gender	Equal	Female > male	Female > male
Seasonality	Seasonal or perennial	Usually perennial, though worse with weather changes	Perennial
Exacerbating factors	Allergen exposure	Irritant exposure, temperature	Allergen, irritants and/or temperature
Symptoms			
Congestion	Common	Common	Common
Rhinorrhea	Common	Less common	Common
Postnasal drip	Less common	Common	Common
Pruritus	Common	Less common	Varies with seasons
Sneezing	Common	Less common	Varies with seasons
Conjunctivitis or itchy eyes	Common	Absent	Varies with seasons

History of atopic disease (e.g., asthma, eczema)	Common	Uncommon	Common
Family history of allergy	Common	Uncommon	Common
Other studies			
Skin-prick/RAST	Common	Uncommon	Common
Cytologic testing			
Eosinophils present	Common	Uncommon except NARES and BENARS	Varies
On nasal scraping			
Peripheral eosinophilia	Common	Absent except for BENARS	Varies

* Abstract demonstrates age less than 20 for AR and more than 20 for NAR, but study has not been reproduced.

AR, Allergic rhinitis; BENARS, blood eosinophilia nonallergic rhinitis syndrome; NAR, nonallergic rhinitis; NARES, nonallergic rhinitis with eosinophilia syndrome; RAST, radioallergosorbent test.

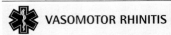

VASOMOTOR RHINITIS

The most predominant chronic etiology of NAR is vasomotor rhinitis (VMR), an autonomic phenomenon thought to be related to vagus nerve stimulation and increased blood flow to the nasal mucosa. An estimated 5% to 10% of individuals have VMR and approximately 65% of NAR patients have VMR. This type of rhinitis can be confused with symptoms of chronic sinusitis and may lead to chronic sinusitis.

VMR is brought on by temperature changes (i.e., cold air), humidity, alcohol, odors (perfumes, tobacco, paint, cleaning solutions), hot or spicy foods, sexual arousal, postural reflexes (e.g., lying flat), and emotional stress.

Comments and Treatment Considerations

Avoidance of the offending trigger is the best course of action. If this is not an option, treatment is based on primary complaints.

For nasal congestion use a topical corticosteroid. This is the most effective treatment for VMR and should be the first-line therapy.

To treat rhinorrhea use a topical anticholinergic such as ipratropium (Atrovent).

For rhinorrhea with sneezing and postnasal drip a topical antihistamine such as azelastine (Astelin) will work.

If the first attempt at treatment fails, switch classes of topical treatments or augment topical corticosteroids with one of the other two classes of nasal sprays.

HORMONAL RHINITIS

There is limited literature on hormonal rhinitis, making diagnosis difficult. A patient will present with hormonal rhinitis as a result of pregnancy, use of OCPs or hormone replacement therapy (HRT), menstruation, or hypothyroidism.

Pregnancy-induced rhinitis is relatively common during pregnancy. It lasts at least 6 weeks, occurs at any time during pregnancy, and usually improves within 2 weeks of delivery. No identifying infectious or allergic cause should be present, though it is often difficult to distinguish hormonal rhinitis from sinusitis. Placental growth hormone is suggested to be involved. Smoking and sensitization to dust mites may be risk factors.

Comments and Treatment Considerations

No specific treatment is particularly effective. Treatment should aim to temporarily relieve troublesome symptoms. Topical nasal decongestants provide temporary relief, but caution should be advised because of the potential overuse leading to rhinitis medicamentosa (discussed later). In one study, external nasal dilators improved subjective complaints of nasal congestion that disrupt sleep. Also, nasal saline can loosen secretions and nasal crusting.

OCP- or HRT-related rhinitis can be relieved by discontinuing the medication. If this is not an option, the temporary alleviation of symptoms described earlier may be helpful. There is insufficient evidence to say if the rhinitis from hypothyroidism improves with correction of the disorder.

 ## DRUG-INDUCED RHINITIS

Drug-induced rhinitis is attributed to the following medications:
- Hypertensive drugs
  - ACE inhibitors
  - Beta-blockers
  - Phentolamine
  - Methyldopa
  - Prazosin
- Topical nasal decongestants
- ASA
- NSAIDs
- Erectile dysfunction medications (i.e., phosphodiesterase inhibitors)
- Chlorpromazine

Comments and Treatment Considerations
Avoidance of the offending medication is the best course of action.

 ## RHINITIS MEDICAMENTOSA

Rhinitis medicamentosa (RM) is the rebound nasal congestion that occurs after repetitive use and withdrawal of topical α-adrenergic nasal decongestant sprays (e.g., oxymetazoline [Afrin] or phenyleph-rine [Neo-Synephrine]) or the abuse of cocaine. The phenomenon is common after 5 to 7 consecutive days of topical nasal decongestant use. Patients affected by RM usually start these OTC nasal sprays for nasal congestion related to URI and AR and continue to use them for their rapid, effective relief.

The physiologic addiction can be unnoticed by the patient at first. When seen at the office, some patients do not realize the degree to which the topical decongestants contribute to their worsening and more frequent nasal congestion. Chronic use of topical nasal decongestant causes red, inflammatory mucosal hypertrophy, loss of cilia, and increased number of mucus-producing glands. Chronic symptoms include increasing nasal congestion, postnasal drip, and epistaxis.

Comments and Treatment Considerations
Treatment aims to discontinue the topical nasal decongestant and replace it with corticosteroid nasal spray. On removal of the topical nasal decongestant, the corticosteroid spray will usually reduce the worst of the nasal congestion within 7 days.

For faster resolution of withdrawal nasal congestion, the corticosteroid spray should be started concomitantly with the nasal decongestant as it is quickly tapered down. The patient should continue the nasal steroid for 4 to 6 weeks. No evidence exists that one corticosteroid spray works better than another. If topical sprays are not tolerated, successful relief of RM has occurred by using systemic treatment with oral decongestants, corticosteroids, and antihistamines.

Education is the key to prevention of RM. Topical decongestants relieve symptoms but not the underlying problem. If treatment is necessary for symptomatic relief, suggest only 3 to 5 days if using twice daily or less than 10 days if used primarily at night before sleep, when symptoms are most problematic. Another creative way to avoid RM is to alternate nostrils with each dose, thereby giving the patient partial relief of symptoms and avoidance of RM. Avoidance of topical decongestant sprays altogether is the best option for prevention.

NONALLEGIC RHINITIS WITH EOSINOPHILIA SYNDROME AND BLOOD EOSINOPHILIA NONALLERGIC RHINITIS SYNDROME

NARES, or eosinophilic rhinitis, accounts for 10% to 33% of those with NAR. Patients typically present with nasal congestion, paroxysm of sneezing, watery rhinorrhea, nasal pruritus, and sometimes hyposmia. Nasal cytology will show eosinophilia with no obvious allergic cause on allergy skin testing.

Though NARES often occurs alone, it is believed to be a precursor to the triad of asthma, nasal polyps, and aspirin intolerance. BENARS is a subset of NARES with similar characteristics, though BENARS also has blood eosinophilia. Its prevalence is approximately 4% of NAR patients.

Comments and Treatment Considerations

The etiology of NARES and BENARS is unknown, and may represent a subset of AR in which potential allergens have eluded scientific detection. It appears they respond well to topical nasal corticosteroid treatment.

OCCUPATIONAL RHINITIS

Occupational rhinitis is under-recognized by physicians and should be suspected if symptoms can be related to the work environment. This condition is often a spectrum disorder, likely an early precursor of respiratory dysfunction and eventually occupational asthma. Some of the common occupations shown to be affected include:
• Construction (dust, solvents, paints)
• Factories (textile, glues, varnish, wood, dust)

- Farmers (wheat, tobacco)
- Laboratories (animal dander, chemical odors)
- Retail (cleaning agents, perfumes, flowers, aerosols)
- Veterinarian offices (animal dander, cleaning products)

Occupational rhinitis can be allergic in nature, or nonallergic resulting from acute or chronic irritation—or a combination of both. Patients usually experience symptoms of mixed rhinitis including nasal and ocular pruritus, nasal congestion, sneezing, and rhinorrhea. Keeping a diary of symptoms or creating a controlled challenge in the office can direct the diagnosis.

Comments and Treatment Considerations

The best management is to avoid the offending substance, ventilate the work environment, decrease exposure time, or wear protective gear. However, this may not be feasible to the patient. Therefore, treatment with antihistamines or topical nasal steroids is effective.

References

Agency for Healthcare Research and Quality: Evidence report/technology assessment No. 54. Management of allergic and nonallergic rhinitis. Available at www.ahrq.gov/clinic/tp/rhintp.htm (accessed Aug 11, 2006).

Arroll B: Non-antibiotic treatments for upper-respiratory tract infections (common cold): evidence based review, *Respir Med* 99:1477–1484, 2005.

Arroll B, Kennedy T: Are antibiotics effective for acute purulent rhinitis? Systematic review and meta-analysis of placebo controlled randomized trials, *BMJ* 33:2790, 2006.

Cory JP, Houser SM, Ng BA: Nasal congestion: a review of its etiology, evaluation and treatment, *Ear Nose Throat* 79:690–702, 2000.

Davis SS, Eccles R: Nasal congestion: mechanisms, measurement and medications. Consideration for the clinician, *Clin Otolaryngol* 29:659–666, 2004.

Dykewicz MS, Fineman D, Skoner DP, et al: Diagnosis and management of rhinitis: complete guidelines of the Joint Task Force on Practice Parameters in Allergy, Asthma and Immunology. American Academy of Allergy, Asthma, and Immunology, *Ann Allergy Asthma Immunol* 81:478–518, 1998.

Ellegard EK: The etiology and management of pregnancy rhinitis, *Am J Respir Med* 2:469–475, 2003.

Gautrin D, Desrosiers M, Castano R: Occupation rhinitis, *Curr Opin Allergy Clin Immunol* 6:77–84, 2006.

Gendo K, Larson EB: Evidence-based diagnostic strategies for evaluating suspected allergic rhinitis, *Ann Intern Med* 140:278–289, 2004.

Graf P: Rhinitis medicamentosa: a review of causes and treatment, *Treat Respir Med* 4:21–29, 2005.

Institute for Clinical Systems Improvement (ICSI): *Rhinitis.* Available at www.icsi.org (accessed Aug 11, 2006).

Long A, McFadden C, DeVine D, et al: *Management of allergic and nonallergic rhinitis,* Agency for Healthcare Research and Quality. Publication No. 02-E024. Available at www.ahrq.gov/downloads/pub/evidence/pdf/rhinitis/rhinitis.pdf (accessed Aug 11, 2006).

Quillen DM, Feller DB: Diagnosing rhinitis: allergic vs. nonallergic, *Am Fam Physician* 73:1583–1590, 2006.

Rabago D, Zgierska A, Mundt M, et al: Efficacy of daily hypertonic saline nasal irrigation among patients with sinusitis: a randomized controlled trial, *J Fam Pract* 51:1049, 2002.

Roth AR, Basello GM, Tullo LG: *Common ear, nose and throat conditions. FP essentials,* ed. 324, Leawood, KS, 2006, AAFP.

Scheid DC, Hamm RM: Acute bacterial rhinosinusitis in adults: part I. Evaluation, *Am Fam Physician* 70:1685–1692, 2004.

Scheid DC, Hamm RM: Acute bacterial rhinosinusitis in adults: part II. Treatment, *Am Fam Physician* 70:1697–1704, 2004.

Settipane GA: Allergic rhinitis—update, *Otolaryngol Head Neck Surg* 94:470–475, 1986.

Settipane RA: Rhinitis: a dose of epidemiological reality, *Allergy Asthma Proc* 24:147–154, 2003.

Settipane RA, Lieberman P: Update on non-allergic rhinitis, *Ann Allergy Asthma Immunol* 86:494–507, 2001.

Slavin RG, Spector SL, Bernstein IL: The diagnosis and management of sinusitis: a practice parameter update, *J Allergy Clin Immunol* 116:S13–S47, 2005.

Wheeler PW, Wheeler SF: Vasomotor rhinitis, *Am Fam Physician* 76:1057–1062, 2005.

Williamson I, Benge S, Moore M, et al: Acute sinusitis: which factors do FPs believe are most diagnostic and best predict antibiotic efficacy? *Fam Pract* 55:789–796, 2006.

Wong DM, Blumberg DA, Lowe LG: Guidelines for the use of antibiotics in acute upper respiratory tract infections, *Am Fam Physician* 79:956–966, 2006.

CHAPTER 16

Cough
Roger Paulman

Coughing is a physiologic response to real or perceived irritation of the respiratory system. It is described as an "explosive expiration" that can be a voluntary act or facilitated by a reflex arc. Irritants, either endogenous or exogenous, such as dust, smoke, secretions, or refluxed gastric acid, stimulate the sensory fibers triggering the cough reflex. Numerous conditions can cause a patient to present to the physician's office with the chief complaint of cough.

As with other conditions in medicine, a good history and physical examination will help sort through the differential diagnosis of cough. Important historical questions to ask include:
- Onset—Is this an acute or chronic problem?
- Associated symptoms—Other URI symptoms, heartburn, wheezing, etc.?
- Seasonality—Is there a certain time of year?
- Sputum production—Quantity, color, or associated hemoptysis?
- Fever?
- Underlying medical conditions—Immunocompromised, medications?
- Associated dyspnea, orthopnea?

Workup
- Complete auscultation of the lungs and heart
- Ear, nose and throat examination
- Lower extremity examination for edema
- Imaging may be of help in determining the etiology of a patient's cough
- Simple PA and lateral chest x-rays may reveal pneumonia, pulmonary edema, lung mass, etc.
- Pulmonary function testing is helpful in the case of chronic lung disease to determine restrictive versus obstructive processes and determine severity of disease.
- Further testing may include chest CT and bronchoscopy when warranted.

ASTHMA

Many patients present for initial visits for asthma complaining only of cough (see Chapter 38).

CANCER

Comprising 28% of all cancer-related deaths, lung cancer is the lead-ing cause of cancer death in the United States. Cigarette smoking is thought to be involved with 87% of cases. Although this is the majority of cases, occupational and environmental exposures, nutri-tion, and genetics are all thought to play a role. Lung cancer can be divided into small-cell, non–small-cell, and miscellaneous cancers. The presentations of lung cancer can vary based on the type and location of the lung mass (Table 16-1).

Symptoms
- Cough
- Hemoptysis
- Dyspnea
- Chest wall pain (peripheral tumors)

Signs
- Pleural effusion
- Pneumonia
- Stridor
- Unilateral wheezing
- Clubbing
- Horner syndrome (apical tumors)
- Paraneoplastic syndromes (Eaton-Lambert syndrome, syndrome of inappropriate antidiuretic hormone [SIADH], parathyroid hormone–like substance secretion, DIC)

Workup
- Lung mass on chest x-ray
- Location and characteristics of mass and associated metastasis on CT scan
- Bronchoscopy with biopsy on central lesions
- Transthoracic needle biopsy under fluoroscopic guidance

Comments and Treatment Considerations
Treatment of lung cancer depends greatly on the type and stage of the tumor. Non–small-cell cancer treatment relies on surgery, with chemotherapy and radiation being adjuncts. Small-cell lung cancer has a poor prognosis, with chemotherapy combined with radiation being mainstays of treatment.

Table 16-1. Classification of Lung Tumors

Small-cell lung cancer	Oat cell, intermediate cell type, and combined oat cell carcinoma
Non–small-cell lung cancer	Squamous cell, adenocarcinoma, large-cell carcinoma
Miscellaneous tumors	Adenosquamous, carcinoid, bronchial gland

Although one's history and physical examination along with diagnostic testing usually lead to a diagnosis, sometimes medications can be the cause of a patient's complaints. Many medications may cause vague symptoms such as cough and one should be aware of a patient's recent changes in pharmaceuticals and over the counter medications (OTC) and supplements. Recent changes in dosing or addition of medicines should be noted. The most notable class of medications to cause chronic coughing is the ACE inhibitors. This class causes a nonproductive, dry cough that resolves with discontinuation of the medication.

CONGESTIVE HEART FAILURE

Heart failure is a broad term that encompasses diastolic, systolic, and high output failure. It is a condition in which the cardiac output cannot keep up with the metabolic needs of the rest of the body. Symptoms of congestive heart failure (CHF) arise from the fluid overload and subsequent pulmonary edema following activation of the renin-angiotensin system, and ensuing fluid retention. Systolic dysfunction arises from the heart's inability to contract properly to circulate adequate volumes of blood. Diastolic failure stems from a stiff, noncompliant ventricle and elevated ventricular filling pressure. High-output heart failure is uncommon and results from shunting or an increase in metabolic needs of the body tissue.

 COMMON CAUSES OF HEART FAILURE

Cardiomyopathies, MI, pericardial effusion, infiltrative disease (amyloid, hemochromatosis), hypertension (systemic and/or pulmonary), valvular disease, anemia, hyperthyroidism, and shunts can cause heart failure.

Heart failure can be further classified as right or left sided. A patient's presenting symptoms and examination can lead the examiner to the diagnosis.

Left–Sided Heart Failure
Symptoms
- Cough +++
- Paroxysmal nocturnal dyspnea
- Orthopnea
- Dyspnea on exertion +++

Signs
- Crackles on auscultation (heard on cardiac auscultator)

Right–Sided Heart Failure
Symptoms
- Leg swelling +++

Signs
- Jugular venous distention
- Enlargement of the liver
- Ascites
- Peripheral edema

Workup
- Laboratory and radiologic testing can lend evidence toward the diagnosis of heart failure.
- Chest x-ray may show fluffy infiltrates of interstitial edema with increased prominence of the cephalad pulmonary vasculature.
- Cardiomegaly, which may also be found on chest x-ray, is defined as a heart size greater than half of the diameter of the thoracic cavity.
- Brain natriuretic peptide (BNP): The ventricles in response to increased stress on the myocardium produce this peptide.
- Echocardiography is the best noninvasive modality for measurement of ventricular size as well as function.

Comments and Treatment Considerations
Although orthopnea can be seen in chronic lung disease, it is caused by increased venous return from the lower extremities and subsequent pulmonary congestion when lying supine. Paroxysmal nocturnal dyspnea can be a sign of poorly compensated heart failure and is characterized by sudden onset of shortness of breath while asleep and is relieved by sitting up or standing.

Treatment of heart failure can take may forms. Lifestyle modification is important. Cessation of smoking, dietary modifications, and cardiac rehabilitation all play a significant role.

Initial treatment of acute decompensation includes diuretics such as furosemide (Lasix). Morphine can be used in the instance of pulmonary edema for vasodilation and as an anxiolytic. Vasodilator medications such as ACE inhibitors and angiotensin receptor blockers have decreased mortality when used in patients with decreased function. ACE inhibitors can also cause cough as a side effect.

Beta-blockers have been shown to decrease mortality in patients with heart failure. Doses should be administered in the "start low and go slow" manner to avoid acute worsening of heart failure.

Inotropic agents like digoxin have long been used to decrease symptoms, but have not shown to decrease deaths from heart failure.

Implantable cardiac defibrillators should be considered in patients with low ejection fractions, because arrhythmias are a large cause of mortality.

GASTROESOPHAGEAL REFLUX DISEASE

Patients experiencing reflux symptoms may come to the physician's office complaining only of chronic cough initially. Refluxed gastric contents cause irritation of the pharynx, and occasional aspiration of the acidic fluid can lead to laryngeal irritation (see Chapter 26).

PNEUMONIA/BRONCHITIS

Pneumonia is an infection of the lung parenchyma. Patients usually complain of fever and cough with or without sputum production. Emerging resistance of bacteria to typical antibiotics has led to classification of the origination of the infection.

Symptoms
- Cough ++++
- Dyspnea ++++
- Sputum production +++
- Chest pain +++
- Hemoptysis ++
- Confusion ++
- Fever

Signs
- Pain may be the only initial complaint, with chest, back, and abdominal pain being common locations.
- Derangements of the vital signs such as tachycardia, tachypnea, and fever may draw your attention toward pulmonary infection.
- Percussion of the chest may reveal dullness over the area of consolidation.
- Auscultation of the chest may show rales or crackles over the infection as fluid collection increases.
- Classic findings such as egophony, whisper pectoriloquy, and tracheal breath sounds may not be initially present, but can develop as the pneumonia progresses.
- Laboratory findings such as elevated WBC counts with bandemia suggest an infectious process.

Workup
- Consider blood cultures on hospitalized patients per some recommended guidelines, though they rarely affect treatment. A basic chemistry panel is helpful to explore electrolyte imbalances.
- Chest radiographs are useful in determining the type and location of community-acquired pneumonia.
- Typical and atypical pneumonias are caused by different organisms and have different presentations (Table 16-2).

Treating patients in the hospital rather than as outpatients requires good clinical judgment along with other evidence such as vital signs, x-ray findings, and laboratory results. Management of community-acquired pneumonia lies with a second-generation cephalosporin plus a macrolide (to cover atypicals) or a respiratory fluoroquinolone. In some areas, vancomycin is required to cover resistant *S. pneumoniae*. Physicians should consult their local laboratory for geographic resistance patterns and their local hospital protocols for treatment of patients who are immunocompromised, older adults, or have hospital- or ventilator-acquired pneumonia.

Table 16-2. Characteristics of Typical and Atypical Pneumonia

	TYPICAL	ATYPICAL
Organisms	*S. pneumoniae* *Haemophilus pneumoniae* *Legionella*	*Mycoplasma* Viral *Chlamydia*
Onset	Sudden	Gradual
Cough	Productive Occasionally bloody	Paroxysmal Nonproductive
X-ray findings	Lobar consolidation	Diffuse involvement

Acute bronchitis shares many of the clinical features of pneumonia, but lacks the radiologic findings. It is thought to be infection or inflammation of the tracheobronchial tree. It is characterized as cough, production of sputum, with normal chest x-rays. Most commonly, bronchitis in adults is caused by viral infection (respiratory syncytial virus [RSV], rhinovirus, adenovirus, coronavirus), but can be caused by bacteria *(Chlamydia pneumoniae, Mycoplasma pneumoniae, Bordetella pertussis)*. Routine use of antibiotics in the treatment of otherwise healthy individuals with acute bronchitis is not recommended. The vast majority of these cases are viral and self-limited. Smokers should be encouraged to stop. Symptomatic treatment is recommended and can include inhaled bronchodilators for bronchospasm. If pertussis is suspected, proper testing should be done for confirmation and antibiotics used for prevention of transmission. Agents effective against pertussis include erythromycin, clarithromycin, and TMP-SMX.

TUBERCULOSIS

A large problem worldwide, tuberculosis infects 8 million new people every year and causes 2 to 3 million deaths yearly. The incidence in the United States is currently 6.5/10,000 with higher incidence in African Americans and Hispanics. One should consider tuberculosis as a diagnosis in the homeless and immigrant population.

Caused by the acid-fast bacillus *Mycobacterium tuberculosis*, this infection begins with inhalation of aerosolized droplets containing the bacteria. Infection initially starts in the lung, but can spread via the bloodstream to the liver, bone, and kidneys among other organs. After an initial asymptomatic infection, most patients will have latent infection in which a skin test will be positive and calcifications of the lung parenchyma can be seen on chest x-ray. Risk factors for active tuberculosis include:

- HIV coinfection
- Recent weight loss (alcoholism, malnutrition)
- Diabetes
- Immunosuppression (medications, cancer, acquired immunodeficiency syndrome [AIDS])

Symptoms
- Cough (productive of purulent sputum)
- Malaise +++
- Weight loss
- Low-grade fever
- Dyspnea
- Chest pain

Signs
- Crackles on lung auscultation
- Tachypnea
- Fever
- Diminished breath sounds (pleural effusion)
- Lymphadenopathy

Workup
- Upper lobe infiltrates
- Cavitary lesions
- Hilar lymphadenopathy
- Positive purified protein derivative (PPD)
- Acid-fast bacilli on sputum smear

Comments and Treatment Considerations
Treatment of patients with active tuberculosis (TB) begins with isolation of the patient in a negative-pressure room. Because tuberculosis can become resistant to monotherapy, treatment with the four-drug regimen listed below takes place for the first 2 months. Then treatment with isoniazid and rifampin continues for a total of 6 months. TB in the immunocompromised patient continues for 9 to 12 months. In noncompliant patients, direct observed therapy can be set up through the health department to ensure treatment. Hepatitis is a major side effect of isoniazid treatment and liver enzymes should be monitored frequently.

For drug tuberculosis treatment, consult infectious disease specialists for local recommendations, follow-up, and dosing:

Isoniazid	5 mg/kg/day (max 300 mg)
Rifampin	10 mg/kg/day (max 600 mg)
Pyrazinamide	15 to 30 mg/kg/day (max 2 g)
Ethambutol	15 to 25 mg/kg/day (max 2.5 g)

References
Barker LR, Fiebach N, Kern D, et al: *Principles of ambulatory medicine*, New York, 2007, Lippincott Williams & Wilkins.

Kasper DL, Brunwald E, Hauser S, et al: *Harrison's principles of internal medicine*, New York, 2005, McGraw-Hill.

Taylor RB: *Family medicine principles and practice*, New York, 2003, Springer.

CHAPTER 17

Depression
Seth Rubin and Stephanie S. Richards

Every year 20.9 million Americans suffer from a depressive illness. Among primary care patients, the incidence of depression may be as high as 8.6%. Depression is a major cause of suicide and disability, and complicates other chronic medical conditions like CAD and diabetes. Because safe, effective, evidence-based treatments are widely available, it is important to identify patients with depressive illnesses. Note that TCAs, once widely used, are rarely indicated as first-line treatment due to severe toxicity in overdose. Classification of depressive disorders is based on the DSM-IV-TR. This chapter reviews important mood disorders seen in primary care.

DEPRESSIVE DISORDERS

There are five depressive illnesses most relevant to primary care: major depression, minor depression, postpartum depression, dysthymia, and seasonal affective disorder (SAD). Each disorder is a syndrome defined by a certain number of depression symptoms occurring with a specific duration or timing (Table 17-1). For each disorder symptoms are present most of the day, nearly every day, and lead to significant distress or impairment in social, occupational, or other areas of functioning.

 MAJOR DEPRESSIVE EPISODE

Symptoms
- Depressed mood (children: may be irritable mood) ++++
- Anhedonia, diminished interest or pleasure in all or almost all activities +++++
- Weight loss (more common) or weight gain (change of more than 5% body weight within 1 month) or change in appetite (decrease more common than increase) (children: failure to achieve expected weight) +++
- Insomnia (most common manifestation), early morning awakening or hypersomnia ++++
- Fatigue, loss of energy or sense of being "slowed down" ++++
- Restlessness ++++
- Feelings of worthlessness or excessive or inappropriate guilt ++++

Table 17-1. Depressive Disorders

SYNDROME	DSM–IV CRITERIA	DURATION, TIMING
Major depressive episode	At least five depressive episode symptoms including depressed mood or anhedonia	Symptom duration at least 2 weeks
Minor depressive episode	Two to four depressive episode symptoms including depressed mood or anhedonia	Symptom duration at least 2 weeks
Postpartum depression	At least five depressive episode symptoms including depressed mood or anhedonia	Symptom duration at least 2 weeks, within four weeks of delivery
Dysthymia	Three or four major depressive episode symptoms including depressed mood; no history of major depressive episode	Symptom duration at least 2 years, no more than 2 months free of symptoms (children, at least 1 year)
Seasonal affective disorder	Depressive episodes with characteristic seasonal pattern	Two episodes with same seasonal timing within last 2 consecutive years

American Psychiatric Association *Diagnostic and statistical manual of mental disorders, IV-R*, 2000, The Association.

- Diminished ability to think, concentrate, or make decisions ++++
- Recurrent thoughts of death, suicidal ideation, or recent suicide attempt +++

Signs
- Flattened affect
- Tearfulness
- Poor eye contact
- Observable psychomotor agitation or retardation ++++

Workup
The clinical interview is used to make a diagnosis of major depression, minor depression, postpartum depression, or dysthymia. Rule out the following before making a diagnosis of major depression, minor depression, dysthymia, or SAD:
- Other psychiatric illnesses, including bipolar disorder (there has never been a manic episode), schizoaffective disorder, schizophrenia, schizophreniform disorder, delusional disorder, and psychotic disorder

- General medical conditions solely responsible for the symptoms (e.g., viral illnesses, hypothyroidism, anemia, Cushing's disease, diabetes mellitus, malignancy, CAD, CHF, and autoimmune disorders)
- Side effects of medications (e.g., glucocorticoids, antihypertensives such as beta-blockers or reserpine), alcohol, or withdrawal from drugs of abuse (alcohol, cocaine, or amphetamine)
- Bereavement

 MINOR DEPRESSIVE EPISODE

Symptoms
- Depressed mood (children: may be irritable mood) ++++
- Anhedonia, diminished interest or pleasure in all or almost all activities ++++
- Weight loss or weight gain (change of more than 5% body weight within 1 month) or change in appetite (children: failure to achieve expected weight) ++
- Insomnia, early morning awakening, or hypersomnia +++
- Fatigue, loss of energy or sense of being "slowed down" ++++
- Restlessness ++
- Feelings of worthlessness or excessive or inappropriate guilt ++++
- Diminished ability to think, concentrate, or make decisions ++++
- Recurrent thoughts of death, suicidal ideation, or recent suicide attempt ++

Signs
- Flattened affect
- Tearfulness
- Poor eye contact
- Observable psychomotor agitation or retardation ++

Work up
The clinical interview is used to make a diagnosis of major depression, minor depression, postpartum depression, or dysthymia. Rule out the following before making a diagnosis of major depression, minor depression, dysthymia, or SAD:
- Other psychiatric illnesses, including bipolar disorder (there has never been a manic episode), schizoaffective disorder, schizophrenia, schizophreniform disorder, delusional disorder, and psychotic disorder
- General medical conditions solely responsible for the symptoms (e.g., viral illnesses, hypothyroidism, anemia, Cushing's disease, diabetes mellitus, malignancy, CAD, CHF, and autoimmune disorders)
- Side effects of medications (e.g., glucocorticoids, antihypertensives such as beta-blockers or reserpine), alcohol, or withdrawal from drugs of abuse (alcohol, cocaine, or amphetamine)
- Bereavement

Special Considerations
Evidence suggests that patients may benefit from antidepressant treatment even if full major depressive episode criteria are not met. There is inadequate evidence to guide therapeutic decision making. Decisions to initiate treatment must involve weighing the degree of functional impairment and duration of minor depression symptoms against the cost and potential side effects associated with the selected treatment.

Medications: Evidence for the efficacy of medication is equivocal. Some studies have demonstrated SSRIs and MAOIs to be effective, whereas others indicated outcomes that were comparable to or worse than placebo. Note potential for drug interactions with MAOIs. SSRIs may improve functional outcomes independent of their effect on minor depression symptoms.

Psychotherapy: Evidence for the efficacy of psychotherapy is also equivocal. Interpersonal psychotherapy and CBT may be effective.

Other interventions: Nonspecific treatments such as empathy from health care clinicians and social involvement may improve symptoms. Large muscle resistance exercise training was effective in one small study.

Authorities in the United States advise caution when prescribing any antidepressant to patients of all age ranges because of the increased risk of suicide (see the following text).

 POSTPARTUM DEPRESSION

Symptoms
- Symptoms of major depressive episode
- Difficulty sleeping, when present, occurs even when the baby is sleeping
- "Baby blues" (sadness, anxiety, irritability, confusion) occurs in the majority of mothers by postpartum day 4 and resolves within 10 days.
- Postpartum psychosis (extreme thought disorganization, bizarre behavior, hallucinations) occurs within 2 weeks of delivery; this is a psychiatric emergency due to risk of suicide and infanticide.

Signs
- Flattened affect
- Tearfulness
- Poor eye contact
- Observable psychomotor agitation or retardation

Workup
The clinical interview is used to make a diagnosis of major depression, minor depression, postpartum depression, or dysthymia.

Rule out the following before making a diagnosis of major depression, minor depression, dysthymia, or SAD:

- Other psychiatric illnesses, including bipolar disorder (there has never been a manic episode), schizoaffective disorder, schizophrenia, schizophreniform disorder, delusional disorder, and psychotic disorder
- General medical conditions solely responsible for the symptoms (e.g., viral illnesses, hypothyroidism, anemia, Cushing's disease, diabetes mellitus, malignancy, CAD, CHF, and autoimmune disorders)
- Side effects of medications (e.g., glucocorticoids, antihypertensives such as beta-blockers or reserpine), alcohol, or withdrawal from drugs of abuse (alcohol, cocaine, or amphetamine)
- Bereavement

Special Considerations
The general treatment recommendations for a major depressive episode apply, except as noted following.

Medication: SSRI treatment is recommended for all patients. Start dosing at one half the usual dose because postpartum patients may be more susceptible to side effects. Increase the dose in increments of the starting dose.

Breastfeeding and medications: Because all antidepressants are excreted in breast milk, use the lowest effective doses. Sertraline (Zoloft) and paroxetine (Paxil) are often used due to case series data indicating that infants breastfed by mothers taking these medications suffered no significant physiologic adverse effects. Children breastfed by mothers taking SSRIs have not exhibited significant developmental delays or neurologic sequelae.

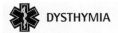 DYSTHYMIA

Symptoms
- Symptoms of major depressive episode
- Feelings of hopelessness
- Low self-esteem

Signs
- Flattened affect
- Tearfulness
- Poor eye contact
- Observable psychomotor agitation or retardation

Workup
The clinical interview is used to make a diagnosis of major depression, minor depression, postpartum depression, or dysthymia. Rule out the following before making a diagnosis of major depression, minor depression, dysthymia, or SAD:

- Other psychiatric illnesses, including bipolar disorder (there has never been a manic episode), schizoaffective disorder, schizophrenia, schizophreniform disorder, delusional disorder, psychotic disorder
- General medical conditions solely responsible for the symptoms (e.g., viral illnesses, hypothyroidism, anemia, Cushing's disease, diabetes mellitus, malignancy, CAD, CHF, and autoimmune disorders)
- Side effects of medications (e.g., glucocorticoids, antihypertensives such as beta-blockers or reserpine), alcohol, or withdrawal from drugs of abuse (alcohol, cocaine, or amphetamine)
- Bereavement

Special Considerations

Medications: SSRIs, TCAs, and MAOIs all have demonstrated efficacy in improving dysthymia symptoms and are considered equally effective. TCAs are highly toxic in overdose and MAOIs have significant drug interactions and therefore are generally not used as front-line agents. Studies indicate pharmacotherapy may be more effective than psychotherapy. The balance between medication side effects and symptom relief may be even more important than for other forms of depression given that dysthymia is chronic and less severe. Therefore, SSRIs are considered to be first-line treatment for dysthymia because TCAs and MAOIs are more likely to cause side effects and adverse events.

Psychotherapy: Psychotherapy has not been proven effective in reducing dysthymia symptoms, whether alone or in combination with medications. Psychotherapy may improve functional capabilities when combined with SSRIs, TCAs, or MAOIs.

Comments and Treatment Considerations for

All Depressive Disorders

Assessment for suicidal ideation is critical. For each patient who has depressive symptoms, determine the following:
- Presence of passive death wish: "Have you been thinking that it would be easier if you were dead, or that life is not worth living?"
- Presence of active suicidality: "Have you been thinking about ending your life?"
- Presence of plans if suicidal ideation is present: "Do you have a plan for ending your life?"
- State of readiness to commit suicide: Possession of weapons or deadly items, possession of items included in the suicide plan, a set timeline for carrying out the plan, or triggers for implementing the plan
- Presence of furtherance of plan: Has the patient taken active steps to obtain items (e.g., weapons) or arrange conditions (e.g., gave away a pet) needed to complete the suicide plan?

A primary care clinician can treat the majority of people with depression. In emergencies or severe cases, specialist evaluation is indicated.

Indications for emergent psychiatrist evaluation or hospitalization: Plans to commit suicide characterized by readiness and/or furtherance, plans to harm others (including the patient's children) (for postpartum depression: postpartum psychosis or inability to care for the infant), life-threatening behaviors (e.g., refusal to eat).

Indications for psychiatric referral: Severe functional impairment, suspicion of mania/bipolar symptoms, psychotic symptoms, suicidal ideation with or without a specific plan, comorbid eating disorder, alcohol abuse or other substance abuse, and treatment-resistant depression.

Treatment phases and monitoring: There are three consecutive treatment phases: acute, continuation, and maintenance.

ACUTE PHASE

- Initial presentation to end of depression: Adjust treatment modalities as needed.
- Failure to treat until complete depression remission results in poorer functional outcomes and increased risk of depression relapses.

Continuation phase: Designed to prevent depression relapse, and involves continued treatment for an additional 4 to 5 months.

Maintenance phase: The maintenance phase involves ongoing treatment with antidepressant medication and/or psychotherapy to prevent depression recurrence. Maintenance treatment is according to patient preference or for patients who have had three or more major depressive episodes, severe depressive episodes, dysthymic symptoms after major depression remission, or comorbid psychiatric illnesses.

Treatment monitoring: Patients should initially be seen every 2 weeks until the depressive symptoms remit. Factors indicating the need for more frequent follow-up include suicidal ideation, more severe symptoms, inadequate social support, and comorbid medical problems.

Selecting treatment modalities: The most commonly applied therapies for depressive episodes are antidepressant medication and psychotherapy, which have comparable efficacy for mild to moderate depressive episodes. Both medication and psychotherapy significantly improve depression severity by 12 months. Although medications lead to more rapid remission, psychotherapy can treat and prevent depressive episodes by helping patients build coping strategies and redirect negative thought processes.

Patients undergoing psychotherapy must be motivated to experience significant reductions in depressive symptoms. The best treatment outcomes are achieved with a combination of medication and psychotherapy. For mild to moderate depression, patients should be encouraged to select from these treatment modalities based on their personal preferences. For patients with moderate to severe depression, medication should be used in nearly all cases, accompanied by psychotherapy for patients who are motivated and/or have prominent interpersonal or psychosocial problems. Consider adding another form of treatment when depression symptoms do not fully respond to the initially selected treatment modalities. Electroconvulsive therapy (ECT) should be considered for patients with severe depression, life-threatening or treatment-resistant symptoms, psychosis, need for rapid improvement, or previous success with the modality.

Initial medication selection: The SSRIs, the serotonin norepinephrine reuptake inhibitors (SNRIs) venlafaxine and duloxetine, the dopamine norepinephrine reuptake inhibitor (DNRI) bupropion, the TCAs, the MAOIs, and the tetracyclic antidepressant mirtazapine have been shown equally effective in promoting remission of depression; all proved more effective than placebo. SSRIs are considered first-line treatment. SSRIs are better tolerated and are associated with less treatment discontinuation than TCAs, which have high risk of morbidity and mortality in overdose. MAOIs have significant side effects, and important (and potentially life threatening) drug and food-drug interactions. Many SSRIs are available as generic formulations. When selecting a medication, incorporate patients' unique needs by considering the following factors: side effect profiles, adverse effect profiles, the medications' relative safety in overdose, the patient's history of success with particular medications, family member's history of success with particular medications, medication cost, dosing frequency, and the patient's preferences. Table 17-2 lists commonly used antidepressants.

Managing medications: Start with half the usual recommended initial dose for older adult patients or patients who have comorbid panic or anxiety symptoms. For patients recently started on a new medication or had a medication dose increase, arrange frequent follow-up (every 2 weeks) to assess for side effects, adherence, emergent suicidality, development of mania, symptom improvement, and functional improvement. Allow 6 to 8 weeks for the patient to experience the full effects of any given dose.

Inadequate medication response: If there is no change or only partial remission of symptoms, first assess adherence to the medication regimen and inquire about medication side effects (see earlier). If adherence is adequate and there are no significant side effects, consider increasing the medication towards its maximum daily dose or to the maximum dose the patient will tolerate. If there is no change in symptoms consider switching to another antidepressant from the same class. If two medications from the same class were both ineffective, consider switching to a medication from a different class. Bupropion or venlafaxine is frequently used when two or more SSRIs have been ineffective. If the symptoms are partly improved and the medication dose is maximal (either at the dose listed in Table 17-2 or limited by side effects), consider augmenting with another medication from a different class. Evidence strongly supports the use of lithium for antidepressant augmentation. Bupropion also has proven

Table 17-2. Commonly Used Antidepressant Medication Adult Doses and Side Effects

MEDICATION	INITIAL DOSE (mg/day)	MAXIMUM DOSE (mg/day)	COMMON SIDE EFFECTS
Selective Serotonin Reuptake Inhibitors (SSRIs)			
Citalopram (Celexa)	20	60	Dry mouth, increased sweating, nausea, somnolence, insomnia, tremor, diarrhea, delayed ejaculation, anorgasmia
Escitalopram (Lexapro)	10	20	Dry mouth, nausea, somnolence, insomnia, diarrhea, delayed ejaculation, anorgasmia
Fluoxetine (Prozac)	20	80	Headache, asthenia, nausea, diarrhea, anorexia, dry mouth, dyspepsia, insomnia, nervousness, anxiety, somnolence, dizziness, tremor, increased sweating, delayed ejaculation, anorgasmia
Paroxetine (Paxil)	Regular: 20 Controlled release: 25	Regular: 50 Controlled release: 65	Headache, asthenia, increased sweating, nausea, dry mouth, constipation, diarrhea, decreased appetite, somnolence, dizziness, insomnia, tremor, delayed ejaculation, anorgasmia, erectile dysfunction
Sertraline (Zoloft)	50	200	Delayed ejaculation, anorgasmia, dry mouth, increased sweating, somnolence, dizziness, headache, tremor, anorexia, constipation, diarrhea, dyspepsia, nausea, fatigue, insomnia, decreased libido

Serotonin Norepinephrine Reuptake Inhibitors (SNRIs)			
Duloxetine (Cymbalta)	40 (divided bid)	60 (may be given daily or divided bid)	Nausea, dry mouth, constipation, diarrhea, vomiting, anorexia, fatigue, dizziness, somnolence, increased sweating, insomnia, anorgasmia
Venlafaxine (Effexor)	Regular: 75 (divided bid-tid) Extended release: 75	Regular: 375 (divided tid) Extended release: 375	Headache, asthenia, infection, increased sweating, nausea, constipation, anorexia, diarrhea, vomiting, somnolence, dry mouth, dizziness, insomnia, nervousness, anxiety, blurred vision, delayed ejaculation/orgasm, erectile dysfunction
Other			
Bupropion (Wellbutrin)	Sustained release: 150 Extended release: 150	Sustained release: 400 (divided bid) Extended release: 450	Headache, infection, dry mouth, nausea, constipation, insomnia, dizziness, tremor, increased sweating, tinnitus, agitation, anxiety, abdominal pain, palpitations, diarrhea, myalgia, pharyngitis
Mirtazapine (Remeron)	15	45	Drowsiness, increased appetite, weight gain, dizziness, anxiety, confusion, dry mouth, constipation, upset stomach, vomiting

efficacy in augmenting partially effective SSRI regimens. Other potential options for antidepressant augmentation include liothyronine (T_3, Cytomel) and psychostimulants such as methylphenidate.

Handling medication side effects: Side effects are the most common reason for antidepressant discontinuation (see Table 17-2). Many patients initially treated with an SSRI will have to switch to another agent due to side effects. If a patient develops mania after starting an antidepressant medication, he or she may have bipolar disorder; the medication should be tapered and the patient should be referred to a psychiatrist immediately for evaluation. Counsel all patients taking antidepressant medications about the side effects they might experience, including suicidality (see following text). Let them know which side effects should be reported immediately. Medication side effects often resolve within 1 to 2 weeks, so watchful waiting is acceptable if the patient is able to tolerate them and they do not pose a medical risk. If the side effects are intolerable, switch to another medication.

Sexual side effects: Sexual side effects are very common and frequently lead to discontinuation of SSRIs and SNRIs. Ask patients directly whether they are experiencing these symptoms. Decreasing the medication dose or instituting drug holidays (e.g., skipping doses on days of sexual activity) can ameliorate sexual side effects, but these strategies should be used with caution because they could lead to poor regimen adherence. Another option is to add a medication that can counteract the sexual side effects such as buspirone or bupropion. Medications such as sildenafil (Viagra), tadalafil (Cialis), and vardenafil (Levitra) can also be effective in treating SSRI-induced sexual dysfunction in men. Finally, the offending medication could be discontinued in favor of another medication that is less likely to cause significant sexual side effects (e.g., a medication from the same class, bupropion, or mirtazapine).

Antidepressants and risk of suicide: The early phases of antidepressant treatment are often activating and may lead to increased agitation and energy relative to the depressed baseline state. Because patients frequently continue to experience a sense of hopelessness during this period, they may be at increased risk for suicidal ideation and suicide attempts. There is not sufficient evidence to rule out the possibility of increased suicide risk. Decisions to institute antidepressant medications should always involve a careful balance of the known benefits and risks. Authorities in the United Kingdom have advised against using the following antidepressants among children: paroxetine, citalopram, venlafaxine, escitalopram, and mirtazapine. Authorities in the United States advise caution when prescribing any antidepressant to patients of all age ranges. During the initial months of treatment with an antidepressant medication, patients must have frequent follow-up visits (e.g., every 2 weeks). Counsel all patients starting antidepressants about the risk of agitation and suicidality, and advise them to seek medical advice immediately if they experience these symptoms. Caregivers and family members must be educated to monitor the patient and immediately seek medical advice if the patient exhibits worsened symptoms, suicidality, or unusual behaviors.

Discontinuation of medications: After the continuation phase of antidepressant treatment, if maintenance treatment is not selected, antidepressant medications should be tapered over at least 1 month to reduce the risk of depression recurrence. Even when they are discontinued prior to depression remission, most antidepressant medications should be tapered to prevent withdrawal symptoms. Withdrawal symptoms may include dizziness, nausea, paresthesia, headache, and vertigo. Because fluoxetine and its metabolites have longer half-lives, this medication may not exhibit as significant withdrawal symptoms when abruptly discontinued.

Selecting psychotherapies: Systematic reviews indicate that both structured and nonstructured psychotherapies achieve better outcomes than placebo or usual care. The best-studied structured psychotherapeutic modalities are CBT and interpersonal therapy; these have comparable efficacy.

Use of ECT: Given the availability of effective antidepressant medications and psychotherapies, use of ECT is limited to patients who cannot take medications, have treatment-resistant depression, have severe or psychotic symptoms, have catatonia, or have life-threatening symptoms such as suicidality or refusal to eat. Compared to medications, ECT is proven to provide more rapid short-term improvement in patients with moderate to severe depression symptoms. ECT may lead to cognitive impairment but this is usually limited to short-term memory loss during treatment.

SEASONAL AFFECTIVE DISORDER

SAD is characterized by the onset and remission of depressive symptoms during specific seasons. SAD is categorized by DSM-IV as a subtype of major depression. Depressive episodes associated with recurrent major depression, or bipolar I or bipolar II disorders (see later discussion about bipolar disorder) can have a seasonal timing. Typically the onset is in the fall and remission is in the spring, but in 10% of cases depression onset may occur in the summer. SAD is more common among women, those living farther from the equator (for winter depression), and those who are 20 to 30 years old. It is important to recognize SAD because the treatment differs from other forms of depression.

Recurrent seasonal onset and seasonal remission of major depression symptoms for at least 2 years in a row defines SAD. Symptoms are generally characteristic of major depressive episodes (see previous section). Winter and summer depression may have a different constellation of symptoms.

 WINTER DEPRESSIVE EPISODES

Symptoms
- Oversleeping
- Daytime fatigue

- Craving carbohydrates (sweets, starches)
- Weight gain
- Irritability
- Heavy feeling in arms and legs
- Symptoms associated with more overcast weather, darkened interior lighting, or working in an office building with few windows

Signs
- Regular temporal relationship between specific time of year and onset of major depressive episodes in recurrent major depressive disorder, bipolar I or bipolar II disorders
- Full remission of depression symptoms (orchange to mania or hypomania) also occurs at predictable times of year.
- Two major depressive episodes in the last 2 years with onset and resolution in characteristic seasons
- No nonseasonal major depressive episodes in the last 2 years
- Lifetime pattern whereby most major depressive episodes were seasonal
- Typically onset in fall and remission in spring

Workup
- Exclude seasonal-related psychosocial factors (e.g., holiday-related stress, losing seasonal work with changing weather).
- Exclude medical conditions solely responsible for the symptoms (e.g., hypothyroidism, hypoglycemia, infectious mononucleosis, other viral illnesses).

Comments and Treatment Considerations
Patients should be encouraged to guide the treatment selection based on their preferences. Patients with mild symptoms may improve with simple adjustments to increase light exposure (e.g., getting more exposure to daylight during winter months, lighting interior spaces with sunlight or bright lights). However, it is light therapy and antidepressant medications that have been proven effective in treating SAD. Fluoxetine and light therapy appear to be equally effective, although patients taking light therapy typically improve more rapidly (within 1 week) and experience fewer side effects. Medication may be more practical than light therapy for certain patients. Patients who have more severe symptoms or other depressive episodes with a nonseasonal pattern may require combination therapy with light and medications.

Light therapy: This modality has been shown to reverse winter depressive episode symptoms in 50% to 80% of patients. The treatment requires special lighting equipment capable of simulating full-spectrum bright light. Symptoms typically resolve within 2 to 4 days of starting treatment, but several weeks may be required.

Implementing light therapy: Effective light boxes deliver light at an intensity of 10,000 lux. Light therapy should occur in the early morning, and be set at eye level or above (and tilted down toward the patient's head). Therapy starts with 10- to 15-minute sessions and is titrated weekly in 15-minute increments up to 30 to 90 minutes per day.

Light therapy must be continued throughout the fall or winter seasons to prevent recurrence of symptoms. It is discontinued in the spring.

Side effects of light therapy: Side effects are relatively common but typically resolve within the first 5 days and may include headache, eyestrain, visual blurring, residual visual glare, insomnia, nausea, vomiting, hypomania, agitation, sedation, dizziness, and irritability.

If light therapy is inadequate or not tolerated: Medication and/or psychotherapy may be initiated (see later).

Medication: Fluoxetine, sertraline, and hypericum extract (e.g., St. John's wort dosed at 900 mg/day) all have demonstrated efficacy in achieving remission of SAD.

Comorbid bipolar I or bipolar II disorder or summer/spring hypomania: Patients must be on a mood stabilizer before SAD treatment is initiated because both light therapy and medications can induce mania or hypomania.

Relapse prevention: Initiate light therapy, bupropion, or CBT prior to the expected onset of SAD symptoms. Citalopram administered immediately following light therapy–mediated remission has been shown to prevent relapse.

 SUMMER DEPRESSIVE EPISODES

- Insomnia
- Decreased appetite
- Weight loss
- Agitation or anxiety

Signs
- Regular temporal relationship between specific time of year and onset of major depressive episodes in recurrent major depressive disorder, bipolar I or bipolar II disorders
- Full remission of depression symptoms (or change to mania or hypomania) also occurs at predictable times of year.
- Two major depressive episodes in the last 2 years with onset and resolution in characteristic seasons
- No nonseasonal major depressive episodes in the last 2 years
- Lifetime pattern whereby most major depressive episodes were seasonal

Workup
- Exclude seasonal-related psychosocial factors (e.g., holiday-related stress, losing seasonal work with changing weather).
- Exclude medical conditions solely responsible for the symptoms (e.g., hypothyroidism, hypoglycemia, infectious mononucleosis, other viral illnesses).

Comments and Treatment Considerations
There is little therapeutic research regarding summer depressive episodes to guide treatment decisions. Medication is typically

prescribed for moderate to severe symptoms (see medication information in "Winter Depressive Episodes").

As noted for the depressive disorders in the previous section, all patients must be assessed for suicidal ideation. Treatment is needed when the symptoms lead to significant distress or impairment in social, occupational, or other areas of functioning. Treatment is different for winter and summer depression episodes.

BIPOLAR DISORDERS AND CYCLOTHYMIA

Bipolar disorder is a syndrome characterized by recurrent episodes of mania/hypomania and depression. Many patients presenting to primary care physicians with depressive symptoms actually have a bipolar disorder. It is crucial for primary care physicians to differentiate between unipolar major depression and bipolar disorder because antidepressant medications can trigger manic/hypomanic episodes in people with bipolar disorder. Bipolar disorder can be difficult to diagnose for two important reasons. First, patients with bipolar disorder frequently present with depressive symptoms as their index episode. Second, many patients do not recognize or report past manic/hypomanic episodes.

Patients with bipolar disorder should be referred to psychiatrists for management. Patients with bipolar disorder are at a higher risk for suicide and tend to exhibit profound impairments in social and occupational functioning. Management of manic and depressive symptoms often requires multiple medications.

Primary care physicians should be aware of the presenting symptoms and management of bipolar illnesses. There are three subtypes of bipolar illness most relevant to primary care: bipolar I, bipolar II, and cyclothymia. Each disorder is defined by a specified pattern of depressive symptoms, full major depressive episodes, manic episodes, or hypomanic episodes occurring during a specific period of time (Table 17-3). For each disorder, symptoms are present most of the day, nearly every day, and lead to significant distress, impairment, or changes in social, occupational, or other areas of functioning.

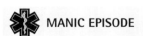 MANIC EPISODE

This is a distinct period of abnormally and persistently elevated, expansive, or irritable mood lasting at least 1 week (a shorter duration is allowed if hospitalization is required). The disturbance is severe, causing at least one of the following: marked impairment in occupational, social, or interpersonal relationship functioning; requirement for hospitalization to prevent harm to self or others; and psychotic features. At least three of the following persistent and significant symptoms are required (four if the mood is only irritable):

Table 17-3. Manic/Hypomanic Disorders

SYNDROME	MANIC SYMPTOM CRITERIA	DEPRESSIVE SYMPTOM CRITERIA	DURATION, TIMING
Bipolar I	One or more manic episodes or mixed depressive or manic episodes	Major depressive episodes	Chronic or episodic Manic episode ≥1 week Major depressive episode ≥2 weeks
Bipolar II	One or more hypomanic episodes; no history of manic or mixed episodes	Major depressive episodes	Chronic or episodic Hypomanic episode ≥4 days Major depressive episode ≥2 weeks
Cyclothymia	Periods of hypomanic symptoms	Periods of depressive symptoms not meeting criteria for major depressive episodes	Chronic or persistent Symptom duration at least 2 years, no more than 2 months free of symptoms (children: at least 1 year)

Adapted from the American Psychiatric Association: *Practice guideline for the treatment of patients with bipolar disorder,* 2nd ed. Available at www.psych.org/psych_pract/treatg/pg/bipolar_revisebook_index.cfm (accessed Oct 17, 2006).

Symptoms*
- Inflated self-esteem ++++
- Decreased need for sleep ++++
- Uncharacteristically talkative or internal pressure to keep talking ++++
- Subjective experience of racing thoughts ++++
- Easy distractibility ++++
- Psychomotor agitation or increase in goal-directed occupational, educational, social, or sexual activity ++++
- Excessive involvement in pleasurable activities with high potential for painful consequences (e.g., shopping sprees, sexual indiscretions) +++

*NOTE: Symptoms must not meet criteria for a mixed episode (see later).

Signs
- Grandiosity
- Pressured speech
- Flight of ideas
- Easy distractibility
- Psychomotor agitation or retardation

Comments and Treatment Considerations
Selecting an initial medication: Bipolar disorder with a current manic episode should always be treated with one or more mood stabilizers. Mild to moderate cases are typically treated with monotherapy using lithium, divalproex, or a second-generation antipsychotic (e.g., olanzapine or risperidone). Any manic episode with psychotic features should be treated with an antipsychotic. Although the three medication types have no significant differences in remission rates (except in bipolar II, mixed episodes, and rapid cycling, in which lithium is less effective), the second-generation antipsychotics more effectively decrease symptom severity and have a shorter time to remission. Thus patients with more severe symptoms are typically treated with a second-generation antipsychotic combined with either lithium or valproate.

Management of persistent or breakthrough manic/hypomanic episodes: Check medication adherence, as this is frequently a problem among patients with bipolar disorder. The serum levels of carbamazepine, divalproex, and lithium can be checked to verify medication adherence and/or absorption (Table 17-4). Next, the medication dose may be increased. Carbamazepine is frequently used when patients do not respond to first-line medications because it has similar efficacy to lithium and divalproex. Second-generation antipsychotics are also frequently prescribed when other first-line medications are not sufficient. If the patient is already on a second-generation antipsychotic, he or she may be switched to another.

Use of antidepressant medication: Antidepressant medications may trigger or exacerbate manic episodes in people with bipolar disorder. Antidepressant medications should therefore never be used to

Table 17-4. Commonly Used Mood Stabilizers: Adult Doses and Side Effects

MEDICATION	INITIAL DOSE (mg/day)	TARGET LEVEL	MAXIMUM DOSE (mg/day)	COMMON SIDE EFFECTS
Antimanic				
Lithium (Eskalith)	Immediate release: 900 (divided tid-qid) Controlled release: 900 (divided bid)	0.7-1.2 mEq/mL	Adjust to target level	Anorexia, nausea, vomiting, diarrhea, abdominal pain, excessive salivation, flatulence, indigestion, tremor, polyuria, polydipsia, weight gain, edema
Anticonvulsants				
Divalproex (Depakote)	750 (divided tid)	60-116 μg/mL	Adjust to target level	Nausea, somnolence, dizziness, ataxia, vomiting, asthenia, abdominal pain, dyspepsia, rash, alopecia, nervousness, tremor
Carbamazepine (Tegretol)	Regular: 200 bid Extended release: 200 bid	7-12 μg/mL	1600 (divided tid-qid) Extended release: 1600 (divided bid)	Dizziness, nausea, somnolence
Oxcarbazepine (Trileptal)	600 (divided bid)	NA	2100 (divided bid)	Fatigue, asthenia, nausea, vomiting, abdominal pain, diarrhea, dyspepsia, headache, dizziness, somnolence, ataxia, nystagmus, abnormal gait, diplopia, vertigo, vision abnormalities
Lamotrigine (Lamictal)	25 *50 †25 qod	NA	200 *400 (divided bid) †100	Back pain, fatigue, abdominal pain, nausea, constipation, vomiting, insomnia, somnolence, dry mouth, rhinitis, cough, pharyngitis, rash

(Continued)

Table 17-4. Commonly Used Mood Stabilizers: Adult Doses and Side Effects—cont'd

Second-Generation Antipsychotics

Aripiprazole (Abilify)	10	NA	Headache, asthenia, accidental injury, nausea, dyspepsia, vomiting, constipation, agitation, anxiety, insomnia, somnolence, akathisia, lightheadedness, extrapyramidal syndrome
Olanzapine (Zyprexa)	Monotherapy: 15 Combination: 10	NA	Accidental injury, asthenia, fever, back pain, dry mouth, constipation, dyspepsia, ecchymosis, weight gain, extremity pain, joint pain, somnolence, insomnia, dizziness, abnormal gait, rhinitis, cough
Quetiapine (Seroquel)	100 (divided bid)	NA	Headache, pain, asthenia, tachycardia, dry mouth, constipation, vomiting, dyspepsia, weight gain, agitation, somnolence, dizziness
Risperidone (Risperdal)	2.5	NA	Dystonia, akathisia, dizziness, parkinsonism, somnolence, agitation, mania exacerbation, dyspepsia, nausea, increased salivation, generalized pain, myalgia, vision abnormalities

*If patient taking carbamazepine, phenytoin, phenobarbital, primidone, rifampin and not on valproate.
†If patient taking valproate.
NA, Not applicable.

treat bipolar disorder without a mood stabilizer, and may need to be discontinued during a manic episode. When patients switch from depression to mania or hypomania in response to an antidepressant, it should be discontinued and a mood stabilizer started instead.

Medication side effects: Lithium, divalproex, and carbamazepine exhibit similar rates of side effects (see Table 17-4). Lithium's side effects are typically dose related. The second-generation antipsychotics exhibit higher rates of side effects, particularly increased appetite, weight gain, and sedation.

Medication adverse effects: Most of the medications commonly used to treat bipolar disorder have been associated with significant adverse effects. Therefore, patients should be monitored periodically with laboratory testing and evaluations for the more common or serious adverse events characteristic for each medication (Table 17-5). Laboratory testing and evaluations should, at minimum, occur at baseline, after 3 months of therapy and periodically thereafter.

Table 17-5. Adverse Effects Associated with Mood Stabilizers, Recommended Evaluations

MEDICATION	ADVERSE EFFECTS	RECOMMENDED EVALUATIONS
Carbamazepine (Tegretol)	Hepatic enzyme elevation, aplastic anemia, agranulocytosis, thrombocytopenia, leukopenia, cortical lens opacities	Hepatic function indices, complete blood count, ophthalmologic examination
Divalproex (Depakote)	Hepatic failure and hepatotoxicity, hyperammonemia, thrombocytopenia, coagulopathy, pancreatitis	Hepatic function indices, ammonia (if indicated), complete blood count, prothrombin time, partial thromboplastin time and INR
Lithium (Eskalith)	Hypothyroidism, renal dysfunction, cardiac conduction delays	Thyroid-stimulating hormone, blood urea nitrogen, creatinine, electrocardiogram
Second-generation antipsychotics (aripiprazole, olanzapine, quetiapine, risperidone)	Metabolic syndrome, extrapyramidal syndrome, hyperglycemia, hyperlipidemia, cortical lens opacities	Fasting serum glucose, fasting lipids, body weight, body mass index, waist circumference, ophthalmologic examination

INR, International normalized ratio.

Maintenance pharmacotherapy: Lithium, valproate, lamotrigine, olanzapine, and aripiprazole are proven to maintain remission. The benefits of maintenance therapy with second-generation antipsychotics should be balanced with the potential for side effects and adverse effects such as risk for metabolic syndrome.

Use of psychotherapy and psychosocial interventions: There is little evidence to support the use of psychotherapy to treat manic symptoms. However, during the maintenance phase of bipolar disorder, counseling should always be combined with pharmacotherapy. Ongoing psychotherapy and other psychosocial interventions may be helpful during maintenance therapy to address issues of treatment adherence, lifestyle adaptations, early recognition of bipolar symptoms, and interpersonal relationships. In particular, the following treatments have proven efficacy in preventing relapse: cognitive therapy, interpersonal social rhythm therapy, education about early recognition of bipolar symptoms, and psychoeducation for patients' families.

 HYPOMANIC EPISODE

This is a distinct period of persistently elevated, expansive, or irritable mood that is different from the patient's usual nondepressed mood, with symptoms lasting at least 4 days. The episode leads to an unequivocal, observable change in functioning that is uncharacteristic of the person when he or she is not symptomatic. However, the disturbance is *not* severe and does *not* cause marked impairment in occupational, social, or interpersonal relationship functioning; requirement for hospitalization; or psychotic features. At least three of the previously noted persistent and significant manic symptoms are required (four if the mood is only irritable).

Signs
• Grandiosity
• Pressured speech
• Flight of ideas
• Easy distractibility
• Psychomotor agitation or retardation

 MAJOR DEPRESSIVE EPISODE

Symptoms
• Depressed mood (children: may be irritable mood) +++++
• Anhedonia, diminished interest or pleasure in all or almost all activities +++++
• Weight gain (more common) or weight loss (change of more than 5% body weight within 1 month), or change in appetite (increase more common than decrease) (children: failure to achieve expected weight) +++

- Hypersomnia (most common manifestation), early morning awakening or insomnia ++++
- Fatigue, loss of energy or sense of being "slowed down" ++++
- Restlessness ++++
- Feelings of worthlessness or excessive or inappropriate guilt ++++
- Diminished ability to think, concentrate, or make decisions ++++
- Recurrent thoughts of death, suicidal ideation, or recent suicide attempt ++

Comments and Treatment Considerations

There is little evidence to guide decisions regarding medication and psychotherapeutic treatment for depressive episodes in bipolar disorder. Mood stabilizers are the primary treatment. Antidepressant medications may trigger or exacerbate manic episodes in people with bipolar disorder. Antidepressant medication should therefore never be used to treat bipolar disorder without one or more mood stabilizers.

Selecting an initial medication: The American Psychiatric Association (APA) recommends initiation of either lithium or lamotrigine. If monotherapy is ineffective, combinations of mood stabilizers are recommended. Typical combinations include lithium and lamotrigine; lithium and second-generation antipsychotics; mood stabilizers and SSRIs; and mood stabilizers and bupropion. Antidepressant medication should only be started in association with one or more mood stabilizers or second-generation antipsychotics. SSRIs or bupropion are preferred because they have lower rates of triggering an episode of mania or hypomania compared with other antidepressants. Lithium is less effective for bipolar II, mixed episodes, and rapid cycling. Any depressive episode with psychotic features should be treated with an antipsychotic.

Treatment for persistent or breakthrough depressive episodes: Check medication adherence, as this is frequently a problem among patients with bipolar disorder. Check the serum levels of carbamazepine, divalproex and lithium (see Table 17-4). Inquire about medication side effects (see Tables 17-2 and 17-4). If adherence is adequate and there are no significant side effects, consider increasing the medications toward their maximum daily dose or to the maximum doses the patient will tolerate. If symptoms remain partially remitted, consider adding another mood stabilizer or adding a second-generation antipsychotic. It is not unusual for a patient with bipolar disorder to require two or three mood stabilizers, or a second-generation antipsychotic. If the depressive symptoms are still inadequately treated, an antidepressant medication may be added.

Maintenance pharmacotherapy: See the manic episode section. Lithium and lamotrigine are proven to maintain depression remission. There are insufficient data to determine whether antidepressant medications should be considered in maintenance treatment.

Use of ECT: Typically ECT is reserved for patients exhibiting suicidal ideation, suicide attempts, psychosis, severe depression, treatment-resistant depression, and depression with catatonic features. Periodic ECT may be continued as maintenance therapy if it was needed to achieve remission.

Use of psychotherapy and psychosocial interventions: See the manic episode section.

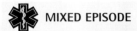

MIXED EPISODE

A mixed episode simultaneously meets criteria for both a manic episode and a major depressive episode (except for duration) every day for at least 1 week. The disturbance is severe, causing one of the following: marked impairment in occupational, social, or interpersonal relationship functioning; requirement for hospitalization to prevent harm to self or others; and psychotic features.

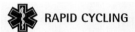

RAPID CYCLING

Rapid cycling is a DSM-IV specifier that can be applied to either bipolar I or bipolar II disorder. It is characterized by rapid alternation between separate mood disturbance episodes. Separate episodes are distinguished by either switches to an episode of opposite polarity (e.g., from a depressive to manic mood disturbance) or 2 months of full or partial remission between episodes. There are at least four separate episodes in a 12-month period.

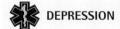

DEPRESSION

Signs
- Flattened affect
- Tearfulness
- Poor eye contact
- Observable psychomotor agitation or retardation

GENERAL WORKUP FOR BIPOLAR DISORDERS

The clinical interview and mental status examination are used to make a diagnosis of a bipolar illness. Exclude the following before making these diagnoses:
- Manic or hypomanic episodes caused by antidepressant treatment (e.g., medication, ECT, light therapy)
- Other psychiatric illnesses, including schizoaffective disorder, schizophrenia, schizophreniform disorder, delusional disorder, and psychotic disorder

- General medical conditions solely responsible for the symptoms (cerebrovascular accident or other CNS lesion, viral illnesses, hyperthyroidism, hypothyroidism, anemia, Cushing's disease, diabetes mellitus, malignancy, CAD, CHF, autoimmune disorders)
- Side effects of medications: steroids or substance abuse, intoxication, or withdrawal (e.g., from alcohol, cocaine, or amphetamines)

Comments and Treatment Considerations

There are two treatment phases: acute and maintenance. The acute phase starts at initial presentation and ends when bipolar symptoms have remitted. During this period treatment modalities are implemented and adjusted until the manic or depressive symptoms resolve. The maintenance phase, designed to prevent or delay recurrence of manic/hypomanic or depressive episodes, involves continued long-term treatment at the effective acute phase dose. Sometimes adjunctive medications can be discontinued in the maintenance phase. However, all patients with bipolar disorder require some form of long-term maintenance treatment. Treatment guidelines have been published by several organizations including the APA and the Canadian Network for Mood and Anxiety Treatments (CANMAT).

Patients with bipolar disorder require pharmacotherapeutic interventions. In fact, most patients require two or more medications to control their symptoms. Psychotherapeutic interventions alone are not proven effective for manic episodes or depressive episodes associated with bipolar disorder. Commonly used medications are listed in Table 17-4.

The treatment modalities in Table 17-5 can be used in bipolar I, bipolar II, and cyclothymia.

References

Ackermann RT, Williams JW: Rational treatment choices for non-major depressions in primary care: an evidence-based review, *J Gen Intern Med* 17:293–301, 2002.

American Academy of Family Physicians: *Seasonal affective disorder*. Available at http://familydoctor.org/267.xml (accessed March 30, 2011).

American Psychiatric Association: *Diagnostic and statistical manual of mental disorders, fourth edition, text revision*, Washington, DC, 2000, American Psychiatric Association.

American Psychiatric Association: *Practice guideline for the treatment of patients with bipolar disorder*, 2nd ed. Available at www.psych.org/psych_pract/treatg/pg/bipolar_revisebook_index.cfm (accessed Oct 17, 2006).

American Psychiatric Association: *Practice guideline for the treatment of patients with major depressive disorder*, 2nd ed. Available at www.psych.org/psych_pract/treatg/pg/Depression2e.book.cfm (accessed Oct 15, 2006).

Arnow BA, Constantino MJ: Effectiveness of psychotherapy and combination treatment for chronic depression, *J Clin Psychol* 59:893–905, 2003.

Barrett J, Williams J, Oxman T, et al: Treatment of dysthymia and minor depression in primary care: a randomized trial in patients age 18-59 years, *J Fam Pract* 50:405–412, 2001.

Benazzi F: Sensitivity and specificity of clinical markers for the diagnosis of bipolar II disorder, *Compr Psychiatry* 42:461–465, 2001.

Benazzi F: Symptoms of depression as possible markers of bipolar II disorder, *Progr Neuropsychopharm Biol Psychiatry* 30:471–477, 2006.

Browne G, Steiner M, Roberts J, et al: Sertraline and/or interpersonal psychotherapy for patients with dysthymic disorder in primary care: 6-month comparison with longitudinal 2-year follow up of effectiveness and costs, *J Affect Disord* 68:317–330, 2002.

Calabrese JR, Bowden CL, Sachs G, et al for the Lamictal 605 Study Group: A placebo-controlled 18-month trial of lamotrigine and lithium maintenance treatment in recently depressed patients with bipolar I disorder, *J Clin Psychiatry* 64:1013–1024, 2003.

Cassidy F, Carroll BJ: Frequencies of signs and symptoms in mixed and pure episodes of mania: implications for the study of manic episodes, *Progr Neuropsychopharm Biol Psychiatry* 25:659–665, 2001.

Cassidy F, Murry E, Forest K, Carroll BJ: Signs and symptoms of mania in pure and mixed episodes, *J Affect Disord* 50:187–201, 1998.

Chilvers C, Dewey M, Fielding K, et al: Antidepressant drugs and generic counseling for treatment of major depression in primary care: randomized trial with patient preference arms, *BMJ* 322:1–15, 2001.

Churchill R, Hunot V, Corney R, et al: A systematic review of controlled trials of the effectiveness and cost-effectiveness of brief psychological treatments for depression, *Health Technol Assess* 5:1–173, 2001.

De Lima MS, Hotopf M: Benefits and risks of pharmacotherapy for dysthymia: a systematic appraisal of the evidence, *Drug Saf* 26:55–64, 2003.

Friedman MA, Detweiler-Bedell JB, Leventhal HE, et al: Combined psychotherapy and pharmacotherapy for the treatment of major depressive disorder, *Clin Psychol Sci Pract* 11:47–68, 2004.

Gartlehner G, Hansen R, Carey T, et al: Discontinuation rates for selective serotonin reuptake inhibitors and other second-generation antidepressants in outpatients with major depressive disorder: a systematic review and meta-analysis, *Clin Psychopharmacol* 20:59–69, 2005.

Geddes JR, Burgess S, Hawton K, et al: Long-term lithium therapy for bipolar disorder: systematic review and meta-analysis of randomized controlled trials, *Am J Psychiatry* 161:217–222, 2004.

Gijsman HJ, Geddes JR, Rendell JM, et al: Antidepressants for bipolar disorder: a systematic review of randomized controlled trials, *Am J Psychiatry* 161:1537–1547, 2004.

Gloaguen V, Cottraux J, Cucherat M, et al: A meta-analysis of the effects of cognitive therapy in depressed people, *J Affect Disord* 49:59–72, 1998.

Goldberg JF, Garno JL, Portera L, et al: Qualitative differences in manic symptoms during mixed versus pure mania, *Compr Psychiatry* 41:237–241, 2000.

Golden RN, Gaynes BN, Ekstrom RD, et al: The efficacy of light therapy in the treatment of mood disorders: a review and meta-analysis of the evidence, *Am J Psychiatry* 162:656–662, 2005.

Goodwin GM, Bowden CL, Calabrese JR, et al: A pooled analysis of 2 placebo-controlled 18-month trials of lamotrigine and lithium maintenance in bipolar I disorder, *J Clin Psychiatry* 65:432–441, 2004.

Hellerstein DJ, Little SAS, Samstag LW, et al: Adding group psychotherapy to medication treatment in dysthymia: a randomized prospective pilot study, *J Psychother Pract Res* 10:93–103, 2001.

Kasper S: Treatment of seasonal affective disorder (SAD) with hypericum extract, *Pharmacopsychiatry* 30:89–93, 1997.

Kogan AO, Guilford PM: Side effects of short-term 10,000-lux light therapy, *Am J Psychiatry* 155:293–294, 1998.

Lam RW, Levitt AJ, Levitan RD, et al: The Can-SAD study: a randomized controlled trial of the effectiveness of light therapy and fluoxetine in patients with winter seasonal affective disorder, *Am J Psychiatry* 163:805–812, 2006.

Lima MS, Hotopf M: Pharmacotherapy for dysthymia, *Cochrane Database System Rev* 3, 2006.

Lynch DJ, Tamburrino MB, Nagel R: Telephone counseling for patients with minor depression: preliminary findings in a family practice setting, *J Fam Pract* 44:293–298, 1997.

Macritchie KAN, Geddes JR, Scott J, et al: Valproic acid, valproate and divalproex in the maintenance treatment of bipolar disorder, *Cochrane Database System Rev* 2, 2004.

Markowitz JC, Kocsis JH, Bleiberg KL, et al: A comparative trial of psychotherapy and pharmacotherapy for "pure" dysthymic patients, *J Affect Disord* 89:167–175, 2005.

Martinez B, Kasper S, Ruhrmann S, et al: Hypericum in the treatment of seasonal affective disorders, *J Geriatr Psychiatry Neurol* 7:S29–S33, 1994.

Martiny K, Lunde M, Simonsen C, et al: Relapse prevention by citalopram in SAD patients responding to 1 week of light therapy: a placebo-controlled study, *Acta Psychiatr Scand* 109:230–234, 2004.

Meehan K, Zhang F, David S, et al: A double-blind, randomized comparison of the efficacy and safety of intramuscular injections of olanzapine, lorazepam, or placebo in treating acutely agitated patients diagnosed with bipolar mania, *J Clin Psychopharmacol* 21:389–397, 2001.

Miranda J, Munoz R: Intervention for minor depression in primary care patients, *Psychosom Med* 56:136–141, 1994.

Modell JG, Rosenthal NE, Harriett AE, et al: Seasonal affective disorder and its prevention by anticipatory treatment with bupropion XL, *Biol Psychiatry* 58:658–667, 2005.

Moscovitch A, Blashko CA, Eagles JM, et al: A placebo-controlled study of sertraline in the treatment of outpatients with seasonal affective disorder, *Psychopharmacology* 171:390–397, 2004.

Mossey J, Knott K, Higgins M, et al: Effectiveness of a psychosocial intervention, interpersonal counseling, for subdysthymic depression in medically ill elderly, *J Gerontol Med Sci* 51a:M172–M178, 1996.

Mynors-Wallis L: Problem-solving treatment: evidence for effectiveness and feasibility in primary care, *Int J Psychiatry Med* 26:249–262, 1996.

Mynors-Wallis L, Gath DH, Day A, Baker F, et al: Randomized controlled trial of problem solving treatment, antidepressant medication, and combined treatment for major depression in primary care, *BMJ* 320:26–30, 2000.

National Alliance on Mental Illness: *Seasonal affective disorder.* Available at www.nami.org/Content/ContentGroups/Helpline1/Seasonal_Affective_Disorder_(SAD).htm (accessed Oct 14, 2006).

National Institute of Mental Health: *Depression.* Available at www.nimh.nih.gov/publicat/depression.cfm (accessed Oct 8, 2006).

Nolen WA, Bloemkolk D: Treatment of bipolar depression: a review of the literature and a suggestion for an algorithm, *Neuropsychobiology* 42:11–17, 2000.

Olfson M, Das AK, Gameroff MJ, et al: Bipolar disorder in a low-income primary care clinic, *Am J Psychiatry* 162:2146–2151, 2005.

Oxman TE, Sengupta A: Treatment of minor depression, *Am J Geriatr Psychiatry* 10:256–264, 2002.

Pampallona S, Bollini P, Tibaldi G, et al: Combined pharmacotherapy and psychological treatment for depression: a systematic review, *Arch Gen Psychiatry* 61:714–719, 2004.

Physicians' desk reference, 60th ed, Montvale, NJ, 2006, Thompson PDR.

Poolsup N, Li Wan Po A, de Oliveira IR: Systematic overview of lithium treatment in acute mania, *J Clin Pharm Ther* 25:139–156, 2000.

Rapaport MH, Judd LL, Schettler PJ, et al: A descriptive analysis of minor depression, *Am J Psychiatry* 159:637–643, 2002.

Ravindran AV, Anisman H, Merali Z, et al: Treatment of primary dysthymia with group cognitive therapy and pharmacotherapy: clinical symptoms and functional impairments, *Am J Psych* 156(10):1608–1610, 1999.

Schulberg HC, Raue PJ, Rollman BL: The effectiveness of psychotherapy in treating depressive disorders in primary care practice: clinical and cost perspectives, *Gen Hosp Psychiatry* 24:203–212, 2002.

Schwartz PJ, Brown C, Wehr TA, et al: Winter seasonal affective disorder: a follow-up study of the first 59 patients of the National Institute of Mental Health Seasonal Studies Program, *Am J Psychiatry* 153:1028–1036, 1996.

Serretti A, Olgiati P: Profiles of "manic" symptoms in bipolar I, bipolar II, and major depressive disorders, *J Affect Disord* 84:159–166, 2005.

Simon GE, von Korff M: Medical co-morbidity and validity of DSM-IV depression criteria, *Psychol Med* 36:27–36, 2006.

Singh N, Clements KM, Fiatarone MA: A randomized, controlled trial of progressive resistance training in depressed elders, *J Gerontol Med Sci* 52a:M27–M35, 1997.

Thase ME, Haight BR, Richard N, et al: Remission rates following antidepressant therapy with bupropion or selective serotonin reuptake inhibitors: a meta-analysis of original data from 7 randomized trials, *J Clin Psychiatry* 66:974–981, 2005.

Tohen M, Ketter TA, Zarate CA, et al: Olanzapine versus divalproex sodium for the treatment of acute mania and maintenance of remission: a 47-week study, *Am J Psychiatry* 160:1263–1271, 2003.

UK ECT Review Group: The efficacy and safety of electroconvulsive therapy in depressive disorders: a systematic review and meta-analysis, *Lancet* 361:799–808, 2003.

Weisler RH, Kalali AH, Ketter TA, SPD417 Study Group: A multicenter, randomized, double-blind, placebo-controlled trial of extended-release carbamazepine capsules as monotherapy for bipolar disorder patients with manic or mixed episodes, *J Clin Psychiatry* 65:478–484, 2004.

Wileman SM, Eagles JM, Andrew JE, et al: Light therapy for seasonal affective disorder in primary care: randomized controlled trial, *Br J Psychiatry* 178:311–316, 2001.

Williams JW, Barrett J, Oxman T, et al: Treatment of dysthymia and minor depression in primary care: a randomized controlled trial in older adults, *JAMA* 284:1519–1526, 2000.

Williams JW, Hitchcock Noël P, Cordes JA, et al: Is this patient clinically depressed? *JAMA* 287:1160–1170, 2002.

Williams JW, Mulrow CD, Chiquette E, et al: A systematic review of newer pharmacotherapies for depression in adults: evidence report summary: clinical guidelines, part 2, *Ann Intern Med* 132:743–756, 2000.

Wisner KL, Parry BL, Piontek CM: Postpartum depression, *N Engl J Med* 347:194–199, 2002.

Yatham LN, Kennedy SH, O'Donovan C, et al: Canadian Network for Mood and Anxiety Treatments (CANMAT) guidelines for the management of patients with bipolar disorder: consensus and controversies, *Bipolar Disord* 7:5–69, 2005.

Young LT, Joffe RT, Robb JC, et al: Double-blind comparison of addition of a second mood stabilizer versus an antidepressant to an initial mood stabilizer for treatment of people with bipolar depression, *Am J Psychiatry* 157:124–126, 2000.

Zisook S, Rush AJ, Haight BR, et al: Use of bupropion in combination with serotonin reuptake inhibitors, *Biol Psychiatry* 59:203–210, 2006.

CHAPTER 18

Diarrhea
Paul Lyons

Few medical conditions are more common than diarrhea, clinically noted as increased quantity or frequency of stool and an associated decrease in solid consistency. Almost all patients will experience diarrhea at some point. Although most of those cases will not require a physician's attention, diarrhea is a significant source of medical morbidity, mortality, and substantial economic expense.

Clinically, diarrhea can be diagnosed in the presence of (1) more than three loose watery stools per day or (2) a significant increase in frequency or decrease in consistency from the patient's baseline bowel function.

Diarrhea can be classified as acute (up to 2 weeks), persistent (2 to 4 weeks), or chronic (greater than 4 weeks). In some instances, diarrhea may last indefinitely, for example in IBS with diarrhea.

Diarrhea is a nonspecific physiologic response that can reflect a variety of underlying etiologies both infectious and noninfectious. The vast majority of infectious cases of diarrhea are secondary to viral disease. A smaller number can be related to bacterial and parasitic infections. Among noninfectious causes of diarrhea, malabsorption and medications are two leading and medically important considerations.

VIRAL GASTROENTERITIS

The vast majority of all cases of diarrhea in the United States can be attributed to viral infection and present a considerable medical and economic challenge. Viral etiologies (most prominently norovirus) are responsible for more than 90% of all gastroenteritis (GE) outbreaks reported to the CDC. Viral GE represents the second most common illness reported among family units in the United States. Although generally self-limited and generally not fatal among immunocompetent adults, viral GE is responsible for approximately 100,000 hospitalizations annually in the United States as well as several hundred deaths. Worldwide viral GE is responsible for 800,000 deaths annually primarily due to dehydration and electrolyte depletion.

The vast majority of all viral GE can be attributed to one of four viral agents: norovirus, rotavirus, enteric adenovirus, or astrovirus. Of these rotavirus and norovirus are by far the most common.

Table 18-1. Endemic versus Epidemic Viral Gastroenteritis

	ENDEMIC	EPIDEMIC
Etiology	Group A rotavirus	Norovirus
Age range affected	4 to 24 months	5 years and up
Peak season (United States)	December through April	Small peak in winter
Transmission	Fecal-oral	Foodborne, fecal-oral
Source or location	Variable but seen within families; community-acquired infection has been reported	Restaurants, hospitals/long-term care facilities, daycare/schools, vacation areas (including cruise ships)

Viral GE can be epidemiologically distinguished as either endemic or epidemic (Table 18-1). Epidemic GE is characterized by distinct outbreaks usually associated with the introduction of the virus into a defined population such as restaurant patrons, long-term care facility residents, or cruise ship passengers. In general epidemic viral GE does not affect young children (<24 months). Although epidemic viral GE shows a small peak in the winter, seasonality is not usually a prominent feature. Most epidemic viral GE is caused by norovirus.

Endemic viral GE is generally characterized by person-to-person infection that may be primary, reinfection, or community acquired. There is distinct seasonality to endemic viral GE with a peak from December through April in the United States. Most cases are caused by rotavirus and most symptomatic illness is confined to young children 4 to 24 months old. Enteric adenovirus and astrovirus are the less common causes of endemic GE.

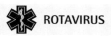 **ROTAVIRUS**

- Leading cause of viral GE worldwide
- Fecal-oral transmission
- Incubation generally less than 48 hours
- Fecal shedding for 10 to 21 days
- Within affected families 50% of exposed children and up to 30% of exposed adults will become infected.
- Peaks December through April in United States; spreads from southwest to northeast

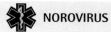 **NOROVIRUS**

- 90% of adults are seropositive
- Only limited immunity associated with seropositivity
- Responsible for two thirds of all foodborne illness
- Fecal-oral transmission
- Incubation 24 to 48 hours
- Fecal shedding 2 to 3 weeks
- Resistant to heating up to 60° C and to chlorine disinfectant

 ENTERIC ADENOVIRUS

- Responsible for 3% to 10% of endemic GE in patients less than 2 years old
- Incubation period is 8 to 10 days

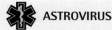 **ASTROVIRUS**

- Responsible for up to 9% of endemic pediatric GE worldwide
- Responsible for up to 7% of daycare center GE
- Responsible for approximately 10% of diarrhea in patients with AIDS

Symptoms
- Frequent loose stools, more than three per day ++++
- Decreased stool consistency ++++
- Vomiting ++++
- Fever is variably present +++
- Bloody stool +

Signs
- Related to dehydration secondary to GI fluid loss
- Frequency is directly related to the degree of dehydration
- Tachycardia
- Skin changes
- Dry mucous membranes
- Hypotension
- Sunken fontanelles (infants)

Comments and Treatment Considerations
Although viral GE is more common than bacterial diarrhea, patient consideration should be given to possible bacterial or parasitic etiologies. Primary evaluation consists of a careful history to identify critical symptoms suggestive of nonviral disease including severity of diarrhea (more than four stools per day for >3 days), blood, limited vomiting, and prolonged incubation periods. The Kaplan criteria

Table 18-2. Kaplan Criteria for Viral Gastroenteritis

- More than 50% of patients experience vomiting
- Mean incubation period 24 to 48 hours
- Mean duration is 12 to 60 hours
- All bacterial cultures are negative

(Table 18-2) have been used to distinguish clinically between viral and bacterial etiologies during outbreaks of diarrhea. The Kaplan criteria have been shown to be 99% specific and 68% sensitive for identifying viral causes of GE.

Serum antibody testing is not generally useful for suspected cases of rotavirus (endemic GE). Greater than 90% of adults demonstrate antibodies. Antibody presence does not confer long-term immunity. In patients with more than four stools per day for more than 3 days' duration, bacterial cultures will be positive in approximately 90% of cases. Visibly bloody diarrhea will demonstrate positive bacterial cultures in approximately 20% of cases.

In critically ill patients with impending or evident organ failure, emergent management is required. In noncritically ill patients, treatment for viral GE is largely directed toward fluid and electrolyte repletion. Oral rehydration therapy (ORT) has been shown to be as effective as IV rehydration in most patients with GE-associated dehydration. ORT for mild (3% to 5% body weight loss) to moderate (6% to 9% body weight loss) dehydration can be used alone for patients who can tolerate oral fluids. IV hydration with or without oral rehydration therapy is recommended for patients with severe dehydration.

BACTERIAL AND PARASITIC INFECTION

Although less common than viral GE, bacterial and parasitic GE remains a medically and economically important source of concern. While there are no well-established criteria for the diagnostic consideration of bacterial or parasitic diarrhea, several key clinical findings should prompt evaluation including fever, blood, severity, or persistence of diarrhea. In addition a history of recent travel, known exposure, or antibiotic use should also prompt consideration of bacterial or parasitic infection (Table 18-3).

Table 18-3. Factors Favoring Bacterial or Parasitic Etiology for Diarrhea

- Marked fever
- Visibly bloody diarrhea or report of bloody diarrhea
- Severe diarrhea defined as more than four stools per day for >3 days
- Persistent (>14 days' duration) or chronic diarrhea (>1 month's duration)
- Recent antibiotic use
- Recent hospitalization
- Recent travel

✢ BACTERIAL INFECTION

The estimated prevalence of bacterial diarrhea, however, is 5% to 7% of all diarrhea cases. Among the bacterial causes of diarrhea a handful of organisms represent the most commonly cultured bacteria. One large study in the early 1990s found positive bacterial cultures in 5.6% of samples. The four most common organisms were *Campylobacter* (2.3%), salmonella (1.8%), shigella (1.1%), and *Escherichia coli 0157:H7* (0.4%). Of note in this study, *E. coli* was found in 7.8% of samples reporting blood and only 0.1% of those not reporting blood. A second large study released in 2005 found similar prevalent organisms but also noted the presence of cryptosporidium at rates in excess of *E. coli*. Less common organisms noted in this study included yersinia, listeria, vibrio, and cyclospora.

Bacterial diarrhea can be usefully categorized as primarily originating in either the small or large bowel.

Clostridium difficile infection results in diarrhea associated with colitis and is usually the result of antibiotic use. The bacterial causes of diarrhea are reviewed under "Medication-Related Diarrhea."

Campylobacter
- Primary source is undercooked infected poultry
- Second leading cause of foodborne illness in the United States
- Incubation period is 3 days (1 to 7 days)
- Prodromal fever often noted +++; abdominal pain more prominent than in most diarrheas; nausea is common +++/++++ but vomiting is less common ++ (≈15%)
- Associated with a watery and/or hemorrhagic diarrhea, large bowel disease ++++/+++++
- Usually self-limited (≈7days) but abdominal pain may persist
- Bacterial shedding persists for approximately 1 month (mean 38 days) but is not clinically important.
- Does not usually require antibiotic therapy but is sensitive to macrolides and fluoroquinolones orally or aminoglycosides parenterally
- Has been associated clinically with reactive arthritis and Guillain-Barré disease

Salmonella
- Non-typhoidal salmonella is the leading cause of foodborne illness.
- Most commonly associated with poultry, eggs, and milk; also found in fresh produce, meats, and pets (notably reptiles)
- Peak incidence in summer and early fall
- Usually presents as small bowel diarrhea (nausea, fever, diarrhea)
- Presentation of salmonella infection may range from asymptomatic to life threatening; patients presenting for evaluation will almost universally present with some combination of nausea, fever, and diarrhea +++++

- Symptoms usually appear 6 to 72 hours after ingestion.
- Antibiotics show little benefit in otherwise healthy adults or children older than 12 months of age.
- Possible indications for antibiotic use in adults include high fever, need for hospitalization, or more than 10 stools per day.
- In infants younger than 3 months of age, antibiotic therapy is recommended to reduce the risk of complications. Some authorities recommend treating all children younger than 1 year of age.
- Treatment is also recommended regardless of age for immuno-compromised individuals including sickle cell disease, AIDS, organ transplant, or vascular/osseous prostheses.
- When indicated, antibiotic choice includes third-generation cephalosporins and fluoroquinolones.

Shigella
- Associated with person-to-person transmission and through contact with contaminated food or water
- Produces classic large bowel diarrhea characterized by small volume bloody +++ (30% to 50%) or mucoid diarrhea ++++ (70% to 85%), associated with high fever ++ (30% to 40%) and abdominal pain ++++ (70% to 90%)
- Disease is self-limited (mean duration ≈7 days) and does not generally require antibiotics for resolution
- Bacterial shedding persists up to 6 weeks without antibiotic treatment.
- Many experts recommend antibiotic treatment to reduce the risk of person-to-person transmission.
- In general, treatment for suspected shigella may be held until culture results are available. For high-risk patients with suggestive clinical presentations, therapy may be considered prior to culture results. At-risk populations include health care workers, food service workers, older adults, malnourished, daycare center participants, and patients with HIV with or without AIDS.

E. coli 0157:H7
- Foodborne diarrhea associated primarily with undercooked ground beef. Has also been associated with other food sources including unpasteurized apple cider.
- Incubation period between exposure and disease is 3 to 4 days.
- Clinical disease is often characterized by bloody diarrhea (by history or visibly bloody sample), elevated white count (>10,000), significant abdominal tenderness and absence of fever. +++ In one study at least three of these five signs/symptoms were present in 65% of all cases of *E. coli.* By contrast at least three were noted in only 19% of cases of shigella, campylobacter, or salmonella.
- The peak incidence of disease in the United States is summer with two thirds of all cases reported in June and September.
- *E. coli 0157:H7* has been associated with hemolytic-uremic syndrome and thrombocytopenic purpura.

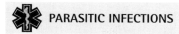 **PARASITIC INFECTIONS**

Parasitic infections may also present clinically with diarrhea. Although generally less common and less clinically significant than either viral or bacterial etiologies within the United States, parasitic infections remain a consideration in patients with diarrhea. Worldwide parasitic infections continue to represent a substantial public health and economic challenge.

Although the number of parasites that may present with GI symptoms is large, the most significant organisms are reviewed below. Parasitic infections resulting in diarrhea may be either foodborne or may arise via exposure to infected individuals or contaminated water supplies.

Cryptosporidium
- Intracellular protozoa that reproduce within epithelial cells of the Gi tract
- Most common parasitic cause of foodborne illness
- Organism is acquired via contact with contaminated food or water (drinking or swimming) or via contact with another affected individual via fecal-oral transmission
- Associated with diarrhea and biliary disease
- In immunocompetent individuals, cryptosporidial disease is associated with diarrhea and dehydration (at times severe) but is generally self-limited.
- In immunocompromised individuals, cryptosporidial disease may be both more severe and more prolonged.
- Diagnosis is via identification of oocysts on microscopic examination of suspected stool sample.

Giardia lamblia
- Giardiasis is the second most common parasitic infection in the United States.
- 2.5 million cases annually
- Animals provide the reservoir and transmission is via the fecal-oral route often from exposure to contaminated water supplies.
- Up to 60% of infected adults remain asymptomatic.
- Symptoms include dyspepsia and typical small bowel diarrhea with associated nausea ++++ (70%), vomiting ++ (30%), cramping ++++ (70%), and weight loss +++ (65%).
- Additional symptoms include steatorrhea/foul-smelling stool ++++ (70%), malaise ++++ (85%), and flatulence ++++ (75%).
- Clinical course is marked by a gradual onset and a prolonged duration (2 to 4 weeks).
- Diagnosis is via stool studies for ova and parasites from three separate samples (85% to 90% sensitive).
- Alternative diagnostic options include antibody studies via ELISA or immunofluorescence (90% to 99% sensitive, 95% to 100% specific).
- Treatment is generally with metronidazole and is outlined in Table 18-4.

Table 18-4. Antibiotic Treatment for Bacterial and Parasitic Gastroenteritis

ORGANISM	TREATMENT
Campylobacter	5 days of treatment with: • Macrolides (e.g., erythromycin 500 mg PO bid) • Aminoglycosides for severe infection
Salmonella	3 to 7 days of treatment with: • Third-generation cephalosporins (e.g., ceftriaxone 2 g IV every day) • Fluoroquinolones (e.g., ofloxacin 400 mg PO bid) • Alternatives include amoxicillin, TMP-SMX
Shigella	5 days of treatment with: • Quinolones (e.g., ciprofloxacin 500 mg PO bid; 1 g PO single-dose therapy is an alternative for mild disease) • Alternative treatments include macrolides and TMP-SMX in patient isolates shown to be sensitive
E. coli 0157:H7	Supportive therapy only. No proven or generally accepted benefit from antibiotic therapy. In patients with hemolytic-uremic syndrome management should be directed to these sequelae of infection.
Cryptosporidium	Treatment in immunocompetent adults is not usually necessary. When indicated (for persistent symptoms), however, may be treated with: • Nitazoxanide, 500 mg PO bid for 3 days Treatment is generally recommended for children with: • Nitazoxanide 100 mg PO bid for 3 days (age 1-3 years old) • Nitazoxanide 200 mg PO bid for 3 days (age 4-11 years old) • 12 years and older as adults Treatment for immunodeficient individuals has shown variable benefit. Recommended treatment is with: • Nitazoxanide 1000 mg bid PO for 2 weeks alone or with azithromycin
Giardia lamblia	Treatment varies by age and pregnancy status. • Nonpregnant adults: metronidazole 250 mg PO tid for 5 to 6 days • Pregnant with mild disease: defer • Pregnant with severe disease: metronidazole as above or paromomycin 500 mg PO qid for 7 to 10 days • Children: albendazole 400 mg PO for 5 days

Table 18-4. Antibiotic Treatment for Bacterial and Parasitic Gastroenteritis—cont'd

ORGANISM	TREATMENT
Entamoeba histolytica	Intestinal disease should be treated for luminal and tissue organisms Luminal disease: • Iodoquinol 650 mg PO tid for 20 days *or* • Paromomycin 500 mg PO tid for seven days *or* • Diloxanide furoate 500 mg PO tid for 10 days Tissue disease: • Metronidazole 750 mg PO tid for 10 days

Entamoeba histolytica
- Protozoa transmitted via fecal-oral route
- 10% of the worldwide population infected, primarily in underdeveloped areas
- 90% of infected patients are asymptomatic
- Responsible for approximately 60 million symptomatic infections and 100,000 deaths annually
- Diagnosis is via stool antigen studies that are 87% sensitive and 90% specific.
- Treatment is dependent on the location of infection (intestinal or liver) and is summarized in Table 18-4.

Cyclospora
- Usually a foodborne pathogen
- Generally presents with small bowel diarrheal symptoms
- Often associated with severe fatigue and malaise as well as diarrhea
- Course may be prolonged (>3 weeks)

Symptoms
- Small bowel disease—High-volume, high-frequency, watery diarrhea with gas, bloating, cramping, and nausea. Generally not associated with reports of bloody diarrhea.
- Large bowel disease—Small-volume, lower-frequency diarrhea with blood or mucus

Signs
- Fever
- Abdominal tenderness
- Visible blood
- Hyperactive bowel sounds

Comments and Treatment Considerations
- Most cases of bacterial GE do not require antibiotic treatment.
- The cornerstone of treatment for bacterial GE is fluid and electrolyte repletion.

- It is generally not cost-effective, or necessary, to send stool cultures on healthy patients with diarrhea because the vast majority are self-limited without specific treatment. When cultures indicate a specific bacterial etiology and the clinical conditions suggest a need for antibiotic treatment, therapy should begin with antibiotics known to be active against the identified organism. Specific treatment recommendations are highlighted in Table 18-4.

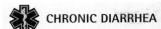 **CHRONIC DIARRHEA**

Although often unpleasant and possibly medically concerning, most diarrhea is relatively brief in duration lasting no longer than a few days to a few weeks. In some instances, however, diarrhea may persist beyond 2 weeks (persistent diarrhea) or even beyond a month (chronic diarrhea). When diarrhea has persisted beyond a relatively brief period, physicians should entertain the possibility of either medication-related diarrhea or a malabsorptive process.

Chronic diarrhea may result from a variety of medical conditions including IBS, functional diarrhea, IBD, systemic disease such as thyrotoxicosis or carcinoid syndrome, and malabsorption syndromes. Although a variety of conditions may be associated with malabsorption, the most common disease processes include chronic pancreatitis, celiac disease, lactose intolerance, and bacterial overgrowth. It should be noted that some infectious etiologies may be associated with chronic diarrhea. In cases of chronic diarrhea, a thorough evaluation including stool cultures for bacteria and ova or parasites may be helpful. The most significant of these are covered earlier.

MALABSORPTION

Malabsorption is defined as dysfunction of nutrient absorption either due to intrinsic GI disease or acquired defects. Although a generally accepted algorithm for evaluation of chronic diarrhea has not been established, the majority of cases ($\approx$90%) eventually yield a specific diagnosis.

History should emphasize the nature, frequency, and duration of diarrhea. Risk factors for HIV should be reviewed. Family history should be reviewed for GI disease processes. Additional non-GI symptoms should be reviewed because patterns may be suggestive of specific disease entities.

Travel, exposures, and occupation should be reviewed. Psychosocial stressors should be identified. All chronic and recent acute medical conditions should be identified as well as any medication use associated with these conditions.

Symptoms
- Symptoms may vary from nearly asymptomatic to fulminant.
- A diagnosis of malabsorption should be prompted by duration of diarrhea because specific symptoms are highly variable in frequency and intensity.

- Classic symptoms include diarrhea, gas, bloating, crampy abdominal pain, flatulence, and excessive bowel noise.
- Patients who present with symptoms consistent with a nutrient deficiency should be evaluated for malabsorption.
- Foul-smelling or greasy-appearing stool
- Weight loss
- Fecal incontinence

Signs
- The physical examination is rarely revealing in patients with chronic diarrhea.
- Note should be made of fever, rash, ulcers, abdominal distention or tenderness, adenopathy, and thyroid size

Comments and Treatment Considerations
Additional testing should be largely directed by the history and physical examination because no generally accepted set of tests can be recommended for all patients with chronic diarrhea.

Evaluation for most patients will include a CBC, thyroid function testing, basic electrolyte levels, serum protein or albumin and fecal occult blood testing. In patients for whom infectious etiologies are considered stool samples for white blood cells, ova and parasite and culture may be appropriate. For patients with suspected malabsorption, fecal fat studies may be indicated. In selected patients endoscopic evaluation may contribute to diagnosis.

Treatment is generally directed toward modification of the underlying disease process or avoidance of the inciting agent (e.g., dairy products in lactose intolerance).

MEDICATION–RELATED DIARRHEA

 MEDICATIONS

Almost any medication may be associated with diarrhea although a few such as metformin and the macrolides have classically been noted to produce diarrhea as a side effect of therapy. A comprehensive review of the patients' medications is warranted in patients who present with chronic diarrhea, who do not manifest other signs or symptoms of infection, or who note an acute change in GI function shortly after initiating a new medication or changing the dose of a previously prescribed medication. In addition to reviewing the timing and nature of the patients' symptoms a review of medication allergies, prior medication reactions, and past or family history of drug sensitivity (such as G6PD deficiency) may help illuminate the connection between medications and diarrhea. In reviewing medications, physicians should take particular care to review possible drug-drug interactions, especially in patients with extensive medication lists.

Symptoms
- Diarrhea with or without additional GI symptoms shortly after medication change or initiation
- Absence of symptoms more consistent with infection (fever, chills, fatigue, malaise)

Signs
- Clinical presentation may be highly variable ranging from no overt physical signs to evidence of acute allergic reaction.
- Signs of infection such as elevated temperature, abdominal pain, or visibly bloody diarrhea should prompt investigation of alternative explanations prior to diagnosing medication-related diarrhea.

 CLOSTRIDIUM DIFFICILE

C. difficile is responsible for significant disease burden associated primarily with colitis and diarrhea in hospitalized patients and in those receiving (or recently received) antibiotics. Physicians should have a high index of suspicion for *C. difficile* in any patient who presents with diarrhea in these circumstances.
- Gram-positive spore-forming rod
- Associated with approximately 3 million cases of diarrhea and/or colitis annually in the United States
- Mortality associated with *C. difficile* infection is 1% to 2.5%.
- Hospitalization and antibiotic use is the most common precedent risk factor.
- Prevalence is rising among population with no precedent risk factors (18:100,000 in 2004).
- Antibiotics classically associated with *C. difficile* colitis include clindamycin, broad-spectrum penicillins and cephalosporins.
- High risk of colitis is also associated with hospital contact with infected individuals; 13% of all hospitalized patients acquire *C. difficile* by 2 weeks; 50% do so by 1 month. Time to acquisition is 18.9 days if not in the same room with an infected patient; it is 3.2 days when in the same room with an infected patient.
- Treatment consists of discontinuation of the inciting antibiotic whenever possible.
- First-line therapy for *C. difficile* diarrhea is metronidazole 500 mg PO three or four times a day for 10 to 14 days.
- Second line therapy consists of vancomycin 125 to 500 mg PO every 6 hours for 10 to 14 days.

Comments and Treatment Considerations
When a diagnosis of medication-related diarrhea is made the physician is faced with the challenge of weighing the necessity of the medication against the severity of the disease. When the medication is easily replaced and/or the symptoms are severe, consideration should be given to discontinuing the medication and replacing it with an alternative. When the medication is not easily replaced and/or the

symptoms are mild, adjustments in dose may be sufficient to ameliorate the diarrhea.

Short-term medications can often be continued while the patient is treated symptomatically for the GI complaints. Diarrhea that presents shortly after the use of antibiotics or hospitalization should prompt consideration of *C. difficile* with appropriate stool studies and treatment as indicated. Treatment of *C. difficile* consists of either metronidazole 500 mg PO three or four times a day for 10 to 14 days or vancomycin 125 to 500 mg PO every 6 hours for 10 to 14 days.

References

Banks J, Meadows S: FPIN Clinical inquiries: Intravenous fluids for children with gastroenteritis, *Am Fam Physician* 71:1, 2005.

Blacklow NR: Epidemiology of viral gastroenteritis in adults, *UptoDate* May 2006.

Blacklow NR, Greenberg HB: Viral gastroenteritis, *N Eng J Med* 325:252, 1991.

Everhart JE, editor: *Digestive disease in the United States: epidemiology and impact*, NIH Pub No. 94-1447, Bethesda, MD, 1994, National Institutes of Health.

Glass RI, Kilgore PE, Holman RC, et al: The epidemiology of rotavirus diarrhea in the United States: surveillance and estimates of disease burden, *J Infect Dis* 174:S5, 1996.

Guerrant RL, Van Gilder T, Steiner TS, et al: Practice guidelines for the management of infectious diarrhea, *Clin Infect Dis* 32:331, 2001.

Hohmann EL: Approach to the patient with nontyphoidal *Salmonella* in a stool culture, *UpToDate*, 2009. Accessed January 28, 2011.

Kucik CJ, Martin GL, Sortor BV: Common intestinal parasites, *Am Fam Physician* 69:1161–1168, 2004.

Preliminary FoodNet data on the incidence of infection with pathogens transmitted commonly through food—10 States, United States, 2007, *MMWR Morb Mortal Wkly Rep* 57(14):366–370, 2008.

Schroeder MS: *Clostridium difficile*–associated diarrhea, *Am Fam Physician* 71:921–928, 2005.

CHAPTER 19

Dizziness
Jeremy Szeto

Dizziness is one of the most common and difficult symptoms to address in the primary care setting. Often the complaint is vague and is extremely subjective from the perspective of the patient. Dizziness may describe everything from feeling faint or lightheaded to feeling weak or unsteady. The workup of this symptom involves considering simple and complex medical illnesses and the list of possible etiologies is vast.

Because dizziness may be used to describe many different sensations, it is imperative that physicians have an exact idea of what is meant by the patient. For example, lightheadedness should be distinguished from vertigo. Lightheadedness may suggest a low blood flow state to the brain, whereas vertigo suggests an inner ear or cerebellar dysfunction. Obtaining an accurate history is a crucial step and allows the physician to work through the different possible causes. This section highlights the most common causes of dizziness: positional vertigo, atherosclerotic vascular disease, cardiac causes, stroke and transient ischemic attacks (TIAs), medications, and anxiety.

LIGHTHEADEDNESS

There are many causes for global hypoperfusion of the brain which may be transient or persistent.

VASOVAGAL EPISODES

Vasovagal episodes are a type of noncardiac syncope usually precipitated by pain, fear, or stress (emotional). These events are most often recurrent and are a reaction to a specific trigger. Younger individuals are more often affected although they may be experienced by individuals of any age. A prodrome, consisting of nausea, vision changes, diaphoresis, and abdominal and chest discomfort, may occur prior to losing consciousness. Treatment of vasovagal episodes is identification and avoidance of certain triggers. Unlike other forms of cardiogenic syncope, vasovagal syncope is benign and is not life threatening.

RUPTURED ABDOMINAL ANEURYSM

An aneurysm is the abnormal bulging of an artery. Aneurysms most commonly occur in the aorta although they may present in any part of the body—brain, intestine, and so on. The defect in the wall of the artery may be caused by atherosclerosis, hypertension, and trauma, or it may be congenital. This condition is worrisome because many people who have aneurysms are asymptomatic until the aneurysm enlarges and is at risk of rupturing.

A ruptured abdominal aneurysm is a medical emergency. Individuals 55 to 60 years of age and older with multiple risk factors (aneurysm >6 cm, uncontrolled blood pressure, smoker, female gender) are more likely to experience rupture. The danger involved is when individuals are asymptomatic when diagnosed. Most of the time these individuals may continue to experience little to no symptoms (up to 75%) associated with the enlarging vessel. Continual expansion will result in rupture, exsanguinations, and death. Treatment of a ruptured abdominal aneurysm is surgical intervention, taking into account the risks and benefits of the particular patient.

THORACIC ANEURYSM

Twenty-five percent of aneurysms occur in the thoracic area. The wall of the aorta in the chest cavity is usually weakened by chronic, uncontrolled high blood pressure although conditions such as Marfan syndrome, smoking, Takayasu arteritis, and syphilis have also been associated with thoracic aneurysms. Imaging modalities useful for diagnosis include x-rays, ultrasound, CT, and MRI. Treatment of thoracic aneurysms is surgical and may include stent grafting.

ANEMIA

Anemia has many causes and is a symptom that increases with age. The World Health Organization has set normal hemoglobin ranges for men and women (lower limit of 12.5 g/dL). Problems with blood loss, blood hemolysis, or diminished production cause a person to become anemic.

ARRHYTHMIAS

Arrhythmias may cause the heart to pump blood less effectively by altering the duration and/or force of the contractions. The ventricles may also not fill completely, leading to suboptimal cardiac output.

Symptoms
- Dizziness ++++
- Feeling faint
- Fatigue

Signs
- Syncope
- Hypotension
- Palpitations

Workup
- Differentiate types of arrhythmias
- ECG
- Stress test
- Electrophysiologic studies (EPS)—Invasive procedure to locate the origin of the arrhythmia via insertion of a catheter
- Holter monitor

Comments and Treatment Considerations (Depending on the Clinical Situation)
- Therapeutic lifestyle modifications
- Medications
- Pacemaker
- Implantable defibrillator
- Ablation—Via catheter
- Surgery—Surgical ablation, more invasive and usually a last resort

THROMBOSIS OR EMBOLISM

Thrombosis, usually referred to in the context of DVT, indicates the presence of a blood clot in a vein. The clot impedes blood flow and may break off (embolize) and lodge in different areas of the body.

Symptoms
- Swelling, pain, tenderness in affected extremity
- Chest pain (embolism)
- Shortness of breath (embolism)

Signs
- Warmth in extremity that is swollen and erythematous
- Color changes in affected leg or extremity

Workup
- Blood work—Including D-dimer
- Ultrasound
- Venography

Comments and Treatment Considerations
- Anticoagulant medication—Warfarin/heparin
- Thrombolytics—To be used in emergencies
- Vena cava filter—Used to filter out blood clots prior to traveling to lungs to prevent pulmonary embolus

MYOCARDIAL INFARCTION

Large MI may lead to hypoperfusion and dizziness.
See Chapter 12, Chest Pain.

CARDIAC CAUSES

Decreased blood flow to the brain causes dizziness that is from a cardiac abnormality. Coronary artery disease (uncontrolled and overcontrolled), blood pressure, and arrhythmias may impede blood perfusion. Coronary artery disease is a condition involving atherosclerosis and arteriosclerosis. Blood pressure abnormalities contribute to CAD because of the effects it has on the arteries. Dysrhythmias are irregular heartbeats cause by some disruption in the electrical activity of the heart.

MEDICATIONS

A wide array of prescription and nonprescription medications may cause symptoms of dizziness. This potential side effect may exert a greater effect on the individual depending on metabolism, body weight or size, dosage of medication, and duration of use. A variety of nonspecific vestibulopathies and related drug-induced ototoxicity may cause an individual to experience a sensation of imbalance, hearing loss, or both. Listed are some of the more common ototoxic agents.
- Aminoglycosides are a class of antibiotics that include streptomycin, gentamicin, and tobramycin. The medications may damage the inner ear permanently and result in imbalance. The medications may also affect vision causing oscillopsia, the perception that objects are swinging.
- Aspirin has potential side effects that may cause tinnitus (ringing in the ears) and problems with balance. Usually the side effects are temporary and resolve when aspirin is stopped.
- Loop diuretics, such as furosemide, may also cause ototoxicity and dizziness that is often reversible.
- Cisplatin is a chemotherapeutic agent that may affect balance and hearing in much the same fashion as aminoglycosides.

VERTIGO

 ARTERIOSCLEROTIC VASCULAR DISEASE

Cerebrovascular accident (CVA) generally presents with focal weakness. Occasionally some cerebrovascular disorders may present with dizziness (vertigo), with stroke and transient ischemic attacks. Interrupted perfusion in the posterior circulation may lead to dizziness, and vascular disease should be suspected in these patients. Atherosclerosis, thrombosis, embolism, and aneurysms are types of disease that must be considered.

POSITIONAL VERTIGO

Vertigo describes a sensation of motion experienced by the patient (self-motion) or the environment. Terms include "spinning," "whirling," or a sensation that the room (your surroundings) is moving. The most frequent cause of vertigo is benign paroxysmal positional vertigo (BPPV). Proposed theories note the imbalance in the vestibular system are due to canalithiasis (canal rocks) that are mobile densities in the semicircular canals that impede or redirect fluid, thus creating symptoms of vertigo. Patients may have a difficult time describing their symptoms. Peripheral causes of vertigo must be distinguished from central causes. In general, peripheral causes are extremely symptomatic with minimal change in head position. Some causes of peripheral vertigo include ear infections, benign positional vertigo, Meniere's disease, and labyrinthitis. Central causes occur in older patients and may be more subtle and be associated with other neurologic findings. In obtaining a history keep these things in mind to help differentiate among other type of dizziness: A description of dizziness with movement is too general and may be due to BPPV or postural presyncope, and head position changes without alterations in blood pressure (i.e., rolling over in bed, looking up, lying down) indicate positional vertigo.

Symptoms
- Dizziness, usually abrupt onset
- Nausea and vomiting with head movement
- Imbalance
- Blurred vision

Signs
- Nystagmus (rotatory—top pole toward affected side)
- Unsteady gait
- Worsening of symptoms with head movement—Patients with vertigo will be still and usually reluctant to move the head

Workup
- The Dix-Hallpike maneuver can be used to diagnose positional vertigo. The patient is moved from a sitting position to a supine position. In the supine position the patient's head is turned 45 degrees to one side and the head is bent backward 20 degrees off the table. Dizzy symptoms and eye movements are then assessed. Vertigo will present within 5 to 10 seconds and nystagmus will be observed in 30 seconds if BPPV is present. This test can differentiate the origin of a patient's vertigo. Central vertigo is caused by a problem in the brain whereas peripheral vertigo is caused by a problem in the ear. A positive Dix-Hallpike maneuver can distinguish which ear is affected.
- No laboratory tests directly confirm the presence of BPPV.

- No specific imaging exists for diagnosing BPPV. Abnormalities in the physical examination should be addressed via MRI to rule out other sources of inner ear pathology if necessary.
- Electronystagmography (ENG) may be used to better assess nystagmus.

Comments and Treatment Considerations

Brandt-Daroff exercise—A patient is initially sitting and then quickly leans to the side which worsens symptoms. The patient ends up lying on their side with that ear down. The patient remains in this position until the vertigo resolves. This is repeated approximately 20 times and done twice a day.

The Epley maneuver—With the patient in the sitting position the physician quickly lays the patient down with the head hanging off the table. The head is rapidly turned to the affected side. The physician then turns the head to the other side and then to the neutral position (ear parallel to the floor). The patient is then returned to the seated position and remains upright for the next 24 hours.

The Semont maneuver—With the patient seated the physician turns the patient's head 45 degrees horizontally to the unaffected ear. The head is then tilted 105 degrees so that the patient is lying on the side of the affected ear, head hanging and nose up. This position is held for 3 minutes, then the physician, while holding the head in place, rapidly moves the patient through a seated position ending when the patient is lying on the side of the affected ear, nose pointed to the ground. This position is held for 3 minutes and then the patient is slowly returned to the seated position.

STROKE AND TRANSIENT ISCHEMIC ATTACK

In terms of peripheral vestibular conditions that cause dizziness, 6% may be attributed to strokes and TIAs. Both stroke and TIAs involve an interruption of blood flow to brain tissue. The difference between the two is in the duration of ischemia.

TIA symptoms usually occur suddenly and resolve within an hour, although they may persist for up to 24 hours. Symptoms of a stroke and TIA are similar, and because of this one should always assume an acute stoke is occurring and should be evaluated as soon as possible. Narrowing of the vessels leading to or located within the brain is the cause of strokes and TIAs.

Other vessels in the vicinity of the occlusion may be able to compensate for the reduced or occluded blood perfusion; however, time is of the essence. Tissue that is oxygen deprived for only a few minutes may recover, but brain tissue starved of blood and oxygen that dies will not regenerate. There are two main types of stroke: ischemic and hemorrhagic.

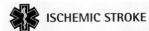 ISCHEMIC STROKE

Ischemic stroke accounts for the majority of strokes. Brain cells are deprived of oxygen and blood and as a result die. The cause of this ischemia may be from a thrombus, an accumulation of plaque within the vessels commonly seen in those with atherosclerosis. Ischemia may also result from an embolus, a blot clot that has dislodged and is trapped in a narrow portion of the vessel. In people with atrial fibrillation (irregular beating of the heart) embolus is of concern.

 HEMORRHAGIC STROKE

Hemorrhagic stroke constitutes approximately 20% of strokes. In this case there is bleeding within the skull, usually from uncontrolled hypertension, aneurysms, or congenital malformations of the vessels, such as arteriovenous malformation (AVM).

Symptoms
- General symptoms can include numbness or weakness, dizziness, or nausea.
- In the majority of patients it depends on location of stroke
  - Lacunar infarct: Contralateral motor and sensory deficit, ipsilateral ataxia, and dysarthria.
  - Anterior cerebral artery: Contralateral leg weakness and sensory deficit, confusion, incontinence
  - Middle cerebral artery: Contralateral hemiplegia, hemisensory loss, homonymous hemianopia, and aphasia. Involvement of posterior branch of middle cerebral artery may cause Wernicke's aphasia.
  - Posterior cerebral artery: Contralateral hemisensory disturbance, macular sparing homonymous hemianopia
  - Vertebral artery: May be asymptomatic due to circulation from other artery. With occlusion of small arteries symptoms such as contralateral hemiplegia and sensory deficit corresponding to ipsilateral cranial nerve
  - Posteroinferior cerebellar artery: Ipsilateral cranial nerve (CN) IX and X lesions, ataxia, Horner syndrome, contralateral spinothalamic sensory loss of limbs

Signs
- Depends on location (see previous)
- Dysarthria
- Dysphagia
- Ataxia
- Ptosis
- Facial droop

Workup
- History and physical examination—Assess risk factors (blood pressure, cholesterol, diabetes)
- Ultrasound of carotids
- CT scans—Used to assess if hemorrhage is present
- MRI—Used to assess area of ischemia

Comments and Treatment Considerations
The risk of stroke increases with patients who have had a TIA. Therefore, the focus of treatment should be to reduce the risk of a stroke via maintaining appropriate blood pressure, controlling cholesterol, managing diabetes, instituting lifestyle changes such as eating healthy, maintaining weight, exercising, smoking cessation, and taking low-dose aspirin or anticoagulants if appropriate.

Individuals should not wait to see if their symptoms resolve because there is no way to differentiate an acute stroke from a TIA. Prompt medical evaluation is absolutely necessary. Specific treatment depends on the type of stroke diagnosed.

Ischemic strokes hinder on correcting the underlying obstruction and restoring blood flow to the brain. Thrombolytics (clot-busting drugs such as tissue plasminogen activator) may be administered within 3 hours. Contraindications include neoplasm, active bleeding, aneurysm, arteriovenous malformations (AVMs), uncontrolled BP, aortic dissection, CVA less than 2 months ago, and allergy to thrombolytics. Procedures including endarterectomy or angioplasty, and stent placement may be used to recannulate the narrowed vessel.

Hemorrhagic strokes, mainly caused by aneurysms or AVMs, may be surgically corrected. Aneurysm clipping places a clamp at the base of the aneurysm in an attempt to keep the aneurysm from bursting or prevent rebleeding. Removal of an AVM depends on size and location. In case an AVM is not able to be removed, focused radiation or embolization interrupts blood supply to the AVM, causing it to decrease in size.

ANXIETY

Psychogenic dizziness refers to any psychologic disorder that causes imbalance or dizziness. The most notable cause of this problem are anxiety disorders, including but not limited to phobias, panic attacks, and chronic anxiety.

Symptoms
- Varied, numerous nonspecific complaints ++++
- Feeling faint
- Dizzy

Signs
- Tachycardia
- Diaphoresis
- Anxious mood ++++
- Syncope

Workup
- History and physical examination—Physical examination to evaluate balance, gait, function
- Psychologic questionnaires, if appropriate

Comments and Treatment Considerations
- Cognitive-behavioral therapy
- Medications (anxiolytics or antidepressants), if applicable
- Referral and evaluation by a psychiatrist

References

Baloh RW: Vertigo in older people, *Curr Treat Options Neurol* 2:88, 2000.

Brown DL, Morgenstern LB: Stopping the bleeding in intracerebral hemorrhage, *N Engl J Med* 352:828–830, 2005.

Lovett D, Newman-Toker V, Stanton Y, et al: Diagnosing dizziness in the emergency department: physicians may rely too heavily on symptom quality: results of a multicenter, quantitative survey, *Ann Emerg Med* 50:S11, 2007.

Dix MR, Hallpike CS: The pathology, symptomatology and diagnosis of certain common disorders of the vestibular system, *Ann Otol Rhinol Laryngol* 61:987–1016, 1952.

Epley JM: New dimensions of benign paroxysmal positional vertigo, *Otolaryngol Head Neck Surg* 88:599–605, 1980.

Hamann K, Arnold W: Menière's disease, *Adv Otorhinolaryngol* 55:137–168, 1999.

Kroenke K, Lucas CA, Rosenberg ML, et al: How common are various causes of dizziness? A critical review, *South Med J* 93:160–167, 2000.

Massoud EA, Ireland DJ: Post-treatment instructions in the nonsurgical management of benign paroxysmal positional vertigo, *J Otolaryngol* 25: 121–125, 1996.

CHAPTER 20

Earache
Michelle Whitehurst-Cook

There is a very long list of differential diagnoses for "otalgia" or painful ear. The most common include neuralgias, otitis, temporomandibular joint (TMJ) syndromes, tooth and oral pathology, cervical adenitis, ear barotraumas, and eustachian tube dysfunction. If the diagnosis is still uncertain after the appropriate history and physical examination, less common diagnoses need to be considered such as tumors in the nasopharyngeal area or in the ear.

Ear pain is characterized as primary or secondary. Those causes associated with ear pathology such as acute otitis media, external otitis, and tympanic membrane perforation are considered primary. Secondary causes are those sources of pain that are referred to the ear from other anatomic sites such as TMJ, cervical adenitis, or a tooth abscess.

It is important to examine the head and neck very methodically in order to identify the source of the pain. Keep in mind the multiple innervations of the ear and the structures which are also innervated by these common pathways.

ACUTE OTITIS MEDIA

Acute otitis media (AOM) is diagnosed when a patient presents with fluid in the middle ear with acute systemic symptoms such as fever, irritability, and pain. AOM occurs when fluid builds up in the eustachian tube causing increase in negative pressure and fluid collection in the middle ear from a URI or allergic rhinitis. This fluid in the middle ear provides the culture medium for bacteria or viral growth and subsequent infection. The most common pathogens are *Streptococcus pneumoniae, Haemophilus influenzae, Moraxella catarrhalis*, and viruses. Viruses were identified in 16% of children diagnosed with AOM using several studies. The most common viruses were RSV, rhinoviruses, influenzaviruses, and adenoviruses.

Symptoms
- Fever
- Irritability
- Pain
- Difficulty hearing

Signs
- Red bulging tympanic membrane
- Otorrhea
- Air fluid level in the middle ear
- Decreased hearing on examination
- Immobile tympanic membrane using the pneumatic otoscope

Workup
- Examination reveals signs of inflammation such as a red bulging tympanic membrane.
- Otorrhea or purulent exudate may be present in the auditory canal.
- Air fluid level and poor mobility of the TMJ by pneumatic otoscopy
- It is important to remember that redness can be caused by trauma and crying and may not be related to an infection.
- If the purulent exudate in the ear from AOM builds up too much pressure, a perforation in the tympanic membrane may occur. In this case pus is observed in the external canal and the perforation is visible with an otoscope.

Comments and Treatment Considerations
The pain can be of varying intensity and responds to acetaminophen (Tylenol), NSAIDs, and local anesthetic drops such as Auralgan (antipyrine, benzocaine, and dehydrated glycerin). Treatment of AOM has gone through dramatic change (Table 20-1). New guidelines recommend treating all children younger than 6 months and all children with severe illness (which includes fever >39° C and severe pain) with antibiotics.

For children older than 6 months and adults, watchful waiting with close follow-up (48 to 72 hours) can be planned. The diagnosis is often difficult because of the difficult use of the pneumatic otoscope; therefore, it is recommended for children less than 2 years that antibiotic treatment be started.

For uncertain cases and less severe symptoms in children older than 2 years of age watchful waiting for 48 to 72 hours before beginning treatment may be a strategy. Treatment of choice with amoxicillin (80 to 90 mg/kg/day) is recommended and macrolides are the second choice for penicillin-allergic patients.

Resistance to sulfa drugs has become a problem. Other drugs recommended as second line therapy are ceftriaxone and amoxicillin-clavulanate (90 mg/kg/day of the amoxicillin component). These should be reserved for children with resistant bacteria. Cefuroxime has been shown in recent studies to have poor activity against penicillin-resistant *S. pneumoniae*.

In children with refractory disease, tympanocentesis may be useful in determining the bacterial cause of disease and evaluating resistance to antimicrobials, though this is rarely performed. Decrease in frequency of AOM caused by *S. pneumoniae* has been seen since the institution of immunizations began against this pathogen.

All children less than 2 years and those at risk for recurrent disease should receive the pneumococcal conjugate vaccine. Children at risk are those in daycare and those with a family history of acute otitis in siblings.

Table 20-1. Medications Used in the Management of Otitis Media

MEDICATION	DOSING RANGE
Antibiotics	
Amoxicillin (Amoxil)	80-90 mg/kg PO daily in divided doses
Amoxicillin-clavulanate (Augmentin)	Amoxicillin 90 mg/clavulanate 6.4 mg/kg PO daily in 2 divided doses
Azithromycin (Zithromax)	10 mg/kg PO on day 1, followed by 5 mg/kg/day as single does for 4 days
Cefdinir (Omnicef)	14 mg/kg PO in 1 or 2 doses
Cefpodoxime (Vantin)	10 mg/kg PO once daily
Ceftriaxone (Rocephin)	50 mg/kg IM or IV once daily
Cefuroxime (Ceftin)	30 mg/kg/day PO in 2 divided doses
Clarithromycin (Biaxin)	15 mg/kg/day PO in 2 divided doses
Clindamycin (Cleocin)	30-40 mg/kg/day PO in 3 divided doses
Levofloxacin (Levaquin)*	10 mg/kg PO every 12 h for 10 days; max 500 mg/day
Topical Antimicrobials	
Ciprofloxacin/dexamethasone otic suspension (Ciprodex)	3 drops instilled into ear canal twice daily for 7 days
Ofloxacin otic solution (Floxin Otic)	AOM: 5 drops instilled into ear canal twice daily for 10 days CSOM: 10 drops instilled into ear canal twice daily for 14 days
Analgesics	
Acetaminophen (Tylenol)	10-15 mg/kg PO every 4-6 h prn; do not exceed 5 doses in 24 hr
Ibuprofen (Motrin)	4-10 mg/kg PO every 6-8 hr prn; max dose 40 mg/kg/day
Antipyrine/benzocaine otic solution (Auralgan)	Fill ear canal with solution every 1-2 hr prn

*Off-label use.
AOM, Acute otitis media; *CSOM,* chronic suppurative otitis media; *max,* maximum.
From Neff, M: Practice Guidelines: AAP, AAFP release guideline on diagnosis and management of acute otitis media *Am Fam Physician* 69:2713-2715, 2004.

Otitis media with effusion is diagnosed with a retracted tympanic membrane, usually with no pain or fever. There is usually an abnormal tympanogram that reveals decreased tympanic membrane movement with pressure gradients. The acute illness that is often associated with AOM and the physical findings of inflammation in the middle ear along with systemic symptoms of illness help to differentiate the two.

EXTERNAL OTITIS

External otitis is usually caused by a disruption in the protective lining of the external canal. Cerumen is produced from gland secretions found in the canal. This ear wax protects the external canal from pathogenic invasion and maintains a pH less than 6, which prevents bacterial and fungal overgrowth. External otitis may be acute or chronic. The acute form is usually bacterial or can be fungal, though rarely. A dermatologic skin disorder is usually the etiology of chronic external otitis.

Symptoms
- Feelings of discomfort or pain and soreness in the ear canal
- Swelling of the soft tissue in the external canal and around the os
- Hearing loss related to decrease in air conduction through the narrowed swollen external canal
- Pruritus

Signs
- Tender external canal on palpation
- Tender ear with manipulation of the pinna
- Edematous soft tissue of the external canal and occasionally the tragus and pinna
- Exudate in the external canal
- Tender lymphadenopathy in the postauricular and preauricular lymph nodes

Workup
- When evaluating the patient consider:
  - Swimming, hair washing, foreign body trauma, or excoriations of the canal can lead to invasion of the skin by common pathogens or fungi.
  - Trauma is commonly caused by hearing aids, cotton-tipped swabs, hairpins, and pencils and may lead to disruption of protective barriers.
  - Environments with high humidity are usually associated with increased incidence of otitis externa.
  - It is most common between the ages of 6 and 12, and less common after age 50.

- *Pseudomonas aeruginosa* and *Staphylococcus aureus* are the most common bacterial pathogens.
- Otitis externa diagnosis requires a careful history to determine the potential cause of the disruption of the protective barrier.
- Educate patients on the causes of this problem.
- It is important to identify patients with skin disease such as eczema for treatment to prevent recurrences.
- If the otitis externa fails to resolve with usual treatments, it is imperative to consider malignant otitis externa.
- Test all patients for diabetes mellitus who are diagnosed with malignant otitis externa.
- Cultures of the exudate should be done in all patients with diabetes mellitus prior to beginning any treatment.

Comments and Treatment Considerations

Topical acidifying solutions (acetic acid) or local antibiotic and steroid solution such as Cortisporin Otic (neomycin/polymixin B/hydrocortisone) can be used. A wick is commonly placed so that the solutions may be successfully placed and maintained in an often swollen external ear canal.

During treatment patients should avoid getting water in the ear. Cotton balls coated with Vaseline can keep water out of the ear while bathing.

Dermatologic conditions such as eczema or contact dermatitis may cause similar presentations. Patients present with itching, dryness, and flaky skin of the external canal. The history usually is important and identifies history of eczema.

Treatment with topical medication like neomycin can cause contact dermatitis reaction and may be mistaken for bacterial otitis externa. Often secondary bacterial infections occur due to chronic scratching with fingernails, hairpins, and so on that cause excoriations of the skin in patients with eczema or contact dermatitis.

Fungal external otitis (up to 10%) may have similar presentations in which there is little to no discharge and usually minimal swelling. The examination reveals tiny black or white spores and filaments. Treatment requires antifungal agents such as clotrimazole or tolnaftate.

Malignant otitis externa occurs in patients with diabetes mellitus and other conditions causing immunocompromised states. *P. aeruginosa* is the most common pathogen. Patients present with several weeks to months of itching, exudate, and decreased hearing. This condition responds well to the fluoroquinolones with 6 to 8 weeks of treatment.

Malignant otitis externa spreads to the underlying bone and into the meninges or vascular system, which can cause severe morbidity and mortality. Any patient whom you suspect has malignant otitis externa should be cultured prior to treatment. Poor response to oral treatment requires hospitalization.

TEMPOROMANDIBULAR JOINT SYNDROME

A diagnosis of TMJ syndrome is considered in patients who present with ear and face pain. Diagnosis is based on the history of pain and functional problems the patient has experienced. TMJ disorders are either intracapsular or extracapsular. Most common are the extracapsular etiologies referred to as myofascial pain of the masticatory muscles, TMJ myofascial pain syndrome, TMJ dysfunction syndrome, or TMJ syndrome.

- Rheumatoid arthritis, osteoarthritis, and articular displacements are causes of intracapsular disease.
- The etiology of TMJ is thought to be due to stress, jaw malocclusion, jaw clenching, bruxism, degenerative joint disease, cervical muscle dysfunction, dental surgery, TMJ intra-articular problems, or trauma.
- Often multiple etiologies are identified in one patient.
- Many patients have a history of grinding their teeth at night (bruxism) or chronic clenching of the jaw.
- Jaw malocclusion may be genetic.
- Malocclusion may also relate to chronic anxiety with chronic masticatory muscle tension.
- Patients with body asymmetry, cervical lordosis, scoliosis, and joint laxity have a higher incidence of developing problems with the TMJ.
- TMJ syndrome is more common in women than in men: 30- to 40-year-old women are more affected by TMJ problems.
- The pain can be in the ear but usually is made worse by chewing. Patients usually present after several months of the painful problem. They note the pain is worse with chewing and stressful and anxiety-producing situations.

Symptoms
- Headache
- TMJ sounds
- Pain in the face and neck
- Feelings of jaw muscle fatigue

Signs
- Masticatory muscle tenderness to palpation (41%) +++
- TMJ clicking sounds (22%) ++
- Dislocation of the joint palpated while the patient opens and closes the mouth
- Limited mobility of the TMJ preventing a wide opening of the mouth

Workup
- The examination is usually consistent with marked tenderness over the joint.
- Joint displacement may be noted on examination when the patient opens the jaw widely.
- Noises such as clicking and excess movements of the jaw are noted by patients especially when there is displacement of the articular disk.

- Physical examination may reveal a narrow chin and asymmetry of the face with the affected side being smaller.
- Ask the patient to open and close the jaw to observe jaw dislocation if present.
- Bilateral palpation of the muscles of mastication (masseter, temporal, pterygoid) is performed to check for tenderness and asymmetry.

Comments and Treatment Considerations

The diagnosis is usually made on the basis of history and physical examination. If patients fail usual treatment strategies, an MRI is the best test to detail the joint anatomy including placement of the disk, disk morphology, and degenerative joint changes.

A nonreducing disk is significant when viewed by MRI. A restricted TMJ condylar movement by physical examination is also significant. Because it involves the muscles of mastication, which include the temporal muscle, temporal arteritis should be included in the differential.

Treatment includes discouraging the patient from eating food that requires opening the jaw widely (biting an apple) and refraining from chewing gum or biting hard substances such as hard candy. NSAIDs may be helpful for pain management.

Jaw exercises help to relax the muscles of mastication. Patients should be screened for physical findings of chronic inflammatory joint disorders such as RA. Tricyclic antidepressants are often used to relieve stress and for pain management.

Muscle relaxants may be used to relive the spasm in the facial muscles. Patients often get relief from the use of mouth guards that relieve nighttime jaw clenching. Injections of steroids and lidocaine (Xylocaine) are used if symptoms continue. Botulinum toxin injections into the muscles of mastication can provide relief if other treatments have not worked.

Some dentists have special interest in caring for patients with TMJ syndrome and will help with prescribing the mouth guards and evaluating patients for treatable malocclusion and other associated dental problems. Beware that occlusal appliances may increase the symptoms of sleep apnea.

Some patients respond well to low laser therapy. Surgery is the last resort but should not be done unless it is preceded by arthroscopy.

Beware of initiating narcotic therapy for this chronic condition. Patients should be warned about the chance of addiction. Consider only when nonaddicting alternatives are contraindicated.

TYMPANIC MEMBRANE PERFORATION

The etiology of tympanic membrane perforation may be related to AOM, may occur after tympanostomy tube placement, or may be caused by a traumatic event. An earache is often relieved when a perforation occurs, which relieves the negative pressure buildup in the middle ear caused by the presence of increasing amounts of purulent exudate.

Traumatic tympanic membrane perforation is associated with sudden onset of ear pain. The etiology of the pain is often associated with the accident but the diagnosis of perforation does not occur until examination of the ear. Water accidents, barotraumas, explosions, penetrating injuries, temporal bone fractures, and being slapped on the ear are common causes of perforated eardrums. Perforations following tympanostomy tube placements occur from nonhealing of the site after the tube is extruded or may be caused by a retained tube.

Perforations of less than 2 mm heal quickly. Central perforations heal better than peripheral perforations. More than 60% of perforations heal in less than 1 month. Greater than 90% of temporomandibular perforations heal in less than 3 months.

Symptoms
- Patients present with sudden onset of pain.
- Bleeding from the ear through the external canal os
- Noises of air in the ear when blowing the nose

Signs
- Examination of the tympanic membrane reveals a disruption or hole.
- Presence of blood on the tympanic membrane
- Purulent exudate in the external canal
- Conductive hearing loss
- Hearing test should always be ordered when there is a history of trauma.
- If sensorineural loss is noted, a concern for inner ear trauma should be explored. A disconnection of the stapes from the other ossicles may have occurred during the trauma and will need attention.

Workup
- Patients who call and complain of sudden ear pain, blood or purulent discharge in the ear should be seen immediately.
- Documentation of hearing should be performed.
- It is important to examine both ears.
- The patients' ears should be examined for any traumatic event that may be associated with perforation.

Comments and Treatment Considerations
A complication may be development of a middle ear infection. It is important that the external canal remain dry and free of water while the perforation is healing. Patients should not swim and may use ear plugs or cotton balls coated with Vaseline to prevent water from getting into the ear while bathing.

If the perforation fails to heal, surgery is an option. A patch using the temporal muscle, gelatin film, a paper patch, or fat can be used by the otolaryngologist for myringoplasty.

References

Brown TP: Middle ear symptoms while flying. Ways to prevent a severe outcome, *Postgrad Med* 96:135, 1994.

Casey JR, Pichichero ME: Changes in frequency and pathogens causing acute otitis media in 1995-2003, *Pediatr Infect Dis J* 23:824, 2004.

Chandler JR: Malignant external otitis, *Laryngoscope* 78:1257, 1968.

Clenney TL, Lassen LF: Recreational scuba diving injuries, *Am Fam Physician* 53:1761, 2006.

Garbutt J, Jeffe DB, Shackelford P: Diagnosis and treatment of acute otitis media: an assessment, *Pediatrics* 112:143, 2003.

Kulekcioglu S, Sivrioglu K, Ozcan O, Parlak M: Effectiveness of low-level laser therapy in temporomandibular disorder, *Scand J Rheumatol* 32:114, 2003.

Netter F: *Atlas of human anatomy*, ed 3, Icon Learning Centers, 2003, *Oral Surgery Oral Med Pathol* 7(2):1180–1183, 1990.

Osguthorpe JD, Nielsen DR: Otitis externa: review and clinical update, *Am Acad Fam Physicians* 74:1510–1516, 2006.

Pelton SI: Otoscopy for the diagnosis of otitis media, *Pediatr Infect Dis J* 17:540, 1998.

Rosenfeld RM, Singer M, Wasserman JM, Stinnett SS: Systematic review of topical antimicrobial therapy for acute otitis externa, *Otolaryngol Head Neck Surg* 134:524, 2006.

Rovers MM, Schilder AG, Zielhuis GA, Rosenfeld RM: Otitis media, *Lancet* 363:465, 2004.

Russell JD, Donnelly M, McShane DP, et al: What causes acute otitis externa? *J Laryngol Otol* 107:898, 1993.

Weinberg LA, Chastain JK: New TMJ clinical data and the implication on diagnosis and treatment, *J Am Dent Assoc* 120:305–311, 1990.

CHAPTER 21

Family Discord
Kathleen Nurena and Heath A. Grames

Family discord can affect the health of individuals as well as the function of family life. Often symptoms and signs of family discord are subtle and manifest as vague illness or behavior in family members. Family discord must be on the differential diagnosis for many behavioral and psychiatric problems. Helping restore families to healthy functioning often improves the health and quality of living for all members of the family.

ADOLESCENT ISSUES

Adolescent medicine presents a unique challenge to the family practitioner. Preventive services have been provided for years, through vaccines and counseling regarding healthy lifestyle choices. It is routine to screen children for cardiovascular risk factors and obesity, as well as for sexual activity and emotional problems (see Chapter 25).

 PSYCHIATRIC ISSUES IN ADOLESCENT MEDICINE

Signs
- Sexual activity as marker: Involuntary sexual activity is reported by 74% of sexually active girls younger than 14 and 60% of sexually active girls 14 and older +++
- Depression
  - Studies have suggested an association between having a sexually transmitted disease (STD) and depression in adolescents. (see http://www.cdc.gov/nchs/data/nvsr/nvsr56/nvsr56_10.pdf).
  - Depression is an important diagnosis in adolescence.
- There has been an association between SSRI use and adolescent suicide.

 SAFETY ISSUES

- Sports evaluation
  - Screen in an attempt to decrease incidence of sudden death or cardiovascular diseases.

- Seatbelt use and helmet use for bicycles and motorcycles should be reinforced.
- Discourage drinking and driving.
- Assess for safety.
  - Screen for weapons use in the home.

 SEXUAL ACTIVITY AND ADOLESCENT HEALTH

- Approximately 45% of high school girls and 48% of high school boys have had sex. +++
- Average age of first intercourse is 17 for females, 15 for males.
- STDs are better prevented than treated.
- Condoms help prevent both pregnancy and STDs.
- Postcoital contraception is an option that can be offered to patients within 72 hours of intercourse.
- There are 900,000 teenage pregnancies per year.
- Approximately 50% of adolescent pregnancies occur within the first 6 months of initiating intercourse. +++
- The United States has the highest adolescent birth rate compared to Europe.

DOMESTIC VIOLENCE

Domestic violence or intimate partner abuse is a pervasive health problem in the United States. In 2000, the CDC reported that 25% of women experience physical and or sexual abuse over a lifetime compared with a 7.6% lifetime prevalence for men. The National Violence Against Women Survey reports 4.8 million women have experienced intimate partner violence compared with 2.9 million men; 6% of all pregnant women experience battering, and approximately 1200 women die in homicides each year.

For the purpose of screening and patient care, domestic violence and intimate partner violence are defined as a pattern of violent and coercive behavior in which one partner in an intimate relationship controls another through force, intimidation, or threat of violence. Practitioners must be attuned and assess for problems related to stalking, intimidation and threats, psychologic abuse including social isolation, and economic deprivation. The patterns include inflicted physical injury and sexual abuse, but are not limited to outward signs of abuse. Indirect health consequences may be related to the psychologic effects of abuse.

Symptoms
- Homicide
- Broken bones
- Injuries often to the head, face, neck, thorax, breast, and abdomen +++
- Contusions, scratches
- Ecchymosis on the neck

- Multiple strangulation attacks lead to injuries to the neck and throat and neurologic disorders.
- STDs, vaginal injuries

Signs
- Suicide attempts
- Anxiety (panic, posttraumatic stress, agoraphobia)
- Depression
- Fatigue
- Somatic complaints (chronic)
- Headaches
- Alcohol and substance abuse
- Abdominal pain (chronic)
- Visits to the physician can range from frequent abundance, to poor, lacking follow-up appointments.
- A partner who appears to be controlling and will not permit the physician to examine the patient alone may be an indication of abuse.

Signs During Pregnancy
- Maternal injury and death
- Late onset to health care and or inadequate follow-up for prenatal care
- Inadequate weight gain
- Placental abruption, preterm labor, fetal injury and fetal demise
- Increased risk for sexual assault and sexually transmitted disease
- Substance abuse

Workup
- Radiographic imaging if suggested by history and if suggestive necessary orthopedic referral
- Genital examination/STD screening
- Careful skin examination (staging of contusions)
- Digital photography for documentation

Comments and Treatment Considerations
Treat all acute injuries. Provide nonjudgmental support; people stay with abusive partners for a variety of complex reasons including fear, positive connection to abuser during times of calmness, financial and cultural reasons, family, hope for change, and isolation.

Have frequent visits: Even if the patient has left an abusive partner continue to inquire about threats and danger. Discuss orders of protection. Provide information about local domestic violence shelters and services. Repeat domestic violence screening more than once during the course of pregnancy any time indicators are present and again at postpartum visit.

Discuss a safety plan. Have the patient pack a bag with clothes, toys, or special items for children to evade imminent danger. Refer to mental health counselor or domestic violence service agency.

- Emergency housing
- Support group
- Legal advocacy

Cautiously provide psychopharmacologic therapy for comorbid mental health problems; symptoms are unlikely to abide until abuse discontinues.

Perpetrator of the violence should be referred to batterers group or individual counseling.

 SCREENING INTERVIEW

RADAR screening method:
- *R*outine screening: ask about domestic violence during:
  - New patient examinations
  - Annual examinations
  - Family planning visits
  - Episodic visits that present indicators of abuse
- *A*sk direct questions about abuse and acknowledge the patient's experience.
- *D*ocument your findings.
- *A*ssess for the patient's safety.
- *R*eview options and make appropriate referrals.

 CHILDREN AND DOMESTIC VIOLENCE

Children who witness domestic violence are prone to adverse psychologic and health consequences. Children who are exposed to domestic violence are at higher risk for smoking, alcoholism, substance abuse, obesity, depression, pulmonary disease, hepatitis, heart disease, and suicide.

Symptoms
- Psychosomatic symptoms
- Depression
- Anxiety
- Low self-esteem
- Eating disorders
- Effect on early brain development

Signs
- Injury ++
- Trauma
- Child abuse or neglect +++
- Fear
- Withdrawal
- Depression
- Suicide tendencies
- Sleeplessness

Workup
- Treat injuries and acute trauma.
- Assess safety and make referral to ensure child is safe; a protection referral is needed if the child is harmed.
- Conduct an in-depth clinical interview to determine if the child has witnessed violence.
- Be acquainted with local laws regarding child abuse. Many states require a report to child protection services when a child witnesses domestic violence.
- Refer to a mental health counselor.

END OF LIFE

End-of-life issues present difficult challenges for patients, family members, family practitioners, and staff. The complex and emotional nature of mortality is further compounded by ethical and legal issues, individual and family preparations for the impending death, and timeframe of onset of terminal illness or condition to death.

Comments and Treatment Considerations
Due to cultural, generational, and age differences and types of illnesses and conditions that patients face at the end of life, there is no absolute formula on what a person's end of life should look like. Patients should be involved in decision making and have the right to refuse care in accordance with law. Pain management is also a goal and right of the patient.

There are several recommendations: relieve suffering, maintain patient dignity, and provide palliative care for dying patients and their families.

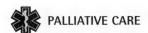 **PALLIATIVE CARE**

The primary goal is to provide comfort and quality of life to patients rather than to cure a disease or prolong life. Dying is regarded as a normal process. However, the patient may be receiving aggressive treatments and therefore may also include care that is disease oriented.

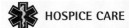 **HOSPICE CARE**

The primary goal is to provide care to dying patients using a multidisciplinary team approach. Such care is appropriate for patients with a life expectancy of less than 6 months and for patients willing to give up disease-focused treatments and aggressive care, including hospitalizations.

When considering hospice care, maximize quality of life offered by using services such as hospice or palliative care. Address safety and comfort with the patient as well as the unique needs of the patient, such as children and the patient's family. Respect cultural, spiritual, and religious preferences.

 ## PAIN AND SYMPTOM MANAGEMENT

The patient has a right to pain and symptom management. Assess for pain and symptoms, including diagnosis, presenting problems, current treatment and medication, existing pain management regimen, patient and family concerns/preferences, and patient/family values concerning pain management. Use a pain assessment scale to record baseline.

Create a pain management plan and educate the patient about pain management, including home care. Monitor the patient's response to medications, pain relief compared to baseline from scale, side effects and reactions, level of sedation, and satisfaction with the intervention. If pain is not satisfactorily managed, refer to other pain management resources.

 ## ADVANCE DIRECTIVES

Advance directives are formal documents that guide health care decisions if a patient becomes sufficiently incapacitated to speak for him- or herself and include a living will, five wishes document, and/or health care proxy (durable power of attorney).

Support patients and their family through communication and presence. Be present through transition: many patients report a lack of physician presence and communication during important end-of-life decisions and discussion.

Have ongoing contact with the patient through scheduled meetings or facilitate meetings between patients and their primary care provider and/or specialist. Communication is vital and a family conference may be appropriate. Address goals of care and changes in patient status. Discuss family conflict surrounding end-of-life issues (patient may need referral to a mental health practitioner). Discuss care options and family beliefs (including spiritual and cultural).

Be available to debrief with the family after the death of the patient.

 ## TREATMENT TEAM CONFERENCE

Discuss coordination of care. Discuss plan for managing the patient or family members who may be seen as "difficult." Discuss other pertinent patient care issues, such as complications due to mental health issues.

GRIEF AND LOSS CONSIDERATIONS

Grief and loss are normal reactions to death and dying. Discuss grief and loss with the patient and family. Refer to a mental health practitioner as needed. Distinguish between normal feelings of grief and clinical depression, anxiety, and other treatable compounding mental health disorders.

 PSYCHIATRIC CONSIDERATIONS

There may be an overlap of symptoms among depression, anxiety, and terminal illness, such as trouble sleeping, fatigue, and poor appetite. Symptoms that are out of proportion given the patient's context should be considered. Refer to a mental health practitioner.

 CHILDREN AND DYING

The event of dying or preparing for death is unique when applied to children in that it is not a normative life-cycle event. Many of the emotions are likely to be more intense for all involved in care.

Due to prognostic ambiguity of childhood illnesses that threaten life, palliative services should be offered early to aid the child and family in experiencing a "good death." Help parents and caregivers understand that palliative care does not necessarily mean that a search for a cure has been abandoned.

Follow pain and symptom relief procedures. As the family physician, support the family and patient and find additional support for the family as needed.

MARITAL STRIFE

According to the CDC, in 2009, the marriage rate was 6.8 per 1000 population, and the divorce rate was 3.4 per 1000 population for the 44 reporting states and Washington, DC.

Overall, 50% of first marriages end in divorce. The rate of divorce for second marriages increases 10%. Couples who experience marital difficulties are more prone to physical illness with an increased rate of 35%. Furthermore, there is a decrease of up to 4 years in life expectancy. Psychologic health for the individuals and the family members is also affected by marital distress.

Children in families with marital strife are more prone to infectious diseases due to elevated stress hormones. Increased depression, substance abuse, increased acting-out behavior, and poor school performance may also occur.

Symptoms
- Depression +++
- Anxiety ++
- High blood pressure
- Heart disease
- Substance abuse
- STDs

Signs
- Tension is high.
- Verbal or physical fights may ensue.
- Lack of regular affection and positive regard
- Decrease in sexual and nonsexual, affectionate contact
- The couple's mode of emotional communication is characterized by:
  - Criticism (feedback is often delivered in a harsh manner right from the start). The individual or pair has global negative critical feelings about the partner's character or personality.
  - Contempt
  - Defensiveness
  - Stonewalling (distance in which an individual ignores the other)

Workup
- Rule out any medical cause for the symptoms (i.e., depressed mood due to thyroid function).
- A sexually transmitted disease screening and examination should be involved for STD symptoms or disclosure of extramarital sexual affairs.
- An in-depth clinical biopsychosocial interview should identify the marital difficulties. Questions should include the following:
  - How do you deal with conflict with your partner?
  - Do you avoid conflict?
  - Do these interactions become destructive and disrespectful?
  - Do you or your partner become physically abusive?
  - Do you think there are differences in your relationship since your marriage or commitment?
  - Is there emotional distance in the relationship? Do you talk with each other about concerns, goals, and aspirations?
  - Do you spend less time with each other? Do you feel taken for granted by your partner?
  - Is the relationship passionate and affectionate? Is there a decrease in sexual desire?
  - Do you and your partner enjoy each other's company? Do you have fun together?
  - As a couple, how have you adjusted to major changes in your relationship? (job loss, illnesses, birth of a child)
  - Are there recent disturbing stressors that have occurred in your relationship? (substance abuse, financial strain, extramarital affair)
  - Do you and your partner agree on child rearing, values, spirituality, finances, and relationships with friends and relatives?

- Do you have a partnership and work together as a team? Is there mutual decision making, planning and sharing responsibilities for household, child care, and family responsibilities?
- Did you have difficulties from your past childhood that interfere with your relationship in the present?

Comments and Treatment Considerations

Efforts to repair distance and tension are often unproductive. These efforts include positive attention measures for the purpose of reconnection such as compliments, humor, and apologies. The couple lacks positive feelings, friendship, respect, affection, and admiration for each other. When inquiring about their dating history and/or wedding memories, the reports are often negative.

Distance prevails as a means of coping with the marital strife. As the couple becomes more distant from each other, it creates a lack of emotional connection, loneliness, and often leads to living separate lives. Consequently, one or both members of the relationship turn toward outside areas for fulfillment. This may take the form of workaholism, alcoholism, substance abuse, and attention only to the children or outside activities and friends. For some, emotional connection and intimacy are sought outside the relationship in extramarital affairs.

References

American College of Obstetricians and Gynecologists: *Guidelines for women's health care*, 2nd ed, Washington, DC, 2002, ACOG.

CDC Injury Fact Book: *Intimate partner violence, 2001-2002.* Available at www.cdc.gov/ncipc/fact_book/16_Intimate_Partner_Violence.htm (accessed December 26, 2006).

Center to Advance Palliative Care: *Crosswalk of JCAHO standards and palliative care with PC policies, procedures and assessment tools.* Available at www.capc.org/support-from-capc/capc_publications/JCAHO-crosswalk.pdf (accessed January 11, 2010).

Felitti V: Relationship of childhood abuse and household dysfunction to many of the leading causes of death in adults. The Adverse Childhood Experiences (ACE) study, *Am J Prev Med* 14:245–258, 1998.

Gazmararian J, Lazorick S, Spitz A, et al: Violence against pregnant women, *JAMA* 275:1915–1920, 1996.

Gelder M, Gath D, Mayou R: *Concise Oxford textbook of psychiatry*, USA, 1994, Oxford University Press, pp. 71–84.

Gottman JM, Katz LF: Children's emotional reactions to stressful parent-child interactions: the link between emotion regulation and vagal tone, *Marriage Fam Rev* 34:265–283, 2003.

Gottman J, Silver N: *The seven principles for making marriage work*, New York, 1999, Three Rivers Press.

Gurman AS, Jacobson NS, editors: *Clinical handbook for couple therapy*, ed 3, New York, 2002, Guilford Press.

Hedin LW, Grimstad H, Möller A, et al: Prevalence of physical and sexual abuse, *Acta Obstet Gynecol Scand* 78:310–315, 1999.

Heise L, Ellsberg M, Gottemoeller M: Ending violence against women, *Popu Rep* 11:1999.

Hinds P, Schum L, Baker JN, Wolfe J: Key factors affecting dying children and their families, *J Palliat Med* 1:70, 2005.

Hornor G: Domestic violence and children, *J Pediatr Health Care* 19:206–212, 2005.

Kaplan DW, Feinstein RA, Fisher MM, et al: Care of the adolescent sexual assault victim, *Pediatrics* 107(6):1476–1479, 2001.

Klein Jonathan D, and the Committee on Adolescence: Adolescent pregnancy: current trends and issues, *Pediatrics* 116:281–286, 2005.

Lyznicki JM, Nielsen NH, Schneider JF: Cardiovascular screening of student athletes, *Am Fam Physician* 62(4):765–774, 2000. Erratum in: *Am Fam Physician* 15:63(12):2332, 2001.

Montalto NJ: Implementing the guidelines for adolescent preventive services, *Am Fam Physician* 57(9):2181–2190, 1998.

Minuchin S: *Families and family therapy*, Cambridge, MA, 1974, Harvard University Press.

Minuchin S, Fishman HS: *Family therapy techniques*, Cambridge, MA, 2004, Harvard University Press.

Munson ML, Sutton PD: *Births, marriages, divorces and deaths: provisional data for 2005*. National vital statistics reports, Hyattsville, MD, 2006, National Center for Health Statistics.

National Crime Victimization Survey (NCVS): U.S. Department of Justice Office of Justice Programs Bureau of Justice Statistics. Available at www.ojp.usdoj.gov/bjs/cvict.htm (accessed December 26, 2006).

Satir V: *Conjoint family therapy*, rev ed, Palo Alto, CA, 1967, Science and Behavior Books.

Titus K: When physicians ask, women tell about domestic abuse and violence, *JAMA* 275:1863–1865, 1996.

Tjaden P, Thoennes N: Extent, nature, and consequences of intimate partner violence: findings from the National Violence Against Women Survey, Rockville, MD, 2000, National Institute of Justice. Available at www.ncjrs.org/pdffiles1/nij/181867.pdf. Accessed March 30, 2011.

Yost NP, Bloom SL, McIntire DD, Leveno KJ: A prospective observational study of domestic violence during pregnancy, *Obstet Gynecol* 106:61–65, 2005.

CHAPTER 22

Fatigue

Todd A. Thames, Larry R. Karrh, Ellen Bajorek,
and Christine C. Higgins

Few clinical complaints can be as frustrating, yet be so common, as that of fatigue. It is estimated that close to 7 million office visits per year are generated for the complaint of fatigue. Further, it has been estimated that of the patients being seen by a primary care provider, up to 33% report fatigue as part of their symptom complex. Patients are often concerned that their fatigue results from a serious organic medical condition. A medical or psychiatric cause is identified in about two thirds of cases of chronic fatigue. In the majority of cases, which can be up to 80% in some studies, a psychiatric illness is found as the underlying cause. Table 22-1 highlights the most common causes of fatigue.

As a clinical syndrome, fatigue generally refers to exhaustion during or after usual activities, or a lack of energy sufficient to begin these activities. Fatigue should be distinguished from weakness, shortness of breath, and hypersomnolence, which are possible markers for other disease processes, though these symptoms may coexist in a patient with fatigue.

Fatigue can be categorized based on the length of time the symptoms have been present. Recent fatigue represents symptoms presenting within 1 month; prolonged fatigue refers to symptoms lasting between 1 and 6 months; and chronic fatigue (not necessarily chronic fatigue syndrome, per se) refers to symptoms of greater than 6 months' duration.

This chapter presents the general approach to a patient with fatigue as a primary complaint, then focuses on the more common clinical syndromes associated with fatigue: anemia, cancer-related fatigue, depression, chronic fatigue and postviral fatigue, HIV, and hypothyroidism.

Symptoms
- Generalized tiredness and weakness ++++
- Depression (often) +++
- Lethargy with increased perceived sleep need

Signs
- Typically none in the setting of idiopathic fatigue with no underlying organic disorder

Workup
Fatigue is an extremely common complaint in primary care, though seldom is a serious organic cause identified. One large study found

Table 22-1. Common Causes of Fatigue

TYPE OF FATIGUE	CAUSES
Cardiopulmonary	Congestive heart failure Chronic obstructive pulmonary disease Aortic stenosis
Endocrine	Hypothyroidism Diabetes mellitus Hypercalcemia Chronic kidney disease Adrenal insufficiency
Infectious	Human immunodeficiency virus infection Tuberculosis Mononucleosis Hepatitis Cytomegalovirus
Medications	Hypnotics Antihypertensives Antidepressants
Neoplastic or hematologic	Occult malignancy Severe anemia Paraneoplastic syndrome
Psychologic	Depression Anxiety Somatization disorder
Rheumatologic	Rheumatoid arthritis Systemic lupus erythematosus Mixed connective tissue disease
Miscellaneous	Sleep apnea Idiopathic chronic fatigue Chronic fatigue syndrome

a prevalence of chronic fatigue, separate from a diagnosis of chronic fatigue syndrome, as between 1700 and 6300 cases per 100,000. Nonetheless, for patients with fatigue the consequences from a quality of life standpoint can be dire.

Patients with primary fatigue generally report being tired all the time, not particularly related to exertion and often not improved with rest. Conversely, patients with fatigue arising from organ-specific disease typically relate that they are unable to complete tasks due to increasing fatigue.

- Thorough history elucidating the specific tasks the patient is unable to perform as a measure of the degree of fatigue
- Investigation of other associated constitutional symptoms such as weight loss, night sweats, persistent fever, and thorough review of systems
- Assessment of psychiatric status through history and by use of an established depression inventory

- Thorough evaluation of prescription and nonprescription medications known to cause fatigue, most notably antihypertensives, hypnotics, antidepressants, neuroleptics, and drugs of abuse
- Physical examination should include: assessment for thyroid disease; full cardiopulmonary examination to detect evidence of CHF, valvular disease, or chronic lung disease; full neurologic examination including muscle strength, bulk, and tone; and examination of the lymphatic system to assess for lymphadenopathy.
- Laboratory studies are generally of low yield in the absence of abnormal findings in the patient history or on physical examination. However, it is reasonable to use laboratory tests to exclude other diseases. The Centers for Disease Control and Prevention (CDC) recommend as an accepted approach the following: CBC; serum chemistry including metabolic panel, creatinine kinase, hepatic function tests, and calcium; TSH; and ESR. Additionally, evaluation of iron studies, including serum ferritin, should be considered if indicated. Finally, targeted tests could include an HIV screen and a PPD based on history and risk profile.
- ECG, chest radiographs, and pulse oximetry are infrequently useful in the setting of a normal physical examination.

Comments and Treatment Considerations

Therapeutic goals for patients with fatigue are best focused on maintaining or reestablishing normal daily living patterns of personal and household duties, work-related activities, and personal relationships.

A prescription for regular exercise should be included in the plan. Maintenance of appropriate sleep hygiene must be emphasized (e.g., normal sleep-wake cycles, avoidance of inappropriate caffeine intake, intentional bedtime routine).

Suggest using an antidepressant agent, especially to patients exhibiting features of depression, but even those who do not may benefit. Consider treatment with oral iron replacement therapy, especially in women still menstruating and who have a low serum ferritin level.

ANEMIA

Anemia is a well-known cause of symptomatic fatigue and should be included in the assessment of the fatigued patient. Fatigue is especially prominent in the patient with a hematocrit of less than 30%, or someone that has a relatively acute anemia. Patients who experience a slowly developing anemia over time are often able to compensate and only in retrospect realize their degree of functional impairment due to fatigue. In patients with an identified anemia, correction of the anemia can lead to dramatic improvement in their fatigue (see Chapter 3 for a full discussion of the evaluation of and therapy for the anemic patient).

CANCER–RELATED FATIGUE

Although fatigue can be associated with the initial presentation of malignancy, fatigue alone as a presenting symptom of malignancy is unusual. Generally, other signs and symptoms, such as fever of unknown cause, diaphoresis, weight loss, respiratory symptoms, GI symptoms, or genitourinary symptoms will be present as well. In patients that do have fatigue as a primary presenting symptom of a malignancy, the cancer is far more likely to be hematologic as opposed to solid organ.

On the other hand, fatigue is extremely common among patients diagnosed with cancer and undergoing therapy, especially for those with metastatic disease. So common, in fact, that a separate clinical entity, known as cancer-related fatigue (CRF) has been defined as persistent tiredness or weakness that interferes with normal functioning, in the setting of known malignancy or cancer therapy. Fatigue is often reported by cancer patients to be one of the most difficult and distressing elements of their cancer and its treatment. CRF often results from many factors, most notably are anemia, chronic pain and pain therapy, emotional distress, poor sleep hygiene or disturbed sleep, poor nutrition (usually due to appetite loss or nausea), and other comorbid conditions. Additionally, disturbance of muscle metabolism and loss of muscle mass contribute to the weakness experienced by these patients. CRF can persist even after completion of the cancer therapy. Evaluation and management of these patients should focus on these potential reversible causes of fatigue.

Symptoms
- Generalized tiredness or weakness ++++
- Lethargy with diminished initiative
- Depression
- Organ-specific symptoms (chronic cough, hemoptysis, chronic dyspepsia)

Signs
- Anemia
- Neutropenia or leukocytosis
- Lymphadenopathy (often diffuse)
- Fever, often with diaphoresis, night sweats
- Unintended weight loss, with or without cachexia
- Organ-specific signs (i.e., hypoxia, hematuria, melena)

Workup
- In the setting of no known cancer:
  - Thorough history investigating associated constitutional symptoms (fever, weight loss, night sweats) and a careful, thorough review of organ systems
  - Physical and laboratory examination as discussed earlier in this chapter. Further evaluation is based on findings.

- In the setting of known cancer:
  - Assessment of severity of fatigue based on functional disability with ADLs
  - Assessment of stage of disease, type and phase of treatment, and response to treatment
  - Use of a standard fatigue inventory, such as the Multidimensional Fatigue Symptom Inventory-Short Form (MFSI-SF)
  - Careful evaluation of sleep history, pain control and current treatment, and depression signs and symptoms
  - Nutritional assessment including both dietary intake and GI symptoms preventing proper eating (e.g., nausea, vomiting, loss of appetite, constipation)
- Thorough physical and laboratory evaluation, which may reveal anemia, kidney or hepatic disease (primary or as an effect of therapy), cardiopulmonary disease (primary or as an effect of therapy), or other comorbid condition

Comments and Treatment Considerations

Treatment of anemia has had the most profound effect on improvement in CRF. Various approaches, depending on the etiology of the anemia, include correction of ongoing blood loss; replacement of iron, vitamin B_{12}, and folate; transfusion of RBCs; and therapy with recombinant erythropoietin or darbepoetin. Target hemoglobin levels to maximize quality of life appear to be between 11 and 13 g/dL.

Other pharmacotherapy approaches for CRF have mixed results when assessed with placebo-controlled studies. Nonetheless, attempts have been made to alleviate symptoms with the psychostimulants methylphenidate, pemoline, and modafinil. These agents may be considered options in selected patients when no other option is available and in patients who experience sedation from opioid analgesics for pain control. Antidepressants are effective in patients with a strong depression component to their fatigue. Low-intensity, regular exercise is typically advised for patients with CRF after careful evaluation for contraindications (lytic bone lesions, thrombocytopenia). The effects of an exercise program appear to be maintenance of muscle mass, improved sleep, improved mental outlook, and improved functional capacity.

Sleep hygiene should be maintained as close to normal as possible. Typical counseling includes avoidance of caffeine, restful activities prior to nighttime sleep, avoidance of afternoon or evening naps, and keeping regular bedtime and wake times.

CHRONIC FATIGUE SYNDROME / POSTVIRAL FATIGUE

Two main subtypes of chronic fatigue have been identified: (1) chronic fatigue syndrome (CFS) and (2) idiopathic CFS or non-CFS. CFS is characterized by unexplained, persistent, or relapsing chronic fatigue, lasting 6 months or more, and ascribed associated symptoms. In idiopathic chronic fatigue, the fatigue is significant but less severe and the associated symptoms may or may not be present. In both syndromes, the fatigue is not exertional, is not alleviated by rest, and results in substantial reduction in functioning. The diagnoses are controversial and complex. Potential etiologies discussed in the literature include infection, immune dysfunction, endocrine-metabolic dysfunction, neurally medicated hypotension, and psychologic distress. Fibromyalgia (FM) and TMJ disorder are generally considered allied conditions.

Contemporary North American literature considers CFS and postviral fatigue (PVF) as the same entity. British literature, however, using the term myalgic-encephalomyelitis considers PVF a distinct entity resulting from viral infection, most often Coxsackievirus or other enteroviruses. This is also separate from the short-term, self-limited fatigue that often accompanies acute viral infections (notably mononucleosis, cytomegalovirus, and hepatitis A and B). Often cited studies demonstrate enteroviral nucleic acid in muscle biopsies and unique enteroviral antigen in serum of up to 65% of patients with PVF. Other studies have shown evidence of Epstein-Barr virus in up to 20% of patients with PVF. Still other researchers have reported evidence that oxidative stress and excess free radical production from viral infection contribute to the chronic fatigue state. In animal studies, infection with one proposed etiologic agent, herpesvirus type I, resulted in significantly elevated F2-isoprostanes.

The CDC defines chronic fatigue syndrome as clinically evaluated, unexplained, persistent or relapsing fatigue with four or more associated symptoms, lasting 6 months or more. No physical findings were required to make the diagnosis. Fatigue, impairment in functioning, associated symptoms and psychological distress tend to be more severe in CFS patients. Psychological factors, primarily anxiety and depression, were present in a majority of CFS patients. Idiopathic chronic fatigue is associated with significant fatigue, but the symptoms are less severe than CFS and the prognosis is better.

The typical patient with CFS has a history of being a highly functional adult, varying in age from young to middle age (ages 20 to 55), who suddenly has significant impairment in functioning. Women are two times as likely to have the disease. The person may have a psychiatric history but she or he tends not to be someone with somatic complaints or who has chronic pain. The relative onset of the severe fatigue is often associated with a typical infection (e.g., a URI or true mononucleosis).

Patients with CFS have severe fatigue with four or more of the following symptoms:

Symptoms
- Substantial impairment of daily functioning* ++++
- Self-reported impairment in short-term memory or concentration*

---

*Symptoms included in the revised CDC criteria (1994) for CFS. Additional symptoms are described in the literature.

- Sore throat and/or muscle aches*
- Tender cervical or axillary lymph nodes*
- Migratory arthralgias without redness or swelling*
- Headaches of a new pattern or severity*
- Unrefreshing sleep*
- Postexertional malaise lasting 24 hours or more*
- Psychiatric problems
- Feverishness, rash, rapid pulse, chest pain, or night sweats
- Allergic rhinitis
- Abdominal cramps, weight changes

Signs
- Muscles are easily fatigued, but muscle strength is not affected.++++
- Excessive physical exercise exacerbates the symptoms.

Workup
CFS is a diagnosis of exclusion. Less than 10% of patients with chronic fatigue have CFS. The CDC and the International Chronic Fatigue Syndrome Study Group recommend the CFS workup to include (1) a thorough history and physical examination; (2) CBC with differential count; (3) ESR; (4) chemistry profile; (5) TSH; and other tests when clinically relevant. Screening tools for evaluating fatigue, anxiety, depression, degree of functional impairment, and illness beliefs may be useful in quantifying the symptom. The diagnosis is made if the patient has a typical history for CFS and no abnormality can be detected on physical examination or in the initial screening tests. Though *not* recommended, muscle biopsy and EMG are normal. Lymph nodes show only reactive hyperplasia if biopsied. Neuroimaging is not routinely performed.

Comments and Treatment Considerations
Beneficial treatments for chronic fatigue syndrome and idiopathic chronic fatigue are CBT and graded aerobic exercise programs. CBT focuses on altering beliefs and behaviors. Graded aerobic exercise programs prevent deconditioning and physical weakness. Both treatments improve scores on measures of fatigue, physical functioning, and quality of life.

Treatments with unknown effectiveness are antidepressants, corticosteroids, oral nicotinamide adenine dinucleotide, prolonged rest, yoga, coenzyme Q10, immunotherapy, dehydroepiandrosterone (DHEA), ginseng, vitamins, dietary supplements, and IM magnesium.

Antidepressants affecting both norepinephrine and serotonin (e.g., bupropion and sertraline) may be more effective than those acting predominantly on one neurochemical pathway. Citalopram (20 to 40 mg/day) when used for patients with idiopathic chronic fatigue, showed significantly and substantially reduced symptoms

---

* Symptoms included in the revised CDC criteria (1994) for CFS. Additional symptoms are described in the literature.

of fatigue, headaches, and muscle aches overall. Depression symptoms were not significantly lower in all subgroups.

Iron supplementation therapy may be beneficial in menstruating female patients with chronic fatigue, who have a baseline serum ferritin concentration less than or equal to 50 µg/mL.

DEPRESSION

In the setting of depression the symptom of fatigue is sustained, not resultant from physical exertion, and limits the patient's activities. Depression can occur by itself (unipolar) or as part of bipolar disorder. Three subtypes of unipolar depression are important to primary care physicians: (1) recurrent, major depressive disorder; (2) single-episode, major depressive disorder; and (3) dysthymia. See the chapter on depression for a full discussion of this topic.

Recurrent, major depressive disorder is the most common subtype seen in primary care and can be divided clinically into two groups: Atypical depression and typical depression. Fatigue tends to be the primary symptom of atypical depression, along with anxiety, anhedonia, and mood reactivity. Typical depression is characterized by dysphoria, tearfulness, low self-esteem, and appetite and sleep changes. Management for typical and atypical depression is generally the same.

Similarly, dysthymia is characterized as chronic, mild to moderate dysphoria, lasting 2 years or more. The vegetative symptoms (fatigue, appetite and weight changes, sleep disturbance, and psychomotor symptoms) in dysthymic individuals appear to be less common than in individuals experiencing a major depressive episode. Management for dysthymia and major depressive disorder is generally the same. Single-episode and recurrent major depressive disorders tend to have higher mortality risks than the dysthymia.

The DSM-IV criteria for the diagnosis of major depressive disorder, both single episode and recurrent, are at least 2 weeks of dysphoria or anhedonia accompanied by at least four additional symptoms of depression that cause significant distress and impairment of functioning.

Symptoms
- Anhedonia or dysphoria (with or without irritability) +++
- Fatigue, general tiredness, loss of energy or weakness +++
- Weight and/or appetite change (increase or decrease)
- Insomnia or hypersomnia ++
- Feelings of worthlessness, hopelessness, low self-esteem, and guilt
- Recurrent thoughts of death or suicidal ideation +
- Psychotic symptoms (hallucinations, delusions, cognitive distortions)

Signs
- Psychomotor retardation or agitation +++
- Diminished ability to think or concentrate, or indecisiveness ++

Workup

- See the chapter on depression for a thorough discussion of the workup.
- In general, limited laboratory testing (CBC, TSH, FSH) is recommended to rule out typical secondary medical causes. No laboratory findings are diagnostic of major depressive disorder or dysthymia.

Comments and Treatment Considerations

Up to 15% of individuals with severe major depressive disorder die by suicide. Monitor for suicidal ideation. Ask the patient about suicidal ideation, means, plan, and reason to live. Treatment for the depression may increase suicide risk.

Evaluate for manic symptoms and mixed episodes to rule out bipolar disorder, which is managed differently from unipolar depression. Watch for onset of depression after a death of a loved one or during the postpartum period. Up to 20% to 25% of individuals with specific medical conditions (e.g., diabetes mellitus, MI, carcinomas, stroke) will develop major depressive disorder during the course of their illness.

SSRIs, SNRIs, or DNRIs are the treatment of choice for mild and moderate depression. Fatigue, along with other physical symptoms, will often improve over the first month with SSRIs. Antidepressants that list fatigue as an adverse reaction are duloxetine, trazodone, and escitalopram oxalate. Watch for a gradual response of the antidepressants. Most take 4 to 6 weeks to show effects.

Some articles support psychotherapy and pharmacologic management as first-line therapy in moderately depressed patients. Some patients benefit from psychotherapy alone, others benefit from medication management alone. For mild to moderate depression, start with medication management and refer for a psychologic evaluation and confirmation of the diagnosis.

The results of a randomized trial of 573 depressed patients in a primary care setting identified no differences in outcome measures between paroxetine, fluoxetine, and sertraline. A systematic review of 46 randomized controlled trials and 26 observational studies noted no significant differences in efficacy, tolerability, and outcome measures between second-generation antidepressants (SSRIs, venlafaxine, duloxetine, mirtazapine, and bupropion). For severe, refractory depression, referral to a psychiatrist is warranted and additional therapies such as antipsychotics, anticonvulsants, and ECT may be indicated.

HUMAN IMMUNODEFICIENCY VIRUS

Up to 60% of patients with HIV and up to 85% of patients with AIDS report moderate to severe fatigue as a problem in the course of their illness. Furthermore, HIV patients with fatigue were significantly more disabled than their nonfatigued counterparts across the whole spectrum of the SF-36 health survey. Overall quality of life was markedly affected by fatigue as a sole factor.

Historically, HIV-related fatigue has been assumed to correlate with stage of disease, relative CD4 count, and viral load. However, evidence has not found this to be the case. Rather, the strongest correlate of fatigue in the HIV-infected patient has repeatedly been shown to be the degree of psychologic distress and depression. Additionally, there does not seem to be a direct association between drug regimen and fatigue. Most HIV patients are treated with highly active antiretroviral therapy (HAART) combinations and although mortality from HIV has dramatically declined, neither the biologic response (decreased viral load, increased CD4 count) nor the taking of these medications seems to directly affect fatigue.

Interestingly, there is evidence that increased fatigue predicts lower adherence to medical therapy. Fatigue is identified as a primary reason for forgetting a dose, oversleeping and missing a dose, and/or resisting intensive medical therapy.

Symptoms
- Nonexertional fatigue, tiredness, general malaise +++
- Depression and anxiety ++
- Chronic pain, either organic from disease process or perceived
- Myalgias, arthralgias
- Sleep disturbance

Signs
- Positive HIV, with or without criteria for AIDS ++++
- Depression, as quantified by any validated depression rating scale
- Lymphadenopathy
- Weight loss and "wasting syndrome"
- Anemia, pancytopenia, or iron deficiency (usually nutritional)

Workup
- In general, no specific workup is required outside that already accomplished as part of the management of HIV infection.
- In the setting of new-onset fatigue in an HIV/AIDS patient, careful evaluation for depression should be done.
- Any additional psychiatric or neurologic signs or symptoms should prompt a more thorough neuropsychiatric evaluation, including neuroimaging as appropriate.

Comments and Treatment Considerations
There is a lack of good evidence regarding treatment of fatigue in the HIV-infected patient. All authors agree that in the patient with depression, standard therapy with antidepressant medications is warranted and generally effective. Additionally, there is growing evidence that CBT and regular graded exercise therapy are effective in treating medically unexplained fatigue and CFS. It is cautiously held that these results should be applicable to the HIV-infected population as well.

Of course, organic disorders such as anemia and iron deficiency should be treated by standard modalities. Finally, nutritional counseling should be considered for all HIV-infected patients, but especially those suffering from fatigue would be well served with a structured dietary education program.

HYPOTHYROIDISM

Fatigue is a prominent presenting symptom of hypothyroidism. Most symptoms of hypothyroidism, such as fatigue, are nonspecific. The onset is often insidious and may be accompanied by other vague symptoms such as weakness, sluggishness, and weight gain. The symptoms of hypothyroidism derive from the deficit in circulating thyroid hormones and can be found in virtually all types of hypothyroidism regardless of the underlying etiology. The lack of thyroid hormones causes a generalized slowing of metabolic processes as well as the accumulation of matrix glycosaminoglycans in the interstitial spaces; either of these effects may induce fatigue depending on the involved organ. The organ systems most responsible for hypothyroidism-induced fatigue include the cardiovascular, respiratory, hematopoietic, and neurologic systems.

Thyroid hormones have both inotropic and chronotropic effects. A decrease in thyroid hormones results in decreased cardiac output at rest due to a reduction in contractility, stroke volume, and heart rate. Reduced cardiac output also contributes to decreased exercise capacity and relative shortness of breath during exercise, which may be perceived as fatigue.

Fatigue can result from impaired respiratory function as well as cardiovascular dysfunction. Although lung volumes usually remain unaffected, maximal breathing capacity and diffusing capacity are reduced due to hypoventilation from respiratory muscle weakness and reduced pulmonary responses to hypoxia and hypercapnia.

Decreased levels of thyroid hormones can also slow the production of erythropoietin resulting in a normocytic, normochromic anemia. In addition but less commonly, a pernicious (macrocytic) anemia may ensue due to atrophy of the gastric mucosa caused by antibodies found in about one third of patients with primary hypothyroidism.

Decreased cerebral blood flow, decreased glucose use, and a general depression of CNS function may cause patients to complain of fatigue and sluggish thought processes.

The clearance of many sedating drugs, including antiepileptics, hypnotics, and opioids is decreased in hypothyroidism. Drug toxicity may present as fatigue, even at minimal dosing.

Symptoms
- Fatigue, sluggishness, difficulty concentrating +++
- Heat or cold intolerance ++
- Constipation
- Peripheral paresthesias

Signs
- Periorbital puffiness, coarse dry skin, patchy hair loss
- Bradycardia, occasionally hypotension

- Slow relaxation phase of deep tendon reflexes
- Hypothermia

Workup
- Emphasis is placed on assessing the TSH level, with subsequent evaluation of the free T_4 and total T_3 levels.
- Further evaluation for Hashimoto's thyroiditis (including antithyroid antibody titer) and subacute thyroiditis (CBC, ESR) may be considered.
- Evaluation of any palpable abnormalities of the thyroid should also be performed via radioactive iodine uptake scanning or ultrasound (or both), or fine-needle biopsy as appropriate.

Comments and Treatment Considerations
Once the diagnosis of hypothyroidism is made, treatment is to replace the diminished circulating thyroid hormone. Levothyroxine is the most commonly used agent, but desiccated thyroid is available and preferred by some physicians and patients. Additionally, liothyronine (synthetic T_3) is at times used as an adjunct. HRT for hypothyroidism should be followed carefully with regular physician visits and serum levels of TSH, T_4, and, when using liothyronine, T_3 to ensure maintenance in the therapeutic range.

References
Aaron LA, Burke MM, Buchwald D: Overlapping conditions among patients with chronic fatigue syndrome, fibromyalgia, and temporomandibular disorder, *Arch Intern Med* 160:221, 2000.

American Psychiatric Association: *Diagnostic and statistical manual of mental disorders (DSM-IV)*, 4th ed, Washington, DC, 1994, American Psychiatric Association.

Bates DW, Schmitt W, Buchwald D, et al: Prevalence of fatigue and chronic fatigue syndrome in a primary care practice, *Arch Intern Med* 153:2759, 1993.

Bentler SE, Hartz AJ, Kuhn EM: Prospective observational study of treatments for unexplained chronic fatigue, *J Clin Psychiatry* 66:625–632, 2005.

Brody DS, Hahn SR, Spitzer RL, et al: Identifying patients with depression in the primary care setting, *Arch Intern Med* 158:2469–2475, 1998.

Buchwald D, Umali P, Umali J, et al: Chronic fatigue and the chronic fatigue syndrome: prevalence in a Pacific Northwest health system, *Ann Intern Med* 123:81, 1995.

Chappert SM: National ambulatory medical care survey: 1989 summary, National Center for Health Statistics, *Vital Health Stat* 13:16, 1992.

Darbishire L, Ridsdale L, Said PT: Distinguishing patients with chronic fatigue from those with chronic fatigue syndrome: a diagnostic study in UK primary care, *Br J Gen Pract*, 53:441–445, 2003.

Deale A, Chadler T, Marks I, Wessley S: Cognitive behavior therapy for chronic fatigue syndrome: a randomized controlled trial, *Am J Psychiatry* 154:408–414, 1997.

Demtri G, Kris M, Wade J, et al: Quality of life benefit in chemotherapy patients treated with epoetin alfa is independent of disease response or tumor type: results from a prospective community oncology study, *J Clin Oncol* 16:3412, 1998.

Fukuda K, Straus SE, Hickie I, et al: The chronic fatigue syndrome: a comprehensive approach to its definition and study. International Chronic Fatigue Syndrome Study Group, *Ann Intern Med* 121:953, 1994.

Greco T, Eckert G, Kroenke K: The outcome of physical symptoms with treatment of depression, *J Gen Intern Med* 19:813–818, 2004.

Hamilton WT, Gallagher AM, Thomas JM, White PD: The prognosis of different fatigue diagnostic labels: a longitudinal survey, *Fam Pract* 22:383–388, 2005.

Hartz AJ, Bentler SE, Brake KA, Kelly MW: The Effectiveness of citalopram for idiopathic chronic fatigue, *J Clin Psychiatry* 64:927–935, 2003.

Harvard Mental Health Letter: *Atypical depression*, Boston, MA, 2005, Harvard Health Publications.

Henderson M, Safa F, Easterbrook P, Hotopf M: Fatigue among HIV-infected patients in the era of highly active antiretroviral therapy, *HIV Med* 6:347–352, 2005.

Jackson JL, O'Malley PG, Kroenke K: Antidepressants and cognitive behavioral therapy for symptom syndromes, *CNS Spect* 11:212–222, 2006.

Klein I, Ojamaa K: Thyroid hormone and the cardiovascular system: from theory to practice, *J Clin Endocrinol Metab* 78:1026, 1994.

Kroenke K, Wood DR, Manglesdorff AD, et al: Chronic fatigue in primary care: prevalence, patient characteristics, and outcome, *JAMA* 260:929, 1988.

Ladenson PW, Goldenheim PD, Ridgeway EC: Prediction and reversal of blunted ventilatory responsiveness in patients with hypothyroidism, *Am J Med* 84:877, 1988.

Laroche CM, Cairns T, Moxham J, et al: Hypothyroidism presenting with respiratory muscle weakness, *Am Rev Respir Dis* 138:472, 1988.

McCrone P, Ridsdale L, Darbishire L, Seed P: Cost-effectiveness of cognitive behavioural therapy, graded exercise and usual care for patients with chronic fatigue in primary care, *Psychol Med* 34:991–999, 2004.

Mock V, Atkison A, Barsevick A, et al: NCCN practice guideline for cancer related fatigue, *Oncology* 14:151, 2000.

Nesse RE, Finlayson RE: Management of depression in patients with coexisting medical illness, *Am Fam Physician* 53:2125–2133, 1996.

Siafakas NM, Salesiotou V, Filaditaki V: Respiratory muscle strength in hypothyroidism, *Chest* 102:189, 1992.

Skapinaski P, Lewis G, Mavreas V: Unexplained fatigue syndromes in a multinational primary care sample: specificity of definition and prevalence and distinctiveness from depression and generalized anxiety disorder, *Am J Psychiatry* 160:785–787, 2003.

Smith TJ, Bahn RS, Gorman C: Connective tissue, glycosaminoglycans, and diseases of the thyroid, *Endocr Rev* 10:366, 1989.

Sovner RD: The clinical characteristics and treatment of atypical depression, *J Clin Psychiatry* (42):285–289, 1981.

Stein K, Jacobsen P, Blanchard C, Thors C: Further validation of the multidimensional fatigue symptom inventory-short form, *J Pain Symptom Manage* 27:14, 2004.

Stone P, Richardson A, Ream E, et al: Cancer-related fatigue: inevitable, unimportant and untreatable? Results from a multi-center patient survey, *Ann Oncol* 11:971, 2000.

Straus SE: The chronic mononucleosis syndrome, *J Infect Dis* 157:405, 1988.

Wearden AJ, Riste L, Dowrick C, et al: Fatigue Intervention by Nurses' Evaluation—the FINE Trial. A randomised controlled trial of nurse led self-help treatment for patients in primary care with chronic fatigue syndrome: study protocol, *BioMed Central Med* 4:9, 2006.

Woeber KA: Thyrotoxicosis and the heart, *N Engl J Med* 327:94, 1992.

CHAPTER 23

Fever
Alan R. Roth and Gina M. Basello

Fever is one of the most common presenting complaints encountered by the family physician during acute office visits in the United States. Fever is generally defined as a temperature higher than 38.3° C (100.9° F). Most cases of fever are secondary to acute viral illnesses and are generally termed upper respiratory infections (URIs). Other common causes of fever include viruses such as GI and influenza, sinusitis, pharyngitis, bronchitis, pneumonia, and urinary tract infections (UTIs).

A careful history and problem-focused physical examination is essential to the accurate diagnosis and management of these conditions. A cost-effective evidence-based approach to the diagnosis and management of febrile illness, including the appropriate use of antibiotic therapy, is the cornerstone of quality medical care.

MEDICATION CAUSES OF FEVER

Fever secondary to many medications is a common cause of prolonged fever or fever of undetermined origin in the adult and pediatric patient. This etiology of fever should be considered in all patients who are taking medications of any kind. If the initial evaluation of a patient fails to reveal a source of the temperature, or if infectious or other etiologies seem unlikely, then medication causes of fever should be considered. Typically fever presents within the first 7 to 10 days of medication use; however, the presentation may be variable and can present even years after initiation of medication.

Symptoms
- Fever +++++
- Chills or rigors +++
- A sense of well-being ++++

Signs
- Usually normal physical examination ++++
- Morbilliform rashes ++

Workup
- The workup should include a thorough history and physical examination. Most patients with drug-induced fever appear well with an absence of physical findings.

- A detailed history of medication use that includes any prescription or nonprescription medications, vitamins, and other herbal agents should be taken.
- Routine laboratory testing including a CBC may reveal the presence of eosinophilia.
- Although any agent may produce a medication-induced fever, the most common agents include antibiotics, antihypertensives, CNS and cardiovascular agents, heparin, and analgesics.

Comments and Treatment Considerations

If the initial evaluation of any patient who presents with a fever fails to reveal an underlying etiology, drug fever should be suspected.

In any patient who presents with a fever 7 to 10 days after starting a new medication, drug fever should be ruled out before beginning any extensive diagnostic evaluation.

A diagnosis of medication-induced fever can only be made if resolution of the fever occurs within 48 hours or three to five half-lives of the drug after discontinuation.

Drug fever may sometimes be associated with serum sickness–like reactions. These patients are usually much sicker and often present with erythema multiforme or exfoliative dermatitis. Resolution of symptoms in these patients is much slower and treatment is symptomatic.

PNEUMONIA

Community-acquired pneumonia (CAP) is the most common of all pneumonias and is a common etiology of febrile illness. The most common include *Streptococcus pneumoniae, Haemophilus influenzae,* and atypical organisms such as mycoplasma, legionella, and influenza. Patients usually present with fever, chills, cough, pleuritic chest pain, and dyspnea. An accurate assessment of the patient is essential in determining the need for hospitalization and appropriate antibiotic selection. The use of evidence-based clinical pathways and consensus guidelines is important for accurate diagnosis and cost-effective management.

Symptoms
- Fever, chills, rigors, generalized malaise ++++
- Dyspnea +++
- Pleuritic chest pain ++
- Cough: dry or productive, colored (green-yellow or rust) sputum ++++
- Hemoptysis ++
- Atypical pneumonias may be associated with generalized constitutional and GI symptoms. ++++

Signs
- Fever ++++
- Tachypnea and tachycardia +++
- Crackles or rales ++++

- Dullness to percussion ++
- Bronchial breath sounds ++
- Tactile fremitus ++

Workup
- Chest radiography (posteroanterior and lateral views) are essential in making a diagnosis of pneumonia. Typical pneumonias present with a lobar consolidation, whereas atypical pneumonia presents with more bilateral and diffuse infiltrates. Chest radiography is also important to rule out complications of pneumonia such as pleural effusion, multilobar disease, and abscess. All infiltrates should be followed until complete resolution. Underlying pulmonary or neoplastic diseases cannot be excluded before 8 to 12 weeks.
- A leukocytosis count ranging between 15,000 and 25,000 cells/µL with increased immature cells is most often seen.
- Sputum Gram stain should be performed but its usefulness is controversial. Contamination, limited sensitivity and atypical organisms limit the benefits of the test.
- Blood cultures (two sets) may be obtained on all patients who require hospitalization but rarely affects treatment. The use of blood cultures in the ambulatory setting is limited and not considered necessary or cost-effective.
- Urinary antigens and PCR testing for common pathogens are important in the diagnosis and management of the critically ill patient.
- Additional testing of the hospitalized patient should include electrolytes, liver function studies, and arterial blood gases.

Comments and Treatment Considerations
Initial treatment of pneumonia is empiric and should be based on a careful history, physical examination, preliminary workup, and patient risk stratification. Following published consensus guidelines from the American Thoracic Society or the Infectious Disease Society of America will guide appropriate antibiotic selection.

The decision to treat a patient in the outpatient setting or admit to the hospital should be based on clinical judgment and the use of clinical pathways such as the pneumonia severity index. Increased risk is associated with factors including age, comorbid illness, smoking history, findings on physical examination, and laboratory workup.

Treatment of CAP should be initiated empirically with the use of antibiotics that will cover streptococcal pneumonia and atypical pathogens. Acceptable first-line agents include macrolides, fluoroquinolones, and doxycycline.

The emergence of increasing resistance of *S. pneumoniae* is of great concern. The prevalence of penicillin-resistant strains of *S. pneumoniae* is as high as 25%. Significant resistance is also seen with macrolides, fluoroquinolones, cephalosporins, and other agents.

Controversy exists and the working group of the CDC recommends limiting the initial use of fluoroquinolones because of concerns of emerging resistance that have occurred following the liberal use of these agents. The CDC recommends that these agents be reserved for second-line therapy or in patients with significant comorbidities. They recommend starting therapy with a macrolide, doxycycline, or an oral β-lactam.

Hospitalized patients should be risk stratified for potential admission to an intensive care unit. Empirical antibiotic therapy should be started with a β-lactam plus macrolide or a fluoroquinolone. Broad-spectrum therapy may be indicated in patients who are from nursing homes, are immunocompromised, have significant comorbidities, or develop hospital-acquired pneumonia. Further therapy should be guided by results of the initial evaluation and patient response to therapy.

Adjunctive therapies may include antipyretics, expectorants and cough suppressants, and oxygen and bronchodilator therapy. The use of circulatory and respiratory support may be necessary in the critically ill patient.

Because of the changing microbiology of pneumonia, clinicians should periodically confirm updated treatment recommendations.

PYELONEPHRITIS

Pyelonephritis is a common cause of febrile illness in both adults and children. Acute pyelonephritis is defined as an uncomplicated infection of the upper urinary tract. More than 100,000 hospitalizations annually are secondary to infections related to the urinary tract. The condition is much more common in women, who are five times more likely than men to require hospitalization. In men, underlying causes such as benign prostatic hypertrophy, prostatitis, or nephrolithiasis are usually evident. *Escherichia coli* accounts for more than 80% of cases of acute pyelonephritis. Other common pathogens include gram-negative bacteria, *Staphylococcus saprophyticus,* and enterococci. Early use of effective antibiotics is essential in reducing morbidity and unnecessary hospitalizations.

Symptoms
- Fever ++++
- Chills ++++
- Nausea and vomiting ++++
- Diarrhea ++
- Back pain ++++
- Suprapubic or abdominal pain ++
- Gross hematuria ++
- Dysuria, urinary frequency and urgency +++

Signs
- Tachycardia, diaphoresis +++
- Costovertebral angle tenderness that may be unilateral or bilateral ++++
- Lower abdominal or suprapubic tenderness and guarding +++
- In older adults, fever and other common symptoms of urinary tract infection may be absent. GI symptoms are most frequently seen. +++

Workup

- Urinalysis is effective using the dipstick method to detect leuko-cyte esterase or nitrate. Microscopic analysis for WBCs, RBCs, WBC casts, and bacteria is also useful.
- Urine culture and sensitivity should be performed on all patients with a differential diagnosis that includes pyelonephritis. Urine cultures are positive in more than 90% of patients with pyelone-phritis. A urine culture is considered positive if it reveals greater than 10,000 colony-forming units (CFUs) and symptoms com-patible with pyelonephritis, whereas in uncomplicated cystitis, counts of 50 to 100,000 CFUs are considered positive. Lower num-bers should be carefully evaluated in males, and in immunocom-promised or pregnant patients. Urine cultures are not necessary in uncomplicated cases of nonfebrile cystitis in the ambulatory setting.
- Blood culture and sensitivity is recommended only for hospital-ized patients and yields are very low.
- Imaging studies including, ultrasonography, IV pyelography, CT scanning, and MRI may be indicated to rule out underlying ana-tomic abnormalities, nephrolithiasis, complications and other coexisting conditions as well as to confirm the diagnosis.
- Hospitalized patients should also receive a CBC and electrolytes to monitor systemic effects of infection and renal function.

Comments and Treatment Considerations

Most patients with acute pyelonephritis can be treated in the ambu-latory setting. Indications for admission include the very young, older adults, diabetic or other immunocompromised patients, intractable vomiting or inability to tolerate oral intake, toxic-appearing patients, or those with progression of uncomplicated infections.

Most consensus guidelines recommend fluoroquinolones as empiric first-line antimicrobial therapy. Resistance to fluoroquino-lones by common pathogens of the urinary tract is increasing. Orally administered ciprofloxacin is considered the drug of choice for uncomplicated infections in nonpregnant individuals. Alternative treatment options include amoxicillin-clavulanate potassium and cephalosporins, particularly with fluoroquinolone resistance.

Patients who require hospitalization should be treated with a fluoroquinolone if hospital resistance rates are low, an aminoglyco-side with ampicillin, or an extended-spectrum cephalosporin with or without an aminoglycoside.

Most patients should be treated for a total of 10 to 14 days. Short regimens of 3 to 5 days are only indicated for cases of uncomplicated cystitis.

Fluoroquinolones are classified as a pregnancy Category C drug and should not be used in pregnant women because of pos-sible teratogenic effects on the fetus. Amoxicillin and amoxicillin-clavulanate potassium are considered agents of choice in pregnant women. All pregnant women who present with pyelonephritis should be hospitalized for IV hydration and antibiotics.

Complications include septicemia, chronic pyelonephritis, hydro-nephrosis, perinephric abscess formation, hypertension, and renal failure.

Treatment failures are usually secondary to resistant organisms, nephrolithiasis, or underlying anatomic abnormalities.

UPPER RESPIRATORY INFECTION

URIs account for almost 50 million visits to primary care physicians each year. Viral infections such as the common cold account for the vast majority of these infections. More than 150 million prescriptions for antibiotics are written for these conditions on an annual basis, many of which are not justified. A careful evidence-based approach using clinical practice guidelines and consensus recommendations is essential for a rational approach to the diagnosis and manage-ment of these conditions. A problem-focused history and physical examination will guide the determination of a specific diagnosis that may require targeted antibiotic therapy. The differential diagnosis of these conditions includes pharyngitis, tonsillitis, otitis media, and sinusitis as well as complications such as abscess formation and disseminated infections.

Symptoms
- Sore throat +++
- Fever +++
- Cough +++
- Nasal congestion, rhinorrhea, sneezing, or postnasal drip ++++
- Headache, facial or dental pain ++
- Pain or fullness in the ear ++
- Systemic symptoms such as nausea, vomiting, or diarrhea ++

Signs
- Erythema of the oropharynx, tonsillar hypertrophy, and/or exudates +++
- Cervical lymphadenopathy +++
- Abdominal tenderness and/or hepatosplenomegaly ++
- Clear or purulent nasal discharge ++++
- Sinus tenderness ++
- Fullness or bulging of the tympanic membrane with distinct erythema and air-fluid levels ++

Workup
- A careful and problem-focused history and physical examination is the key to accurate diagnosis.
- Acute pharyngitis is most often secondary to viral pathogens. The presence of tonsillar erythema, exudates, and anterior cervical lymphadenopathy raises the suspicion for group A beta-hemolytic streptococcus (GABHS) infection. Predicting which patients have GABHS infection is essential. Using a clinical scale such as the McIsaac Prediction System can allow for a treatment decision in

many cases without laboratory tests. In equivocal cases, rapid antigen detection tests with culture may help guide appropriate therapy.

- If concern for mononucleosis is present or if symptoms persist, a diagnosis of infectious mononucleosis should be considered. A CBC revealing the presence of atypical lymphocytes and a positive heterophile test will confirm the diagnosis.
- AOM manifests as an acute onset febrile illness with localized symptoms of ear pain. Mobility of the tympanic membrane should be evaluated with the use of pneumatic otoscopy, tympanometry, or acoustic reflectometry.
- Acute rhinosinusitis is a clinical diagnosis that is made when symptoms of an acute URI do not remit after 7 to 10 days. Purulent nasal discharge and unilateral pain are the typical symptoms most predictive of acute sinusitis. The use of CT scanning can be used to diagnose difficult cases or help with management decisions in persistent cases.

Comments and Treatment Considerations

Most cases of URIs can be treated with watchful waiting along with symptomatic treatment such as antipyretics, analgesics, antihistamines, decongestants, nasal saline sprays, expectorants, and cough suppressants.

GABHS infection should be treated with antimicrobial therapy. The use of oral penicillin four times daily for 10 days remains the treatment of choice. Some clinicians prefer amoxicillin due to the better taste and dosing schedule. Macrolides such as clarithromycin or azithromycin can be used in patients with penicillin allergy. Studies have shown that 5-day courses of advanced-generation cephalosporins or macrolides are effective therapy.

Documented cases of acute otitis media and sinusitis may be treated with antimicrobial therapy aimed at the most common organisms including *S. pneumoniae, H. influenzae,* and *Moraxella catarrhalis.* First-line therapy remains amoxicillin. Alternative therapy in very ill or nonresponsive cases includes amoxicillin-clavulanate, advanced-generation cephalosporins, or macrolides, and sulfa-based combinations. Adults may be treated with doxycycline or advanced generation fluoroquinolones, but their use should be limited due to the emergence of resistance. Careful follow-up should be arranged with patients with unusual sinus infections such as frontal and ethmoid sinusitis because serious complications may be seen. Adjunctive therapy should include analgesic and antipyretic medications. The use of nasal saline and inhaled steroids may be effective in the treatment of sinusitis.

VIRAL SYNDROME

Viral infections are the underlying etiology in most patients who present with febrile illness. Common viral infections include upper and lower respiratory tract infections including the "common cold," gastroenteritis, and influenza. Diagnosis of most viral infections is based on the clinical presentation, physical examination, and the exclusion of bacterial etiologies. Knowledge of the common outbreaks and pathogens of the local community is helpful in the diagnosis of viral infections. Rapid-antigen testing is becoming increasingly available and cost-effective in the management of the patient with "viral illnesses." The use of consensus recommendations and clinical practice guidelines, including the judicious use of antibiotics for patients only with clearly documented bacterial infection, is important in the prevention of emerging resistant bacterial pathogens.

Symptoms
- Fever and chills +++++
- Fatigue and weakness ++++
- Coryza ++++
- Sneezing, congestion, sore throat +++
- Headache +++
- Myalgia, arthralgia +++
- Anorexia, nausea, vomiting, and diarrhea +++
- Rashes ++

Signs
- Absence of toxic-appearing clinical features ++++
- Diaphoresis ++
- Tachycardia +++
- A physical examination that does not reveal the presence of other etiologies such as acute otitis media, sinusitis, pneumonia, or pyelonephritis ++++

Workup
- The initial approach to the patient with fever should include a careful history, physical examination, and appropriate laboratory testing.
- Patients who are very ill or toxic appearing should have a laboratory workup. Admission to the hospital should be based mainly on clinical judgment.
- First-line testing should include a CBC. An increase in lymphocytes in the differential suggests a viral etiology for the condition.
- Serum electrolytes are indicated in the presence of possible dehydration.
- Liver function studies may be helpful but are nonspecific findings if elevated and may require the use of additional studies for the presence of acute hepatitis.
- Blood culture and sensitivity (two sets) to rule out bacterial pathogens is indicated in the acutely ill or toxic-appearing patient.
- Urinalysis and culture is indicated in the evaluation of a patient with a possible asymptomatic UTI, which occurs especially in infants and older adults.
- Chest radiography may be indicated in the presence of adventitious sounds on auscultation.

- Additional studies may include nasopharyngeal cultures, throat cultures, stool cultures, and rapid antigen testing. Rapid antigen testing is readily available for the diagnosis of common viral pathogens such as influenza A and B or rotavirus infections.

Comments and Treatment Considerations

A careful history and physical examination are essential for the accurate diagnosis of viral infections as well as the exclusion of bacterial pathogens that may require antimicrobial therapy.

Close monitoring of local community or hospital pathogen prevalence data is important to aid in diagnosis, guide appropriate therapy, and prevent the outbreak of disease.

Prevention using handwashing, isolation of infected individuals, vaccination of appropriate individuals, and use of prophylactic antiviral agents is important in decreasing morbidity and mortality.

Amantadine and rimantadine are antiviral agents indicated for the prophylaxis and treatment of influenzavirus. The agents are inexpensive but are only effective against influenzavirus A and resistance is high. The agents must be given within 48 hours of symptoms to be effective.

Oseltamivir is a neuraminidase inhibitor indicated for the treatment of influenza A or B in patients more than 1 year of age within the first 48 hours of symptoms. The drug is administered orally. The drug may also be used for prophylaxis in individuals older than the age of 13. Studies show that the medication may reduce the duration of symptoms by up to one and one half days as well as decrease the morbidity and mortality associated with the disease.

Symptomatic therapy of all patients should include antipyretics, analgesics, antidiarrheal agents, and cough and cold medications as indicated. Adequate hydration is essential in maintaining fluid volume and preventing hospitalization.

Antibiotics should be used only in those patients who develop secondary bacterial infections.

References

Goetz MB, Rhew DC, Torres A: Pyogenic bacterial pneumonia, lung abscess, and empyema. In Mason RJ, Murray JF, Broaddus VC, Nadel JA, eds: *Murray and Nadel's textbook of respiratory medicine*, 4th ed, Philadelphia, 2005, Saunders.

Llenderrozos HJ: Urinary tract infections: management rationale for uncomplicated cystitis, *Clin Fam Pract* 6:157–171, 2004.

Lutfiyya MN, Henley E, Chang LF: Diagnosis and treatment of community-acquired pneumonia, *Am Fam Physician* 73:442–450, 2006.

Mackowiak PA, LeMaistre CF: Drug fever: a critical appraisal of conventional concepts, *Ann Intern Med* 106:728–733, 1987.

McKinnon HD, Howard T: Evaluating the febrile patient with a rash, *Am Fam Physician* 62:804–813, 2000.

Melio FR: Upper respiratory tract infections. In Marx JA, Hockberger RS, Wallis RM et al, eds: *Rosen's emergency medicine: concepts and clinical practice*, 7th ed, Philadelphia, 2006, Mosby.

Montalto NJ, Gum KD, Ashi JV: Updated treatment for influenza A and B, *Am Fam Physician* 62:2467–2474, 2000.

Ramakrishnan K, Scheid DC: Diagnosis and management of acute pyelonephritis in adults, *Am Fam Physician* 71:933–943, 2005.

Roth AR, Basello GM: Approach to the adult patient with fever of unknown origin, *Am Fam Physician* 68:2223–2229, 2003.

Tabor P: Drug-induced fever, *Drug Intell Clin Pharm* 20:414–416, 1986.

Walsh P, Retik A, Vaughn E, et al, editors: *Campbell's urology*, 8th ed, Philadelphia, 2002, Saunders.

Whitman JH: Upper respiratory tract infections, *Clin Fam Pract* 6:35–74, 2004.

Wong DM, Blumberg DA, Lowe LG: Guidelines for the use of antibiotics in acute upper respiratory tract infections, *Am Fam Physician* 74:956–966, 2006.

CHAPTER 24

Headache

Kathryn A. Seitz and Stephen W. Cobb

Headache, or cephalgia, is pain or discomfort perceived in the head, neck, or both. Many patients who complain of headache have more than one headache syndrome; therefore, precise definition of these symptoms is essential for an accurate diagnosis. Although there are many classification systems for headache disorders, the International Headache Society (IHS) offers a functional taxonomy (ICHD-II). In this system headache disorders are defined as primary or secondary. In a primary headache disorder there is no other causative disease present. A secondary headache disorder has a separate identifiable cause.

This tool focuses the clinician's diagnostic approach on the patient with cephalgia. First, determine how many headache types are present. Second, determine if worrisome symptoms or signs are present (Table 24-1). Third, determine if the headache is a primary headache disorder, and which one. If there is more than one headache disorder, define the diagnosis for each one. It is common for a clinician to encounter acute, distinct cephalgia symptoms in a patient with a history of a completely different headache disorder.

Once the clinician forms an initial diagnosis, further diagnostic workup may be indicated and treatment initiated, with refinement of the diagnosis based on results and response to treatment. This chapter elucidates the diagnostic approach for cephalgia and treatment for the most common and serious etiologies of both primary and secondary headaches.

PRIMARY HEADACHE DISORDERS

The diagnosis of each of these disorders is based primarily on the clinical features elicited on a careful history, and the absence of worrisome symptoms and signs. There should be no other cause identified for the headache. Features such as the quality of the pain, its effect on patient function, and associated symptoms (nausea, photophobia, and phonophobia) are keys to making the diagnosis. When present, symptoms such as an aura or prodrome and signs such as autonomic manifestations can be very helpful.

Table 24-1. Worrisome Symptoms and Signs

Symptoms

Focal neurologic symptoms	Neuroimaging, consider LP
Persistent or progressive pain	Neuroimaging
Abrupt or sudden onset	Neuroimaging, LP
Awakes from sleep	Neuroimaging
Exertional headache	Neuroimaging
Weight loss	Neuroimaging, consider LP
History of cancer, coagulopathy, or immunocompromise	Neuroimaging, consider LP
Older or very young age at onset (<5 years; >50 years)	Neuroimaging

Signs

Fever	Sinus plain films, sinus CT, LP
Severe hypertension	Neuroimaging, consider LP
Meningeal signs	LP
Palpable, tender temporal artery	ESR, TA biopsy
Papilledema	Neuroimaging, consider LP after imaging
Globe tenderness	Intraocular pressures
Focal neurologic deficits	Neuroimaging
Confusion, change in level and alertness	Neuroimaging

CT, Computed tomography; *ESR,* erythrocyte sedimentation rate; *LP,* lumbar puncture.

 CLUSTER HEADACHE

Although not common in the primary care office, cluster headaches are recognized as one of the more common headache disorders in some population studies, with a lifetime prevalence of 0.1%. Males are affected more commonly than females, and the onset of symptoms occurs between the ages of 30 to 50 years. There is a positive association with smoking tobacco. The pain pattern is most distinctive. This pattern of cluster headaches may accelerate in intensity and frequency over the years. Most headaches last between 15 and 180 minutes, with pain-free intervals that are variable in length.

Symptoms
• Pain is sharp and excruciating, with a quick rise to peak pain after onset. +++++

- Headaches are clustered over weeks and months, often in distinct seasons. +++++
- Location is unilateral: supraorbital, orbital, or temporal. +++++
- Nausea +++
- Frequency of one every other day to eight per day +++

Signs
- Autonomic ipsilateral signs:
  - Conjunctival injection and/or lacrimation ++++
  - Nasal congestion or rhinorrhea ++++
  - Eyelid edema, forehead and facial sweating +
  - Miosis or ptosis +++
- Agitation and restlessness; patient often cannot sit still ++++
- Bradycardia and/or hypertension ++

Workup
- If the headache is typical for cluster headache, further workup is rarely indicated.
- A headache diary can be an effective tool in the confirmation of initial diagnosis and evaluation of response to therapy.

Comments and Treatment Considerations
Acute therapy with 7 to 10 L of oxygen by mask, intranasal ergotamine, intranasal topically applied capsaicin or lidocaine, verapamil, and sumatriptan have each shown some efficacy. Indomethacin is particularly effective for benign paroxysmal hemicrania, a condition similar to cluster headache.

Preventive strategies are indicated once clusters begin. Oral corticosteroids, lithium, inhaled ergotamines, certain antiepileptic drugs, and calcium channel blockers have shown benefit. Avoidance of alcohol and tobacco may be beneficial during the cluster periods. Invasive treatments that have been studied include nerve ablation surgery, local nerve injections, and deep brain electronic stimulation.

 MIGRAINE HEADACHE

Migraine affects 18.2% of U.S. women and 6.5% of men each year. Onset of symptoms is usually between adolescence and adulthood. A strong correlation with family history has been observed. The diagnosis of episodic migraine headache is made when there have been at least five episodes lasting 4 to 72 hours, but the headache is present fewer than 180 days in a year and is associated with the following symptoms. If the headache is present more than 180 days per year, this is chronic migraine; successful treatment is much more difficult. Migraine without aura is far more common, but the presence of a typical aura can be diagnostic, as can consistent prodromal symptoms.

A typical aura is fully reversible, and may include positive or negative symptoms. Positive symptoms include visual flickering spots or lines, and cutaneous sensations of pins and needles; negative symptoms include visual field loss, numbness, or speech disturbance. The onset of headache usually occurs within an hour of the aura, and each symptom of the aura lasts between 5 and 60 minutes.

The differential diagnosis of migraine, particularly without aura, should include sinus pain with or without infection, trigeminal neuralgia, and TMJ disorder.

Symptoms
- Unilateral location +++
- Pulsating quality +++
- Moderate or severe pain intensity +++
- Aggravation or causing avoidance of routine physical activity +++
- Nausea during headache ++++
- Photophobia or phonophobia during headache ++++
- Aura ++
- Prodrome +++

Signs
- The physical examination is usually normal with the exception of pain behavior. +++++
- Patients with complicated migraines may have focal neurologic findings (hemiparesis, visual field defect) that are temporally associated with the headache and completely resolve.
- Absence of reproducible pain and dysfunction of the TMJ +++++
- Absence of papilledema on funduscopic examination ++++++
- Cutaneous hypersensitivity is not common, but is positively associated with migraines. ++

Workup
- When the headache is typical for migraine, further workup is rarely indicated.
- A headache diary can be the most effective tool for the confirmation of the initial diagnosis and evaluation of response to therapy.
- If sinusitis is in the differential diagnosis, imaging with plain films or a focused sinus CT may be helpful.

Comments and Treatment Considerations
Treatment goals include reduction in the number and severity of migraines and maximization of functional days. Explicitly communicating treatment goals is essential to success. There are nonpharmacologic interventions that are effective. A nonpharmacologic and three primary pharmacologic strategies for treating migraine—prevention, acute abortive, and rescue—are as follows:
- Nonpharmacologic: Identifying and avoiding triggers, such as certain foods, alcohol, lack of sleep, and estrogen withdrawal can moderate symptoms. Relaxation therapy, thermal biofeedback, and CBT have some beneficial evidence.
- Prevention: Patients with two to four or more headaches per month, or particularly disabling and severe symptoms may benefit from preventive medicines. Beta-blockers, calcium channel

blockers, antidepressants, and antiepileptic drugs have been found to be effective. An herb, feverfew, has some evidence to support its use. Riboflavin has been used with modest success.

- Acute abortive: General analgesics, alone or combination with caffeine and sedative hypnotics, have been useful. Ergot alkaloids and triptan drugs have a theoretic advantage focusing on specific serotonin receptors thought to be involved in the neurogenic inflammatory cascade responsible for migraine. There are many triptans available on the market; efficacy is similar, and the drugs share more similarities than differences. Understanding the differences between onset and duration of action, and the delivery system (tablet, injectable, nasal) may help the provider customize treatment for an individual patient.
- Rescue: If the goal of using abortive drugs is to preserve the function of the patient, the goal of rescue therapy is to provide the patient the power to terminate the headache without having to seek further care. Antiemetics and narcotics are often used alone or in combination.

Treating concomitant disorders, such as mood disorders is essential to success. Recent concerns of increased risk of serotonin syndrome with combined use of SSRI antidepressants and triptans should be noted.

 TENSION-TYPE HEADACHE

Onset occurs at any age. Duration is from 30 minutes to 7 days. If fewer than 15 per year, it is defined as episodic tension headache. If more, it is defined as chronic, and may be much more difficult to treat effectively. The differential diagnosis should include medication-associated headache, headaches caused by medications and substances, and those caused by their withdrawal (rebound headache). Many headaches previously thought to be tension actually meet diagnostic criteria for migraine.

Symptoms
- Bilateral location ++++
- Pain is dull, pressing, or tightening; bandlike pressure ++++
- Mild or moderate intensity ++++
- Not aggravated by routine activity ++++
- Nausea not severe and less common +++
- Rarely associated with phonophobia or photophobia +++
- Often associated with a concomitant mood disorder ++++

Signs
- Palpable muscle tightness in the posterior occipital and cervical areas +++
- Palpable "trigger points" in the same area +++
- Normal examination, including neurologic examination, with the exception of pain behavior +++++

Workup
- When the headache is typical for tension type, further workup is rarely indicated.
- A headache diary can be the most effective tool in the confirmation of initial diagnosis and evaluation of response to therapy.
- If sinusitis is the differential diagnosis, imaging with plain films or a focused sinus CT may be helpful.

Comments and Treatment Considerations
There is evidence of benefit in a number of nonpharmacologic and pharmacologic interventions.

Nonpharmacologic: Biofeedback, stress management, exercise programs, and dietary changes have shown benefit.

Pharmacologic: General analgesics such as ibuprofen and acetaminophen are often effective. Judicious use of muscle relaxants has had mixed results, but may be helpful if limited to a few weeks' duration. Narcotics should generally be avoided. Overuse of any of these agents may lead to rebound headache. TCAs, specifically amitriptyline and mirtazapine, have been used for chronic tension headache with modest success.

A supportive, continual physician-patient relationship may be beneficial in more severe or frequent tension headaches. Treating concomitant mood disorders is essential for success. Effective management of sleep disorders is important.

SECONDARY HEADACHE DISORDERS

Secondary headaches result from an underlying pathology caused by a distinct condition (e.g., aneurysm, infection, inflammation, neoplasm). Less than 0.4% of headaches in primary care are from serious intracranial disease. Though there is a multitude of secondary headache disorders, here are a few of the more common and critical etiologies that should not be missed and others that are more common.

 ## ACUTE BACTERIAL MENINGITIS

CSF infection may occur from various pathogens: viral, bacterial, or fungal. The most serious of these is bacterial. Bacterial meningitis affects more than 1.2 million patients worldwide and is one of the 10 most common infectious causes of death. In the United States frequency has been decreasing.

Risk factors include immunocompromised status (asplenia, complement deficiency, corticosteroid excess, HIV), IV drug use, travel, recent head trauma or neurosurgery, otorrhea and rhinorrhea, but meningitis occurs not infrequently in immunocompetent hosts. There are many different pathogens; age of the patient, risk factors, and recent hospitalizations are predictive and guide therapy.

The most common pathogens are *Streptococcus pneumoniae, Neisseria meningitidis, Haemophilus influenzae, Listeria monocytogenes,* and group B streptococci. The headache is usually generalized, severe, and often the first presenting symptom. It is uncommon that patients have all three signs and symptoms of the classic triad of fever, nuchal rigidity, and change in mental status, but the absence of all of these has a high negative predictive value.

Symptoms
- Headache ++++
- Fever (usually greater than 38° C) ++++
- Neck pain or stiffness ++++
- Fatigue or malaise
- Altered mental status +++
- Rash (meningococcal) +++
- Photophobia
- Nausea and vomiting

Signs
- Fever ++++
- Decreased consciousness (occasionally coma) ++
- Nuchal rigidity (Kernig's and Brudzinski's signs) +++
- Focal neurologic deficits ++
- Seizure ++
- Petechiae or palpable purpura (meningococcal) +++
- Papilledema

Workup
- Head CT: if abnormal neurologic exam or if concerned about mass and herniation prior to lumbar puncture (LP), though this is not absolutely necessary. CT is recommended if immunocompromised state, history of CNS disease, new-onset seizures, papilledema, abnormal level of consciousness, or focal neurologic deficits
- CSF with opening pressure, Gram stain and culture, cell count (leukocytes often >1000/µL); glucose and protein: glucose usually decreased (<45 mg/dL) and protein is increased (>500 mg/dL) but not absolute
- CBC is generally not helpful because CSF is required. WBCs are usually elevated with increased immature forms though leukopenia may instead be present.
- Electrolytes, renal function tests, liver function tests, and coagulation panel are usually not helpful unless there is concern for sepsis or DIC.
- Blood culture (two): positive in 50% to 75% of patients

Comments and Treatment Considerations
Administer resuscitative support as indicated. CSF should be obtained as soon as possible but if there is any delay (unable to obtain CSF or waiting for CT) begin IV antibiotics immediately without waiting for CSF results. Attempt to obtain blood cultures if possible before beginning antibiotics. Antibiotics should be bactericidal and able to penetrate the blood-brain barrier. A third-generation cephalosporin

and vancomycin (plus or minus ampicillin) are usually recommended until the pathogen is identified. Mortality rate approaches 100% if untreated and there is a high failure rate even with treatment.

Consider beginning IV corticosteroids with antibiotics if patient's Glasgow Coma Scale score is 8 to 11 (especially in children). Data are conflicting but have been shown to decrease morbidity. Three features associated with adverse outcomes include seizures, hypotension, and altered mental status.

Neurologic sequelae are common, including hearing loss and focal deficits. Chemoprophylaxis is recommended for close contacts of patients with invasive *N. meningitidis,* and close contacts who are unvaccinated children younger than 4 years of age, or of patients with *H. influenzae* (www.cdc.gov/mmwr/preview/mmwrhtml/rr5407a1.htm).

Prevention
Vaccines are available for pneumococcal and meningococcal disease and *H. influenzae.*

 # CERVICOGENIC HEADACHE

There is considerable overlap of symptoms with cervicogenic headache and migraine, tension, and cluster headaches. Cervicogenic headache is far more common than cluster in primary care. Symptoms such as nausea, photophobia, and phonophobia may be present, but less so than in migraine.

Symptoms
- Mild to moderate headache pain (neck pain may range from severe to absent)
- Pain is nonthrobbing and usually unilateral, but may be in one or more regions of the head or face.
- Referred pain from an ipsilateral source in the neck may be radiculopathic to shoulder and arm. ++++
- Headache may be precipitated by neck movement.
- Valsalva maneuver, cough, and sneeze may initiate or exacerbate pain.
- Resolution of headache after treatment of cause

Signs
- Restricted and/or painful ROM in the neck
- Muscle spasm and tenderness in the cervical spine
- Reproduction of headache with palpation in the occipital area or over C1-C3 +++

Workup
- Neck radiographs demonstrating arthritic change may be supportive, but are not specific for cervicogenic headache.
- MRI showing disorder or lesion in spine or soft tissues of the neck. MRI often reveals disk disease in asymptomatic patients, thus not considered diagnostic.
- Abolition of headache following local nerve block is very supportive of the diagnosis. ++++

Comments and Treatment Considerations

Treating the cause of nerve root irritation is optimal, but given the limits of diagnostic accuracy, a secure diagnosis is often evasive. Physical modalities such as neck-strengthening exercises, physical therapy, osteopathic manipulation, and acupuncture all have evidence for benefit. There is evidence of efficacy for biofeedback, relaxation, and CBT. Pharmacologic modalities are aimed at increasing functionality and participation in physical modalities. They are limited in their efficacy for the headache. General analgesics, TCAs, and muscle relaxants are commonly used. The use of opioid narcotics should be limited. Antiepileptic drugs such as divalproex sodium, gabapentin, topiramate, and carbamazepine have been used with some success.

Nonsurgical Interventions

Injection of trigger points and local nerve blocks can provide temporary relief. Epidural steroid injection can provide longer-lasting relief if anatomic pathology is amenable, for example, disk disease. The efficacy of local injections of botulinum toxin is being studied. Surgical treatment of underlying pathology may help these headaches; however, there should be great anatomic agreement between clinical suspicion and the findings of any diagnostic studies.

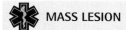 **MASS LESION**

Any condition that elevates intracranial pressure may cause headache. Mass effect from neoplasia may be the most relevant for the family physician. A mass lesion can cause symptoms directly from the neoplasm or can be a result from increased intracranial pressure or hydrocephalus caused by the neoplasm. If the patient is more than 50 years of age with a new headache or a change in pattern, this should be of concern. The headache is usually the worst symptom in about half of patients. It can be localizing or diffuse and usually is not extremely severe. The classic worse-in-the-morning headache is actually not a common presentation. The headaches are usually more of a tension-type pattern than migraine.

Symptoms

- Headache, often worse with positional changes or Valsalva maneuver +++
- Nausea and vomiting +++
- Fatigue
- Weight loss
- Visual changes
- Cognitive dysfunction, such as memory difficulties or mood and personality changes
- Weakness or sensory loss
- Difficulties with speech

Signs

- Change in level of consciousness
- Focal neurologic deficits ++
- Seizures ++
- Papilledema ++
- Hemianopsia

Workup

- Basic laboratory evaluation is not absolutely required for diagnosis of brain lesion but is warranted if other systemic concerns are present.
- If a careful neurologic examination is negative it is very unlikely to find an abnormality on neuroimaging.
- Neuroradiologic imaging: MRI (gadolinium-enhanced) is superior in evaluation when compared with CT, although CT can be used if there is a question of bone or vascular involvement or in an emergent situation.
- Various types of tumor will enhance differently in T1/T2 and FLAIR images. MRI spectroscopy, functional MRI, perfusion MR imaging, and PET scanning are increasingly being used.
- Specialist referral for tissue biopsy

Comments and Treatment Considerations

Resuscitative methods and support if necessary (including sedation, raising of head, mannitol, hyperventilation if herniation is occurring and surgical management is pending) though most patients will not present acutely decompensated. Rarely, patients undergoing Valsalva maneuvers can cause brief acute elevations of intracranial pressure (ICP) leading to seizures.

- Corticosteroids: those patients who have elevated ICP causing seizures, cerebral edema, decreased consciousness, and so on need urgent steroids. Usual starting dose is 10 mg of dexamethasone followed by 4 mg four times per day but can use smaller doses for milder symptoms.
- Anticonvulsants for seizures related to the tumor (unrelated to elevated ICP)
- Neurosurgical referral for urgent ventriculostomy (if acute elevation of ICP) and for further evaluation and definitive treatment of mass lesion.

 MEDICATION OVERUSE HEADACHE

Medication overuse headache (also called rebound, drug-induced) is a very common headache disorder thought to affect 1% of the population with a female predominance, though there are few data on the subject. It is often variable in nature and has shifting characteristics, even within the same day, from migraine-like to those of tension-type headache.

Making the diagnosis is critical because patients rarely respond to preventive medications while overusing acute medications. It is difficult to make the diagnosis because it usually requires avoidance of medication for at least 2 months.

Common medications include acetaminophen, triptans, ergot alkaloids, opioids, NSAIDs, butalbital, midrin, and other combination analgesics. The IHS classification includes taking the medication more than 10 days per month for at least 3 months' duration. Some studies have found a higher prevalence of underlying personality disorders and family history of substance abuse.

Symptoms
- Headache (greater than 15 times per month) that has developed or markedly worsened during medication overuse
- Resolves or remits to its previous pattern within 2 months of medication withdrawal

Signs
- Absence of findings on physical examination, including neurologic

Workup
- Little workup is usually necessary other than a thorough history and physical ruling out of any other etiologies of the headache.
- A headache diary with specific detail to medications, dosage, and frequency is often helpful.

Comments and Treatment Considerations
Withdrawal of medications for at least 2 months is the usual therapy. Avoiding using acute medications more than 10 times per month is recommended for prevention. Some advise a detoxification period in the hospital using parenteral DHE-45 plus or minus metoclopramide. Benzodiazepines and ademetionine (an herbal used in Europe) have also been used in a recent study. Often after the detoxification period patients revert back to an episodic headache pattern. Depending on the type of headache present (migraine, tension, or cluster), prophylactic treatment directed at the specific type may be beneficial as well as exploring nonpharmacologic therapies. Assessment and modification of underlying psychologic factors are important.

 ## SUBARACHNOID HEMORRHAGE

Subarachnoid hemorrhage (SAH) is the most common cause of intense and incapacitating headache of abrupt onset (thunderclap), though it is rare in the practice of a family physician. The incidence is about 8 per 100,000 per year. About 30% to 50% of patients die (often before they arrive to the hospital) and 50% of the survivors are disabled; 80% of cases are from ruptured saccular aneurysms, excluding trauma. Sentinel headaches (prior to rupture) have been reported to be present in 15% to 60% of patients and may be severe at onset and resolve. Diagnosing SAH is life-saving because a sentinel headache ("warning leak") may proceed significant aneurysmal bleed.

The headache is often unilateral and extremely severe with associated neurologic symptoms or signs. However, headaches may be less severe and have no associated signs. Even though sudden, severe headache is the cardinal symptom, the positive predictive value is only 39%. A low threshold for CT scanning of patients with mild symptoms that are suggestive of SAH may reduce the frequency of misdiagnosis.

Symptoms
- Sudden, severe headache (maximal within minutes, lasts for more than an hour) ++++
- Nausea and vomiting +++
- Photophobia ++
- Neck pain or stiffness ++

Signs
- Decreased level of consciousness +
- Nuchal rigidity ++
- Epileptic seizures +
- Focal neurologic symptoms ++
- Cardiac dysrhythmia (late finding) +

Workup
- Noncontrast CT of the brain: ++++ (performed as soon as possible after the onset of the headache, with interpretation by an experienced radiologist. Delays in scanning allow the blood time to degrade and increase possibility of the CT appearing normal).
- Lumbar puncture. ++++ If CT result is normal (CT misses up to 10% of bleeds), an LP should be performed when SAH is suspected. Lack of clearing of RBCs in an atraumatic LP suggests SAH. Xanthochromia may not occur for several hours after bleeding occurs. In addition to looking for RBCs, CSF bilirubin and oxy-hemoglobin may help discern the source of the blood.
- Cerebral angiography if the suspicion for SAH is still considerable and the CT and LP are normal, though this can be nonemergent if the patient is stable. ++++
- FLAIR and T2 sequences on MRI can be used to evaluate for subacute SAH, more than 4 days after onset of symptoms.
- CT angiography or MR angiography may be helpful in evaluating the cause of SAH.

Comments and Treatment Considerations
Administer resuscitative measures as indicated. Refer to a neurosurgical unit for supportive management and interventions. Almost all deaths occur within the first 3 weeks, most due to rebleeding.

Three strongest predictors of death or dependence are impaired consciousness on admission, increasing age, and large volume of blood on initial CT. There is a grading system by the World Federation of Neurological Surgeons that can assist with estimation of prognosis (Table 24-2).

Frequent monitoring of Glasgow score, papillary responses, and focal neurologic deficits is important. Blood pressure, fluid balance, cardiac monitoring, and respiratory function should be closely followed because there are risks of cardiac dysrhythmia and pulmonary edema. Nimodipine has reduced poor outcomes in some studies but good evidence for other medical interventions is limited. Endovascular coiling is superseding neurosurgical clipping for the occlusion of many ruptured aneurysms.

 TEMPORAL ARTERITIS

Temporal arteritis (also called giant-cell arteritis) is a chronic vasculitis affecting medium-size and large vessels usually of the cranial branches of the aortic arch. Its prevalence is approximately 200 per 100,000 persons older than age 50. Persistent headache, temporal headache, or headache with visual changes in a patient older than 50 should prompt consideration of temporal arteritis because there is such variability of presentation and associated symptoms. The headache is usually localized to the temporal regions, although it can be frontal and occipital as well.

Symptoms
- Headache +++
- Fever (usually low grade) +++
- Fatigue, malaise +++
- Weight loss+++
- Visual impairment ++
- Jaw claudication +++
- Polymyalgia rheumatica (PMR) +++
- Tongue or throat pain ++
- Arm claudication +
- Cough ++
- Nonspecific musculoskeletal pain and swelling ++

Signs
- Mild to moderately ill appearing +++
- Tender, swollen temporal artery (other cranial arteries may be involved) sometimes with decreased pulse +++
- Bruits over carotid or subclavian areas ++
- Limited active ROM of neck, shoulders, hips due to pain (with PMR)
- Synovitis (usually wrists and knees) ++
- Abnormal ophthalmoscope exam (swollen pale disk with blurred margins) ++

Table 24-2. World Federation of Neurological Surgeons (WFNS) Grading System for Subarachnoid Hemorrhage Scale

Overview: The clinical grading system proposed by the WFNS is intended to be a simple, reliable, and clinically valid way to grade a patient with subarachnoid hemorrhage. This system offers less interobserver variability than some of the earlier classification systems.

GLASGOW COMA SCORE	MOTOR DEFICIT	GRADE
15	Absent	1
13 or 14	Absent	2
13 or 14	Present	3
7-12	Present or absent	4
3-6	Present or absent	5

Interpretation:
Maximum score of 15 has the best prognosis
Minimum score of 3 has the worst prognosis
Scores of 8 or more have a good chance for recovery
Scores of 3 to 5 are potentially fatal, especially if accompanied by fixed pupils or absent oculovestibular responses
Young children may be nonverbal, requiring a modification of the coma scale for evaluation

In assessing outcome of subarachnoid hemorrhage, the WFNS recommends using the Glasgow Coma Scale:

Eye Opening	Score
Spontaneously	4
To verbal stimuli	3
To pain	2
Never	1

Best Verbal Response	
Oriented and converses	5
Disoriented and converses	4
Inappropriate words	3
Incomprehensible sounds	2
No response	1

Best Motor Response	
Obeys commands	6
Localizes pain	5
Flexion withdrawal	4
Abnormal flexion (decorticate rigidity)	3
Extension (decerebrate rigidity)	2
No response	1

Workup
- ESR is almost always elevated, CRP; ESR is +++++
- Temporal artery biopsy: ideally the procedure should be done prior to beginning corticosteroids but if there will be a delay then steroid therapy should be initiated. ++++

Comments and Treatment Considerations
Corticosteroid therapy is usually 40 to 60 mg of prednisone or equivalent (single daily dose or divided), although as low as 20 mg can be used. Oral is equal to parenteral route of administration. If there is no clinical response initially, increase dose until it is seen and CRP and ESR fall. If the patient appears resistant to the therapy, consider another diagnosis.

Initial steroid dose should be continued until symptoms resolve and ESR and CRP return to normal. Then a slow withdrawal period can begin, decreasing the dose by 10% every 1 to 2 weeks. Steroids are often required for several months to years. If symptoms return, increase the steroid dose until they resolve.

If any visual loss is present, consult ophthalmology and give an IV pulse of methylprednisolone followed by oral therapy; 15% to 20% of all patients experience permanent partial or total visual loss.

Though there is limited evidence, low-dose aspirin is recommended to reduce the risk of complications. GI protection should also be considered with the use of both corticosteroids and aspirin.

With the likely long-term usage of steroids, bone protection needs to be addressed. Bone mineral testing should be considered. Calcium and vitamin D should be prescribed and bisphosphonates may be warranted.

Aortic aneurysms and dissection can be late complications and an annual abdominal ultrasound, chest x-ray, and transthoracic echocardiogram for up to 10 years are recommended. CT can help further evaluation. If the patient is at very high risk, consider annual thoracic CT or MRI along with abdominal ultrasound.

Generally the course of temporal arteritis is self-limited after several months to 1 to 2 years although a few patients will continue to require low doses of corticosteroids for persistence of symptoms.

References
Al-Shahi R, White PM, Davenport RJ, et al: Subarachnoid haemorrhage, *BMJ* 333:235–240, 2006.

Antonaci F, Bono G, Chimento P: Diagnosing cervicogenic headache, *J Head Pain* 7:145–148, 2006.

Beck E, Sieber WJ, Trejo R: Management of cluster headache, *Am Fam Physician* 71:717–724, 728, 2005.

Bensten L, Jensen R: Tension type headache: the most common, but also the most neglected, headache disorder, *Curr Opin Neurol* 19:305–309, 2006.

Bigal ME, Lipton RB: The preventive treatment of migraine, *Neurologist* 12:204–213, 2006.

Biondi D, Mendes P: Treatment of primary headache: cluster headache. In *Standards of care for headache diagnosis and treatment*, Chicago, 2004, National Headache Foundation, pp 59–72.

Biondi DM: Physical treatments for headache: a structured review, *Headache* 45:738, 2005.

Bogduk N: Cervicogenic headache, *Cephalgia* 24:819, 2004.

Bondi DM: Cervicogenic headache: a review of diagnostic and treatment strategies.

Bongartz T, Matteson E: Large-vessel involvement in giant cell arteritis, *Curr Opin Rheumatol* 18:10–17, 2006.

Bronfort G, et al: Non-invasive physical treatments for chronic/recurrent headache, *Cochrane Database Syst Rev* (3):2004.

Capobianco DJ, Dodick DW: Diagnosis and treatment of cluster headache, *Semin Neurol* 26:242–259, 2006.

Clinch CR, Herbert FE: Evaluation of acute headache in adults, *Am Fam Physician* 63:685–692, 2001.

Colas R, Munoz P, Temprano R, et al: Chronic daily headache with analgesic overuse: epidemiology and impact on quality of life, *Neurology* 62:1338, 2004.

Detsky ME, McDonald DR, Baerlocher MO: Does this patient with headache have a migraine or need neuroimaging? *JAMA* 10:1274–1282, 2006.

Forsyth PA, Posner JB: Headaches in patients with brain tumors: a study of 111 patients, *Neurology* 43:1678–1683, 1993.

Goadsby PJ: Recent advances in the diagnosis and management of migraine, *BMJ* 332:25–29, 2006.

Goadsby PJ, Lipton RB, Ferrari MD: Migraine—current understanding and treatment, *N Engl J Med* 346:257–270, 2002.

Huynh C, Rajagopalan S, Scheld MW: Bacterial meningitis in adults, *Top Emerg Med* 25:101–105, 2003.

Kowalski RG, Claassen J, Kreiter KT, et al: Initial misdiagnosis and outcome after subarachnoid hemorrhage, *JAMA* 291:866–869, 2004.

Lenaerts ME: Alternative therapies for tension-type headache, *Curr Pain Headache Rep* 8:484–488, 2004.

Maizels M: The clinician's approach to the management of headache, *West J Med* 168:203, 1998.

Mariano de Silva H Jr, Bordini CA: Cervicogenic headache, *Curr Pain Headache Rep* 10:306–311, 2006.

May A: The role of imaging in the pathophysiology and diagnosis of headache, *Curr Opin Neurol* 18:293–297, 2005.

Millea PJ, Brodie JJ: Tension type headache, *Am Fam Physician* 66:797–805, 2002.

Nordborg E, Nordborg C: Giant cell arteritis: strategies in diagnosis and treatment, *Curr Opin Rheumatol* 16:25–30, 2004.

Rains JC, Penzien DB, McCrory DC, Gray RN: Behavioral headache treatment: history, review of the empirical literature, and methodological critique, *Headache* 45:S92, 2005.

Rozen TD: Acute therapy for migraine headaches, *Semin Neurol* 26:181–187, 2006.

Rozen TD: Cluster headache: clinical presentation, lifestyle features, and medical treatment, *Headache* 46:1246–1254, 2006.

Schwartz BS, Stewart WF, Simon D, Lipton RB: Epidemiology of tension type headache, *JAMA* 279:381–383, 1998.

Silberstein SD, Schulman EA, Hopkins MM: Repetitive intravenous DHE in the treatment of refractory headache, *Headache* 30:334, 1990.

Smetana GW, Shmerling RH: Does this patient have temporal arteritis? *JAMA* 287:92, 2002.

Takahashi M, Macdonald RL: Subarachnoid hemorrhage, *Contemp Neurosurg* 28:1–7, 2006.

The International Classification of Headache Disorders, 2nd ed, Cephalgia, 2004; 24(suppl 1):1–160.

Van de Beek D, de Gans J, McIntyre P, Prasad K: Corticosteroids for acute bacterial meningitis, *The Cochrane Library*, volume (3):2006, CD004405.

Van de Beek D, de Gans J, Spanjaard L, et al: Clinical features and prognostic factors in adults with bacterial meningitis, *N Engl J Med* 351:1849, 2004.

Wen PY, Marks PW: Medical management in patients with brain tumors, *Curr Opin Oncol* 14:299–307, 2002.

Weyand CM, Goronzy JJ: Giant cell arteritis and polymyalgia rheumatica, *Ann Intern Med* 139:505–515, 2003.

Zeeberg P, Olesen J, Jensen R: Probable medication-overuse headache: the effect of a 2-month drug-free period, *Neurology* 66:1894–1898, 2006.

CHAPTER 25

Health Maintenance
Sherry Huang and Sherri L. Morgan

Stedman's Medical Dictionary defines screening as "examination of a group of usually asymptomatic individuals to detect those with a high probability of having a given disease, typically by means of an inexpensive diagnostic test."

Talking to patients about health maintenance and screening tests should occur at any given opportunity, whether in acute, chronic, or preventive service visits. The clinician's role is to present the recommendations, potential benefits, possible harms, and limitations of the tests. Different organizations have varying recommendations. This chapter focuses on the guidelines developed by the USPSTF with input from other organizations. The task force evaluates the evidence along with the risks and benefits (Table 25-1). An Interactive Preventive Services Selector (IPSS) allows clinicians to identify screening tests needed while face to face with the patient in the office. The IPSS in a web form or PDA download can be obtained from the Agency for Healthcare Research and Quality (AHRQ) website (www.ahrq.gov). A chart of common screening tests for adults with average risk is shown in Table 25-2. Deciding whether to screen is based on patient preferences, medical contraindications, and available resources for testing and follow-up. If the test is declined, the discussion should be documented in the chart along with the patient's decision.

ADULT FEMALE

 SCREENING FOR BREAST CANCER

The USPSTF recommends routine screening every 1 to 2 years for women between the ages of 40 and 70 with mammography (with or without clinical breast examination) (B recommendation). The USPSTF recommends referral for genetic counseling and *BRCA* testing for women whose family history is associated with an increased risk for mutations in *BRCA1* or *BRCA2* genes (B recommendation). The age to initiate screening in patients with average risk is 40 years.

Risk Factors
- Family history of breast or ovarian cancer in a first-degree female relative (especially if diagnosed before menopause)
- Previous breast biopsy revealing atypical hyperplasia

Table 25-1. The U.S. Preventive Services Task Force (USPSTF)

The U.S. Preventive Services Task Force (USPSTF) grades its recommendations based on the strength of evidence and magnitude of net benefit (benefits minus harms).

A. The USPSTF strongly recommends that clinicians provide [the service] to eligible patients. The USPSTF found good evidence that [the service] improves important health outcomes and concludes that benefits substantially outweigh harms.

B. The USPSTF recommends that clinicians provide [the service] to eligible patients. The USPSTF found at least fair evidence that [the service] improves important health outcomes and concludes that benefits outweigh harms.

C. The USPSTF makes no recommendation for or against routine provision of [the service]. The USPSTF found at least fair evidence that [the service] can improve health outcomes but concludes that the balance of benefits and harms is too close to justify a general recommendation.

D. The USPSTF recommends against routinely providing [the service] to asymptomatic patients. The USPSTF found at least fair evidence that [the service] is ineffective or that harms outweigh benefits.

I. The USPSTF concludes that the evidence is insufficient to recommend for or against routinely providing [the service]. Evidence that [the service] is effective is lacking, of poor quality, or conflicting, and the balance of benefits and harms cannot be determined.

From www.ahrq.gov/clinic/pocketgd/gcps1.htm#Overview.

- Previous chest radiation
- Early menarche or late menopause
- Diethylstilbestrol (DES) exposure
- Long-term HRT
- Having no children or having a first child after age 30
- Having more than one alcoholic beverage a day
- Being overweight

Referral for counseling and *BRCA* testing is recommended for those with specific family history associated with the *BRCA1* or *BRCA2* genes. The USPSTF recommends against routine referral for women whose family history is not associated with the genetic mutations (D recommendation).

- Frequency: every 12 to 33 months. The American College of Obstetricians and Gynecologists (ACOG) recommends testing every 1 to 2 years between ages 40 to 49 and annually after age 50. The USPSTF cites little evidence showing annual screening to be more effective than biennial screening at more than 50 years of age.
- Age to discontinue screening: unknown. Very little evidence available beyond age 70. Factor in comorbid conditions in decision process.
- Evidence on breast self-examinations and routine clinical breast examinations: evidence is sufficient to determine the effect on breast cancer mortality

Table 25-2. Preventive Services and USPSTF Grades by Gender and Age for Persons of Average Risk*

TEST (MALE, FEMALE)/AGE	18	20	21	35	40	45	50	60	65	70	≥75
Alcohol misuse (M&F)	B (frequency individualized)										
Blood pressure (M&F)	A (every 2 years if normal blood pressures)										
Colorectal cancer (M&F)							A (frequency depends on the test used and risk)				
Depression (M&F)	B (frequency individualized)										
HIV (M&F)	A (frequency individualized)										
Obesity (M&F)	B (frequency individualized)										
Tobacco use (M&F)	A (frequency individualized)										
Lipid disorder (M)		B (if higher risk)		A (consider every 5 years if average risk)							
Prostate cancer (M)											
Breast cancer (F)					B (every 1-2 years)						
BRCA mutation (F)	B (once only if applicable)										
Cervical cancer (F)			A (see section)								
Chlamydia (F)	A (frequency individualized)										
Gonorrhea (F)	B (frequency individualized)										
Lipid disorder (F)		B (if higher risk)				A (consider every 5 years if average risk)					
Osteoporosis (F)									B (no more than once every 2 years)		

*See specific topic sections for higher-risk persons.

F, Female; *HIV*, human immunodeficiency virus; *M*, male.

SCREENING FOR CERVICAL CANCER

The USPSTF strongly recommends screening sexually active women for cervical cancer (A recommendation). The age to initiate screening is approximately 3 years after onset of vaginal intercourse or age 21, whichever is first. This is a deviation from the previous recommendation to start screening by age 18. This recommendation is based on the course of human papillomavirus (HPV) infection, its transient nature in young women with normal immune systems, and the usually slow progression to high-grade lesions and cervical cancer. Screening women who have never been sexually active by age 21 has minimal value, but it addresses the concern that accurate sexual history may not always be attainable.

Risk Factors
- History of cervical neoplasia
- Infection with HPV or other sexually transmitted diseases
- High-risk sexual behavior
- History of DES exposure
- HIV infection
- A weak immune system

Frequency of screening is variable. The American Cancer Society (ACS) recommends yearly conventional Papanicolaou (Pap) test or every 2 years with a liquid-based Pap test up to age 30. After age 30 and having had three normal consecutive tests, screening may be lengthened to every 2 to 3 years or, alternatively, a Pap test plus high-risk HPV deoxyribonucleic acid (DNA) testing every 3 years. Annual screening should be done in high-risk women. High-risk HPV DNA testing with Pap smear as primary screening for women under age 30 is not appropriate because many infections are transient in this age group.

The age to discontinue screening is between 65 and 70, if there were previous normal tests. The ACOG does not recommend an age to stop screening. Factors to consider are adequacy of prior screening, test results, and absence of risk factors. For women who are older than 70 and never had testing, screening is appropriate if comorbid conditions do not limit benefit of testing.

For women who have confirmed total hysterectomy for benign disease (e.g., without history of cancer or precancer), discontinuation of vaginal cytological screening is appropriate.

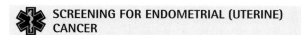 ## SCREENING FOR ENDOMETRIAL (UTERINE) CANCER

The USPSTF makes no recommendation on screening for endometrial cancer. The ACS recommends all women be informed about endometrial cancer at menopause, and to report any unexpected bleeding or spotting. Annual screening with endometrial biopsy should be offered at age 35 for women with or at high risk for hereditary nonpolyposis colon cancer.

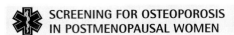

SCREENING FOR OSTEOPOROSIS IN POSTMENOPAUSAL WOMEN

The USPSTF recommends routine screening for osteoporosis in women ages 65 and older, and earlier screening at age 60 for women with increased risk (B recommendation).

Risk Factors for Low Bone Mineral Density
- Lower body weight (weight <70 kg)
- No current use of estrogen therapy

Other Risk Factors That Have Less Supporting Evidence
- Smoking
- Weight loss
- Family history
- Decreased physical activity
- Alcohol or caffeine use
- Low calcium and vitamin D intake

White and Asian women are more likely to develop osteoporosis.
- Frequency of screening: no studies available. A minimum of 2 years may be needed to reliably measure a change in bone mineral density.
- Age to stop screening: no data available. Limited data on women more than 85 years old.

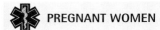

PREGNANT WOMEN

- Alcohol use: screen and inform of harmful effects on fetus (B recommendation)
- Asymptomatic bacteriuria: routine screen using urine culture at 12 to 16 weeks' gestation (A recommendation)
- Chlamydia infection: routine screen if ages 25 years and younger or if at increased risk (B recommendation)
- Gonorrhea infection: screen if high risk (B recommendation)
- Hepatitis B virus infection: routine screen (A recommendation)
- HIV infection: routine screen (A recommendation)
- Iron deficiency anemia: routine screen (B recommendation)
- Rh(D) incompatibility: blood typing and antibody testing at first pre-natal visit (A recommendation); repeat Rh(D) antibody testing for all Rh(D)-negative women at 24 to 28 weeks' gestation (unless bio-logic father is known to be Rh(D)-negative) (B recommendation)
- Syphilis infection: routine screen (A recommendation)
- Tobacco use: routine screen (A recommendation)

ADULT MALE AND FEMALE

 SCREENING FOR ALCOHOL MISUSE

The USPSTF recommends screening for alcohol misuse in adults (B recommendation).

Definitions
- "Risky/hazardous" alcohol misuse is having more than 14 drinks per week or more than 4 drinks per occasion for men and having more than 7 drinks per week, or more than 3 drinks per occasion for women.
- "Harmful drinking" occurs when there is harm from alcohol use but drinker has not yet met criteria for dependence.
- "Alcohol abuse" and "dependence" are associated with repeated negative effects from alcohol.
- "Binge drinking" occurs when five or more alcoholic beverages are consumed by a male, or four or more alcoholic beverages by a female, on at least one occasion during the past month.

The "5-A" behavioral counseling can be implemented: Assess for alcohol abuse or dependence; Advise to reduce consumption; Agree on goals; Assist to achieve behavior change; and Arrange follow-up. Assessment can be made with a quick screening tool, the CAGE questions—feeling the need to Cut down, feeling Annoyed by criticism, feeling Guilty about drinking, and needing an Eye-opener in the morning. A study of 518 patients using a cutoff score of 2 showed the CAGE questions had 75% sensitivity and 96% specificity.

 SCREENING FOR COLORECTAL CANCER

The USPSTF strongly recommends screening adults ages 50 and older for colorectal cancer.

Five screening options are available:
- Home FOBT using two samples from three consecutive stools without rehydration or dietary restriction; a single FOBT from a digital rectal examination is not adequate screening
- Flexible sigmoidoscopy
- Home FOBT plus flexible sigmoidoscopy (if FOBT is heme positive, refer directly for colonoscopy)
- Double-contrast barium enema (DCBE)
- Colonoscopy

The combination of FOBT and flexible sigmoidoscopy is regarded as better than either modality alone. Choosing the mode for screening is based on patient preference and type of testing available.

Risk should be assessed well in advance, as early as 20 years of age, to assess patients with high risk. Patients with increased risk include those who have a personal history of colorectal cancer or adenomatous polyps, or have a first-degree relative diagnosed before age 60, or have two or more relatives diagnosed at any age that is not part of a hereditary syndrome. High-risk patients are those with a family history of familial adenomatous polyposis or hereditary nonpolyposis colorectal cancer, or have a personal history of IBD.

- Age to initiate screening depends on risk. For patients with average risk, begin screening at age 50. If at increased risk, begin at age 40 or 10 years prior to the age of the youngest relative when diagnosed, whichever is first. If at high risk, refer to a center with experience in managing these disorders; screening may start as early as puberty in certain disorders.
- Frequency of screening (for patients with average risk): depends on the test. FOBT annually, flexible sigmoidoscopy or double-contrast barium enema every 5 years, and colonoscopy every 10 years is recommended.
- Age to discontinue screening (for patients with average risk): unknown. Studies are limited to patients younger than 80 years of age. Factor in comorbid conditions and life expectancy in the decision process.

 ## SCREENING FOR DEPRESSION

The USPSTF recommends screening adults for depression (B recommendation). Commonly used screening tools include the Zung Self-Assessment Depression Scale and the Beck Depression Inventory. Whooley and associates found that simply asking two questions about mood and anhedonia, "Over the past 2 weeks, have you felt down, depressed, or hopeless?" and "Over the past 2 weeks, have you felt little interest or pleasure in doing things?" may be as effective. The screening tool used depends on clinician preference and the appropriate population.

- Frequency of screening: unknown. Rescreen in patients with a history of depression, unexplained somatic symptoms, comorbid psychologic conditions, substance abuse, or chronic pain.

 ## SCREENING FOR HIGH BLOOD PRESSURE

The USPSTF strongly recommends screening adults ages 18 and older for high blood pressure (A recommendation).

The sixth report of the Joint National Committee on Prevention, Detection, Evaluation, and Treatment of High Blood Pressure (JNC 6) recommends screening every 2 years for average-risk patients whose systolic blood pressure is less than 130 mm Hg and diastolic blood pressure is less than 85 mm Hg. More frequent screening intervals are recommended for those with higher blood pressures.

SCREENING FOR INFECTIOUS DISEASES

- Chlamydia infection: routine screen in sexually active women age 25 and younger, and other asymptomatic women at increased risk (A recommendation); no conclusion on routine screening in asymptomatic men (I recommendation)
- Gonorrhea infection: screen sexually active women if at increased risk (B recommendation); no conclusion on routine screening in high-risk men (I recommendation)
- HIV infection: screen if at increased risk (A recommendation); CDC recommends offering routine screen for all persons ages 13-64
- Syphilis infection: screen if at increased risk (A recommendation)
- Tuberculosis infection: screen if at increased risk (CDC recommendations)

 SCREENING FOR LIPID DISORDERS

The USPSTF strongly recommends routine screening of men ages 35 years and older and women 45 years and older for lipid disorders (A recommendation). Earlier screening is recommended for men ages 20 to 35 and for women ages 20 to 45 who have diabetes, family history of cardiovascular disease before age 50 in male relatives or age 60 years in female relatives, family history suggestive of familial hyperlipidemia, and/or multiple coronary heart disease risk factors (e.g., tobacco use, hypertension) (B recommendation).

- Frequency of screening: unknown. One option includes testing every 5 years. Age to discontinue screening: unknown. Lipid levels are less likely to increase after age 65.

 SCREENING FOR OBESITY IN ADULTS

The USPSTF recommends screening of all adults for obesity (B recommendation). Measuring body mass index (BMI, calculated as weight in kilograms divided by height in meters squared) and measuring central adiposity (usually waist circumference) are two simple and popular methods for screening for obesity. Increased BMI and central adiposity are independently associated with an increase in adverse health effects.

Definitions
- BMI between 25 and 29.9 is overweight
- BMI of 30 and above is obese. Three classes of obesity are as follows:
  - Class I (BMI 30 to 34.9)
  - Class II (BMI 35 to 39.9)
  - Class III (BMI 40 and above)

- Men with waist circumferences greater than 102 cm (>40 inches) and women with waist circumferences greater than 88 cm (>35 inches) are at increased risk for cardiovascular disease.
- When a BMI is greater than 35, waist circumference values are not reliable. Counseling to promote sustained weight loss should be provided.

 ## SCREENING FOR TOBACCO USE

The USPSTF strongly recommends screening adults for tobacco use (A recommendation). The 5-A behavioral counseling method can be implemented for positive screens.

CHILDREN (BIRTH TO 11 YEARS OF AGE)

The well-child visit is an opportunity for both the primary care physician and patient's caregivers to work together to optimize a child's physical and emotional potential. This provides the caregivers an opportunity to ask questions related to the child's health and developmental process and the provider an opportunity to perform appropriate screening and physical assessment, administer immunizations, and provide adequate education to the family.

Recommendations for preventive pediatric health care have been developed by the USPSTF and the American Academy of Pediatrics (AAP).

- History—Review specific body systems when indicated by age with special attention to family history and concerns. Review information on prenatal history (newborn visit), feeding and nutrition, elimination, sleep, family relationships, school, high-risk behaviors (tobacco, alcohol and/or substance abuse, sexual activity), and activities or interests.
- Measurements—Weight, height/length, head circumference (to age 24 months), blood pressure (measured at least once during each health care visit starting at age 3 years; hypertension is defined as average systolic blood pressure [SBP] and/or diastolic blood pressure [DBP] >95th percentile for gender, age, and height on more than three occasions; prehypertension in children is defined as average SBP or DBP >90th percentile but <95th percentile). Calculate BMI starting at age 2 years (overweight is defined as BMI for age >95th percentile and at risk for overweight is defined as BMI for age >85th and <95th percentiles). Suspect an eating disorder with weight loss more than 10% of previous weight and/or BMI for age less than the 5th percentile.
- Sensory screening—The USPSTF recommends screening to detect amblyopia, strabismus, and visual acuity younger than age 5 years. Screening for hearing in asymptomatic children older than 3 years is not recommended. Screening should be conducted prior to age 3 years because adequate hearing is essential for normal speech and language development.

- Development/behavioral assessment—Regular and specific developmental screening of gross motor function, fine motor skills, and speech milestones should be performed so that delays can be identified as soon as possible. Research shows that parental developmental reports are as accurate as more time-intensive screening tools.
- Physical assessment—The assessment must be comprehensive and include components relevant to the patient's age, chronic conditions, or risks due to family health history.

ADOLESCENTS

Adolescence is a time of transition, affecting the teen, the family, and the health care provider. During this transition adolescents progress through different stages of development with variations in their level of cognition and developmental tasks. These variations affect how adolescents respond to health care providers during their health maintenance services.

The adolescent period is divided into three stages: early (ages 11 to 13 years) when concrete thinking leads to information being taken literally; midadolescence (ages 14 to 16 years) with increased capacity for abstract thinking with self-focused value system; and late adolescence (ages 17 to 20 years) when abstract thinking ability is fully developed, which allows them to reflect on things objectively. This can lead to a high level of self-confidence in one's reasoning ability, which in turn can lead to risk-taking behaviors.

Various guidelines for preventive and health maintenance services for adolescents have been developed by the USPSTF, the American Medical Association (AMA), and the AAP. The purpose of preventive and maintenance services is to reduce serious morbidity and premature mortality.

- Screening and history—Adolescents should be screened at least annually for the following medical conditions:
  - Hypertension: Defined as average SBP and/or DBP greater than the 95th percentile for gender, age, and height on more than three occasions. Adolescents with BP more than 120/80 are considered prehypertensive.
  - Weight: Overweight is defined as BMI for age greater than the 95th percentile; at risk for overweight is defined as BMI for age greater than the 85th and less than the 95th percentile; suspect an eating disorder with weight loss more than 10% of previous weight and/or BMI for age less than the 5th percentile.
  - Hyperlipidemia if patient and/or family has a history of premature CAD, obesity, hypertension, diabetes mellitus, or a total cholesterol greater than 200 mg/dL.

Screening should also cover activities related to high-risk behaviors (tobacco use, alcohol and drug use, unprotected sexual activity), abuse (physical, sexual, and emotional), violence, and school performance. Table 25-3 lists useful mnemonics.

Table 25-3. Mnemonics Useful in Evaluating Adolescent Patients

HEADS

Home, habits
Education, employment, exercise
Accidents, ambition, activities, abuse
Drugs (tobacco, alcohol, others), diet, depression
Sex, suicide

SAFE TEENS

Sexuality
Accident, abuse
Firearms/homicide
Emotions (suicide/depression)

Toxins (tobacco/alcohol, others)
Environment (school, home, friends)
Exercise
Nutrition
Shots (immunization status, school performance)

From Montalto N: Implementing the guidelines for adolescent preventive service, *Am Fam Physician* 57, 1998.

 PHYSICAL ASSESSMENT

Recommendations regarding the frequency of routine physical examinations for adolescents have varied from annually to once every 2 to 3 years. Most of the literature recommends at least one comprehensive assessment during each stage of adolescence.

Tests and Diagnostic Studies

- Fasting lipids performed annually if patient and/or family history of premature coronary artery disease, obesity, hypertension, diabetes mellitus, or a total cholesterol greater than 200 mg/dL
- Tuberculosis if there is exposure to active TB or if patient lives or works in high-risk situation
- Gonorrhea, chlamydia, syphilis, and HPV screen annually if sexually active
- HIV screen if high risk for infection through behavior or exposure. The CDC recommends offering routine screening to all starting at age 13.
- Pap smear annually if high risk for cervical abnormalities and/or high-risk behavior
- Immunizations
- Anticipatory guidance—All adolescents should receive annual health guidance to promote a better understanding of their physical growth, psychosocial and psychosexual development, and the importance of becoming actively involved in decisions regarding their health care. This guidance should also cover dietary habits

including healthy diet, benefits of physical activity and exercise, responsible sexual behaviors including abstinence, and promotion of the avoidance of tobacco, alcohol, and other abusable substances including OTC medications and sports-enhancement drugs.

Anticipatory guidance should also be provided to parents or other adult caregivers at least once during each stage of the child's adolescence about adolescent development (including physical, sexual, and emotional), signs and symptoms of disease and emotional distress, parenting behaviors that promote healthy adolescent adjustment, methods for helping their adolescent avoid high-risk behaviors and ways to discuss health-related behaviors with their adolescent.

 ## TESTS AND DIAGNOSTIC STUDIES

- Anemia—The USPSTF does not recommend screening in asymptomatic low-risk children beyond infancy (15 months).
- Lead—The AAP recommends screening children between ages 6 months and 6 years who have not been screened previously if they live or spend time in buildings built before 1950 or have damaged paint, receive government assistance (Medicaid), live in areas with a high or unknown prevalence of elevated childhood lead levels, or have a housemate or playmate with elevated serum lead level. Additionally, screening should be done in accordance to state law when applicable.
- Lipids—Universal screening in children is not recommended. Screening is recommended in high-risk children ages 2 to 20 years who have a parent with total cholesterol level greater than 200 mg/dL or a first-degree relative with premature CAD.
- Tuberculosis—Recommended only in high-risk children (exposure to active tuberculosis, has HIV, incarcerated or lives or works in high-risk situation)
- Pelvic examination—The USPSTF recommends screening for cervical cancer in females who are sexually active annually along with screening for STDs (chlamydia, gonorrhea).
- Immunizations
- Anticipatory guidance—Provide to the caregivers at each appointment age-appropriate, evidence-based guidelines on healthy diet, feeding and nutrition, sleep habits, oral health, safety issues, illness prevention and recognition, and developmental stages and milestones.

References

American Academy of Pediatrics (AAP): Recommendations for Pediatric Preventive Health Care 1995/2000.

American Cancer Society Guidelines on Screening and Surveillance for the Early Detection of Adenomatous Polyps and Colorectal Cancer. Reprinted from CA – A Cancer Journal for Clinicians 51:44–54, 2001.

American Cancer Society: *Cancer facts & figures 2006, screening guidelines for the early detection of cancer in asymptomatic people*, Atlanta, 2006, ACS.

American Medical Association (AMA): Guidelines for adolescent preventive services (GAPS), 1992.

Behrman RD, Kliegman RM, Jenson HB: *Nelson textbook of pediatrics*, 17th ed, Philadelphia, 2003, Saunders.

Centers for Disease Control and Prevention: Recommended childhood and adolescent immunization schedule—United States, 2006, *MMWR* 54:Q1–Q4, 2005.

Centers for Disease Control and Prevention. Revised recommendations for HIV testing in health-care settings and for screening of pregnant women *(MMWR)*. September 22, 2006.

Clark WD: Alcoholism: blocks to diagnosis and treatment, *Am J Med* 71:275–286, 1981.

Ferris DG, Cox JT, O'Connor DM, et al: *Modern colposcopy textbook and atlas*, 2nd ed, 2004, American Society for Colposcopy and Cervical Pathology, Dubuque, IA, pp 533–542.

Grenz K: *Health care guideline: preventive services for children and adolescents*, Bloomington, MN, 2004, Institute for Clinical Systems Improvement.

Rakel RE: *Textbook of family practice*, 6th ed, Philadelphia, 2002, Elsevier.

Spraycar, Marjory: *Stedman's medical dictionary*, 26th ed, Baltimore, 1995, Williams and Wilkins.

Whooley MA, Avins AL, Miranda J, Browner WS: Case-finding instruments for depression: two questions are as good as many, *J Gen Intern Med* 12:439–445, 1997.

CHAPTER 26

Heartburn

Joel J. Heidelbaugh and Dean Thomas Scow

Heartburn is the most common symptom of GERD, a chronic and relapsing condition that carries a significant risk of morbidity and the potential for resultant complications. It is defined by symptoms related to mucosal damage produced by abnormal reflux of gastric contents into the esophagus. Population-based studies demonstrate that 40% of U.S. adults experience heartburn monthly, with a 20% age- and sex-adjusted prevalence of weekly symptoms. It is important to also consider emergent causes of heartburn, such as MI in addition to GERD and more chronic conditions.

Most patients with GERD self-treat with OTC medications and do not initially seek medical attention for their symptoms. Health-related quality-of-life surveys reveal that patients with GERD have lower symptomatic assessment scores than patients with CHF, CAD, and diabetes mellitus. GERD is responsible for the highest annual direct costs related to all GI disorders, estimated at more than $10 billion per year, with the largest component of these costs attributable to antireflux medications, approaching $6 billion annually.

The vast majority (>90%) of patients with GERD evaluated in primary care practices have nonerosive reflux disease (NERD), whereas a minority will progress to develop erosive esophagitis, and even fewer will develop esophageal strictures, Barrett's esophagus, and adenocarcinoma of the esophagus. Patients with NERD are prone to develop extraesophageal/atypical manifestations (Table 26-1), yet given a small risk of disease progression, they generally do not require long-term surveillance despite persistent reflux symptoms. Symptom relapse rates in patients with NERD are similar to those in patients with erosive esophagitis, and although many patients will require daily pharmacologic treatment to control heartburn, less than 10% will develop erosive esophagitis on upper endoscopy over time.

When a patient exhibits the classic symptoms of heartburn and acid regurgitation, the diagnosis of GERD can be made with high specificity, yet the sensitivity remains low. Evidence for the positive predictive value of heartburn for accurately diagnosing GERD is suboptimal due to the lack of a diagnostic gold standard. Intensity and frequency of reflux symptoms are poor predictors of the presence or severity of reflux esophagitis. The diagnostic workup for determining GERD includes:

Table 26-1. Extraesophageal or Atypical Manifestations of GERD

- Aspiration
- Asthma
- Chronic cough
- Dental enamel loss
- Globus sensation
- Noncardiac chest pain
- Recurrent laryngitis
- Recurrent sore throat
- Subglottic stenosis

Adapted from Heidelbaugh JJ, Nostrant TT: Medical and surgical management of gastroesophageal reflux disease, *Clin Fam Pract* 6:547-568, 2004.

- The Bernstein test—A test infusion into the distal esophagus of either 0.1N HCl or 0.9% NaCl in a single-blinded fashion with an assessment of the patient's response can be used to detect GERD, if a patient's symptoms are directly related to acid reflux (not widely used).
- The 24-hour pH probe—Accepted as the standard for establishing or excluding the presence of GERD, but is often inconvenient to the patient, and lacks the sensitivity and specificity (70% to 96%) required to be a gold standard; more often used in infants and children to accurately diagnose GERD
- Double-contrast barium radiography—Has limited usefulness in making an accurate diagnosis of GERD, but may be useful in defining the presence of anatomic abnormalities, including pyloric stenosis, malrotation, and annular pancreas in the vomiting infant, and hiatal hernia and esophageal strictures in children and adults
- Upper endoscopy or EGD with or without biopsy—The gold standard in assessing esophageal complications of GERD (e.g., erosive esophagitis and Barrett's esophagus), yet lacks an appreciable sensitivity and specificity for identifying pathologic reflux

Symptoms
- Acid regurgitation +++++
- Burning sensation in the throat ++++
- Sour or bitter taste in the mouth (water brash) +++
- Swallowing can be difficult ++
- Belching ++
- Wheezing +

Table 26-2 lists alarm symptoms of GERD that suggest complicated disease and warrant referral to gastroenterology for evaluation.

Signs
- Commonly, none are present in NERD and uncomplicated disease. +++++
- Physical manifestations may include extraesophageal/atypical manifestations (see Table 26-1) ++ and alarm symptoms of complicated disease (see Table 26-2). +

Table 26-2. Alarm Symptoms of GERD Suggesting Complicated Disease

- Black or bloody stools
- Choking
- Chronic coughing
- Dysphagia
- Early satiety
- Hematemesis
- Hoarseness
- Iron deficiency anemia
- Odynophagia
- Weight loss

Adapted from Heidelbaugh JJ, Nostrant TT: Medical and surgical management of gastroesophageal reflux disease, *Clin Fam Pract* 6:547-568, 2004.

Workup

- If suggested by history and physical examination, CAD should first be ruled out in patients presenting with heartburn.
  - ECG and cardiac enzyme testing initially
  - Stress testing as indicated
- Differential diagnosis
  - CAD—Myocardial infarction and angina pectoris
  - Other acid-related illnesses—Peptic ulcer disease, gastritis, and non-ulcer dyspepsia
  - Esophageal motility disorders—Spasm, achalasia, scleroderma, and radiation injury
  - Infectious esophagitis—*Candida*, herpes, HIV, and cytomegalovirus (CMV)
  - Pill-induced esophagitis—Doxycycline, ascorbic acid, quinidine, potassium chloride, and bisphosphonates
  - Anatomic problems of the esophagus—Strictures, webs, rings, diverticula, atresia, and fistulas
  - Esophageal carcinoma
  - Chemical esophagitis (i.e., lye ingestion)
  - Crohn's disease of the esophagus
  - Biliary tract disease
  - Other esophageal-related problems—Eosinophilic esophagitis, alkaline reflux, Mallory-Weiss syndrome, and Chagas disease
  - Nonesophageal or indirect problems—Myasthenia gravis, pulmonary embolus, muscle strain, asthma, and pregnancy
- History will often reveal causes such as ingestions, medications, or radiation.
- Infectious causes can be suggested by history and physical examination and confirmed by endoscopic visualization and, in some cases serology, or culture.
- Esophageal manometry is useful in confirming motility disorders.
- Abdominal or biliary ultrasonography, double contrast barium swallow, 24-hour esophageal pH monitoring, radionuclide scintigraphy, and EGD complete the diagnostic armamentarium.

Table 26-3. Pharmacologic Therapy for the Treatment of GERD

- Histamine-2 receptor antagonists (H_2RAs)
  - Cimetidine (Tagamet)
  - Famotidine (Pepcid)
  - Nizatidine (Axid)
  - Ranitidine (Zantac)
- Proton pump inhibitors (PPIs)
  - Esomeprazole (Nexium)
  - Lansoprazole (Prevacid)
  - Omeprazole (Prilosec)
  - Pantoprazole (Prevacid)
  - Rabeprazole (Aciphex)

- Diagnostic testing is recommended in patients with GERD who:
  - Have an inadequate response to an empiric trial of antisecretory therapy (e.g., on-demand treatment with PPIs taken 15 to 30 minutes prior to the first meal of the day or histamine-2 receptor antagonists [H_2RAs] taken daily to twice daily during symptom exacerbations [Table 26-3])
  - Require continuous chronic antisecretory therapy to control frequent GERD symptoms
  - Have chronic reflux symptoms lasting more than 5 years and are thus at an increased risk for esophageal strictures and Barrett's esophagus
  - Have extraesophageal/atypical manifestations suggesting complicated disease (see Table 26-1)
  - Have alarm symptoms suggesting complicated disease or cancer (see Table 26-2)
- In the absence of alarm signs or symptoms, the diagnosis of GERD can be made with high sensitivity and specificity based on clinical presentation without the need for testing or gastroenterology referral.
- In the presence of alarm signs or symptoms or extraesophageal/atypical manifestations, upper endoscopy is recommended to rule out complicated or advanced disease.
- In observational studies, the progression from NERD to severe esophagitis has not occurred in patients with an initial normal endoscopy whose symptoms have remained unchanged during 10-year follow-up, arguing against repeat endoscopy during that time period, in the absence of alarm symptoms.

Comments and Treatment Considerations

Initial empiric pharmacotherapy for treatment of GERD should consist of either a PPI or H_2RA, and is reasonable without the need for immediate diagnostic testing in the vast majority of cases (Fig. 26-1). In patients who incompletely respond to a trial of either OTC or prescription H_2RAs, PPIs taken once daily are preferred over continuing H_2RA therapy due to their greater efficacy and faster symptom control, as well as the limited additional benefit gained from extending

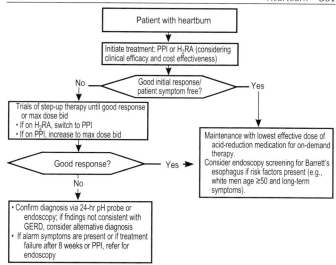

FIGURE 26-1 Algorithm for the diagnosis and treatment of GERD. *(Adapted from Heidelbaugh JJ, Gill A, Nostrant TT, Harrison RV:* Gastroesophageal reflux disease (GERD), *Ann Arbor, MI, 2006, Office of Clinical Affairs, University of Michigan Health System.) H₂RA,* Histamine-2 receptor antagonist; *PPI,* proton pump inhibitor.

therapy with the same or higher-dose H₂RA. Additional benefit may be obtained by extending treatment for another 4 to 8 weeks with either the same or double-dose PPI.

An inadequate response to a 4- or 8-week trial of standard dose PPI may indicate longer treatment is needed, more severe disease, or an incorrect diagnosis. Evidence from RCTs demonstrated improved control of GERD symptoms over a 4- to 8-week period in patients treated with PPIs (83%) compared with those given H₂RAs or placebo (60% and 27%, respectively). A greater percentage of patients treated with PPIs has been found to be in symptomatic remission at 12 months compared with patients who received either H₂RAs or placebo.

In the treatment of erosive esophagitis, faster healing rates have been achieved in patients who received PPI therapy for 4 to 8 weeks (78%) than in patients given H₂RAs or placebo (50% and 24%, respectively) for the same period; at 1 year, patients treated daily with a PPI were significantly less likely to relapse than those who received an H₂RA. Economic analyses of various empiric treatment strategies revealed that an 8-week course of PPIs for initial symptom relief taken on demand is more cost-effective than continuous, step-up/step-down, or intermittent strategies with either H₂RAs or PPIs.

Expert opinion states that lifestyle modifications should be recommended as adjunctive therapy in all patients with GERD (Table 26-4).

Table 26-4. Suggested Lifestyle Modifications for the Treatment of GERD

- Avoid acidic foods (citrus and tomato-based products), alcohol, caffeinated beverages, chocolate, onions, garlic, salt, and peppermint
- Avoid large meals
- Avoid medications that may potentiate GERD symptoms: calcium channel blockers, β-agonists, α-adrenergic agonists, theophylline, nitrates, and sedatives
- Avoid recumbency 3 to 4 hours postprandially
- Avoid tight clothing around the waist
- Decrease dietary fat intake
- Elevate the head of bed 4 to 8 inches
- Lose weight
- Smoking cessation

Summarized from DeVault KR, Castell DO: Updated guidelines for the diagnosis and treatment of gastroesophageal reflux disease. The practice parameters committee of the American College of Gastroenterology, *Am J Gastroenterol* 94:1434-1442, 1999.

References

DeVault KR, Castell DO: Updated guidelines for the diagnosis and treatment of gastroesophageal reflux disease. The practice parameters committee of the American College of Gastroenterology, *Am J Gastroenterol* 94:1434–1442, 1999.

DeVault KR, Castell DO: Updated guidelines for the diagnosis and treatment of gastroesophageal reflux disease, *Am J Gastroenterol* 100:190–200, 2005.

Heidelbaugh JJ, Nostrant TT: Medical and surgical management of gastroesophageal reflux disease, *Clin Fam Pract* 6:547–568, 2004.

Heidelbaugh JJ, Gill A, Nostrant TT, Harrison RV: *Gastroesophageal reflux disease (GERD)*, Ann Arbor, MI, 2006, Office of Clinical Affairs, University of Michigan Health System. Available at www.guideline.gov.

Heidelbaugh JJ, Nostrant TT, Kim C, Harrison RV: Management of gastroesophageal reflux disease, *Am Fam Physician* 68:1311–1318, 1321–1322, 2003.

CHAPTER 27

Hypertension
Bradford S. Volk, David D. Proum, and Michael J. Polizzotto

HYPERTENSIVE URGENCY AND EMERGENCY

Hypertensive urgency is defined as a BP greater than 180/120 mm Hg. BPs in this range causing impending or progressive organ dysfunction are hypertensive emergencies. The distinction is an important one because hospitalization and parenteral antihypertensive agents are typically recommended for a hypertensive emergency, whereas with hypertensive urgency, one can modify the oral antihypertensive regimen and provide close outpatient follow-up over the following few days.

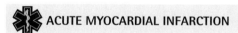 ACUTE MYOCARDIAL INFARCTION

See "Acute Coronary Syndromes."

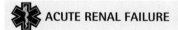 ACUTE RENAL FAILURE

Symptoms
- Generally asymptomatic
- Oliguria or anuria
- Flank pain
- Anorexia, nausea, vomiting

Signs
- Confusion, generalized weakness
- Edema, rales, jugular venous distention

Workup
- BMP: look for elevations in serum creatinine suggestive of compromised renal function, as well as hyperkalemia or hyponatremia
- Urinalysis
  - Presence of proteinuria suggests renal insufficiency but will not differentiate acute from chronic

- If prominent RBCs or casts are present, a separate renal process must be considered because this is a rare finding in cases of solely hypertensive nephrosclerosis.
- Chest x-ray: to assess pulmonary edema

Comments and Treatment Considerations
Goal of treatment is to reduce systemic vascular resistance without compromising glomerular filtration rate.

Specific electrolyte abnormalities should be managed as needed. A nephrology consultation for possible dialysis in cases of uremic symptoms (encephalopathy, pericarditis), severe volume overload, severe acid-base imbalance, uncontrollable severe hyperkalemia, or hyponatremia should be considered.

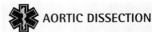 AORTIC DISSECTION

Symptoms
- Sudden tearing posterior chest, back, or abdominal pain, typically excruciating
- Syncope, lightheadedness

Signs
- Pulse deficits in the carotid, brachial, femoral, or dorsalis pedis arteries
- Variations in pulse or blood pressure, including between the left and right arms
- New murmur of aortic insufficiency: low pitched, short early diastolic murmur

Workup
- Chest x-ray: looking for widened mediastinum
- ECG and cardiac enzymes to help rule out ischemic causes of chest pain
- Echocardiography: transesophageal is preferred because of its higher sensitivity and specificity. Chest CT with IV contrast and MRI are alternatives.

Comments and Treatment Considerations
Type A, involving the ascending aorta, requires immediate surgical referral. Type B, or descending ruptured aneurysms, can typically be treated medically.

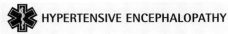 HYPERTENSIVE ENCEPHALOPATHY

Symptoms
- Nonfocal neurologic deficits including headache (typically insidious onset), delirium or disorientation, and speech disturbances. Seizure and coma are late findings.

- Visual changes
- Nausea and vomiting

Signs
- Brisk tendon reflexes
- Papilledema, with retinal hemorrhages and exudates

Workup
- Head CT without contrast, or MRI with T2 weighting: Cerebral edema involving white matter of the posterior portions of both cerebral hemispheres, especially the parieto-occipital regions

Comments and Treatment Considerations
Consider alternative causes for neurologic symptoms. If hypertensive in origin, BP control alone should improve or resolve symptoms. The lower limit of cerebral blood flow autoregulation is reached when BP is reduced by 25%, and cerebral ischemia can be precipitated with rapid reductions more than 50%. The goal is to reduce mean arterial pressure (MAP) by no more than 25% within the first hour, and if stable, to 160/100 mm Hg over the next 2 to 6 hours.

Use caution with sodium nitroprusside as it may cause a precipitous lowering of BP. Other reasonable choices include fenoldopam and labetalol.

 # ILLICIT DRUG USE

See Chapter 41.

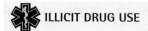 # POORLY CONTROLLED ESSENTIAL HYPERTENSION

Due either to lack of compliance with treatment or previously undiagnosed disease; this is a diagnosis of exclusion, so patients presenting with new onset severe hypertension should have other hypertensive emergency diagnoses considered and ruled out.

Symptoms
- Chronically uncontrolled hypertension is largely an asymptomatic disease ++++

Signs
- Grades III and IV hypertensive retinopathy (hemorrhages, exudates, or papilledema)

Workup
- Review medical records for prior BPs.
- ECG: left ventricular hypertrophy suggests chronically uncontrolled hypertension.

- Consider echocardiography if any clinical suspicion for heart failure
- Serum creatinine and urine microalbumin, indicating underlying renal disease

Comments and Treatment Considerations
- In the absence of hypertensive emergency, the patient can be started on appropriate oral antihypertensive medication and sent home with close follow-up.

 PREECLAMPSIA/ECLAMPSIA

Symptoms
- Edema (especially of the face) ++++
- Epigastric pain, nausea, or vomiting
- Visual changes

Signs
- Sudden and rapid weight gain
- Oliguria
- Seizure

Workup
- Labs: CBC (checking for hemoconcentration or hemolysis, as well as thrombocytopenia), liver function tests (LFTs), serum creatinine (to evaluate renal function), uric acid, urinalysis, and/or 24-hour urine for proteinuria
- Ultrasound to evaluate for growth restriction and oligohydramnios

Comments and Treatment Considerations
Treatment of BP generally not recommended if SBP is less than 160. If BP control is indicated, consider labetalol, hydralazine, or methyldopa. Avoid use of ACE or angiotensin-receptor blocker (ARB) due to teratogenic risk.

Magnesium infusion may be indicated for seizure prophylaxis.

Consult with an obstetrician about the proper management of pregnancy/labor (including possible induction or cesarean delivery).

SECONDARY HYPERTENSION

Secondary hypertension should be considered in a patient with elevated BP (≥140/90 in adults and >95th percentile for age and height in children) along with symptoms, signs, or laboratory tests that suggest an identifiable etiology. The following situations should raise the clinician's index of suspicion:
- Hypertension before age 30 (especially with a negative family history) or after age 55
- Resistant or refractory hypertension despite good compliance with three or more antihypertensive agents (including a diuretic)

- Malignant hypertension (severe hypertension and signs of end-organ damage)
- Acute rise in BP in a previously stable, well-controlled hypertensive patient
- Acute rise in creatinine concentration after starting an ACE-I inhibitor or ARB-II

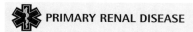

PRIMARY RENAL DISEASE

Primary renal disease, renal parenchymal disease, and renal artery stenosis (RAS) are common causes of secondary hypertension in adults and children.

Symptoms
- Edema, especially flash pulmonary edema
- Dyspnea
- Leg claudication (with RAS)

Signs
- Acutely elevated BP above baseline
- Abdominal bruit
- Decreased/nonpalpable ankle pulses

Workup
- BMP and complete urinalysis, looking for elevated creatinine concentration (estimate glomerular filtration rate [GFR]), as well as proteinuria, hematuria, casts, etc.
- Renal ultrasonography (with Doppler evaluation of renal vasculature) is a good initial imaging study; follow-up CT, MRI, or magnetic resonance angiography (MRA) may be required.

Comments and Treatment Considerations
In most patients with renal disease and diabetes or significant cardiovascular risk factors, use of ACE inhibitors reduces both renal and cardiovascular risk. A trial of medical therapy can be appropriate for many patients with RAS, but renal angioplasty (with possible stent placement) should be considered in certain subgroups, including patients with poorly controlled hypertension, patients with only one functioning kidney, and patients with recurrent CHF.

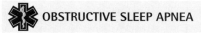

OBSTRUCTIVE SLEEP APNEA

Obstructive sleep apnea (OSA) is a mechanical obstruction of the upper airway that is an independent risk factor for hypertension.

Symptoms
- Daytime somnolence ++++
- Snoring or irregular nocturnal breathing patterns (often noticed by bed partners) ++++

Signs
• Obesity

Workup
• Sleep study with oxygen saturation

Comments and Treatment Considerations
Primary treatment of OSA with continuous positive airway pressure (CPAP) can result in improved BP. Beta-blockers may be more effective than other medications.

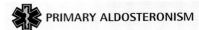 PRIMARY ALDOSTERONISM

Primary aldosteronism is suggested by the combination of hypertension, hypokalemia, and metabolic acidosis.

Symptoms
• Often asymptomatic, but can have headaches, easy fatigue, and weakness

Signs
• Rare and nonspecific

Workup
• Plasma aldosterone (high) and plasma renin activity (low)
• CT scan of adrenal glands (looking for unilateral adenoma versus bilateral hyperplasia)

Comments and Treatment Considerations
Adrenalectomy is the treatment of choice for unilateral adenomas, but results in blood pressure control in only one third of patients. Mineralocorticoid receptor blockers (such as spironolactone or eplerenone) should be used in patients with adrenal hyperplasia.

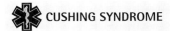 CUSHING SYNDROME

This etiology will include Cushing syndrome and other excess glucocorticoid states, such as chronic steroid use.

Symptoms
• Proximal weakness
• Depression or anxiety

Signs
• Cushingoid facies
• Central obesity
• Hyperpigmentation (purple striae and ecchymoses) and hirsutism

Workup
- Low-dose dexamethasone suppression test or 24-hour urinary free cortisol

Comments and Treatment Considerations
Surgery is the primary treatment for pituitary and adrenal adenomas. If long-term steroid use is unavoidable, the minimum effective steroid dose should be used.

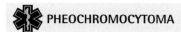 PHEOCHROMOCYTOMA

Pheochromocytoma is often listed in the differential of secondary hypertension, but accounts for only about 0.2% of cases. It is more common in children than adults.

Symptoms
- Classic triad of paroxysmal headaches, palpitations, and diaphoresis

Signs
- Labile hypertension

Workup
- 24-hour urinary vanillylmandelic acid, metanephrine, and normetanephrine

Comments and Treatment Considerations
Surgery is the treatment of choice. Hypertensive crises are effectively treated with IV nitroprusside.

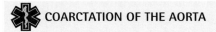 COARCTATION OF THE AORTA

Coarctation of the aorta, more commonly encountered in children, is a congenital, varying constriction of the aorta at any point from the transverse arch to the iliac bifurcation.

Symptoms
- Usually asymptomatic; weakness or leg pain after exercise

Signs
- Delayed femoral pulse and decreased femoral blood pressure
- Heart murmur (variable types)

Workup
- Four-point pulses and BP
- Echocardiogram

Comments and Treatment Considerations
Surgical correction is essential. Patients require lifelong follow-up. Hypertension may recur, even after surgery.

Table 27-1. Drug and Supplement Causes of Hypertension

DRUG CLASS	EXAMPLE
Antiparkinsonian agents	Bromocriptine
Food	Licorice (carbenoxolone), alcohol
Heavy metals	Lead, mercury
Illicit drugs	Phencyclidine (PCP), cocaine, MDMA (Ectasy)
Immunosuppressants	Cyclosporine, tacrolimus, corticosteroids
Monoamine oxidase inhibitors	Phenelzine, tyramine foods
NSAIDs (including COX-2 inhibitors)	Ibuprofen
Oral contraceptives	Estrogen
Stimulants	Nicotine, amphetamines, caffeine
Sympathomimetics	Pseudoephedrine, bronchodilators
Tricyclic antidepressants	Amitriptyline
Weight loss agents	Phentermine, sibutramine, ma huang

COX, Cyclooxygenase; *NSAIDs,* nonsteroidal antiinflammatory drugs.

Drugs and supplements that cause hypertension and their associated symptoms/signs are extensive and varied. History is key. See Table 27-1 for a partial list of potential offenders.

References

Aggarwal M, Khan IA: Hypertensive crisis: hypertensive emergencies and urgencies, *Cardiol Clin 24*:135–146, 2006.

Arnaldi G, Angeli A, Atkinson AB, et al: Diagnosis and complications of Cushing's syndrome: a consensus statement, *J Clin Endocrinol Metab* 88:5593–5602, 2003.

Baillargeon J, McClish D, Essah P, Nestler J: Association between the current use of low-dose oral contraceptives and cardiovascular arterial disease: a meta-analysis, *J Clin Endocrinol Metab* 90:3863–3870, 2005.

Becker C, Jerrentrup A, Ploch T, et al: Effect of nasal continuous positive airway pressure treatment on blood pressure in patients with obstructive sleep apnea, *Circulation* 107:68–73, 2003.

Bhat MA, Neelakandhan KS, Unnikrishnan M, et al: Fate of hypertension after repair of coarctation of the aorta in adults, *Br J Surg* 88:536–538, 2001.

Chin K, Nakamura T, Fukuhara S, et al: Falls in blood pressure in patients with obstructive sleep apnoea after long-term nasal continuous positive airway pressure treatment, *J Hypertens* 24:2091–2099, 2006.

Chobanian AV, Bakris GL, Black HR, et al: Seventh report of the Joint National Committee on Prevention, Detection, Evaluation, and Treatment of High Blood Pressure, *Hypertension* 42:1206–1252, 2003.

Chobanian AV, Bzkris GL, Black HR, et al: The seventh report of the Joint National Committee on Prevention, Detection, Evaluation, and Treatment of High Blood Pressure: the JNC 7 report, *JAMA* 289:2560–2571, 2003.

Dosh SA: The diagnosis of essential and secondary hypertension in adults, *J Fam Pract* 50:707–712, 2001.

Duley L, Henderson-Smart DJ, Meher S: Drugs for treatment of very high blood pressure during pregnancy. Cochrane Pregnancy and Childbirth Group, *Cochrane Database of Systematic Reviews* 3, 2006.

Gerstein H: Effects of ramipril on cardiovascular and microvascular outcomes in people with diabetes mellitus: results of the HOPE study and MICRO-HOPE substudy. Heart Outcomes Prevention Evaluation Study Investigators, *Lancet* 355:253–259, 2000.

Erbel R, Alfonso F, Boileau C, et al: Diagnosis and management of aortic dissection, *Eur Heart J* 22:1642–1681, 2001.

Flynn JT: Hypertension in adolescents, *Adolesc Med* 16:11–29, 2005.

Guller U, Turek J, Eubanks S, et al: Detecting pheochromocytoma: defining the most sensitive test, *Ann Surg* 243:102–107, 2006.

Hirsch AT, Haskal ZJ, Hertzer NR, et al: American Association for Vascular Surgery. ACC/AHA Task Force on Practice Guidelines, *Circulation* 113: e463–e654, 2006.

Kraiczi H, Hedner J, Peker Y, Grote L: Comparison of atenolol, amlodipine, enalapril, hydrochlorothiazide, and losartan for antihypertensive treatment in patients with obstructive sleep apnea, *Am J Respir Crit Care Med* 161:1423–1428, 2000.

Lip GY, Beevers M, Beevers DG: Does renal function improve after diagnosis of malignant phase hypertension? *J Hypertens* 15:1309–1315, 1997.

Nordmann AJ, Woo K, Parkes R, Logan AG: Balloon angioplasty or medical therapy for hypertensive patients with atherosclerotic renal artery stenosis? A meta-analysis of randomized controlled trials, *Am J Med* 114:44–50, 2003.

Onusko E: Diagnosing secondary hypertension, *Am Fam Physician* 67:67–74, 2003.

O'Rorke JE: What to do when blood pressure is difficult to control, *BMJ* 322:1229–1232, 2001.

Rey E, LeLorier J, Burgess E, et al: Report of the Canadian Hypertension Society Consensus Conference: 3. Pharmacologic treatment of hypertensive disorders in pregnancy, *CMAJ* 157:1245–1254, 1997.

Sawka SM, Young WF, Thompson GB, et al: Primary aldosteronism: factors associated with normalization of blood pressure after surgery, *Ann Intern Med* 135:258, 2001.

Tisdale JE, Huang MB, Borzak S: Risk factors for hypertensive crisis: importance of out-patient blood pressure control, *Fam Pract* 21:420–424, 2004.

Tumlin JA, Dunbar LM, Oparil S, et al: Fenoldopam, a dopamine agonist, for hypertensive emergency: a multicenter randomized trial, *Acad Emerg Med* 7:653–662, 2000.

Vora CK, Mansoor GA: Herbs and alternative therapies: relevance to hypertension and cardiovascular diseases, *Curr Hypertens Rep* 7:275–280, 2005.

Wilson SL, Poulter NR: The effect of non-steroidal anti-inflammatory drugs and other commonly used non-narcotic analgesics on blood pressure level in adults, *J Hypertens* 24:1457–1469, 2006.

Zampaglione B, Pascale C, Marchisio M, Cavallo-Perin P: Hypertensive urgencies and emergencies: prevalence and clinical presentation, *Hypertension* 27:144–147, 1996.

CHAPTER 28

Jaundice
Catherine McCarthy and Marcia M. Lu

Jaundice (icterus) is a yellowing of the skin, sclerae, and mucous membranes resulting from elevated circulating bilirubin from the breakdown of hemoglobin. Mild elevation in the serum bilirubin (2 to 2.5 mg/dL) is first noted as mild jaundice when the sclerae are viewed in natural light. Yellow skin coloring also occurs with elevated serum carotene, but the sclerae will be anicteric.

Hyperbilirubinemia can be divided into unconjugated (indirect) and conjugated (direct) types. The unconjugated type occurs from overproduction of bilirubin or defects in liver uptake or conjugation (hemolysis, ineffective erythropoiesis, or Gilbert syndrome). The conjugated type occurs from intra- or extrahepatic cholestasis, resulting in decreased excretion of conjugated bilirubin. An unconjugated hyperbilirubinemia occurs when the indirect fraction is 85% of the total. A conjugated hyperbilirubinemia occurs when the direct fraction is more than 30% of the total measured bilirubin.

Because jaundice is a symptom and not a specific disorder, it is important to identify its etiology, and then to identify any treatment that may be indicated. It is always important to obtain a complete history, and with the workup of jaundice this may provide important clues to the etiology.

GALLBLADDER DISEASE OR OBSTRUCTIVE JAUNDICE

Gallstones are the most common cause of blocked bile ducts and cancer is a much less common cause, but together these are the most common extrahepatic etiologies of jaundice. Stones typically form in the gallbladder (cholelithiasis) and can block the common bile duct (choledocholithiasis). Obstruction of the biliary system causes cholestasis or "obstructive jaundice" and may lead to cholecystitis, or inflammation of the gallbladder.

Symptoms
- Abdominal pain
- Jaundice
- Loss of appetite (anorexia)
- Weight loss
- Pruritus
- Dark urine

- Pale stools
- Vomiting
- Fever

Signs
- Xanthelasmas
- Murphy's sign—Pain with palpation of right upper quadrant on exhalation in the setting of cholecystitis

Workup
- Alkaline phosphatase and gamma-glutamyl transpeptidase (GGT)—Both increase disproportionately with cholestasis
- LFTs—May be markedly elevated with a common duct stone
- Ultrasound—Good screening tool for biliary tree dilation and gallstone identification; may also detect parenchymal disease
- CT—Best for evaluation of parenchymal liver disease; also good for evaluating the pancreas; can evaluate for biliary tree dilation
- ERCP—Dye is instilled into the biliary tree and is most useful after initial screening with ultrasound (US), CT, or MRI in the identification of biliary abnormalities; good for evaluating intraductal stones; provides direct visualization of the biliary tree; useful for extra hepatic obstruction.
- MRI imaging of the biliary tree may detect stones or ductal lesions and is a noninvasive alternative to ERCP.
- Consider liver biopsy.

Comments and Treatment Considerations
There is a risk of nutritional deficiencies and fat malabsorption. For diarrhea, a trial of a low-fat diet can be considered. Patients with steatorrhea may have a deficiency in the fat-soluble vitamins (A, D, E, K). Gallstones that are impacted require either endoscopic removal or cholecystectomy.

ERCP can be used to remove stones, perform papillotomy, or to place stents or drainage catheters to improve bile flow, for symptomatic choledocholithiasis. Percutaneous transhepatic biliary drainage can be tried if ERCP fails.

Cholecystectomy should be considered for symptomatic gallstone disease. Chemotherapy may be tried in the case of biliary tract tumors. Pruritus may be treated with cholestyramine, a bile acid sequestrant resin, at a dose of 4 g mixed with water before meals.

Monitor for osteoporosis in patients with cholestatic liver disease, supplement calcium, and vitamin D and screen with bone densitometry.

GILBERT SYNDROME

Gilbert syndrome is a common, hereditary, mild disorder of the liver. In this syndrome the liver improperly processes bilirubin produced from the breakdown of RBCs. There is decreased activity of the enzyme UDP glucuronosyltransferase, which causes an increase in the indirect fraction of serum bilirubin.

Approximately 3% to 10% of the U.S. population have Gilbert syndrome, with men affected more than women (2 to 7:1). Most often people discover that they have Gilbert syndrome when routine blood testing reveals elevated unconjugated hyperbilirubinemia with other liver function values unaffected.

Jaundice or increased bilirubin levels may occur or become more pronounced during periods of stress or illness. The condition is benign and typically does not require any treatment. There is no indication for liver biopsy.

Symptoms
• May have mild jaundice, especially of sclera

Signs
• Elevated indirect bilirubin ++++

Workup
• LFTs normal ++++
• No signs of hemolysis ++++
• No biopsy indicated ++++
• Important to rule out other causes of elevated serum bilirubin

Comments and Treatment Considerations
It is normally a benign condition with excellent prognosis, and usually no treatment is indicated. Jaundice or bilirubin level may increase with illness or stress (transient).

HEMOLYSIS

RBCs typically have a life span of 120 days. When they are destroyed prematurely it is called hemolysis. The bone marrow typically reacts by increasing the production of red cells to prevent the development of anemia. If the production cannot keep up with the rate of destruction, anemia develops. The symptoms of hemolytic anemia vary according to the speed at which the anemia develops. If the anemia is mild or develops slowly, the patient may remain asymptomatic. If the process is more moderate the patient may complain of dyspnea with exertion. The possible etiologies include spherocytosis, G6PD deficiency, sickle cell disease, microangiopathic hemolytic anemia, autoimmune disorders, and drugs.

Symptoms
• Jaundice—Usually mild
• Fatigue
• Weakness
• Dizziness
• Diaphoresis
• Dyspnea
• Chest pain
• Leg cramps with exercise
• Abdominal fullness or discomfort

Signs
- Jaundice
- Pallor
- Tachycardia
- Tachypnea
- Hypotension
- Splenomegaly

Workup
- Bilirubin level—Usually only mildly elevated (3 to 5 mg/dL); may be within normal range if mild
- LDH elevated with hemolysis
- CBC—Evaluate for schistocytes (fractured RBCs) and reticulocyte count; CBC usually increased; indicates increased erythropoiesis
- Direct antiglobulin test (DAT; direct Coombs' test) to detect the presence of IgG and complement (C3) on the RBCs; differentiates immune from nonimmune hemolysis
- LFTs and alkaline phosphatase usually within normal limits
- Haptoglobin levels are decreased as protein binds hemoglobin.
- Urinalysis—Elevated urobilinogen, even without hyperbilirubinemia

Comments and Treatment Considerations
For mild symptoms no treatment may be needed. Monitor hemoglobin and the potential for transfusion. For more advanced symptoms, a steroid such as prednisone is the treatment of choice. Doses are usually started high and then followed by a gradual taper over months.

For patients with an inadequate response to steroids, splenectomy may be an option. If symptoms continue after splenectomy, immunosuppressive therapy may be indicated with cyclophosphamide or azathioprine. Plasmapheresis is another option.

HEPATITIS

Hepatitis is an inflammation of the liver with hepatocellular necrosis that results most commonly from viral infection, alcoholism, toxins, or autoimmune disorders. Inflammation within the liver is the most common intrahepatic cause of jaundice. The manifestations vary depending on whether the clinical scenario is acute or chronic. When considering the potential etiologies, it is important to assess the risk factors (foreign travel, alcoholism, history of IV drug use, blood transfusions before 1992, high-risk sexual behavior, hemodialysis, raw seafood ingestion, tattoos or body piercing, needle punctures, or close contact with infected individual). Both viral- and toxin-induced hepatitis may lead to fulminant hepatic failure, chronic liver disease or end-stage liver disease (ESLD). In the United States more than 50% of ESLD results from alcoholism.

Symptoms
- Jaundice ++++
- Abdominal pain +++
- Nausea +++

- Emesis (nausea and vomiting preceding jaundice may indicate hepatitis or common bile duct obstruction)
- Anorexia (loss of appetite)
- Fever
- Fatigue
- Malaise
- Diarrhea
- Headache
- Dark urine ++++
- Joint pain
- Depression
- Altered taste
- Pruritus ++++

Signs
- Jaundice +++++
- Spider angiomas*
- Bruising
- Gynecomastia*
- Palmar erythema*
- Ascites*
- Testicular atrophy*
- Caput medusae*
- Hepatomegaly
- Splenomegaly
- Tenderness of liver to palpation

Workup
- Bilirubin (direct and indirect)—To determine conjugated or unconjugated, direct fraction of 30% or higher consistent with viral hepatitis, persistent elevation of total bilirubin greater than 20 mg/dL indicates poor prognosis
- Serum transaminase levels (LFTs): aspartate transaminase (AST) or serum glutamic-oxalo-acetic transaminase (SGOT), alanine transaminase (ALT) or serum glutamate pyruvate transaminase (SGPT), GGT—markers of hepatocellular injury, elevations suggestive of hepatitis (less helpful in chronic disease, because may be normal or mildly elevated), acute viral hepatitis causes LFTs to rise from several hundred to several thousand units per liter, with the AST:ALT ratio less than 1; in alcohol-induced hepatitis the AST greater than ALT, often a 2:1 ratio
- Serum alkaline phosphatase: If elevated more than threefold, consider cholestasis rather than hepatocellular process
- Hepatitis A IgM, hepatitis B surface antigen and core antibody, hepatitis C antibody
- Low albumin with high globulin level indicates chronic rather than acute liver disease.
- Prothrombin time (PT) or partial thromboplastin time (PTT) may be elevated in chronic hepatitis; prolonged PT indicates poor prognosis.

---

*Signs of portal hypertension or endocrine findings usually indicate chronic process.

- CBC may have a lymphocytosis with viral hepatitis; anemia may indicate GI bleeding or hemolysis
- Urinalysis—If positive for bilirubin, indicates conjugated bilirubinemia (water soluble)
- Viral hepatitis panel—Serologies including hepatitis A IgM, hepatitis B surface antigen and core antibody, and hepatitis C ribonucleic acid (RNA)
- Toxicology screen—Acetaminophen level
- Ceruplasmin (consider in patient <40 years of age)
- US—Good first test; inexpensive, quick and easy; no radiation; safe in pregnancy
- CT—Good for identifying infiltrative process (i.e., metastatic disease, but less helpful for evaluating hepatocellular disorders [too nonspecific])
- Liver biopsy—For evaluating liver architecture and determining prognosis; may also aid in diagnosis
- Differential diagnosis—Alcohol-induced hepatitis, toxin-induced hepatitis, mononucleosis, cholecystitis, ascending cholangitis, lymphoma, sarcoidosis, metastatic liver disease, pancreatic or biliary tumors

Comments and Treatment Considerations

Patients with any of the following symptoms should be considered for admission to the hospital: age more than 45, encephalopathy, vomiting, hypoglycemia, immunosuppression, volume depletion, electrolyte abnormalities, and coagulopathy. Treatment is generally supportive with IV fluids, correction of hypoglycemia, electrolyte abnormalities, and coagulopathies. Patients should abstain from alcohol and potentially hepatotoxic medications, and vaccinations should be updated.

Hepatitis A—Fecal-oral transmission. There is no treatment. Avoid alcohol because it can worsen liver disease. Hepatitis A vaccine is recommended for all children older than 2 years and anyone at risk (travel, exposure, men who have sex with men, drug abusers, recipients of clotting factor replacement, immunocompromised, chronic liver disease). Practice handwashing and careful food handling.

Hepatitis B—Generally acquired percutaneously via exposure to infected blood or body fluids. Often subclinical, but in symptomatic patients may be severe and protracted. Chronic HBV occurs in 6% to 10% and may cause cirrhosis, ESLD, and hepatocellular carcinoma (HCC). Antiviral treatment may be effective in up to 40% of patients with chronic infection. Regular medical surveillance is recommended, and liver transplant if indicated (availability issues). Avoid alcohol.

Hepatitis C—Most common of all blood infections in the United States may be contracted parenterally, sexually, or perinatally. Most patients are asymptomatic, but 85% become chronically infected. As much as 70% of chronic HCV progress to cirrhosis and ESLD, with an increased risk of HCC. Chronic infection may respond to interferon, pegylated interferon, or ribavirin. Combination therapy may eliminate the virus in 50% of patients with genotype 1. Vaccinate against hepatitis A or B, and avoid alcohol.

NEONATAL JAUNDICE

Neonatal jaundice is the most commonly encountered medical condition during the care of term, healthy newborns. Fortunately, neonatal unconjugated hyperbilirubinemia is most commonly a transitional physiologic condition that resolves without the need for medical treatment. Physiologic jaundice is caused by a combination of factors including increased turnover of fetal erythrocytes (due to higher erythrocyte mass and shortened life span of fetal erythrocytes), and decreased hepatic excretory capability due to low levels of ligandin in hepatocytes and low activity of bilirubin-conjugating enzyme glucuronyltransferase. In physiologic jaundice, total serum bilirubin levels peak at a level of 5 to 6 mg/dL on the third to fourth day of life and then declines over the first week after birth.

Pathologic jaundice should be suspected when jaundice occurs within the first 24 hours of life, with rapidly rising levels of total serum bilirubin concentration (more than 5 mg/dL increase per day), with total serum bilirubin levels higher than 17 in a full-term newborn, and with direct-reacting conjugated hyperbilirubinemia or jaundice that persists beyond 3 weeks of life. Causes of pathologic jaundice can be classified in the following manner:

 UNCONJUGATED HYPERBILIRUBINEMIA

- Increased bilirubin load
  - Hemolytic causes
    - G6PD deficiency
    - Rh factor incompatibility
    - ABO incompatibility
    - Spherocytosis
  - Nonhemolytic causes
    - Cephalhematoma
    - Bruising
    - CNS hemorrhage
    - Polycythemia
    - Twin-twin transfusion
- Decreased bilirubin conjugation and clearance
  - Crigler-Najjar syndrome, types 1 and 2
  - Gilbert syndrome
  - Hypothyroidism
  - Breast milk jaundice

 CONJUGATED HYPERBILIRUBINEMIA

- Biliary obstruction or cholestasis
  - Biliary atresia
  - Choledochal cyst

- Hepatocellular injury
  - Intravenous hyperalimentation
  - Viral infection (cytomegalovirus, hepatitis B)
  - Septicemia
  - α-1 Antitrypsin deficiency
  - Dubin-Johnson syndrome
  - Rotor syndrome

In very rare instances elevated bilirubin levels may lead to acute bilirubin encephalopathy or kernicterus. This condition occurs when neurotoxic unconjugated bilirubin is deposited into brain tissue. Bilirubin is bound to albumin during transport in the plasma.

When unconjugated bilirubin levels exceed the binding capacity of albumin, unbound bilirubin can more readily cross the intact blood-brain barrier. Albumin binding of bilirubin is also impaired in ill infants. There are several phases of bilirubin encephalopathy including intermediate, advanced, and chronic phases. Once it has progressed to the advanced phase, irreversible CNS damage has likely occurred.

Symptoms
- Jaundice or yellow discoloration of the skin ++++
- Yellow staining of the sclera +++++
- Poor feeding, lethargy, high-pitched cry, and decreased tone may be seen with acute bilirubin encephalopathy or kernicterus.
- Pathologic causes may present with specific symptoms such as lethargy and fever in a septic newborn, or decreased voiding and stooling with significant dehydration.

Signs
- Jaundice starts on the face and progresses in a cephalocaudal direction. ++++
- Icteric sclera +++++
- Excessive weight loss may occur with inadequate feeding and dehydration.
- Kernicterus or acute bilirubin encephalopathy can present with the following signs:
  - Early phase—Lethargy, poor suck, hypotonia
  - Intermediate phase—Moderate stupor, irritability, hypertonia, fever, high-pitched cry, retrocollis (backward arching of the neck), opisthotonos (backward arching of the trunk)
  - Advanced phase—Pronounced retrocollis-opisthotonos, shrill cry, no feeding, apnea, fever, deep stupor or coma, seizures, death
  - Chronic form—Athetoid cerebral palsy, auditory dysfunction, dental-enamel dysplasia, paralysis of upward gaze, mild intellectual deficit
  - Other signs are largely dependent on the cause. Observe for signs of possible causes of pathologic jaundice such as pallor, hepatosplenomegaly, dehydration, cephalhematoma, lethargy.

Workup

- Noninvasive transcutaneous bilirubinometry (TcB) can be used in mild jaundice to ensure that levels are safely below those requiring intervention. TcB is accurate to within 2 to 3 mg/dL of the total serum bilirubin (TSB) particularly for TSB levels less than 15 mg/dL. TcB cannot be used to monitor infants undergoing phototherapy because phototherapy "bleaches" the skin.
- Capillary total serum bilirubin and direct bilirubin levels should be ordered if TcB levels are elevated. A conjugated hyperbilirubinemia is present if the direct bilirubin level is more than 20% of the TSB. Always interpret TcB/TSB levels based on the infant's age in hours.
- Blood type (ABO, Rh)
- Direct antibody test (Coombs')
- Serum albumin
- CBC with differential
- If history or presentation suggests hemolysis, order reticulocyte count and smear for RBC morphology.
- If history or presentation suggests sepsis, perform septic workup.
- Other tests may be warranted based on history and presentation including urine for reducing substances (for galactosemia), LFTs and ultrasound (for cholestasis), thyroid function tests (for hypothyroidism), TORCH titers (for congenital infections).

Comments and Treatment Considerations

Intensive phototherapy should be initiated based upon the TSB level interpreted according to the infant's age in hours. Intensive phototherapy should be used when the TSB exceeds the line indicated for each category. Phototherapy causes a rapid configurational isomerization that changes the bilirubin isomer to a water-soluble isomer and does not allow it to cross the blood-brain barrier.

Phototherapy is most effective when more of the infant's body surface area is exposed to the phototherapy unit. Adverse effects may include insensible water loss (not as relevant as previously thought), risk of retinopathy (routine eye patches help prevent this), and decreased parental bonding time. Monitor TSB levels every 6 to 12 hours in moderate jaundice. Phototherapy is discontinued once the TSB level is less than 13 to 14 mg/dL. A follow-up TSB level measured 6 to 24 hours after discontinuation of phototherapy may be ordered to assess for rebound.

Poor response to phototherapy strongly suggests the presence of hemolysis. Exchange transfusion should be considered in infants when TSB levels rise 5 mg/dL or more above the lines (guidelines for exchange transfusion) or if the TSB rises to these levels despite intensive phototherapy. It should also be considered if there are clinical signs of acute bilirubin encephalopathy.

Bilirubin/albumin ratios can be used in conjunction with TSB levels in determining whether to perform an exchange transfusion. Exchange transfusion should only be performed by experienced personnel in a neonatal intensive care unit with full monitoring and resuscitation capabilities. Significant morbidity (apnea, bradycardia, cyanosis, vasospasm, thrombosis, necrotizing enterocolitis) occurs in as many as 5% of exchange transfusions. Risks associated with use of blood products must also be considered.

IVIg (0.5 to 1 g/kg over 2 hours) can be administered in isoimmune hemolytic disease if intensive phototherapy is ineffective and the TSB is approaching 2 to 3 mg/dL of the exchange level. The dose can be repeated in 12 hours. IVIg has been shown to reduce the need for exchange transfusion in Rh and ABO hemolytic disease.

Hydration with IV fluid is only indicated when there is clinical evidence of dehydration. No evidence exists to show that excessive hydration affects TSB level. The best approach is to have infant breastfeed or bottle-feed (formula or expressed breast milk) every 2 to 3 hours.

Treat any underlying pathologic cause of jaundice as indicated. Empiric antibiotic therapy should be initiated once neonatal sepsis is suspected. Home phototherapy should only be used when an infant's TSB level is in an "optional" range. It is not appropriate for infants in whom serial TSB levels should be followed more regularly. Sunlight exposure should no longer be recommended because it is unsafe to expose an unclothed infant to the sun and risk sunburn or overheating.

References

AAP Clinical Practice Parameter Subcommittee on Hyperbilirubinemia: Management of hyperbilirubinemia in the newborn infant 35 or more weeks gestation, *Pediatrics* 114:297–316, 2004.

Behrman RE, Kliegman RM, Jenson HB, editors: *Nelson textbook of pediatrics*, 16th ed, Philadelphia, 2000, Saunders, pp. 511–528.

Bergasa NV: Medical palliation of the jaundiced patient with pruritus, *Gastroenterol Clin North Am* 35:113–123, 2006.

Brundage SC, Fitzpatrick AN: Hepatitis A, *Am Fam Physician* 73:12, 2006.

Crump WJ: New guidelines for managing neonatal jaundice: a case-based report, *Fam Pract Recent* 27:40–46, 2005.

Dennery PA, Seidman DS, Stevenson DK: Neonatal hyperbilirubinemia, *N Eng J Med* 344:581–590, 2001.

Hansen TWR: *Neonatal jaundice.* Available at www.emedicine.com/PED/topic 1061htm (accessed June 8, 2006).

Jensen DM: Cholestasis, *Clin Liver Dis* 8:41–54, 2004.

Maisels MJ: The contribution of hemolysis to early jaundice in normal newborns, *Pediatrics* 118:276–279, 2006.

Naithani R: Autoimmune hemolytic anemia in India, *Hematology* 11:73–76, 2006.

Roche SP, Kobos R: Jaundice in the adult patient, *Am Fam Physician* 69:2, 2004.

Rogoveanu I: The role of imaging methods in the identification of jaundice, *J Gastrointest Liver Dis* 15:265–271, 2006.

Ruiz-Arguelles GJ: Gilbert's syndrome disclosed during the treatment of hematological malignancies, *Hematology* 10:59–60, 2005.

CHAPTER 29

Lower Extremity Pain and Swelling
Tina M. Flores

The patient presenting with lower extremity pain and swelling in the clinical setting can pose a diagnostic challenge because the differential diagnosis is extensive. Causes of lower extremity swelling could be related to musculoskeletal, vascular, or systemic diseases. This broad differential can be narrowed down by first taking a history, which may help elucidate an etiology such as a prior injury, severe sprain, or a chronic illness such as liver or renal disease.

The next step is to determine whether the extremity swelling is acute or chronic (Table 29-1). Patients with acute swelling should be evaluated for conditions that have the potential to be limb or life threatening.

ACUTE

 COMPARTMENT SYNDROME

Compartment syndrome (CS) is a painful limb- and life-threatening condition that results when perfusion pressure falls below tissue pressure in a closed anatomic space (e.g., muscle groups in the hands, arms, feet, legs, and buttocks). Acute CS is a medical emergency that requires a fasciotomy to lower the pressure within the compartment of the affected muscle group. Left untreated, acute CS leads to tissue necrosis, permanent functional impairment, infection, myoglobinuria, renal failure, and death.

Compartment syndrome can be either acute or chronic. Acute CS can be triggered by a traumatic injury, such as a contusion. Tibial fractures account for the cause of nearly 45% of CS. Acute CS usually requires a surgical intervention to preserve the muscle. Chronic CS, on the other hand, is characterized by pain and swelling caused by activity. Chronic CS improves with rest.

Many things can cause CS. Causes include intensive muscle use, snakebite, surgery, fractures, burns, intra-articular injections, infiltrated infusion, hemorrhage (especially in patients being treated with anticoagulants), and casts.

Symptoms
- Unilateral extremity swelling +++
- Always suspect CS when a patient complains of severe pain in an extremity.

Table 29-1. Differential Diagnosis of Lower Extremity Swelling

ACUTE SWELLING	CHRONIC SWELLING
Baker's cyst	Congenital vascular abnormality
Cellulitis	Congestive heart failure
Compartment syndrome	Hypoproteinemia
Deep vein thrombosis/superficial thrombophlebitis	Lymphedema
	Venous stasis
Ruptured gastrocnemius muscle	
Sprain or fracture	

- Tightness or burning sensation in an extremity following an injury
- Paresthesia

Signs
- Pain, severe and increasing and out of proportion to the apparent injury, especially when the muscle is stretched (passive or active)
- Increased intracompartmental pressure is the sole objective criterion for diagnosing CS. Physicians have used absolute values of intracompartmental pressure ranging between 30 and 45 mm Hg to indicate the need for a fasciotomy, but others have urged prophylactic fasciotomy with symptomatic patients who have normal pressures to prevent CS. Recently, the perfusion pressure (Δ P), the patient's diastolic blood pressure minus intracompartmental pressure of 30 to 40 mm Hg, has been suggested to be used for the threshold for fasciotomy.

Workup
- Closely observe and frequently examine the patient for muscle strength and sensory changes until swelling begins to subside. Sensory changes (e.g., loss of feeling, numbness) usually indicate the onset of decreased tissue perfusion.
- Use radiography of the affected extremity and ultrasonography to help eliminate other diagnoses.

Comments and Treatment Considerations
Pallor, poikilothermia, and pulselessness are *not* good tools for diagnosing CS, so they should not affect management.

If the affected area becomes numb or paralyzed, cell death has begun and efforts to lower the pressure in the compartment may not restore function.

Measuring intracompartmental pressure is a critical step in evaluating a patient who is suspected of having CS. However, intracompartmental pressure does *not* measure nerve and muscle ischemia because ischemia depends on the magnitude *and* duration of the elevated pressure.

A patient's comorbidities (e.g., shock and compensatory hypertension) may affect the outcome of CS. Acute compartment syndrome is a medical emergency. Immediately refer any patient with suspected CS to an orthopedic surgeon for a possible fasciotomy.

Administer supplemental oxygen to the patient to decrease tissue damage by increasing the partial pressure of oxygen in the injured muscle. Administer appropriate antivenom in cases of venomous snake bites: antivenom reverses hypoperfusion and increases oxygenation while controlling the direct toxic effect of the venom and the accompanying inflammatory response. Mannitol and hyperbaric oxygen therapy can also benefit patients with CS.

Do *not* elevate the injured extremity in cases of suspected CS because elevation decreases arterial perfusion and results in decreased oxygenation of tissue.

In the case when a patient has a cast in place and complains, in nearly all cases the cast should be "bivalved" to relieve constricting pressure.

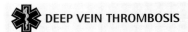 DEEP VEIN THROMBOSIS

DVT occurs most frequently in the lower extremities but can also occur in the inferior vena cava, the upper extremities, and the portal venous system. There are a number of risk factors for DVT (Table 29-2). Early diagnosis and management of DVT is important to avoid complications, particularly pulmonary embolism. The Wells Clinical Prediction Rules helps assess the likelihood that a patient has a DVT and guides decisions about further workup.

Table 29-2. Risk Factors for Deep Vein Thrombosis

- Recent surgery, especially orthopedic, neurosurgical, and vascular procedures
- Recent long travel
- Immobilization
- Malignancy
- Family history of thrombosis
- Acute decompensated illness (MI, acute CHF, stroke, sepsis)
- Oral contraceptive use (3 times the risk of nonusers)
- Hormone replacement therapy use (2 to 4 times the risk of nonusers)
- Pregnancy (2 times the risk of nonpregnant female)
- Postpartum (14 times the risk of average female)
- Trauma, particularly spinal cord injuries, burns, and fractures
- Coagulopathies
- Myeloproliferative disorders
- Medications: tamoxifen, chemotherapeutics, thalidomide
- Central venous catheters
- Vena cava filters
- Intravenous drug abuse
- Inflammatory bowel disease

CHF, Congestive heart failure; *MI,* myocardial infarction.

Symptoms
- No symptoms +++
- Unilateral extremity pain
- Unilateral extremity swelling
- Sometimes present with symptoms of pulmonary embolism

Signs
- Unilateral extremity edema
- Reddish purple, blanchable discoloration of affected extremity (phlegmasia cerulea dolens)
- Homans' sign (calf pain when foot is forcefully dorsiflexed with knee extended): present in about one third of patients with DVT and in about half of all patients without ++
- Prominence of superficial veins or superficial thrombophlebitis

Workup
- Wells Clinical Prediction Rules criteria (Box 29-1) +++++
- D-dimer—A negative D-dimer is useful as a "rule-out" DVT. False-positive D-dimers are seen in patients with cancer, extensive inflammation, trauma, recent surgery, or pregnancy. There are many different types of D-dimer assays; the ELISA tests are most reliable because they are more specific (have fewer false positives) +++++
- Doppler ultrasound—Safe, noninvasive, and reliable. A technician looks to see whether the veins can be compressed; first-line imaging test. Very accurate for proximal veins; less accurate for calf veins. May choose to repeat a negative test 1 week later to ensure no proximal spread from an undetected calf vein thrombus (serial ultrasonography). Difficult to perform on very obese patients or with profound edema. +++++
- MRI—Newest imaging modality currently being studied; may prove to be more accurate than ultrasound, but more expensive and less widely available
- Contrast venography—Gold standard with nearly 100% sensitivity and specificity. Expensive, invasive, and higher risk of complications, so not a first-line test. Not as accurate in patients with history of prior thrombosis.

Comments and Treatment Considerations
Anticoagulation with warfarin (Coumadin) should typically last for 6 months. If there was a transient risk factor likely responsible for the DVT (e.g., long travel), it may be reasonable to stop anticoagulation after 3 months in most patients older than 50, and in all more than 70 years old. Treat for longer duration, or even for lifetime, if patient has multiple risk factors for recurrence.

Initiate treatment using warfarin concurrently with either IV heparin or subcutaneous LMWH until a goal INR of 2 to 3 is reached.

Warfarin is contraindicated in pregnancy; LMWH is the preferred treatment.

Inferior vena cava filters are indicated to prevent PE in patients who have contraindications to anticoagulation or who have failed anticoagulation therapy, though they can increase risk of future DVT.

BOX 29-1   WELLS CLINICAL PREDICTION RULE FOR DEEP VEIN THROMBOSIS

Most reliable if combined with a negative D-dimer to rule out the possibility of deep vein thrombosis (DVT)
Add one point for each of the following that is applicable to the particular patient:

- Active cancer
- Paralysis or recent plaster immobilization of lower extremities
- Recently bedridden more than 3 days and/or major surgery within the past 4 weeks
- Localized tenderness along distribution of deep venous system
- Entire leg swelling
- Calf swelling more than 3 cm compared with asymptomatic leg
- Pitting edema greater than asymptomatic leg
- History of documented DVT
- Dilated collateral superficial veins (not varicose)

Subtract 2 points for any alternative diagnosis that is as likely or more likely than DVT.

Total score:
High probability: ≥3
Moderate probability: 1-2
Low probability: ≤0

Interpretation:
High probability: need imaging to rule out DVT regardless of D-dimer results; if imaging is negative, consider repeating ultrasound in 1 week to confirm negative results, particularly if D-dimer positive.
Moderate probability: if D-dimer is negative, can usually follow clinically; ultrasound might help establish an alternate diagnosis.
Low probability: no imaging necessary if D-dimer is negative; DVT essentially ruled out (<1% chance of DVT).

In order to prevent DVT in hospitalized patients, use compression stockings or automated cycling compression devices/intermittent pneumatic compression devices. Medications can include heparin 5000 units subcutaneously two or three times a day depending on risk or LMWH—enoxaparin (Lovenox) 40 mg subcutaneously daily (different dosing perioperatively). Aspirin alone is *not* effective prevention for DVT.

Workup for recurrent DVTs: more than one DVT in a patient is indicative of a possible coagulopathy. Workup should include investigation for inherited clotting disorders such as lupus anticoagulant, protein C or S deficiency, or factor V Leiden mutations.

Postthrombotic syndrome occurs in up to one third of patients after a first DVT. Symptoms include prolonged pain, swelling, and skin changes. Risk of developing postthrombotic syndrome can be lowered by wearing compression hose for 2 years after diagnosis.

CHRONIC SWELLING

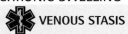 **VENOUS STASIS**

Venous stasis (also called venous insufficiency and venous edema) is characterized by chronic, lower extremity pitting edema, and is most often bilateral. Venous stasis is usually accompanied by skin induration, varicosities, fibrosis, and hyperpigmentation.

The incidence of venous stasis in the general population can be as high as 30%. The condition is caused by chronic venous valvular incompetence leading to peripheral venous hypertension, although the central venous pressure remains normal. About 50% of patients with venous stasis have a history of a leg injury. The most common cause of venous vascular incompetence is prior DVT, but only one third of patients with venous stasis will give a history of DVT. As the thrombosis heals, the normal venous valvular and wall structure are destroyed, leading to incompetence.

The signs and symptoms of venous stasis range from mild to severe and can be debilitating. Heat and prolonged sitting or standing may worsen the symptoms. Skin ulcers that usually develop over the medial malleoli are the most serious complication and can be very challenging to manage.

Symptoms
- Pain or dull aching ++
- Sensation of leg fullness
- Nocturnal leg cramps

Signs
- Lower extremity pitting edema (usually bilateral, but may be asymmetric and occasionally unilateral) +++++
- Varicosities
- Subcutaneous fibrosis
- Hyperpigmentation
- Cellulitis
- Skin ulcers (usually over the medial malleoli) +

Workup
- CBC (to rule out systemic infection or anemia)
- Urinalysis and a BMP (assess for renal disease)
- TSH (to rule out hypothyroidism)
- Albumin (low albumin may be a sign of liver disease, nephrotic syndrome, or protein-losing enteropathy)
- ECG, chest x-ray, CHF peptide and echocardiogram should be obtained only if a cardiac etiology for the edema is suspected by history and exam.
- If sudden, unilateral leg swelling, obtain lower-extremity Doppler studies to rule out DVT

Comments and Treatment Considerations

Venous stasis and its complications are difficult to treat, and patients usually require several treatment modalities to achieve satisfactory results. Leg elevation: simply elevating the legs above heart level for 30 minutes three or four times daily reduces edema and improves circulation.

Compression stockings: a variety of compression stockings are available, but knee-high stockings are usually sufficient for most patients. The stockings should exert at least 20 mm Hg at the ankle and less at the knee. Thigh-high stockings should be avoided because they limit venous return.

Aspirin at doses of 325 mg/day has been shown to improve ulcer healing and should be used unless contraindicated in the patient. Systemic antibiotics should only be used in cases of cellulitis or ulcer infection.

Horse chestnut seed extract has been shown to reduce leg volume and edema. Topical emollients and steroids should be used to treat stasis dermatitis. Diuretics should be avoided in patients with venous stasis because they can lead to hypoperfusion and volume depletion and generally do not relieve the edema.

Dressings, usually occlusive and with compression, should be used to cover venous stasis ulcers. Superficial venous surgery may improve symptoms and ulcer recurrence in patients with severe symptoms. Topical antibiotics, antiseptics, debriding enzymes, growth factors, and silver sulfadiazine have not been shown to be effective treatment options.

CONGESTIVE HEART FAILURE

See Chapter 16, Cough.

LYMPHEDEMA

Lymphedema is a chronic debilitating and often disfiguring condition. It is an uncommon cause of both unilateral and bilateral lower extremity swelling that results from an incompetent lymphatic system. Early in its course, this disease can be difficult to distinguish from venous stasis. It differs from venous stasis in that it is comprised of protein rich fluid in the subcutaneous tissue.

There are two types of lymphedema: primary (congenital) or secondary (acquired). Secondary lymphedema is more often observed than primary. Worldwide the most common cause of secondary lymphedema is related to the parasitic infection, filariasis. However, secondary lymphedema needs to be considered as a possible diagnosis of leg swelling in those patients with a history of pelvic malignancy, radiation therapy, or prior pelvic surgery.

Symptoms

- Unilateral or bilateral extremity swelling present for greater than 3 months
- No improvement in edema with elevation of the affected limb

- May cause aching of the affected extremity, but usually not acute pain
- Heavy sensation of the affected limb

Signs
- Nonpitting edema
- Positive Kaposi-Stemmer's sign (inability to pinch a fold of skin at the base of the second toe) ++++
- Thickening of the skin
- Warty or cobblestone appearance of the skin
- Enhanced skin creases at the toes or ankles
- Lymphorrhea (weeping of lymph fluid on to skin)
- No response to diuretics

Workup
- Evaluation to rule out more probable cause of edema (see workup for venous stasis)
- Obtain limb volume measurements of the affected and unaffected limb for comparison.
- Obtain CT or MRI only if concerned about possible pelvic malignancy
- Lymphoscintigraphy and evaluation of the lymph system may be beneficial in making the diagnosis in difficult cases. ++++

Comments and Treatment Considerations
Lymphedema is not curable and is notoriously difficult to treat. Treatment requires a lifelong commitment and often requires multiple modalities to control the symptoms; proper skin care, which may include emollients, steroid creams, or antifungal creams; and elevation of the affected limb. Lymphorrhea can promote bacterial growth on the skin. Prompt diagnosis and treatment of secondary bacterial and fungal infections are necessary to prevent further complications.

Compressive garments can be used after initial evaluation for arterial insufficiency. Manual lymphatic drainage, a form of massage, has proven to be a mainstay of treatment. Multilayer bandaging can help significantly decrease swelling. Pneumatic compression has also shown some benefit.

Regular exercise and weight management may help improve symptoms because obesity can contribute to lymphedema. Surgical intervention is rarely indicated.

References
Alguire PC, Mathes BM: Treatment of chronic venous insufficiency. In Rose BD, editor: *UpToDate*, Waltham, MA, 2006.
Cho S, Atwood JE: Peripheral edema, *Am J Med* 113:580–586, 2002.
de Araujo T, Valencia I, Federman DG, Kirsner RS: Managing the patient with venous ulcers, *Ann Intern Med* 138:326–334, 2003.
Ely JW, Osheroff JA, Chambliss ML, Ebell MH: Approach to leg edema of unclear etiology, *J Am Board Fam Med* 19:148–160, 2006.
Geerts WH, Pineo GF, Heit JA, et al: Prevention of venous thromboembolism, *Chest* 126:338S–400S, 2004.
Hardy D: Managing long-term conditions: non–cancer-related lymphoedema, *Br J Nurs* 15:444, 2006.

Kostler W, Strohm PC, Sudkamp NP: Acute compartment syndrome of the limb, *Injury* 35:1221–1227, 2004. Erratum in *Injury* 36:992–998, 2005.

Kyrle PA, Eichinger S: Deep vein thrombosis, *Lancet* 365:1163–1174, 2005.

Langer RD, Ho E, Deneberg JO, et al: Relationships between symptoms and venous disease: the San Diego population study, *Arch Intern Med* 165: 1420–1424, 2005.

Mithoefer K, Lhowe DW, Vrahas MS, et al: Functional outcome after acute compartment syndrome of the thigh, *J Bone Joint Surg Am* 88:729–737, 2006.

Mortimer P: Swollen lower limb-2: lymphoedema, *BMJ* 320:1527, 2000.

O'Brien JG, Chennubhotla SA, Chennubhotla RV: Treatment of edema, *Am Fam Physician* 71:2111–2118, 2005.

Ozkayin N, Aktuglu K: Absolute compartment pressure versus differential pressure for the diagnosis of compartment syndrome in tibial fractures, *Int Orthop* 29:396–401, 2005.

Paula R: Compartment syndrome, extremity (update June 22, 2006). Available at www.emedicine.com/emerg/topic739.htm.

Pittler MH, Ernst E: Horse chestnut seed extract for chronic venous insufficiency, *Cochrane Database Syst Rev* (1), 2006.

Stein PD, Hull RD, Patel KC: D-dimer for the exclusion of acute venous thrombosis and pulmonary embolism, *Ann Intern Med* 140:589–602, 2004.

Swain R, Ross D: Lower extremity compartment syndrome. When to suspect acute or chronic pressure buildup, *Postgrad Med* 105:159–162, 165, 168, 1999.

Tamariz LJ, Eng J, Segal JBP, et al: Usefulness of clinical prediction rules for the diagnosis of venous thromboembolism: a systematic review, *Am J Med* 117:676–684, 2004.

Tornetta P 3rd, Templeman D: Compartment syndrome associated with tibial fracture. Instructional course lectures, *J Bone Joint Surg Am* 78:1438–1444, 1996.

Wells PS, Owen C, Doucette S, et al: Does this patient have deep vein thrombosis? *JAMA* 295:199–207, 2006.

CHAPTER 30

Lymphadenopathy
David S. Gregory

Lymphadenopathy, or abnormal enlargement of lymph nodes, is a common presenting finding in several diseases, occurring in approximately 0.5% of the general population each year. Lymph nodes enlarge due to normal reaction to infection, abnormal inflammatory response, or neoplasia (Table 30-1). The differential diagnosis for lymphadenopathy is very broad and requires an initial thorough history and physical examination, followed by indicated testing.

Signs
- In children, palpable lymph nodes are common, even without evidence of disease.
- In healthy infants, lymph nodes greater than 0.3 cm in diameter are palpated in either cervical, axillary, or inguinal sites. ++++
- Healthy children 3 weeks to 6 years old may have palpable lymph nodes 0.5 cm or larger in cervical, occipital, submandibular, or postauricular sites (descending order of prevalence). ++++
- Patients older than 40 to 50 years are much more likely than those younger to have a neoplastic cause for lymphadenopathy.

Workup
- Detailed history and physical examination
  - Attention to constitutional, respiratory, dermatologic, and neurologic symptoms
  - Investigate medications, history of travel, HIV risk factors, or animal exposures.
  - Measure weight and height (in children plot against growth curves).
  - Note number, size, location, consistency, tenderness, and mobility of palpable nodes.
- Investigations to consider
  - Basic screening labs—CBC with differential, ESR, LDH, uric acid, and LFTs
  - Epstein-Barr virus (EBV), CMV, HIV and/or *Bartonella henselae* titers (if initial workup suggests)
  - Chest x-ray
  - PPD
  - US—To define suppurative lymphadenitis and select aspiration or biopsy
  - CT scan—To distinguish head and neck congenital cysts from lymphadenopathy

Table 30-1. Lymphadenopathy Differential Diagnosis and Lymph Node Acuity

	ACUTE LYMPHADENOPATHY (<3 WK)	CHRONIC LYMPHADENOPATHY (>6 WK)
Normal reaction to infection	Bacterial lymphadenitis • *Staphylococcus aureus* • Streptococcal • Peptostreptococci • Gram-negative rods • Tuberculosis • Atypical Mycobacterium • Tularemia Reactive lymphadenitis • Viral URIs • Group A streptococcal pharyngitis Mononucleosis • EBV • CMV Cat scratch disease	Viral • EBV • CMV • HIV Bacterial • Tularemia • *Yersinia* • Tuberculosis • Atypical Mycobacterium • Cat scratch disease Fungal • Histoplasmosis • Coccidioidomycosis Other • Toxoplasmosis
Abnormal response to inflammation	Kawasaki's disease (children) Serum sickness Vaccination reactions Drug hypersensitivities • Allopurinol • Aspirin • Anticonvulsants (phenytoin) • Antibiotics (sulfa, PCN)	Autoimmune disorders • Sarcoid • Systemic lupus erythematosus • Rheumatoid arthritis • Sjögren syndrome • Amyloidosis Vaccination reactions Drug hypersensitivities
Neoplasia	Acute leukemias	Lymphoma • Hodgkin's • Non-Hodgkin's Lymphoproliferative disorders Leukemia (acute or chronic) Solid tumor metastasis

CMV, Cytomegalovirus; *EBV,* Epstein-Barr virus; *HIV,* human immunodeficiency virus; *PCN,* penicillin; *URI,* upper respiratory infection.

- Needle aspiration—To evaluate fluid with Gram stain, acid-fast stain, and aerobic/anaerobic culture
- Lymph node biopsy—The definitive test to evaluate for neoplastic causes
  - Consider if lymphadenopathy is extensive (generalized or >2 cm in diameter) or associated with other concerning findings on history and physical examination (Table 30-2)

Table 30-2. Concerning ("Red Flag") Findings with Lymphadenopathy

SIGNS AND SYMPTOMS	ASSOCIATED DISORDER(S)
Splenomegaly	Mononucleosis Neoplasia (lymphoma, leukemia)
"B" symptoms Fever Night sweats Weight loss (>10% unexplained)	Tuberculosis HIV Neoplasia (lymphoma, leukemia, solid tumor metastasis)
Pruritus	Neoplasia (lymphoma, leukemia) Autoimmune disorders (SLE, RA)
Chest/hilar lymphadenopathy	Community-acquired pneumonia Tularemia Psittacosis Pertussis Tuberculosis Coccidioidomycosis Histoplasmosis Neoplasia (lymphoma, lung, breast, gastrointestinal)
Abdominal lymphadenopathy	Neoplasia (lymphoma, leukemia, gastric, or bladder) Tuberculosis

HIV, Human immunodeficiency virus; *RA,* rheumatoid arthritis; *SLE,* systemic lupus erythematosus.

- Available prediction rules for the need of biopsy require further validation.
- Nonspecific or nondiagnostic results are common; sometimes repeat biopsy is indicated.

Comments and Treatment Considerations

With only a few exceptions, a lymphadenopathy site does not predict etiology. Head and neck nodes are more frequently associated with localized infectious or inflammatory conditions than malignancy. Extremity nodes often occur in response to peripheral infections (i.e., cellulitis). Supraclavicular, mediastinal, or abdominal lymphadenopathy, however, should be considered neoplastic until proven otherwise.

Based on size alone, lymph node diameter does not reliably distinguish neoplastic or inflammatory causes from more common infectious causes, although lymph nodes less than 1 cm in size are rarely from neoplastic causes. A study of healthy infants found no lymph node enlarged more than 1.2 cm in diameter in neonates or 1.6 cm in older infants. In adults, large lymph nodes are less common but are more likely associated with malignancy. One study found that 8% of adults with unexplained enlarged lymph nodes between 1.0 and 2.25 cm in diameter were eventually found to have a neoplastic cause.

The acuity of lymph node enlargement may suggest certain diseases. Lymphadenopathy has been defined as acute if it lasts less than 3 weeks and chronic if lasting longer than 6 weeks. Acute lymphadenopathy is commonly caused by a normal reaction to localized infection (i.e., pharyngitis), generalized infection (i.e., EBV), or primary lymph node infection (i.e., bacterial lymphadenitis) (see Table 30-1). Chronic lymphadenopathy has a very broad differential diagnosis, sometimes resulting in lymph node biopsy to diagnose. Significant overlap in the duration of the various causes does not reliably distinguish a cause based solely on lymph node acuity. Still, when significant lymph node enlargement is found in its early stages, the more common infectious causes should be considered and if not resolved in an expected duration, chronic causes should also be considered.

CAT SCRATCH DISEASE

Symptoms
- Fever—Sometimes prolonged
- Painful lymph nodes draining from extremity of exposure to cat scratch or bite

Signs
- Lymphadenopathy
  - Starts about 1 to 2 weeks after cat exposure, lasts 2 to 3 weeks and shrinks over 1 to 2 months
- Hepatosplenomegaly in severe cases

Workup
- Antibodies to *B. henselae*
- Polymerase chain reaction (PCR) to *B. henselae*

Comments and Treatment Considerations
Usually a self-limited disease—Antibiotic treatment (e.g., rifampin, azithromycin, ciprofloxacin, and TMP-SMX) is not routinely advised unless hepatomegaly exists, nodes are exquisitely tender, or the patient is immunocompromised. Control fever and lymph node pain with antipyretics and analgesics. Exquisitely tender nodes may require needle aspiration or excision.

HUMAN IMMUNODEFICIENCY VIRUS

Symptoms
- "B symptoms"
  - Weight loss
  - Fever
  - Night sweats
- Opportunistic infections (e.g., mycobacterial, fungal)
- Recurrent infections

Signs
- Generalized lymphadenopathy
- Mediastinal or abdominal lymphadenopathy

Workup
- ELISA and Western blot antibody testing
- CD4 counts and HIV viral load assays
- Lymph node biopsy if dominant lymphadenopathy found
  - HIV infection increases risk of mycobacterial infections and lymphomas

Comments and Treatment Considerations
The goal of treatment is early and total suppression of viral replication with HAART using protease inhibitors (PIs), nucleoside and nucleotide reverse transcriptase inhibitors (NRTIs), nonnucleoside reverse transcriptase inhibitors (NNRTIs), and entry inhibitors (EIs).

CD4 counts and viral loads are followed periodically. Antimicrobial prophylaxis is no longer routinely used.

Patients with HIV often develop a nonspecific generalized lymphadenopathy that is chronic and asymptomatic. If lymphadenopathy progresses or "B symptoms" are present, evaluation for coexisting infections or neoplasia may be needed.

Evaluate and treat HIV patients in conjunction with specialist who is expert and up-to-date on HIV treatments.

LYMPHADENITIS/LYMPHANGITIS

Symptoms
- Rapid onset of painful isolated mass ++++
- Fever
- Associated infection in region of lymph drainage ++++
- With lymphangitis—Radiation of pain from site of infection to lymph node

Signs
- Isolated, tender, and enlarged lymph node +++++
  - Overlying erythema and warmth
- With lymphangitis—Red streaking from infection site toward lymph drainage

Workup
- Physical examination for site of originating infection
- US of mass if suppurative node suspected
- CT of neck if suppurative node confirmed on head or neck to distinguish from other head or neck masses
- Needle aspiration and analysis if suppurative node confirmed

Comments and Treatment Considerations
If symptoms and signs in children are consistent with lymphadenitis, treat with antibiotics because lymphadenitis is the most common

cause for these findings. Choose antibiotics covering a spectrum of the originating source of infection. An initial complete evaluation with further investigations is indicated in adults because other infectious, inflammatory, and neoplastic causes are more common than in children, even while treatment with antibiotics is underway. Lymphangitis may be caused by malignant cells obstructing lymphatic flow; close follow-up and investigation for metastatic neoplasia are suggested if treatment is not effective.

MONONUCLEOSIS

Symptoms
- Fatigue ++++
- Sore throat +++

Signs
- Anterior and posterior lymphadenopathy (one fourth lasting as long as 6 months)
- Pharyngitis
- Splenomegaly

Workup
- Heterophile antibody test (i.e., Monospot) in those older than 4 years
- EBV serology in those less than 4 years old
- Lymph node biopsy may be needed with significantly large or hard nodes; lymphoma can be associated with EBV infection

STREPTOCOCCAL PHARYNGITIS

See Chapter 40, Sore Throat.

References
Allhiser JN, McKnight TA, Shank JC: Lymphadenopathy in a family practice, *J Fam Pract* 12:27–32, 1981.

American Academy of Pediatrics: Cat scratch disease *(Bartonella henselae)*. In Pickering LK, editor: *2000 Red book: report of the committee on infectious disease*, 25th ed, Elk Grove Village, IL, 2000, American Academy of Pediatrics, p. 201.

American Academy of Pediatrics: Chronic lymphadenopathy. In Woodin KA, editor: *PREP 1997 Self-Assessment Exercise American Academy of Pediatrics* SA97:17, 1997.

Bamji M, Stone RK, Kaul A, et al: Palpable lymph nodes in healthy newborns and infants, *Pediatrics* 78:573, 1986.

Fijten GH, Blijham GH: Unexplained lymphadenopathy in family practice. An evaluation of the probability of malignant causes and the effectiveness of physicians' workup, *J Fam Pract* 27:373–376, 1988.

Glaser C, Lewis P, Wong S: Pet-, animal-, and vector-borne infections, *Pediatr Rev* 21:219, 2000.

Habermann TM, Steensma DP: Lymphadenopathy, *Mayo Clin Proc* 75:723–732, 2000.

Herzog LW: Prevalence of lymphadenopathy of the head and neck in infants and children, *Clin Pediatr* 22:485, 1983.

Knight PJ, Mulne AF, Vassy LE: When is lymph node biopsy indicated in children with enlarged peripheral nodes? *Pediatrics* 69:391, 1982.

Nield LS, Kamat D: Lymphadenopathy in children: when and how to evaluate, *Clin Pediatr* 43:25–33, 2004.

Pangalis GA, Vassilakopoulos TP, Boussiotis VA, Fessas P: Clinical approach to lymphadenopathy, *Semin Oncol* 20:570, 1993.

Slap GB, Brooks JSJ, Schwartz JS: When to perform biopsies of enlarged peripheral lymph nodes in young patients, *JAMA* 252:1321–1326, 1984.

Vassilakopoulos TP, Pangalis GA: Application of a prediction rule to select which patients presenting with lymphadenopathy should undergo a lymph node biopsy, *Medicine* 79:338–347, 2000.

CHAPTER 31

Menopause
Debra A. Ahern

The World Health Organization, as well as the Stages of Reproductive Aging Workshop (STRAW), define menopause as the permanent cessation of menstrual periods that occurs naturally or is induced by surgery, chemotherapy, or radiation. Natural menopause is recognized only after 12 months of amenorrhea that is not associated with either a pathologic (e.g., Sheehan syndrome) or physiologic cause (e.g., lactation). Most women achieve natural menopause between the ages of 47 and 55. Perimenopause, a time of hormonal fluctuations, with or without menstrual irregularities, may precede the final menses by 2 to 8 years.

Menopause is a gradual, physiologic process that occurs as part of natural aging and frequently does not require medical intervention. Many women make the transition from regular menses to menopause with little difficulty and few symptoms. For others symptoms such as hot flashes, vaginal dryness, and dyspareunia significantly affect their quality of life. As life expectancy increases, women may spend greater than one third of their life in the postmenopausal years. Issues associated with aging and health maintenance, such as osteoporosis prevention and cardiovascular risk reduction, are addressed elsewhere.

Symptoms
- Hot flashes—Sudden intense sensation of heat, usually starting with the scalp, face, neck, or chest and lasting 2 to 10 minutes +++
- Nocturnal hyperhydrosis—Awakening to damp clothing, sheets, hair +++
- Diaphoresis ++
- Chills

Workup
- History: personal
  - Age at menarche
  - Length of cycle
  - Duration and quantity of flow
  - First day of last menses
  - Menstrual irregularities
  - Obstetric history
  - Surgical history
  - Thromboembolic disorders
  - Cardiovascular disease, HTN, diabetes, dyslipidemia

- Mood disorders—Depression or anxiety, postpartum depression, premenstrual syndrome
- Cancer
- Medications—Prescription, nonprescription, and herbal
- History: family
  - Age of menopause of first-degree relatives
  - Cancer—Breast, uterus, ovarian
  - Osteoporosis
  - Cardiovascular disease
- History: social
  - Tobacco, alcohol, recreational drugs
  - Marital status
  - Children—Empty nest
  - Aging parents
  - Employment or financial
- Physical examination
  - Pelvic and breast examination
  - Vital signs, including height and weight
  - Examination of other systems as directed by history

Comments and Treatment Considerations

Laboratory tests are seldom helpful due to cyclic hormonal fluctuations as well as variations from person to person. Neither the American Academy of Family Practice, the American College of Physicians, or the American College of Obstetricians and Gynecologist (ACOG) make recommendations regarding the diagnosis of menopause. The North American Menopause Society states that FSH and estradiol levels are of limited value in confirming perimenopause but *consistently* elevated FSH levels greater than 30 are indicative of menopause. The American Association of Clinical Endocrinologists recommends measurements of FSH and states that levels greater than 40 are diagnostic of menopause but caution that during perimenopause, levels may be intermittently elevated.

Consider urinary chorionic gonadotropin (UCG), FSH, LH, prolactin, CBC, TSH, and PPD as directed by your history and examination. Inhibin levels and vaginal ultrasounds to measure ovarian volumes and number of antral follicles lack the sensitivity and specificity of less invasive and less costly measures. Other studies may include Papanicolaou (Pap), mammography, DEXA, coagulation studies, lipid profile, glucose, and urodynamic assessments, as indicated by history and examination.

Lifestyle modifications are necessary. Avoid triggers including warm air and hot, spicy food and beverages. Dress in layers and remove to cool off as necessary. Focus on paced respirations (slow deep, diaphragmatic breathing at a rate of 6 to 10 respirations per minute). Exercise-active women report fewer hot flashes; make a daily exercise regimen part of your routine. Quit smoking; smokers experience more hot flashes than nonsmokers.

When lifestyle modifications are not enough, consider supplementing with the following:

- Estrogen (with progesterone as needed): start with low dose
  - 0.3 mg conjugated equine estrogen
  - 0.5 mg micronized estradiol
  - 25 µg transdermal estradiol
  - 2.5 µg ethynyl estradiol
  - Low-dose birth control pills (nonsmokers only)
  - 50 to 100 µg estradiol vaginal ring (Femring)
- Progesterone alone (not FDA approved for this indication)
  - 400 mg medroxyprogesterone acetate (Depo-Provera)
  - 20 to 80 mg/day micronized megestrol acetate (Megace)
- Other
  - 37.5 to 150 mg venlafaxine (Effexor) (FDA approved)
  - Fluoxetine (Prozac) (FDA approved)
  - 12.5 to 25 mg paroxetine (Paxil)
  - 300 to 900 mg gabapentin (Neurontin)
  - 0.1 to 0.3 mg/day transdermal patch clonidine
- Herbal—Supported by randomized controlled studies
  - Black cohosh (8 mg/day). Caution with breast cancer patients—ACOG states that black cohosh may be helpful in the short term.
- Conflicting studies
  - Soy—Patients should be advised to consider the caloric intake of soy supplements
- Not supported by randomized controlled studies
  - Dong quai
  - Evening primrose oil
  - Red clover
  - Ginseng
  - Wild yam
  - Ginkgo biloba
  - Valerian root
  - Flaxseed

The exact etiology of hot flashes is unknown. Although estrogen has been shown to be the most effective treatment for hot flashes, research has failed to demonstrate a difference in estrogen levels between those who suffer from hot flashes and those who do not. Left untreated, the majority of hot flashes stop spontaneously within 5 to 6 years, but in up to 10% of women they may last well into the eighth decade. In women with an intact uterus, estrogen should always be given with progestin to prevent endometrial hyperplasia. Changing the route of estrogen from oral to transdermal may help ameliorate intractable hot flashes by bypassing the liver. Estrogen should always be prescribed for the shortest time possible at the lowest effective dose and serious consideration should be given to stopping it within 5 years. Data from the Women's Health Initiative did show an increase in the rate of breast cancer when both estrogen and progesterone were used (38 versus 30 per 10,000 person-years) but not with unopposed estrogen. The Nurses' Health Study found a 30% higher rate of breast cancer in women taking estrogen alone for 10 years. Low-dose estrogen regimens (e.g., 0.3 mg of conjugated equine estrogen) have not been adequately studied. Other risks of hormonal therapy include an increase in strokes, venous thromboembolism, coronary events, and worsening of lipid profiles. For nonsmokers requiring birth control, low dose OCPs may be considered. Periodically, patients may be withdrawn from the pills and an FSH level drawn 1 to 2 weeks later. A low level indicates that a patient is not yet menopausal, but a high level does not confirm menopause. Patients should be advised to use alternative forms of birth control until 12 months after the last menses.

Contraindications to hormone replacement therapy include vaginal bleeding of unknown etiology, active liver disease, coronary heart disease, history of endometrial cancer, history of thromboembolic disease, and history of breast cancer (controversial). Relative contraindications include migraine headaches, triglycerides in excess of 400, active gallbladder disease, fibroids, atypical ductal hyperplasia of the breast, and more than one first-degree relative with breast cancer.

MENSTRUAL IRREGULARITIES/ POSTMENOPAUSAL BLEEDING

The hallmark of the perimenopausal years is the unpredictability of the intermenstrual cycle length and the variability of the volume and pattern of flow. Few studies are available that have addressed this issue. Bleeding that occurs in women not on hormone replacement therapy after 1 year past the final menses requires evaluation. Although most postmenopausal bleeding is due to benign processes (e.g., vaginal or endometrial atrophy, submucosal fibroids, polyps or endometrial hyperplasia), endometrial carcinoma is found approximately 10% of the time.

Symptoms
- Missed menses
- Frequent menses
- Changes in length of flow and/or quantity of flow
- Menorrhagia
- Postmenopausal bleeding ++

Signs
- Pallor
- Irregular uterine contour
- Enlarged or atrophied uterus
- Atrophic vaginal mucosa

Workup
- History
  - LMP
  - Length and quantity of flow
  - Precipitating factors—Trauma, postcoital
  - Associated symptoms—Pain, fever, vaginal discharge, urinary symptoms, rectal bleeding, vasomotor symptoms

- Age at menarche
- Obstetric history
- Cycle length and regularity
- Presence of vasomotor symptoms
- Medications—Prescribed (OCPs, HRT, warfarin, psychotropics), OTC (ASA, NSAIDs), herbal
- Coagulopathies
- Smoking, alcohol, recreational drugs
- Medical history with emphasis on hepatic, renal, and thyroid disorders
- Physical examination
  - Vital signs
    - Pelvic examination—Assess size, contour, and tenderness of uterus, and note any suspicious lesions, lacerations, or foreign bodies. Assess the mucosa for atrophy and determine the origin of bleeding (rectal, urethral, genital).
    - Cardiovascular
    - Skin examination with emphasis on ecchymosis and petechia
    - Examination of nailbeds, conjunctiva for pallor
- Lab tests
  - Pap should be done in all women with unexplained bleeding with colposcopy and biopsy of any suspicious lesions
  - CBC with differential
  - Reticulocyte count
  - Iron studies
  - Coagulation studies
  - TSH
- Transvaginal ultrasound—Often the initial test in women with unexplained postmenopausal bleeding, an endometrial stripe of more than 5 mm has a 96% sensitivity and 61% specificity for the detection of cancer. Endometrial biopsy (Do indications need to be checked? Is there any postmenopausal bleeding?) is required if the stripe exceeds 5 mm or there is diffuse or increased echogenicity or inadequate visualization of the endometrium. For women on HRT, the sensitivity is similar, but there is a higher false-positive rate due to an average greater endometrial thickness.
- Endometrial biopsy—Less invasive and costly than a dilation and curettage (D&C), endometrial biopsy has about the same sensitivity and specificity. However, only about 5% to 15% of the endometrial surface is sampled and up to 70% of the samples are nondiagnostic
- Hysteroscopy—More costly and invasive than other evaluations, provides direct visualization of the endometrium and allows for targeted biopsy or excision of lesions
- Saline infusion sonography—May detect small lesions missed by transvaginal ultrasound, but provides no tissue for pathology
- MRI may be helpful in further evaluating lesions found initially on sonography (e.g., fibroids, adenomyosis)

Comments and Treatment Considerations
Treatment of vaginal bleeding, whether perimenopausal or postmenopausal, is dependent on the underlying diagnosis. Perimenopausal

woman who require contraception and who do not smoke may be placed on low-dose OCPs. The Mirena intrauterine device (IUD) has also been proven to substantially decrease bleeding. Smokers should be encouraged to stop but may be cycled on progesterone.

Evaluation of postmenopausal bleeding in women on HRT depends on the regimen. Women on cyclic therapy may continue to bleed. No evaluation is needed for women on continuous regimens whose bleeding begins and resolves within 6 to 9 months of initiation of therapy.

PSYCHOSOCIAL ISSUES

Natural menopause occurs at a time of life when many other changes are occurring. Many symptoms commonly associated with menopause are not due to the decline in ovarian function but to the aging process and the social changes accompanying midlife.

Signs
- Insomnia increases in both genders. +++
- Decline in memory, difficulty in thinking or other cognitive disturbances +++

Comments and Treatment Considerations
The relationship of changing hormones and mood disorders (28% to 41%) is unclear. A history of depression, anxiety, premenstrual disorder, life stresses, and general health are the major predictors of psychiatric problems during midlife. Evidence that hormone replacement improves mood is weak. No correlation has been found between menopausal status and the prevalence of arthralgias, joint stiffness, fatigue, and other somatic complaints.

SEXUAL DYSFUNCTION

Although studies have shown that approximately 40% of women stop sexual activity between the ages of 40 and 60, the association of sexual dysfunction and declining hormone levels has not been clearly established. Evidence is strong that vaginal dryness increases in many women as the menopausal transition proceeds.

Symptoms
- Decreased libido +++
- Vaginal dryness +++
- Dyspareunia ++

Signs
- Thin friable atrophic vaginal mucosa
- Caruncle
- Vaginal stenosis

Workup
- History
  - Pain or burning with urination

- Frequent urinary tract infections
- Painful intercourse
- Feeling of vaginal dryness
- Laboratory
  - Seldom helpful—Consider biopsy as needed

Comments and Treatment Considerations

With low-dose vaginal estrogen therapy, systemic absorption is minimal. Progesterone should be considered for women with an intact uterus but is usually not necessary. Small studies involving only 20 women found endometrial hyperplasia in only 1 after 6 months of 0.3-mg Premarin cream therapy. None of 10 women using Estring with vaginal bleeding demonstrated hyperplasia on endometrial biopsy.

The use of testosterone for sexual dysfunction is controversial and not FDA approved. Women who have undergone surgical menopause are most likely to benefit from androgens. Potential side effects include hirsutism, acne, and decreasing high-density lipoprotein (HDL) levels.

Sexual intercourse improves vaginal blood flow, thus maintaining an acidic vaginal pH, promoting normal vaginal flora and a healthy mucosal epithelium. Vaginal weights strengthen pelvic floor musculature and may improve awareness of sexual arousal in women with orgasmic disorders.

Nonpharmacologic lifestyle changes can include frequent intercourse and increased tactile stimulation, smoking cessation, strength training and aerobic exercise, vaginal moisturizers (e.g., Replens), vaginal lubricants (water-soluble preferable, e.g., Astroglide), vaginal weights, and a clitoral suction device (Eros-Clitoral Therapy Device, UroMetrics, Inc., St. Paul, MN).

Pharmacologic therapies can include systemic estrogen therapy (see vasomotor instability); low-dose vaginal conjugated estrogen (0.3 mg of conjugated estrogen daily intravaginally for 3 weeks, twice weekly thereafter); 0.5 g crystalline estradiol (Estrace); 25 µg estradiol tablet intravaginally twice weekly; estradiol vaginal ring (Estring), which releases 6 to 9 mcg estradiol daily for 3 months; testosterone 1.22 to 2.5 mg/day methyltestosterone; combinations estrogen/methyltestosterone 5 mg twice daily of micronized oral testosterone.

References

Buckler H: The menopause transition: endocrine changes and clinical symptoms, *J Br Menopause Soc* 11(2):61–65, 2005.

Carroll DG: Nonhormonal therapies for hot flashes in menopause, *Am Fam Physician* 73(3):457–464, 2006.

Castelo-Branco C, Palacios S, Calaf J, et al: Available medical choices for the management of menopause, *Maturitas* 52(Suppl 1):S61–S70, 2005. Epub Oct 4, 2005.

Deeks AA: Is this menopause? Women in midlife—psychosocial issues, *Aust Fam Physician* 33(11):889–893, 2004.

Dijkhuizen FP, Brolmann HA, Potters AE, et al: The accuracy of transvaginal ultrasonography in the diagnosis of endometrial abnormalities, *Obstet Gynecol* 87(3):345–349, 1996.

Gracia CR, Sammel MD, Freeman EW, et al: Defining menopause status: creation of a new definition to identify the early changes of the menopausal transition, *Menopause* 12(2):128–135, 2005.

Huntzinger A: Practice guidelines: AHRQ releases evidence report on managing menopause-related symptoms, *Am Fam Physician* August 25, 2005.

Iatrakis G, Diakakis I, Kourounis G, et al: Postmenopausal uterine bleeding, *Clin Exp Obstet Gynecol* 24(3):157, 1997.

Kahwati LC, Haigler L, Rideout S, Markova T: What is the best way to diagnose menopause? *J Fam Pract* 54(11):1000–1002, 2005.

Karlsson B, Granberg S, Wikland M, et al: Transvaginal ultrasonography of the endometrium in women with postmenopausal bleeding—a Nordic multicenter study, *Am J Obstet Gynecol* 172(5):1488–1494, 1995.

Landgren BM, Collins A, Csemiczky G, et al: Menopause transition: annual changes in serum hormonal patterns over the menstrual cycle in women during a nine-year period prior to menopause, *J Clin Endocrinol Metab* 89(6):2763–2769, 2004.

Lobo RA, Rosen RC, Yang HM, Block B, Van Der Hoop RG: Comparative effects of oral esterified estrogens with and without methyltestosterone on endocrine profiles and dimensions of sexual function in postmenopausal women with hypoactive sexual desire, *Fertil Steril* 79(6):1341–1352, 2003.

Low Dog T: Menopause: a review of botanical dietary supplements, *Am J Med* 118(Suppl)12B:98–108, 2005.

McKee J, Warber SL: Integrative therapies for menopause, *South Med J* 98(3):319–326, 2005.

Melby MK, Lock M, Kaufert P: Culture and symptom reporting at menopause, *Hum Reprod Update* 11(5):495–512, 2005. Epub May 26, 2005.

Menopause: a guide to management. Brigham and Women's Hospital (Boston) Hospital/Medical Center. 2005. Available at www.brighamandwomens.org/medical/HandbookArticles/Menopause.pdf.

Morelli V, Naquin C: Alternative therapies for traditional disease states: menopause, *Am Fam Physician* 66(1):129–134, 2002.

National Institutes of Health, National Institutes of Health State-of-the-Science Conference statement: management of menopause-related symptoms, *Ann Intern Med* 142(12 Pt 1):1003–1013, 2005. Epub May 27, 2005.

Neff MJ: NAMS releases position statement on the treatment of vasomotor symptoms associated with menopause, *Am Fam Physician* 70(2):393–394, 396, 399, 2004.

Nelson HD, Haney E, Humphrey L, et al: Management of menopause-related symptoms, *Evid Rep Technol Assess* (summ) (11201–6), 2005.

Perimenopause: rocky road to menopause. Symptoms we call "menopausal" often precede menopause by years, *Harv Womens Health Watch* 12(12):1–4, 2005.

Phillips NA: Female sexual dysfunction: evaluation and treatment, *Am Fam Physician* 62(1):127–136, 141–142, 2000.

Reddish S: Assessment of women in midlife, *Aust Fam Physician* 33(11):883–887, 2004.

Reddish S: Menopause—a treatment algorithm, *Aust Fam Physician* 33(11):900–901, 2004.

Shifren JL, Braunstein GD, Simon JA, et al: Transdermal testosterone treatment in women with impaired sexual function after oophorectomy, *N Engl J Med* 343(10):682–688, 2000.

Smith-Bindman R, Kerlikowske K, Feldstein VA, et al: Endovaginal ultrasound to exclude endometrial cancer and other endometrial abnormalities, *JAMA* 280:1510–1517, 1998.

Soares CN, Prouty J, Born L, Steiner M: Treatment of menopause-related mood disturbances, *CNS Spectr* 10(6):489–497, 2005.

Xu J, Bartoces M, Neale AV, et al: Natural history of menopause symptoms in primary care patients: a MetroNet study, *J Am Board Fam Pract* 18:374–382, 2005.

CHAPTER 32

Neck Pain
Kaye B. Carstens

CERVICAL DISK DISEASE

Neck pain is a common problem encountered by the physician. Ten percent of the adult population has neck pain at any given time. In most cases a careful history and physical examination of the neck can lead to the diagnosis of cervical disk disease. One must differentiate between articular and nonarticular causes, which can be lengthy. Articular structures include synovium, synovial fluid, articular cartilage, intra-articular ligaments, joint capsule, and juxta-articular bone. Nonarticular structures are: supportive extra-articular ligaments, tendons, bursa, muscle, fascia, bone, and skin.

Cervical disk disease can be thought of as two forms: soft-disk and hard-disk disease. Soft-disk disease is an acute herniation of gelatinous nucleus pulposus into or through the annulus of the cervical disk and the absence of previous or more chronic symptoms. Patients tend to be younger and usually have an identifiable event such as trauma.

The second most common form of cervical disk disease is hard disk. Due to mechanical forces over the years, intervertebral disk disease occurs leading to loss of normal production of disk components. This includes loss of annular elasticity, extracellular matrix, desiccation of the nucleus pulposus, and formation of osteophytes. Symptoms of hard disk disease tend to be found in patients 50 years of age and older, insidious in onset, and present with episodic neck stiffness and pain that tend to wax and wane.

Symptoms
- Pain of insidious or acute onset ++++
- Isolated episodic neck stiffness +++
- Waxing and waning pain ++
- Posterior neck pain ++++
- Nerve root pain is usually brief, sharp, and shooting. Pain is increased by coughing, straining, standing or sitting, and head tilting and is usually relieved by lying down with the neck in a neutral position. +++
- Sense of muscular weakness ++
- Nerve root pain proximal and around shoulders; radiates to arms with paresthesias distally +++

Signs

- Pain with neck motion +++++
- Lhermitte's sign (urgent consult) ++
- Disturbances in balance or gait (urgent consult) +
- Lower extremity weakness (urgent consult) ++
- Babinski's sign +
- Hoffman's reflex ++
- Ankle clonus +
- Alterations in bowel/bladder function indicate an urgent consult. +
- Spurling's sign +++
- Specific findings can localize the level of nerve root involvement by deficiencies in motor function.
  - C5 — Arm abduction: deltoid and biceps
  - C5, C6, C7 — Arm adduction, wrist extensors and abduction, extension of thumb
  - C5, C6, C7 — Flexion of elbow, wrist flexors, and finger extensors pronate and supinate forearm
  - C7, C8 — Extend elbow, flex and extend fingers, and T1 intrinsic hand muscles
- Biceps and brachioradialis reflex mediated by C5-C6 nerve roots
- Triceps reflex mediated by C6-C7 nerve roots

Workup

- CBC, urinalysis (UA), erythrocyte sedimentation rate (sed rate) (if sed rate is high, look for infectious etiology)
- Complete set of plain films (AP, lateral, oblique, and open-mouth [odontoid]) if indications are as follows:
  - Neck trauma
    - Age older than 50 years
    - Conservative treatment failed
    - All patients presenting with symptoms and signs of radiculopathy
  - Lateral flexion/extension films if previous criteria negative
  - EMG
  - MRI of cervical spine (provides superior delineation of soft-tissue anatomy and is the preferred method for visualizing the intervertebral disk and surrounding structures)

Comments and Treatment Considerations

Treatment includes the following:

 PASSIVE MODALITIES

- Rest
  - Immobilization for short-term soft cervical collar
  - Antiinflammatory medication
  - Local modalities (i.e., heat, ice, and massage)
  - Physical therapy (cervical isometrics, restore ROM)

- Active modalities
  - Exercise programs with dynamic and isometric neck strengthening
  - Neck and shoulder stretching
  - Aerobic activities
  - Selective nerve root injections with local anesthetic and epidural
  - Long-acting corticosteroids (under fluoroscopy and technical expertise)
  - Neuropathic pain treatment with TCAs and gabapentin
- Surgical indications
  - Persistent or recurrent radicular pain
  - Progressive or persistent neurologic deficit
  - Cervical myelopathy (usually associated with central disk herniation)

OTHER CAUSES OF NECK PAIN

- Rheumatoid arthritis (gradual onset, symmetric polyarthritis, morning stiffness lasting 1 hour, swelling in three or more joints, distal to proximal involvement, rheumatoid subcutaneous nodules, migratory and intermittent)
- Ankylosing spondylitis (stiffness of spine and sacral areas on first arising in the morning, low back pain, enthesitis, extra-articular involvement such as anterior uveitis)
- Diskitis (fever, chills, diaphoresis, insidiously and progressive over several weeks, painful tender neck, elevated sed rate and CRP, which can exceed 100 mm/hr)
- Herpes zoster (rash and acute neuritis, unilateral radicular symptoms without neurologic findings, rash quickly evolves into vesicles, pain, burning, throbbing, and allodynia)
- Neoplasms (nocturnal awakenings, gnawing, unremitting pain, sensory dysesthesias, muscular weakness, usually unilateral)
- Coronary artery disease (CAD)
- Thoracic outlet syndrome (triad of numbness, weakness, and sensation of swelling of upper limbs, positive Roos sign, Adson's sign, slow and progressive weakness of intrinsic hand muscles and numbness in distribution of ulnar nerve; EMG and chest x-ray may reveal cervical rib)
- Rotator cuff tendinitis and/or tendinopathy (shoulder pain with overhead activity, localized pain to lateral deltoid, night pain and while lying on shoulder, atrophy of supraspinatus and infraspinatus, sunken appearance, asymmetric motion of scapula, pain with more than 90 degrees abduction, pain with internal rotation, painful arc from 60 to 120 degrees, positive Jobe's sign)
- Carpal tunnel syndrome (pain, paresthesias, and hypoesthesias in the first three fingers and radial half of ring finger, night pain, repetitive shaking of hand returns normal feeling, atrophy of thenar eminence, thumb weakness, positive Tinnel and Phalen signs)
- Brachial neuritis (sensory loss, motor dysfunction, and weakness, isolation to single nerve unlikely of plexus origin)

- Polymyalgia rheumatica (aching, morning stiffness lasting 30 minutes, usually symmetric involvement of neck, shoulders, hip girdle, and torso, malaise, fever, fatigue, decreased ROM, weight loss, anorexia, muscle strength normal and muscle tenderness not prominent feature, increased CRP, sed rate)
- Rule out metastatic disease (bone pain, gout, many rheumatologic symptoms; most common causes are lymphomas, leukemias, and paraneoplastic syndrome)
- TMJ syndrome (pain exacerbated by jaw movement; pain in muscles of mastication; nocturnal bruxism; unilateral; pain radiates to jaw, ear, and posterior cervical region; clicking; jaw deviation on opening and closing; pain with anterior forward pressure in external acoustic meatus; malocclusion)

MECHANICAL NECK PAIN

One third of the adult population reports neck pain each year. Multiple etiologies can give rise to neck pain. However, mechanical neck pain is a common problem especially in the young and a common reason for medical consultation. Sporting accidents are second only to motor vehicle accidents as the leading cause of emergency department (ED) visits involving neck injuries. Mechanical neck pain is limited to injuries of the soft tissues such as anterior and posterior longitudinal ligaments, ligamentum flavum, interspinous ligaments, and supraspinous ligaments, considered stabilizing structures. Other stabilizers consist of cervical spine muscles—the sternocleidomastoid, trapezius, strap, and paracervical spine muscles—which can also be involved with mechanical neck pain. Injury to the head such as a blow causes microscopic or gross tensile failure, often where the tendon joins the muscle (myotendinous junction). Whiplash injury is one of the most common mechanical injuries to the neck. Cervical spine capsules, ligaments, and muscle structures can experience microtears as well as occasional complete rupture of ligaments. Sports injuries, primarily in contact sports, lead to mechanical pain and occasionally more serious states. Certain occupations are prone to neck pain because of poor posture and prolonged immobility such as dentistry. Simple awkward neck positions during the nocturnal hours while sleeping can cause neck pain on awakening (torticollis). In addition, emotional and physical stress can be causative agents. Findings of fever, radiculopathy, or Lhermitte's sign (long tract signs), should prompt the examiner to look for more serious etiologies.

Symptoms
- Neck pain at base of cervical spine or upper border of trapezius muscles +++++
- Limited ROM ++++
- Tingling or numbness (paresthesias) limited to the neck and trapezius ++
- Musculoskeletal pain following unaccustomed exercise on arising in the morning +++
- Dizziness +
- Nausea +

Signs
- Possible normal ROM and no tenderness +
- Tactile trigger points +++
- Pain with motion ++++
- Limited ROM ++++
- Normal neurologic examination +++++

Workup
- Immobilization of spine (if concern for more than muscle or ligamentous injury)
- AP, lateral, and obliques of cervical spine including C7-T1 junction
- Flexion and extension views
- CT and MRI of cervical spine (usually not necessary)
- Rest for acute phase then maintain normal activities
- Continue work (if not possible, engage in active exercise program immediately)
- Avoid cervical collar if possible
- Heat and/or ice
- Ultrasound
- Traction of cervical spine
- IV injection of methylprednisolone within 8 hours of injury
- IM lidocaine injection for chronic mechanical neck pain

Comments and Treatment Considerations
Mechanical neck pain usually responds to conservative treatments. With proper rest and care, recovery usually occurs within 1 to 2 weeks. If symptoms are not subsiding, investigate for other significant causes.

MENINGITIS

Annually, 1.2 million cases of meningitis occur, resulting in 135,000 deaths. The serious nature of this disease and its consequences require physicians to be well acquainted with the signs and symptoms. The clinical signs and symptoms occurring at presentation may predict prognosis and early diagnosis may also decrease the number of adverse outcomes. Unfortunately, the symptoms and signs may vary a great deal depending on the age of the patient and other health problems.

Community-acquired meningitis is more likely to occur in higher-risk groups such as those with alcoholism, asplenia, complement deficiency, corticoid excess, HIV, pneumonia, otitis media, diabetes mellitus, and those who are malnourished and unimmunized. Other factors that place patients at increased risk for meningitis include recent travel (sub-Saharan Africa), recent infection, IV drug use, head trauma, and otorrhea or rhinorrhea. The signs and symptoms of meningitis can be nonspecific. However, an accurate history and physical examination can lead to the diagnosis of meningitis. Findings may significantly differ depending on the age of the patient (Table 32-1). Early symptoms and signs of meningitis in the infant

Table 32-1. Meningitis Treatments by Age Group

Preterm to <1 month	Group B streptococci	49%	Ampicillin + cefotaxime *or*
	Escherichia coli	18%	ampicillin + gentamicin
	Listeria	7%	
	Gram negative	10%	
	Gram positive	10%	
1 month to 50 years	Meningococcus		Streptococcal pneumonia
	Haemophilus influenzae Listeria unlikely		Cefotaxime *or* ceftriaxone + Dexamethasone + vancomycin
>50 years	*Streptococcus pneumoniae*	70 %	Ampicillin+ ceftriaxone *or*
	Listeria	20 %	Cefotaxime + vancomycin +
	Gram-negative bacilli	9 %	IV dexamethasone

may be very subtle; older adults commonly have neck stiffness secondary to cervical disk disease. The most common cause of meningitis is viral followed by bacterial etiologies.

Symptoms
- Neck pain +++
- Fever (95% of patients) +++++
- Myalgia ++
- Nonpulsatile headache +++
- Generalized headache ++++
- Nausea and vomiting ++
- Tachypnea +

 ADULT

Signs

- Rash +
- Kernig's +++
- Brudzinski's +++
- Opisthotonos: late sign +++++

- Mental status change (85% of patients) +++
- Seizure +
- Nuchal rigidity (88% of patients) ++++

✴ INFANT

- Irritability +++++
- Poor feeding and poor muscular tone ++++
- Diarrhea +
- Altered sleep pattern +++
- Hypothermia or hypoxia ++
- Paradoxical irritability ++
- Seizure ++
- Jaundice +
- Bulging anterior fontanelle ++
- Opisthotonos: late sign +++++
- Skin or mucous membrane lesions +
- Nuchal rigidity 27% in 0 to 6 months ++

Workup
- CBC with blood cultures
- UA with urine culture
- Chemistry profile
- Lumbar puncture with opening and closing pressures
- Spinal fluid for cell count, Gram stain (Table 32-2), protein, sugar, cryptococcal stain, acid-fast stain, rapid antigen disclosure by latex agglutination culture, and PCRs for viral assessment
- CT indications—Immunocompromised, HIV, immunotherapy, after transplantation, new onset seizure, papilledema, abnormal level of consciousness, focal neurologic deficit

Comments and Treatment Considerations
Further choices of antibiotics are influenced by patient's history of ventriculoperitoneal shunts, post neurosurgery, post head trauma, post cochlear implant, and AIDS. If physical findings of herpes simplex II are found, acyclovir (Zovirax) should be administered.

Meningitis can be a rapidly fulminant and fatal disease. Expedient evaluation and early treatment are imperative to optimize good

Table 32-2. Gram Stain (May Give Direction to Etiology)

Gram-positive + diplococci	Streptococcal pneumonia
Gram-negative diplococci	Meningococcal
Gram-negative small pleomorphic coccobacilli	*Haemophilus influenzae*
Gram-positive rods and coccobacilli	*Listeria*

outcomes. If delay in results is anticipated, treatment should be empirically given on the basis of the mostly likely bacterial infection according to age group.

SOFT-TISSUE PAIN DISORDERS

Soft-tissue pain refers to the large number of painful conditions that interfere with mechanical function but are not due to arthritis. There are three subdivisions: local (bursitis, tenosynovitis), regional (myofascial pain syndrome, referred pain), and generalized (fibromyalgia, chronic fatigue, osteomalacia, hypermobility syndrome). This chapter addresses fibromyalgia and myofascial pain syndrome.

Differential diagnoses for soft-tissue pain disorders include:
- Joint disorders: osteoarthritis, loss of joint motion
- Inflammatory disorders: rheumatoid arthritis; polymyositis; polymyalgia rheumatica
- Neurologic disorders: radiculopathy; nerve entrapment
- Regional soft-tissue disorders: bursitis, tendinitis, cumulative trauma
- Diskogenic disorders: degenerative disk disease; annular tears; herniation
- Visceral referred pain: GI, cardiac, pulmonary, renal
- Mechanical stress: scoliosis, leg-length discrepancy
- Metabolic conditions: alcoholic or toxic myopathy; hypothyroidism; deficiency of vitamin B_1, B_{12}, folic acid, calcium, or magnesium
- Infectious diseases: viral illnesses, especially chronic hepatitis
- Psychologic disorders: depression, anxiety, disordered sleep

 FIBROMYALGIA SYNDROME

Signs
- Widespread pain of at least 3 months' duration
- Pain on palpation over at least 11 of 18 paired trigger points (above and below the waist) ++++
  - Occiput
  - Cervical (anterior C5-C7)
  - Trapezius (midpoint of upper border)
  - Supraspinatus (upper medial border)
  - Second rib (costochondral junction)
  - Lateral epicondyle
  - Gluteal (upper outer buttock)
  - Greater trochanter
  - Knee (medial condyle)

Symptoms
- Female gender ++++
- Musculoskeletal pain and stiffness in the low back and/or neck (shoulder and pelvic girdle areas)

- General fatigue
- Poor sleep
- Paresthesias (which may mimic nerve root compression)
- Migraine headaches
- IBS
- Restless leg syndrome

Workup

- The pressure applied by the examiner to the trigger point should blanch half of the fingernail bed.
- Neurologic and orthopedic examinations are normal (despite complaints of feeling swollen in the joints). ++++
- Lab tests are normal and are done to rule out other causes of the pain: CBC, sed rate, chemistry profile, TSH
- Radiologic studies may show incidental osteoarthritis or diskogenic changes.
- Electromyography, nerve conduction studies, and muscle biopsies are normal.
- It is known that people with these pain conditions do not sleep well. However, sleep studies should be ordered only if other problems are suspected such as sleep apnea or restless leg syndrome.

Comments and Treatment Considerations

There is no significant peripheral pathology. However, in the spinal fluid there is increased substance P (which mediates pain transmission) and decreased serotonin (which mediates pain inhibition).

As the pathophysiology has been identified, treatments and medications have been devised to address specific aspects of these syndromes. One mnemonic is ADEPT:

Attitude: The attitudes of the patient, family and coworkers, and health care providers are all important. The patient needs empathy.

Diagnosis: Treat comorbid conditions.

Education: CBT is helpful.

Physical: Low-impact aerobic exercise is beneficial for reducing pain, improving sleep, and balancing mood. Consider starting with walking in place in a swimming pool. As the fear of pain related to exercise decreases, the person will increase activity. The patient needs to balance the amount of exercise and rest.

Treatments: Select medications to treat the primary complaints. Pain responds well to tramadol with acetaminophen; nonsteroidals are not effective. Insomnia has been treated in the past with tricyclics and cyclobenzaprine. Benzodiazepines such as clonazepam reduce anxiety and nocturnal myoclonus (if also present). Two medications that treat both pain and insomnia are pregabalin and gabapentin. These correct the non–rapid-eye movement sleep pattern abnormalities. Duloxetine treats both pain and depression. Fatigue decreases with improved sleep, treatment of comorbid conditions such as depression, and balance between exercise and rest.

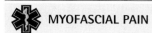 **MYOFASCIAL PAIN**

Signs
- Pain originates from myofascial trigger points in skeletal muscle. ++++
- Trigger points are identifiable by taut bands of muscle that are painful to palpation and cause referred pain in a characteristic pattern.

Symptoms
- Equal male/female distribution ++++
- May begin after a discrete trauma or start insidiously
- Deep aching sensations that fluctuate in intensity
- Each myofascial trigger point has its own characteristic pain pattern.
- Accompanying problems include autonomic dysfunctions (abnormal sweating, vasomotor and temperature changes); neuro-otologic symptoms (dizziness, tinnitus) related to cervical myofascial irritation; and impaired muscle coordination, stiff joints, weakness, paresthesias, and blurred vision.

Workup
- The myofascial trigger point can be identified by gentle palpation across the muscle fibers. ++++
- It is usually accompanied by restricted ROM due to pain from the trigger point. ++++

Comments and Treatment Considerations
These patients have abnormal motor endplates that release excessive amounts of acetylcholine. This results in sustained contraction of the muscle fibers. The local ischemia from chronic contraction stimulates the release of substances that sensitize afferent nerve fibers. In the dorsal horn of the spinal cord these pain signals are referred to adjacent spinal segments. When there is persistent pain, the second-order neurons in the dorsal horn develop a long-lasting increase in excitability of nociceptor pathways.

Trigger-point injections, acupuncture, botulinum toxin injections, and massage therapy are useful. TENS units and ultrasound have yielded mixed results.

References
Andersen B, Sheon RP: Evaluation of the patient with neck pain. *2006 Up To Date*, Meningitis, Sheldon L. Kaplan, M.D.

Binder A: *Neck pain*, Stevenage, UK, 2004, BMJ Publishing Group Ltd.

Borg-Stein J: Treatment of fibromyalgia, myofascial pain, and related disorders, *Phys Med Rehabil Clin North Am* 17:491–510, 2006.

Aminoff MJ: Mechanical and other lesions of the spine, nerve roots, and spinal cord. In Goldman L, Ausiello D, editors: *Cecil textbook of medicine,* 22nd ed, Philadelphia, 2004, Saunders.

Harrison's on line: *Back and neck pain,* 2005, John W. Engstrom.

Huffman GB: Diagnosis of acute meningitis in adult patients, *Am Fam Physician* 2000.

Medicinal and Injection therapies for mechanical neck disorders (Review) The Cochrane Library 2006, Issue 2

Russell IJ: Fibromyalgia syndrome: approach to management, *Primary Psychiatry* 13:76–84, 2006.

Russell IJ: Fibromyalgia syndrome: presentation, diagnosis, and differential, *Prim Psychiatry* 13:40–45, 2006.

Scherping SC Jr: Cervical disc disease in the athlete, *Clin Sports Med* 21(1): 27–37, 2002.

Smith L: Management of bacterial meningitis: new guidelines from the IDSA, *Am Fam Physician* 71(10):2003–2008, 2005.

The Cochrane Database of Systemic Reviews 2006. Issue 2 Copyright 2006 Exercises for mechanical neck disorders. The Cochrane Collaboration Publishers by John Wiley & Sons.

Young WF: Cervical spondylotic myelopathy: a common cause of spinal dysfunction in older persons, *Am Fam Physician* 62(5):1064–1070, 1073, 2000.

Zepf W: Review of bacterial meningitis in the older patient, *Am Fam Physician* 65(6):1173–1176, 2002.

Zmurko MD, Matthew G, Tony Y, et al: *Cervical sprains, disc herniations, minor fractures, and other cervical injuries in the athlete,* Philadelphia, Saunders.

CHAPTER 33

Pelvic or Genital Pain
Mark K. Huntington

Genital pain is one of the most personally distressing symptoms a patient can experience. Because the potential psychosocial implications inherent to certain etiologies of these symptoms, they may generate greater anxiety for patients than less morally charged symptoms such as crushing chest pain or severe dyspnea. For similar reasons, patients may be reluctant to seek timely care in spite of their high level of concern. A number of causes of genital and pelvic pain may be life threatening; delays in seeking care increase this risk. The family physician's approach to a patient presenting with genital or pelvic pain must be thorough yet sensitive, addressing the patient's concerns as well as those of the physician.

APPENDICITIS

A presentation of pelvic pain may in fact represent abdominal pain. As such, intra-abdominal processes such as appendicitis must be considered. These are discussed in Chapter 1.

DYSURIA

Dysuria, painful urination, is another symptom that may appear as a presenting complaint of genital pain. This symptom of urethritis and other urinary tract infections is covered in detail in Chapter 42.

ECTOPIC PREGNANCY

Ectopic pregnancy is a medical—and possibly surgical—emergency. Untreated it can result in the rupture of the fallopian tube, which may be accompanied by significant bleeding. It is the leading cause of first-trimester maternal mortality. Because of these potentially dire consequences, it is imperative that the physician recognize and appropriately treat ectopic pregnancy.

Ectopic pregnancy refers to any pregnancy outside the uterine cavity. Implantation and subsequent development may occur in the fallopian tubes, within the cervix, or a variety of other intra-abdominal and pelvic locations. Risk factors identified for ectopic pregnancy include prior ectopic pregnancy, history of reproductive system infection, history of infertility, induced ovulation, current IUD usage, prior cesarean section, multiple sexual partners, and cigarette smoking at the time of conception.

Symptoms
- Typically appear 6 to 8 weeks after the last menstrual period ++++
- Abdominal and/or pelvic pain +++++
- Amenorrhea prior to onset of symptoms ++++
- Vaginal bleeding +++
- Shoulder pain (from blood irritating the diaphragm) +++
- An urge to defecate (from blood in the cul-de-sac) +++
- Lightheadedness or even shock (in case of rupture) ++
- More than half of patients are asymptomatic prior to rupture. +++

Signs
- Variable, and may range from a normal examination to that of an acute abdomen to complete hemodynamic collapse
- Tachycardia ++
- Orthostatic hypotension ++
- Adnexal and cervical motion tenderness +++
- Uterine enlargement ++
- Adnexal mass ++
- Abdominal/pelvic pain +++++
- Fever +

Workup
- Pregnancy test +++++
- Ultrasonography (generally transvaginal) ++++
- Quantitative chorionic gonadotropin (β-hCG) should be checked if ultrasound is equivocal. +++++
- Laparoscopy is generally not necessary for diagnostic purposes, but is essential for surgical treatment of tubal rupture and is the visualization modality of choice in unstable patients.
- Culdocentesis is of little value.
- MRI, although capable of identifying the location of the pregnancy, is not cost-effective.

Comments and Treatment Considerations
Because of the variability in the clinical presentation of ectopic pregnancy, a high index of suspicion must be maintained. Ultrasonography (generally transvaginal) must be undertaken in all pregnant women with pelvic pain and vaginal bleeding to confirm intrauterine or extrauterine location of the gestational sac. Heterotropic pregnancies (i.e., one twin intrauterine, the other ectopic) are rare, but should be kept in mind if the patient clinically looks like an ectopic pregnancy but has an intrauterine gestational sac demonstrated. This is especially true of assisted reproduction patients.

A β-hCG value greater than 1500 IU/L in the presence of an adnexal mass and absence of an intrauterine gestational sac is generally diagnostic (specific cutoff is institution specific). If no adnexal mass or intrauterine gestational sac is present, repeat the quantitative β-hCG and ultrasound in 2 days. If the β-hCG has risen or plateaued, but no intrauterine sac is yet visible, a presumptive diagnosis of ectopic pregnancy may be made and appropriate treatment instituted. If the β-hCG is declining, no intervention is necessary, but levels should be monitored until they return to negative. In cases in which the level is less than 1500 IU/L, it should be rechecked along with another ultrasound in 3 days. A normally rising β-hCG level should be followed by ultrasound until either an intrauterine or ectopic pregnancy is visualized, then treated accordingly. An abnormal increase (less than doubling in 3 days) coupled with an absence of an intrauterine gestational sac on ultrasound, indicates a viable intrauterine pregnancy is not present.

Methotrexate is the most widely used medication for nonsurgical treatment of ectopic pregnancy; other agents such as misoprostol and mifepristone have been investigated. Methotrexate is most successful in patients whose β-hCG is less than 5000 IU/L at the time of diagnosis, with an ectopic sac of less than 3 cm. There are both single- and multiple-dose regimens.

The single-dose methotrexate regimen is frequently used, though multi-dose regimens are available.

Surgical treatment of ectopic pregnancy has become less common with the advent of good diagnostic ultrasound and the therapeutic use of methotrexate. Still, there remains a vital role. Surgery is the preferred treatment for ruptured ectopic pregnancies and patients with hemodynamic instability. Indications vary and surgery is strongly considered in patients with anemia, pain longer than 24 hours, β-hCG greater than 5000 IU/L, or ectopic gestational sacs measuring more than 3.5 cm on ultrasound. Laparoscopic procedures are typically the first-line approach, though laparotomy may be needed for cases of extensive intraperitoneal bleeding, adhesions, and other special circumstances.

One final but important aspect of the treatment of ectopic pregnancy to remember is the use of RhoGAM to all Rh-negative women to prevent sensitization and related complications in future pregnancies.

The differential diagnosis for ectopic pregnancy includes conditions such as threatened abortion, ruptured corpus luteum cyst, urinary tract infection, appendicitis, diverticulitis, ovarian torsion, endometriosis, dysfunctional uterine bleeding, and pelvic inflammatory disease. Once ectopic pregnancy is excluded via a negative pregnancy test, these other potential etiologies for pelvic pain may be evaluated.

ENDOMETRIOSIS

Endometriosis, the presence of endometrial glands and stroma outside the uterine cavity, is a common cause of pelvic pain. Half of adolescents, and up to one third of all women of reproductive age who undergo laparoscopy for pelvic pain are found to have endometriosis.

Symptoms
- May range from asymptomatic to debilitating.
- Pelvic pain (worse during menses or at ovulation) +++
- Dysmenorrhea ++++
- Dyspareunia on deep penetration +++
- Cyclic bowel or bladder symptoms ++
- Dysfunctional uterine bleeding ++
- Infertility +++
- Chronic fatigue ++
- Depression ++

Signs
- Often no physical findings on examination ++++
- The most common finding is tenderness when palpating the posterior fornix. +++
- Localized tenderness in the cul-de-sac or uterosacral ligaments ++
- Palpable, tender intrapelvic nodules ++
- Cervical motion tenderness ++
- Adnexal tenderness ++
- Adnexal masses ++
- Fixation of adnexa +
- Fixed, retroverted uterus +

Workup
- Visualization of the implants via laparoscopy is the only way to make a definitive diagnosis. +++++ Other studies are undertaken to rule out other pathologies.
- Urinalysis and culture
- Cervical culture and wet mount
- CBC

Comments and Treatment Considerations
Many cases of endometriosis may be managed expectantly, after ruling out other pathologies, using NSAIDs for symptomatic relief. Oral contraceptives have shown some symptomatic benefit, as well, and may slow the progression of the disease.

For those with more severe disease, a number of medical and surgical options exist. The medical approach essentially seeks to simulate the hormonal milieu of pregnancy or menopause, using progestins, androgens (i.e., danazol), GnRH analogs (e.g., leuprolide, nafarelin, and goserelin), and aromatase inhibitors (e.g., anastrozole, letrozole). Data for superiority of one regimen over another are lacking, but 80% to 90% of women will experience improvement—though not complete resolution—of their symptoms with medical management.

Surgery is reserved for the more severe cases. Modalities include both laparoscopy and laparotomy and may be definitive (removal of uterus and ovaries) or more conservative (focusing on destruction of the implants). Neurectomy in association with the conservative approach may be beneficial in select cases, but is not without adverse effects.

EPIDIDYMITIS

As its name implies, epididymitis is an inflammatory process affecting the epididymis. Presentations may be acute, subacute, or chronic. Sexual activity, heavy physical exertion, and bicycle/motorcycle riding have all been found to increase the risk for developing this condition. Infectious epididymitis is most commonly caused by *Chlamydia* or gonococci in men younger than age 35; coliforms in those who are older. A wide variety of other organisms have also been implicated less frequently. Older men are at higher risk for developing an acute presentation, in conjunction with severe urinary symptoms and prostatitis; younger men generally have a more insidious onset.

Symptoms
- Scrotal pain ++++ This may appear abruptly or insidiously.
- Urinary symptoms +++ (present in acute epididymitis; absent in subacute or chronic presentations)
- Rigorous chills (acute epididymitis) ++

Signs
- Varying degrees of epididymal induration and tenderness on palpation ++++
- Severe swelling of affected side (acute epididymitis) ++
- Fever (acute epididymitis) ++
- Inflammatory nodule may be palpable +++
- Reactive hydrocele may be present +++ (common in acute epididymitis, less frequent in subacute or chronic presentations)

Workup
- Ultrasound generally reveals no anomalies.
- Urinalysis is generally negative; culture may be helpful. ++
- Blood count and cultures may be of value in patients with systemic signs (acute epididymitis). ++

Comments and Treatment Considerations
In making the diagnosis of epididymitis, it is critical to differentiate it from torsion of the testes or the testicular appendix. These conditions are presented later in this chapter. Other conditions that may appear clinically similar to epididymitis include orchitis, which is usually viral (though *Brucella* may be a bacterial cause), in which the tenderness tends to be more diffuse; trauma, which can generally be derived from the history; and systemic conditions, like Henoch-Schönlein purpura, which may include scrotal pain as a manifestation.

Treatment varies with severity and suspected etiology. Septic presentations should be treated as inpatients with IV antibiotics and fluids. Less ill individuals may be treated as outpatients with oral antimicrobials. Generally, men younger than 35 years of age should be treated for gonorrhea and chlamydia using agents such as ceftriaxone 250 mg IM once plus azithromycin 1g PO once. Alternatively, a fluoroquinolone (e.g., levofloxacin 500 mg PO daily for 10 days) and doxycyline (100 mg PO twice a day for 10 days) may be used. For those older than 35 years, enteric bacteria are more likely and a 21-day course of a fluoroquinolone is recommended.

Noninfectious epididymitis is attributed to urine reflux and is associated with prolonged sitting (travel, sedentary jobs), cycling, and vigorous exercises such as lifting and others that involve Valsalva-type straining. Noninfectious epididymitis may also result from certain medications such as amiodarone and autoimmune disease. Antibiotics are not indicated in these cases.

Regardless of the etiology, scrotal elevation, cold compresses, and NSAIDs may provide symptomatic relief.

INGUINAL HERNIA

Hernias are the result of weakness or disruption of the fibrous tissues and the resultant protrusion of the internal structures through the defect. Groin hernias can be either inguinal or femoral, and inguinal hernias may be either direct or indirect. Ninety-six percent of groin hernias are inguinal, with a 9:1 male preponderance. Conversely, the less common femoral hernias are four times more common in women than men, and 40% present as strangulated. Hernias move from being merely inconveniences (albeit significant ones) to potentially life threatening when they become strangulated.

Symptoms
- May be asymptomatic +++
- "Heaviness" or dull pain in low abdomen or scrotum when straining (Valsalva maneuver), lifting, or standing for a prolonged time. ++ The discomfort may resolve when the patient stops straining or lies down
- Groin mass +++
- May have severe focal progressing to diffuse pain, nausea and vomiting, diarrhea, and even fever if strangulated ++

Signs
- Palpable (or even visible) mass in inguinal canal or femoral triangle, ++++ most easily detected with the patient in an upright posture. It may extend into the scrotum.
- May be reducible if not incarcerated +++
- Exquisite local pain (if strangulated ++++)
- Peritoneal signs (if strangulated ++++)

Workup
- Diagnosis is based on clinical examination and history in the majority of cases.
- Occasionally imaging may used for equivocal presentations. MRI, ultrasound, and herniography have demonstrated efficacy.
- If strangulation is suspected, preoperative laboratory work should be initiated.
- Remember, hernias may occur bilaterally: examine both the presenting and the contralateral sides!

Comments and Treatment Considerations

Other conditions that may present in a fashion similar to hernia include muscle strains, epididymitis, hydrocele, spermatocele, varicocele, testicular or appendiceal testis torsion, epididymal cysts, or neoplasms. If possible, these should be ruled out prior to surgery.

Definitive treatment of hernia is surgery. However, watchful waiting is reasonable in minimally symptomatic patients. In deciding whether to manage surgically, bear in mind that the risk of strangulation is greatest shortly after the hernia manifests itself, and diminishes with time. Risk is also lower for larger hernias than for small ones. Surgical repair of hernia may use either open or laparoscopic approaches. Though there are strong proponents of each technique, negligible differences in outcomes have been demonstrated.

Historically, trusses have been used as an alternative to surgery. However, there is no evidence of benefit, and there is the potential for the truss to compress the hernia, producing a strangulation-type injury. Truss use should generally be discouraged.

SALPINGITIS AND TUBO–OVARIAN ABSCESS

These conditions usually arise as complicated manifestations of pelvic inflammatory disease (PID), which may less commonly also include endometritis, oophoritis, peritonitis, and perihepatitis (Fitz-Hugh–Curtis syndrome). The progression of PID to salpingitis and tubo-ovarian abscess (TOA) represents a continuum rather than discrete, quantal steps in the disease process. Though PID is the primary antecedent, TOA may occasionally be seen as a complication of surgery, in association with malignancy, or from the spread of other infectious processes such as appendicitis and diverticulitis.

Symptoms
- Low abdominal and pelvic pain, often beginning around the time of menses (the most reliable symptom) ++++
- Fever and chills (not always present) +++
- Vaginal discharge (not always present) ++

Signs
- Palpable, tender adnexal mass (in 90% of TOA [Landers and Sweet, 1985]) ++++
- Peritoneal signs such as rebound tenderness +++
- Fever +++
- Toxic appearance +++
- Cervical motion tenderness +++
- Exquisite adnexal tenderness, ++++ which may preclude a thorough examination
- Purulent discharge from the cervix ++
- Decreased bowel sounds and other signs of ileus ++

Workup
- Thorough history, including sexual history
- Complete examination, including pelvic examination

- Ultrasound is the modality of choice to confirm clinical suspicion of TOA.
- CBC (but leukocytosis is present in only 60% to 80% of TOA) ++++
- hCG (to rule out ectopic pregnancy, an important consideration in the differential diagnosis)

Comments and Treatment Considerations

The differential diagnosis for TOA is broad, including ectopic pregnancy, torsion of the ovaries, other abdominopelvic abscesses, and both benign and malignant neoplasms.

One important distinction to make is that of the tubo-ovarian complex. Another complication of PID, this painful adnexal mass develops as the result of adherence of the inflamed pelvic tissues to one another. It appears clinically very similar to TOA, but has the important difference in that it does not consist of the devitalized tissue and pus collection present in the latter and is thus conducive to medical rather than surgical treatment. Ultrasound is quite useful in differentiating these two entities and directing the physician to institute the appropriate therapeutic intervention.

Treatment of TOA is controversial. Historically, TOA, as virtually every other abscess, was considered a surgical disease. Certainly, the rupture of a TOA may be a life-threatening event. A trial of broad-spectrum antibiotics, targeting the anaerobe-predominant polymicrobial mix present in PID and TOA, is advocated in most cases and supported by reasonable evidence. The online reference, *UpToDate,* takes the middle road and suggests that individuals not responding to medical management within 4 days require surgical drainage.

Whether medical or surgical modalities are used, individuals with TOA should be treated as inpatients. If the surgical approach is chosen, drainage may be accomplished via the transvaginal, transgluteal, laparoscopic, or surgical routes. Medically, two regimens are suggested: (1) cefoxitin 2 g IV every 6 hours (or cefotetan 2 g IV every 12 hours) plus doxycycline 100 mg PO every 12 hours, for at least 48 hours, followed by oral doxycycline for 2 weeks after discharge; *or* (2) clindamycin 900 mg IV and gentamicin 1.5 mg/kg PO every 8 hours (following a 2 mg/kg bolus of the gentamicin) with discharge medications of either oral doxycycline (100 mg daily) or clindamycin (450 mg five times daily) for 2 weeks.

TESTICULAR TORSION

Affecting up to two in five patients presenting with acute scrotal pain, torsion of the testis is a surgical emergency. Untreated, it can result in infarction and loss of the testis. Neonates and adolescent boys are most commonly affected, but it can occur at any age.

Symptoms

- Sudden onset of scrotal pain developing several hours after vigorous exercise or minor testicular trauma ++++
- May present as awakening with scrotal pain +++
- Nausea and vomiting +++

Signs
- Asymmetric, high-riding testis on the affected side with a "bell-clapper" deformity +++
- Testicular swelling is typical early; +++ later there may be a reactive hydrocele.
- Erythema of the scrotum +++
- Exquisite tenderness (may be distinguishable from the point tenderness of epididymitis) +++++
- Absent cremasteric reflex ++++
- Prehn's sign (worsening pain with elevation of the scrotum) may be present but cannot distinguish between torsion and epididymitis. +++

Workup
- Usually the diagnosis can be made clinically ++++; based on this, emergent surgery is arranged.
- Color Doppler ultrasonography is useful if clinical examination is equivocal. +++++
- If color Doppler is unavailable, use of a Doppler stethoscope may demonstrate lack of arterial pulses in the affected hemiscrotum. ++++

Comments and Treatment Considerations
Surgery is the definitive treatment, and should be undertaken once the diagnosis is made. The procedure consists of detorsion and bilateral fixation of the testes. Timing is critical because the duration of vascular compromise determines the clinical outcome. If more than 12 hours have elapsed, damage is considered permanent and orchiectomy may be required. Because no test is definitive, consideration of urologic consultation/surgery should be given for suspect cases.

If surgery is not available in a timely fashion, manual detorsion may be attempted by rotating the affected testis outward toward the thigh. Success is indicated by resolution of both the pain and the bell-clapper deformity. In these cases, Doppler pulses will be detectable in the scrotum, where they were absent prior to detorsion. Manual detorsion attempts should never delay surgery; even when successful, surgical orchiopexy must be performed to prevent recurrence.

The differential for testicular torsion includes epididymitis (managed medically, as noted previously), traumatic rupture (which requires surgical repair), and torsion of the testicular appendix, the last of which can present in a fashion very similar to that of testicular torsion and deserves a brief review.

The torsion of this müllerian duct remnant has a more gradual onset of pain than torsion of the testis. It may be accompanied by a reactive hydrocele, but the bell-clapper deformity is absent. One important distinguishing physical finding is an intact cremasteric reflex, which is typically absent in testicular torsion. A "blue dot" sign may be observed on the anterosuperior scrotal wall. On palpation, pain may be localized to this same region, with the epididymis and the testis itself being nontender. Diagnosis of this disorder is primarily clinical, though ultrasonography is a useful confirmatory test. Treatment of appendiceal torsion is medical via rest, ice, and antiinflammatory drugs. Surgical management may speed the resolution of the symptoms, but is not essential as it is in the case of testicular torsion.

References

Anderson FW, Hogan JG, Ansbacher R: Sudden death: ectopic pregnancy mortality, *Obstet Gynecol* 103:1218, 2004.

Centers for Disease Control and Prevention: Sexually transmitted diseases treatment guidelines 2002, *MMWR* 51:1, 2002.

Cheek CM, Williams MH, Farndon JR: Trusses in the management of hernia today, *Br J Surg* 82:1611, 1995.

Gianom D, Schubiger C, Decurtins M: Trusses in the current management of hernia, *Chirurgie* 73:1105, 2002.

Ginsburg DS, Stern JL, Hamod KA, et al: Tubo-ovarian abscess: a retrospective review, *Am J Obstet Gynecol* 138:1055, 1980.

Hamlin JA, Kahn AM: Herniography: a review of 333 herniograms, *Am Surg* 64:965, 1998.

Karaer A, Avsar FA, Batioglu S: Risk factors for ectopic pregnancy: a case-control study, *Aust N Z J Obstet Gynaecol* 46:521, 2006.

Khan KS, Wojdyla D, Say L, et al: WHO analysis of causes of maternal death: a systematic review, *Lancet* 367:1066, 2006.

Kirk E, Bourne T: The nonsurgical management of ectopic pregnancy, *Curr Opin Obstet Gynecol* 18:587, 2006.

Landers DV, Sweet RL: Current trends in the diagnosis and treatment of tuboovarian abscess, *Am J Obstet Gynecol* 151:1098, 1985.

Landers DV, Sweet RL: Tubo-ovarian abscess: contemporary approach to management, *Rev Infect Dis* 5:876, 1983.

McIntosh A, Hutchinson A, Roberts A, Withers H: Evidence-based management of groin hernia in primary care—a systematic review, *Fam Pract* 17:442, 2000.

McNeeley SG, Hendrix SL, Mazzoni MM, et al: Medically sound, cost-effective treatment for pelvic inflammatory disease and tuboovarian abscess, *Am J Obstet Gynecol* 178:1272, 1998.

Menon S, Colins J, Barnhart KT: Establishing a human chorionic gonadotropin cutoff to guide methotrexate treatment of ectopic pregnancy: a systematic review, *Fertil Steril* 2006; prepublication print of doi:10.1016/j.fertnstert.2006.10.007.

Missmer SA, Hankinson SE, Spiegelman D, et al: Incidence of laparoscopically confirmed endometriosis by demographic, anthropometric, and lifestyle factors, *Am J Epidemiol* 160:784, 2004.

Moir C, Robins RE: Role of ultrasound, gallium scanning, and computed tomography in the diagnosis of intra-abdominal abscess, *Am J Surg* 143:582, 1982.

Mosteller RD: Simplified calculation of body surface area (letter), *N Engl J Med* 317:1098, 1987.

Neumayer L, Giobbie-Hurder A, Jonasson O: Veterans Affairs Cooperative Studies Program, 456 Investigators. Open mesh versus laparoscopic mesh repair of inguinal hernia, *N Engl J Med* 350:1819, 2004.

Ramakrishnan K, Scheid DC: Ectopic pregnancy: expectant management or immediate surgery? *J Fam Prac* 55:517, 2006.

Reed SD, Landers DV, Sweet RL: Antibiotic treatment of tuboovarian abscess: comparison of broad-spectrum beta-lactam agents versus clindamycin-containing regimens, *Am J Obstet Gynecol* 164:1556, 1991.

Rein DB, Kassler WJ, Irwin KL, Rabiee L: Direct medical cost of pelvic inflammatory disease and its sequelae: decreasing but still substantial, *Obstet Gynecol* 95:397, 2000.

Ringdahl E, Teague L: Testicular torsion, *Am Fam Physician* 74:1739, 2006.

Roper RJ, Doerge RW, Call SB, et al: Autoimmune orchitis, epididymitis, and vasitis are immunogenetically distinct lesions, *Am J Pathol* 152(5):1337, 1998.

Sadek I, Biron P, Kus T: Amiodarone-induced epididymitis: report of a new case and literature review of 12 cases, *Can J Cardiol* 9:833, 1993.

Sangi-Haghpeykar H, Poindexter AN: Epidemiology of endometriosis among parous women, *Obstet Gynecol* 85:983, 1995.

Seeber GE, Barnhart KT: Suspected ectopic pregnancy, *Obstet Gynecol* 107:399, 2006.

Sessions AE, Rabinowitz R, Hulbert WC, Goldstein MM: Testicular torsion: direction, degree, duration and disinformation, *J Urol* 169:663, 2003.

Stovall TB, Ling FW: Single dose methotrexate: an expanded clinical trial, *Am J Obstet Gynecol* 168:1759, 1993.

Stovall TG, Kellerman AL, Ling FW, Buster JE: Emergency department diagnosis of ectopic pregnancy, *Ann Emerg Med* 19:1098, 1990.

Vandenberg JC, DeValois JC, Go PM, Rosenbusch G: Detection of groin hernia with physical examination, ultrasound, and MRI compared with laparoscopic findings, *Invest Radiology* 34:739, 1999.

Wiesenfeld HC, Sweet RL: Progress in the management of tuboovarian abscesses, *Clin Obstet Gynecol* 36:433–444, 1993.

Wilbert DM, Schaerfe CW, Stern WD, et al: Evaluation of the acute scrotum by color-coded Doppler ultrasonography, *J Urol* 149:1475, 1993.

Zullo F, Palomba S, Zupi E, et al: Effectiveness of presacral neurectomy in women with severe dysmenorrhea caused by endometriosis who were treated with laparoscopic conservative surgery: a 1-year prospective randomized double-blind controlled trial, *Am J Obstet Gynecol* 189:5, 2003.

CHAPTER 34

Polyuria
Elisabeth L. Backer

Polyuria can be defined as urine output exceeding 3 L/day in adults, and 2 L/m^2 in kids. Polyuria needs to be differentiated from frequency and nocturia, which are not associated with an increase in total urine output.

Causes of polyuria include glucose-induced osmotic diuresis (e.g., uncontrolled diabetes mellitus), conditions associated with a defect in water balance leading to the excretion of large volumes of diluted urine (e.g., primary/psychogenic polydipsia, central diabetes insipidus, and nephrogenic diabetes insipidus), osmotic diuresis (e.g., postobstructive diuresis, high-protein feedings, saline loading/volume expansion), prostatic hypertrophy and associated nocturia, medications (e.g., diuretics, lithium), hyperparathyroidism, and renal disease. This section focuses on selected, common causes of polyuria—other causes may be described elsewhere.

The diagnosis is often suggested through the history (age/rate of onset, family history) and by the plasma sodium concentration. In most cases the diagnosis can be confirmed by examining the response (urine volume and osmolality) to water restriction, and if appropriate, by administration of exogenous antidiuretic hormone (ADH) once plasma osmolality exceeds 295 mOsm/kg. Plasma ADH levels at baseline and post-water restriction may be helpful if the response to water restriction is equivocal.

Certain specific tests may be useful in evaluating the etiology of polyuria. These include a fasting glucose level to screen for diabetes mellitus, the exclusion of potential polyuria-inducing medication, a calcium and parathyroid hormone (PTH) level to look for hyperparathyroidism, renal functions to exclude renal diseases, a TSH to screen for hyperthyroidism, and a urine and plasma osmolality (a low urine osmolality/specific gravity and normal serum osmolality and hypernatremia point to diabetes insipidus).

DIABETES INSIPIDUS

Diabetes insipidus (DI) is an uncommon disease marked by increased thirst and passage of a large quantity of urine with a low specific gravity, usually less than 1.006. The urine is otherwise normal. The volume of ingested fluid varies from 2 to 20 L daily, with corresponding large urine volumes. Diabetes insipidus is caused by a lack of or resistance to vasopressin. ADH deficiency causes central DI with polyuria and polydipsia; hypernatremia occurs if fluid intake is inadequate.

 TYPES OF DIABETES INSIPIDUS

Primary/Central Diabetes Insipidus
If no lesion of the pituitary/hypothalamus is visible, then autoimmunity against the hypothalamic vasopressin secreting cells or genetic causes (familial DI) should be considered.

Secondary Diabetes Insipidus
Damage to the hypothalamus or pituitary stalk secondary to a tumor, anoxia, trauma, infection or metastasis may cause this to occur.

Vasopressinase–Induced Diabetes Insipidus
This occurs during the last trimester of pregnancy and puerperium. It *is* associated with oligohydramnios, preeclampsia, and hepatic dysfunction.

Nephrogenic Diabetes Insipidus
This is a defect in the renal tubules that hinders water reabsorption. The polyuria is unresponsive to vasopressin.

Symptoms
- Intense thirst, craving for ice
- Polyuria ++++
- Nocturia
- Headache
- Visual disturbance

Signs
- Hypernatremia and dehydration (if damage to hypothalamic thirst center or no access to free water)

Workup
- Clinical judgment essential
- No single lab test sufficient
- Accurate 24-hour urine collection measured for volume and creatinine (volume <2 L/24 hr in absence of hypernatremia rules out DI)
- Other screening tests
  - Fasting plasma glucose level (to rule out diabetes mellitus [DM])
  - BUN (to assess for dehydration and azotemia)
  - Calcium level (to exclude hypercalcemia, which causes polyuria)
  - Potassium level (to exclude hypokalemia, which causes polyuria)
  - Sodium level (to screen for dehydration)
  - Uric acid level (hyperuricemia can occur in patients with DI)
- Supervised vasopressin challenge test (measures urine output for 12 hours before and after administration of vasopressin; thirst and polyuria decreases and sodium stays normal in patients with central DI)

- MRI of pituitary gland/hypothalamus (to exclude mass lesions in nonfamilial DI)
- Vasopressin levels (should be elevated during modest fluid restriction in nephrogenic DI)

Comments and Treatment Considerations

Central DI post pituitary surgery may be temporary (lasting days to weeks), or permanent (if upper pituitary stalk is cut). Chronic central DI is more inconvenient than medically dangerous. Treatment with desmopressin allows normal sleep and activity. Hypernatremia can occur, especially when the thirst center is damaged, but life expectancy is not reduced, and the overall prognosis reflects that of the underlying disorder.

- Desmopressin
  - Treatment of choice for central DI
  - Also useful in pregnancy- or puerperium-related DI
  - Available in tablet form 0.05 mg twice a day to 0.4 mg three times a day; as a nasal preparation 0.05 to 0.1 mL every 12 to 24 hours; and in a parenteral form (IM, IV, subcutaneous) 1 to 4 µg every 12 to 24 hours.
  - Possible adverse reactions: nasal irritation, agitation, erythromelalgia, hyponatremia
- Mild cases of DI: adequate fluid intake may suffice
- Avoidance of aggravating factors (such as steroids) reduces polyuria.

Additional Therapies

- Hydrochlorothiazide 50 to 100 mg/day PO (with potassium supplementation) is helpful in both central and nephrogenic DI.
- Indomethacin (50 mg PO every 8 hours)—alone or in combination with hydrochlorothiazide, desmopressin or amiloride—can be effective.
- Psychotherapy is required in patients with compulsive water intake.

DIABETES MELLITUS

Increased urination arises as a consequence of osmotic diuresis secondary to sustained hyperglycemia. This results in a loss of glucose and free water and electrolytes in the urine, creating a hyperosmolar state.

Symptoms

- Polyuria ++++
- Thirst or polydipsia
- Blurred vision
- Weakness or fatigue (due to potassium loss and muscle protein catabolism)
- Paresthesias (peripheral neuropathy)
- Anorexia, nausea and vomiting (linked to ketoacidosis and hyperosmolality)
- Pruritus/vulvovaginitis

Signs

- Weight loss in spite of polyphagia (caused by the depletion of water, glucose, triglycerides, and protein) associated with random plasma glucose 200 mg/dL or more
- Fasting plasma glucose of 126 mg/dL or higher
- Nocturia
- Ketonemia, ketonuria, or both (rare in type 2 diabetes)
- Dehydration
- Postural hypotension (due to decreased plasma volume)

When an absolute insulin deficiency arises acutely, symptoms may arise abruptly (type 1 DM). Although many individuals with type 2 diabetes may present with increased urination and thirst, others may have an insidious onset of hyperglycemia and may be asymptomatic initially.

Workup

- Urine analysis for the detection of glucosuria and ketonuria
- Elevated fasting plasma glucose (normal <100; impaired glucose tolerance between 100 and 125; diabetes at or >126)
- Glycosylated hemoglobin (reflects metabolic control over 3-month period; use for screening controversial)
- Glucose tolerance test (helpful in suspected cases in which the plasma glucose <126)
- Serum fructosamine (used in cases with abnormal hemoglobins or hemolytic states)
- Fasting lipid profile
- ECG
- Renal function studies (screening for microalbuminuria)
- Evaluation of peripheral pulses
- Neurologic, podiatric, and ophthalmologic assessments

Exclusion of secondary causes of hyperglycemia (such as Cushing syndrome, medications, liver diseases, hormonal tumors, pancreatic diseases)

Comments and Treatment Considerations

- Patient education/self-management training
- Diet and weight loss
  - Carbohydrate counting (individual goal setting)
  - Cholesterol limitation (≤300 mg daily)
  - Protein intake of 10% to 20% of total calories
  - Decreased saturated fat intake (≤8% to 9% of total calories)
  - Increased dietary fiber (20 to 35 g daily)

ADA exchange lists available for meal planning (www.eatright.org)

- Oral drugs for treatment of hyperglycemia
  - Sulfonylureas, meglitinide analogs, D-phenylalanine derivates (stimulate insulin secretion)
  - Biguanides, thiazolidinediones (alter insulin action)
  - Alpha glucosidase inhibitors (affect glucose absorption)
  - Combination medications such as glyburide/metformin, rosiglitazone/metformin)
- Incretins (glucagon-like peptide analogs)

• Insulins (rapid, short, intermediate, long acting and pre-mixed preparations)

Optimal care has a marked influence on the disease prognosis, limiting complications such as microvascular disease.

Additional Therapies
• Antihypertensive management (BP goal <130/80 mm Hg)
• Treatment of dyslipidemia (LDL goal <100)
• Monitoring of renal functions and proteinuria (considering ACE-inhibitor therapy)
• Regular podiatric and ophthalmologic evaluations
• Aggressive wound care and treatment of infections such as candidiasis
• Treatment of autonomic neuropathies and erectile dysfunction
• Vaccinations (influenza, pneumovaccine)

MEDICATION–INDUCED POLYURIA

Diuretics are a common cause of polyuria. Polyuria also occurs in up to 20% of patients on chronic lithium therapy; an additional 30% have subclinical impairment in concentration ability, explained by either the decreased density of the ADH receptors or the decreased expression of aquaporin-2.

Symptoms
• Moderate polyuria ++++
• Polydipsia

Signs
• Moderate polyuria
• Polydipsia

The polyuria may be blunted by potassium administration and by once daily dosing of lithium. Nephrogenic DI may resolve about 8 weeks after cessation of lithium therapy.

Certain other medications including demeclocycline, cidofovir, foscarnet, amphotericin B, ifosfamide, ofloxacin, and orlistat can cause nephrogenic DI.

POLYURIA ASSOCIATED WITH INTERSTITIAL CYSTITIS

Patients with interstitial cystitis experience pain with bladder filling/distention, which is relieved by voiding. It is often associated with urinary urgency and frequency. Interstitial cystitis is a diagnosis of exclusion, and requires negative urine cultures as well as negative urine cytology. Other etiologies such as pelvic radiation or chemical cystitis, vaginitis, genital herpes, and urethral cancer or diverticula need to be excluded.

The majority of cases occur in women, ages 40 years and older. Fifty percent of patients experience spontaneous remissions of symptoms; the mean duration of the disease is 8 months without treatment. The exact etiology of interstitial cystitis in unknown.

It may represent several diseases with similar symptomologies. Possible causes include increased epithelial permeability, autoimmunity, and neurogenic factors. Interstitial cystitis may be associated with severe allergies, IBS, and IBD.

Symptoms
- Pain with bladder filling; relieved with urination ++++
- Urinary urgency and frequency +++
- Dyspareunia
- Urge incontinence (if bladder capacity is small)

Signs
- Frequency ++++
- Nocturia

Workup
- Urine analysis and culture to exclude infectious causes
- Urine cytology to exclude malignancy
- Urodynamic testing to assess bladder sensation and compliance, and to exclude detrussor instability
- Cystoscopy: glomerulations (submucosal hemorrhages) detected with bladder filling
- Biopsies to exclude malignancy, eosinophilic cystitis, tuberculous cystitis

Comments and Treatment Considerations
There is no specific cure for interstitial cystitis. Most patients achieve symptomatic relief from one or more of the following approaches:
- Hydrodistention (patients with a bladder capacity of <200 mL are unlikely to respond to medical therapy)
- Oxybutynin, hyoscyamine, or doxepin to decrease frequency
- Amitriptyline therapy
- Nifedipine/calcium channel blockers
- NSAIDs for pain relief and antiinflammatory effect
- Pentosan polysulfate sodium (Elmiron)—Helps restore epithelial integrity
- Intravesical instillation of dimethyl sulfoxide (DMSO), heparin, bacille Calmette-Guérin (BCG)
- Surgery (augmentation cystoplasty or cystourethrectomy with urinary diversion) as a last resort

Additional Therapies
- TENS and acupuncture may be useful. In milder cases exacerbations are followed by remissions. In severe cases, progressive disease usually requires surgery for symptom control.

References
Rose BD, Post TW: *Clinical physiology of acid-base and electrolyte disorders*, 5th ed, New York, 2001, McGraw-Hill, pp 748–757, 767–772.

Tierney LM, et al: *Current medical diagnosis and treatment*, 45th ed, New York, 2006, McGraw-Hill, pp 949–950, 1108–1109, 1198.

CHAPTER 35

Rashes

Richard Stringham, Evan Sihotang, John Cheng,
Himadri M. Patel, and Elizabeth Eddy-Bertrand

At least 30% of outpatient visits to family physicians involve a dermatologic issue. It is helpful to organize skin conditions in terms of their appearance and cause. The appearance of skin changes can be organized based on the primary skin lesions present (e.g., macule, patch, papule) and secondary skin lesion characteristics (scales, crusts, lichenification). The distribution pattern of skin rashes can often help in narrowing the differential diagnosis. Broad categories for causes of skin conditions include infections, immunologic causes, dermatitis conditions, and cancers. We have attempted to include the most recent treatment recommendations in the Comments and Treatment Considerations sections.

ACNE

Acne is one of the most common skin conditions seen by family physicians. Acne vulgaris and rosacea are its two main subgroups. Acne vulgaris affects more than 20 million Americans including more than 85% of adolescents. Rosacea affects mainly middle-aged and older adults.

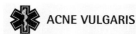 **ACNE VULGARIS**

Symptoms
- Pain, pressure-like feeling, pruritus +++++

Signs
- Acne affects those areas with the most number of sebaceous glands which includes the face, neck, chest, upper arms, and upper back. +++++
- With mild acne, patients have occasional small inflamed papules or pustules. The papules are called comedones and may appear as whiteheads (closed comedones) or blackheads (open comedones).
- As the acne progresses, the comedones and pustules become more prominent and scarring can develop (Fig. 35-1).
- With more severe acne, numerous large cysts can develop along with surrounding erythema and ultimately significant scarring (Fig. 35-2).

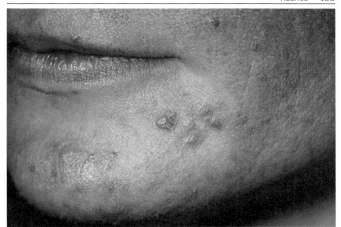

FIGURE 35-1 Chin acne. *(From Schwarzenberger K, Werchniak AE, Ko C:* Requisites in dermatology, *Philadelphia, 2009, Saunders.)*

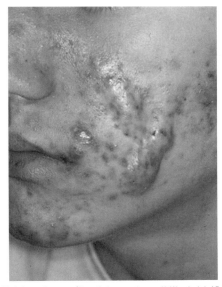

FIGURE 35-2 Nodulocystic acne. *(From Schwarzenberger K, Werchniak AE, Ko C:* Requisites in dermatology, *Philadelphia, 2009, Saunders.)*

Workup
- Acne vulgaris is diagnosed clinically, but a complete history is important especially in the nonadolescent patient or a patient with rapidly progressive acne. These situations may indicate a systemic cause such as PCOS or an adrenal tumor. +
- Other PCOS signs may include menstrual irregularities (most commonly oligomenorrhea), hirsutism, ovarian cysts, and acanthosis nigricans. +++
- Signs of elevated androgen levels other than progressive acne include deepening voice, decreased breast size, alopecia, oligomenorrhea, and hirsutism. ++++
- An evaluation for these conditions may include a pelvic ultrasound, hormone levels, and possibly an endocrinology consult.

Comments and Treatment Considerations
There are no definitive guidelines for acne treatment, but it should be based on the type of lesion present. It is important to note that it takes 8 weeks for microcomedones to mature, so any treatment adjustment must be continued for at least that long to see an effect.

For comedonal or mild inflammatory acne, topical preparations are best. These include the topical retinoids tretinoin (Retin A), adapalene (Differin), and tazarotene (Tazorac). Results of multiple studies do not definitively argue for one of these retinoid creams over the others. It is best to start with lower doses of the creams to minimize skin sensitivity and to apply at night to lessen photosensitivity. Other topical agents that can be used include benzoyl peroxide and topical antibiotics.

For moderate to severe inflammatory acne oral antibiotic treatment should be considered. These include tetracycline, doxycycline, and minocycline among others. It is generally recommended for oral antibiotic treatment to begin with higher doses and then to decrease the dose over time.

Oral isotretinoin (Accutane) can be considered for severe acne that has not responded to other treatments. Due to significant potential adverse effects, the FDA has placed restrictions on prescribing Accutane.

CONTACT DERMATITIS

 ALLERGIC CONTACT DERMATITIS

Allergic contact dermatitis is an acquired inflammatory reaction of the skin. It represents a delayed hypersensitivity reaction. Common causes include poison ivy, poison oak, nickel, hair dyes, soaps, detergents, and cleaning agents.

Symptoms
- Pruritus ++++

Signs

- Papules, vesicles, bullae with surrounding erythema, localized to the site of the allergen contact +++++
  - Crusting and oozing may be present (Fig. 35-3). ++
  - Scaling +++
  - Thickening and lichenification +++

Workup

- Clinical diagnosis—Configuration and location often are clues to the allergen. ++++
  - Patch testing—If unclear

Comments and Treatment Considerations

- Identify and avoid allergens.
- Corticosteroids

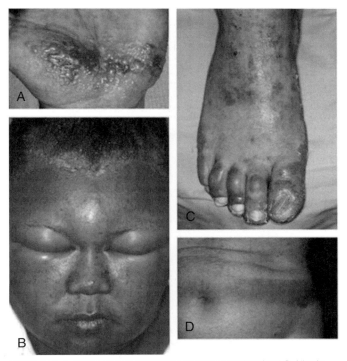

FIGURE 35-3 A, Allergic contact dermatitis to neoprene in keyboard pad. B, Allergic contact dermatitis to paraphenylenediamine. C, Allergic contact dermatitis. D, Bleached rubber dermatitis.

- Topical—Caution in using high potency especially on the face and skinfolds
- Oral—When dermatitis involves greater than 10% of skin surface
- Antihistamines: oral and topical
- Aveeno bath
- Wet dressings soaked in Burow's solution help relieve itching, reduce redness, and debride crusts.

 IRRITANT CONTACT DERMATITIS

Irritant contact dermatitis results from exposure to substances that cause physical, mechanical, or chemical irritation of the skin. Common causes include frequent soaping of skin, lip licking, and thumb sucking.

Symptoms
- Pruritus ++++

Signs
- Skin is dry, cracked, and chapped with macular erythema (Fig. 35-4). +++++

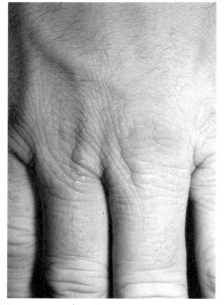

FIGURE 35-4 Irritant dermatitis. *(From Schwarzenberger K, Werchniak AE, Ko C: Requisites in dermatology, Philadelphia, 2009, Saunders.)*

Workup
• Clinical diagnosis

Comments and Treatment Considerations
Identify and avoid the irritant. Recommend applying moisturizers at least twice per day and avoiding excessive washing.

ROSACEA

Symptoms
• Burning and stinging of skin with facial flushing and can have pain or pressure with cystic lesions ++++

Signs
• Variable presentation depending on subtype present, but most patients initially have facial erythema and telangiectasias ++++
• Patients may have recurrent episodes of flushing especially on the face in response to exercise or embarrassment.
• A large subgroup has the papulopustular type with small papules and very small pustules with a red central portion of the face (Fig. 35-5). ++++
• A smaller subgroup has the phymatous subtype that has skin thickening and nodularities especially on the nose. ++

Workup
• Clinical diagnosis

Comments and Treatment Considerations
Treatment of mild rosacea can include topical antibiotics (metronidazole) and benzoyl peroxide. When symptoms worsen tretinoin (Retin A) and/or oral antibiotics (tetracycline, erythromycin, minocycline) can be used.

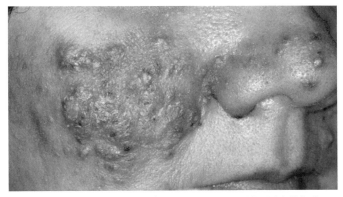

FIGURE 35-5 Papulopustular rosacea. *(From Schwarzenberger K, Werchniak AE, Ko C: Requisites in dermatology, Philadelphia, 2009, Saunders.)*

It is important to note that rosacea is a chronic condition with no curative treatment that has periods or exacerbations and remissions.

CHILDHOOD EXANTHEMS

Although the significant majority of children with exanthems have benign, self-limiting illnesses, more serious conditions can present with similar signs and symptoms. The appearance, distribution, and progression of the rash are very helpful in making an accurate diagnosis. Also, an awareness of associated symptoms including cough, conjunctivitis, arthralgias, and fever and their temporal association with the rash can assist in making the diagnosis. A history of exposure to infectious illnesses and the age of the patient may help narrow the differential.

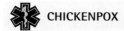 **CHICKENPOX**

Symptoms
- No prodrome in young children; low-grade fever, malaise with rash onset +++++
- Older children and adults—Fever, chills, headache, cough may precede rash by 2 to 3 days +++
- Rash very pruritic ++++
- Rarely CNS complications (i.e., transverse myelitis) 11 to 20 days after rash +

Signs
- Unique feature—Exanthem has lesions in different stages at same time +++++
- Rash begins on face or scalp, then spreads to trunk, relatively sparing extremities +++++
- Rapid progression of lesions 2 to 3 mm in size from rose colored macules, to papules, to vesicles, to pustules, to crusts (Fig. 35-6) +++++
- Early vesicle surrounded by irregular area of erythema ("dew drop on a rose pedal") ++++
- New lesions appear in crops or clusters. ++++
- Crusts fall off in 1 to 3 weeks. Healing lesions may hypopigment for weeks to months. ++++

Workup
- Clinical diagnosis is available by testing with direct fluorescence assay (DFA) or PCR testing. ++++
- A fourfold increase in varicella IgG level is also confirmatory.

Comments and Treatment Considerations
Treatment—Acyclovir is effective for primary varicella infections in both healthy and immunocompromised patients. Acyclovir

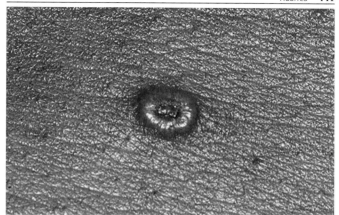

FIGURE 35-6 Varicella (chickenpox). *(From Schwarzenberger K, et al:* Requisites in dermatology, *Philadelphia, 2009, Saunders.)*

is not currently approved for children less than 2 years of age. Valacyclovir safety has not been assessed in prepubertal children. There is a significantly decreased incidence with widespread use of vaccine.

 ## ERYTHEMA INFECTIOSUM

Symptoms
- Healthy appearing with nonspecific signs of headache, coryza, low-grade fever for 2 days prior to rash onset ++++
- 10% have arthralgias; large joints more commonly affected ++

Signs
- Rash begins with confluent, erythematous edematous plaques on cheeks ("slapped cheeks") that fades in 1 to 4 days +++++
- Rash spreads rapidly to trunk and extensor surfaces of proximal extremities but spares the palms and soles +++++
- Rash can be morbilliform, confluent, or annular with central clearing of lesions causing a lacy reticulated appearance ++++
- The rash can wax and wane for 1 to 3 weeks. ++

Workup
- Clinical diagnosis

Comments and Treatment Considerations
The treatment is symptomatic. There can be a transient aplastic crisis in patients with hemolytic anemias (SS disease).

HAND–FOOT–MOUTH DISEASE

Symptoms
- Brief prodrome of 12 to 24 hours of low-grade fever, malaise, and abdominal pain ++++
- Oral lesions usually painful and can interfere with eating +++
- Skin lesions may be asymptomatic, tender, or painful.

Signs
- Oral lesions begin as macules (2 to 8 mm), then progress to gray thin-walled rounded vesicles surrounded by erythema, then erythematous erosions. Lesions resolve in 5 to 10 days. +++++
- Cutaneous lesions appear together with or shortly after oral lesions. ++++
- Each skin lesion begins as an erythematous macule or papule 2 to 10 mm and then develops into gray round/oval vesicle (Fig. 35-7). ++++
- Dorsal surfaces of hand and sides of fingers are more affected than feet. ++++
- Its peripheral distribution is unique for childhood exanthems.

Workup
- Clinical diagnosis

Comments and Treatment Considerations
Treatment is symptomatic. The cause is by enteroviruses, most commonly coxsackievirus A16.

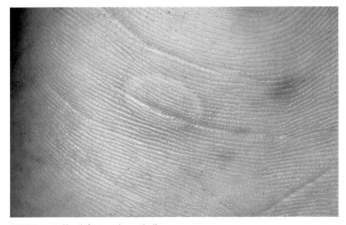

FIGURE 35-7 Hand, foot, and mouth disease.

KAWASAKI'S DISEASE

Symptoms
- Irritable and feverish in acute febrile stage ++++
- Anorexia, urethritis, arthritis/arthralgia, abdominal pain, or vomiting may occur. +++

Signs
- Must have fever of 5 or more days' duration without other explainable cause +++++
- And must have at least four of the five following signs:
  - Bilateral nonexudative conjunctivitis ++++
  - Oropharynx change (injected fissured lips, pharyngitis, strawberry tongue) ++++
  - Extremity changes (erythema or edema palms/soles, or periungual desquamation) (Fig. 35-8) ++++
  - Polymorphous exanthema can be quite variable but is not vesicular. ++++
  - Acute, nonsuppurative cervical lymphadenopathy +++

Workup
- No specific laboratory tests exist but can have elevation of ESR, CRP, or platelets +++
- Echocardiogram is important to evaluate for coronary artery aneurysms.

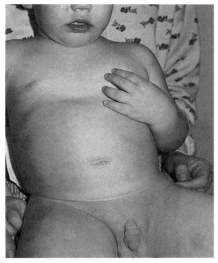

FIGURE 35-8 Kawasaki's disease. *(From White G: Color atlas of dermatology, 3rd ed, Philadelphia, 2004, Mosby.)*

Comments and Treatment Considerations

Treatment is IVIg and high-dose aspirin (80 to 100 mg/kg/day orally divided four times daily) to reduce cardiac complications.

 MEASLES

Symptoms
- High fever (104° F), cough, coryza, conjunctivitis that precedes rash and lasts 3 to 4 days +++++

Signs
- Oral lesions—Koplik's spots are small, irregular, bright red spots that appear within 24 to 48 hours of symptoms and precede rash by about 1 day. ++++
- Rash—Erythematous, discrete maculopapular lesion that starts behind ears and forehead, spreads down over neck and trunk (Fig. 35-9), then spreads distally to arms and legs including hands and feet. Rash worse on third day. +++++
- Face/trunk—Rash confluent; arms/legs; lesions discrete +++++

Workup
- Clinical diagnosis +++++
- Can obtain measles IgM titer or check for rise in measles IgG

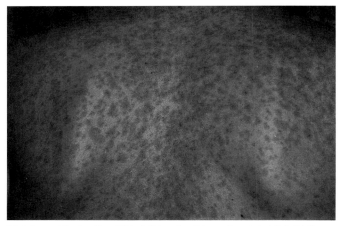

FIGURE 35-9 Measles. *(From White G: Color atlas of dermatology, 3rd ed, Philadelphia, 2004, Mosby.)*

Comments and Treatment Considerations
Symptomatic Treatment
The incidence has significantly decreased since the 1963 vaccine but outbreaks have occurred since that time. Complications are encephalitis and secondary bacterial infections—subacute sclerosing panencephalitis (SSPE)—which results in rapid motor and mental deterioration.

 ## MENINGOCOCCEMIA

Signs
- Caused by *Neisseria meningitidis*
- Adolescent patient with an initial maculopapular rash who develops serious signs including meningitis and septic shock
- May rapidly develop extensive petechiae and purpura (purpura fulminans)

 ## ROCKY MOUNTAIN SPOTTED FEVER

Signs
- Children who are ill appearing
- Maculopapular rash starting in the extremities
- Involves the palms and soles that becomes petechial or hemorrhagic

 ## ROSEOLA

Symptoms
- Fever (102° to 105° F) for 3 to 5 days then rapid defervescence ++++
- Frequently mild URI symptoms but most children are very healthy appearing

Signs
- Rash onset usually correlates with fever subsiding ++++
- Rash is erythematous and macular or maculopapular lasting 1 to 2 days with 2- to 5-mm lesions that blanch under pressure, often with a surrounding whitish ring +++++
- Most prominent on neck and trunk, but proximal extremities and face may be affected +++
- Can have oral lesions: ulcers or erythematous macules ++

Workup
- Clinical diagnosis

Comments and Treatment Considerations
Roseola is caused by HSV-6 and the illness is also known as fifth disease or exanthem subitum. Treatment is supportive; the peak incidence occurs between 7 and 13 months of age and is rare beyond 4 years of age.

 RUBELLA

Symptoms
- Young children—Minimal if any constitutional symptoms ++++
- Older children—Low-grade fever, headache, cough for 1 to 4 days prior to rash +++
- Rash often pruritic ++++

Signs
- Lymphadenopathy precedes rash and is significant especially in posterior cervical region.++++
- Rash—Pink-red discrete macules and papules that appear on trunk and coalesce and give it a uniform red blush; rapid disappearance of rash is in contrast to measles ++++

Workup
- Clinical diagnosis with rubella IgM or IgG titer rise being confirmatory ++++

Comments and Treatment Considerations
The treatment is symptomatic. If the patient is pregnant, a perinatology evaluation and high level ultrasound is indicated. 50% of infants with acquired rubella in the first trimester show signs of fetal damage, and the earlier the exposure the more severe the damage.

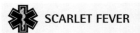 **SCARLET FEVER**

Symptoms
- Onset of sore throat and fever precedes rash. ++++

Signs
- Rash appears 12 to 48 hours after onset of pharyngitis symptoms. ++++
- Rash is a diffuse finely papular, erythematous eruption producing bright red discoloration that feels rough ("sandpaper rash"). ++++
- Rash is more intense along creases of elbows, axillae, and groin (Pastia's lines). ++
- Rash fades in 3 to 4 days then desquamates, first on face then downward ("sunburn"). +++
- Oropharynx examination consistent with strep throat and often has "strawberry tongue" +++

Workup
- Clinical diagnosis but can do strep culture for confirmation ++++
- Rapid strep test has poor sensitivity (around 85%)

Comments and Treatment Considerations
This condition is highly sensitive to penicillin and thus it is the first-line medication. It is also sensitive to azithromycin and other macrolides. There is generally no need for antibiotics with broader coverage such as Augmentin or cephalosporins. The differential diagnosis includes Kawasaki's disease, drug eruptions, rubella, and measles.

 TOXIC SHOCK SYNDROME

Signs
- Abrupt onset of high fever
- Ill-appearing patient with a diffuse erythematous rash that is sunburn-like

 WINTER EXANTHEMS

Symptoms
- Nasal congestion, cough usually preceding rash ++++
- Rash—Usually asymptomatic ++++

Signs
- Rash usually mildly erythematous and maculopapular, and of short duration ++++
- Variable presentations due to many different viruses causing winter exanthems

Workup
- Clinical diagnosis

Comments and Treatment Considerations
The treatment is symptomatic. 5% to 10% of these infections are caused by parainfluenza viruses, RSV, and influenza A and B. These are frequently confused with drug rashes, particularly amoxicillin.

 ZOSTER

Symptoms
- Pain and paresthesias precede rash in affected dermatome ++++
- Pain quality and severity varies. May simulate appendicitis, pleurisy, etc. +++++

Signs

- Dermatomal distribution of rash is distinctive, usually unilateral and involving only one dermatome ++++
- T3-L2 most common dermatomes affected
- 10% of zoster involves ophthalmic division of trigeminal nerve. Of these 30% have involvement of tip of nose (nasociliary branch) and can have potential complications in the eye (keratosis, scleritis). ++

Workup

- This is a clinical diagnosis but can do testing as described in chickenpox workup section. +++++

Comments and Treatment Considerations

Start antivirals if less than 72 hours since rash first appeared. If more than 72 hours and new lesions appear consider starting treatment. See chickenpox section for comments on acyclovir and valacyclovir. Simultaneous prednisone treatment may be considered if initial symptoms are severe. Steroids speed lesion healing, decrease pain, but do not affect postherpetic neuralgia. Prednisone dose is 1 to 2 mg/kg/day PO with 7- to 10-day taper.

DIAPER DERMATITIS

Diaper rash is a general term for various inflammatory conditions in the diaper area, but its common starting point is wet skin under a diaper. Prevention involves frequent diaper changes, leaving the diaper off as much as possible, and gentle skin care. Breastfed babies have a lower incidence of diaper rash.

Signs

- The irritative pattern ("the hills"), a mild red peeling rash on the convex surfaces that touch the diaper, sparing the inguinal folds ++
- The skinfold pattern ("the valleys"), moist macerated symmetric rashes in skinfolds and creases. This is often due to *Candida* and may follow oral antibiotic use. +++

Workup

- A thorough history of the rash
- Generally, tests are not indicated.

Comments and Treatment Considerations

To treat the irritative rash, stop using harsh soaps, detergents, or products with fragrances or alcohol; recommend mild fatty soap or non-soap cleansers for bathing. Use only water-based alcohol and fragrance-free diaper wipes. Use a barrier cream or ointment (NOTE: these may worsen candida). Use disposable diapers with absorbent gel material that wicks away moisture; vapor-permeable coverings have also been shown to be helpful. If using cloth diapers, wash at high temperature using fragrance-free and enzyme-free detergents. Do not use plastic pants.

If rash has been present for more than 72 hours, the presence of *Candida* is likely. If rash is moderate to severe, consider using hydrocortisone 1% for the first day or two of treatment. Do not use longer than 2 weeks. If rash does not respond, alternative diagnoses in the same distribution are:

- Atopic dermatitis (uncommon in infants younger than 6 months)
- Bacterial superinfection: impetiginous pattern with thin-walled blisters
- Zinc deficiency, either inherited (acrodermatitis enteropathica) or acquired
- Kawasaki's disease
- Wiskott-Aldrich syndrome: X-linked, with severe eczema and petechiae

To treat the skinfold rash (or rash lasting more than 72 hours), in addition to treatments for the irritative rash, use topical antifungals. Creams or ointments have better penetration and effectiveness than powders. Simultaneous use of hydrocortisone 1% hastens healing. No greater strength should be used because of local and systemic side effects. Steroid-antifungal mixes contain stronger steroids than are safe. If rash does not respond, alternative diagnoses in the distribution as the skinfold pattern rash are:

- Seborrheic dermatitis—Salmon-colored, greasy lesions with yellowish scale in skinfolds; look for similar rash on scalp, face, neck, behind ears
- Psoriasiform dermatitis—Beefy red, confluent, silvery scales, involving the entire diaper area but with skinfold areas more prominent
- Letterer-Siwe disease (histiocytosis)—More papular and more likely to be ulcerated than *Candida*. Look for constitutional symptoms and abnormal examination findings such as hepatosplenomegaly.
- HIV or DM may rarely present as severe persistent or recurrent *Candida* infections resulting from immunosuppression.

DRUG RASHES

Drug rashes manifest through two mechanisms: immunologic and nonimmunologic. Immunologic mechanisms present as one of the following four types: type I, IgE-dependent reactions; type II, cytotoxic reactions; type III, immune complex reactions; and type IV, delayed-type reactions. Nonimmunologic drug rashes present as an accumulated, direct release of mast cell mediators, overdosage, and/or phototoxicity.

Signs
- Most reactions occur within 1 to 2 weeks.

Workup
- Skin examination
- Medication list including dose, route, frequency, and when started
- Recent changes in medications
- Relation to when medications started or stopped
- Biopsy if needed

Comments and Treatment Considerations
Epidemiology for drug rashes includes a higher female-to-male ratio and higher risk for older adult patients.

Treatment should include any of the following as necessary: stop affecting agent; administer antihistamines (i.e., Benadryl, Claritin, Atarax); supportive treatment; steroids: topical (symptomatic relief) or systemic (if severe); epinephrine and hospitalization for severe cases; immunoglobulins if appropriate.

Symptoms
- Inflammatory papules
- Pustular lesions

Common Drug Associations
- Amoxapine
- Corticosteroids
- Halogens
- Haloperidol
- Hormones
- Isoniazid
- Lithium
- Phenobarbital
- Phenytoin
- Trazodone

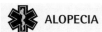 **ALOPECIA**

Symptoms
- Hair loss

Common Drug Associations
- ACE inhibitors
- Allopurinol
- Anticoagulants
- Azathioprine
- Bromocriptine
- Beta-blockers
- Cyclophosphamide
- Didanosine
- Hormones
- Indinavir
- NSAIDs

- Phenytoin
- Methotrexate (MTX)
- Retinoids
- Valproate

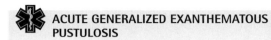 ## ACUTE GENERALIZED EXANTHEMATOUS PUSTULOSIS

Symptoms
- Small, sterile, nonfollicular pustules
- Generalized scarlatiniform erythema
- Fever

 ## BULLAE

Symptoms
- Bullous, blister-like lesions

Common Drug Associations
- Ampicillin
- D-penicillamine
- Captopril
- Chloroquine
- Ciprofloxacin
- Enalapril
- Furosemide
- Neuroleptics
- Penicillins
- Phenacetin
- Psoralen plus UVA
- Salicylazosulfapyridine
- Sulfasalazine
- Terbinafine

 ## DERMATOMYOSITIS-LIKE RASHES

Symptoms
- Violet-colored or dusky red rash
- Usually in areas of the skin that are sensitive to the sun

Common Drug Associations
- BCG vaccine
- Hydroxyurea ++++
- Lovastatin
- Penicillamine
- Simvastatin
- Tegafur

ERYTHEMA MULTIFORME

 ERYTHEMA MULTIFORME MINOR

Symptoms
• Target lesions distributed on the extremities
• Mucous membranes

Comments and Treatment Considerations
Most cases are due to infection with herpes simplex virus, and treatment and prophylaxis with acyclovir is helpful.

 STEVENS–JOHNSON SYNDROME

Symptoms
• Widespread skin involvement
• Large and atypical targetoid lesions
• Significant mucous membrane involvement
• Constitutional symptoms are present
• Sloughing of the skin may develop

Common Drug Associations
• Allopurinol
• Anticonvulsants
• Aspirin/NSAIDs
• Barbiturates
• Carbamazepine
• Cimetidine
• Ciprofloxacin
• Codeine
• Didanosine
• Diltiazem
• Erythromycin
• Furosemide
• Griseofulvin
• Hydantoin
• Indinavir
• Nitrogen mustard
• Penicillin
• Phenothiazine
• Phenylbutazone
• Phenytoin
• Ramipril
• Rifampicin
• Saquinavir
• Sulfonamides
• Tetracyclines
• TMP-SMX

TOXIC EPIDERMAL NECROLYSIS

Symptoms
- Severe skin reaction +++
- Prodrome of painful skin quickly followed by rapid, widespread, full-thickness skin sloughing
- Affects 30% or more of the total body surface area
- Secondary infection is a major concern.

Common Drug Associations
- Allopurinol
- Anticonvulsants
- Aspirin/NSAIDs
- Sulfadoxine and pyrimethamine (Fansidar)
- Isoniazid
- Penicillins
- Phenytoin
- Prazosin
- Sulfonamides
- Tetracyclines
- Thalidomide
- TMP-SMX
- Vancomycin

 ERYTHEMA NODOSUM

Symptoms
- Reactive red nodules
- Usually appear on the anterior part of the lower legs

Common Drug Associations
- Echinacea
- Halogens
- Oral contraceptives ++++
- Penicillin
- Sulfonamides
- Tetracycline

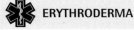 **ERYTHRODERMA**

Symptoms
- Inflammation of a large portion of the body's skin

Common Drug Associations
- Allopurinol
- Anticonvulsants

- Barbiturates
- Captopril
- Carbamazepine
- Cefoxitin
- Chloroquine
- Chlorpromazine
- Cimetidine
- Diltiazem
- Griseofulvin
- Lithium
- Nitrofurantoin
- Omeprazole
- Phenytoin
- St John's wort
- Sulfonamides
- Thalidomide

 FIXED DRUG ERUPTIONS

Symptoms
- Skin lesions that occur in the same area every time the offending drug is taken
- Circular
- Violaceous
- Edematous plaques that resolve and cause some macular hyper-pigmentation
- Sites commonly affected are the hands, feet, and genitalia

Common Drug Associations
- Acetaminophen
- Ampicillin
- Anticonvulsants
- Aspirin/NSAIDs
- Barbiturates
- Benzodiazepines
- Butalbital
- Cetirizine
- Ciprofloxacin
- Clarithromycin
- Dapsone
- Dextromethorphan
- Doxycycline
- Fluconazole
- Hydroxyzine
- Lamotrigine
- Loratadine
- Metronidazole
- Oral contraceptives
- Penicillins
- Phenacetin
- Phenolphthalein

- Phenytoin
- Piroxicam
- Saquinavir
- Sulfonamides
- Tetracyclines
- Ticlopidine
- Tolmetin
- Vancomycin
- Zolmitriptan

 HYPERSENSITIVITY SYNDROME

Symptoms
- Fever
- Sore throat
- Skin rash
- Lymphadenopathy
- Hepatitis
- Nephritis
- Leukocytosis with eosinophilia
- Potentially a life-threatening reaction

Common Drug Associations
- Allopurinol
- Amitriptyline
- Carbamazepine
- Dapsone
- Lamotrigine
- Minocycline
- NSAIDs
- Olanzapine
- Oxcarbazepine
- Phenobarbital
- Phenytoin
- Saquinavir
- Spironolactone
- Sulfonamides
- Zalcitabine
- Zidovudine

 LICHENOID RASHES

Symptoms
- Extremely pruritic reaction that looks similar to lichen planus

Common Drug Associations
- Amlodipine
- Antimalarials
- Beta-blockers

- Captopril
- Diflunisal
- Diltiazem
- Enalapril
- Furosemide
- Glimepiride
- Gold
- Leflunomide
- Levamisole
- L-thyroxine
- Penicillamine
- Phenothiazine
- PPIs
- Rofecoxib
- Salsalate
- Sildenafil
- Tetracycline
- Thiazides
- Ursodeoxycholic acid

 LUPUS

Symptoms
- Annular psoriasiform
- Nonscarring lesions in a photodistributed pattern

Common Drug Associations
- Drug-induced systemic lupus erythematosus (SLE)
  - Hydralazine
  - Procainamide
  - Minocycline
  - Beta-blockers
  - Chlorpromazine
  - Cimetidine
  - Clonidine
  - Estrogens
  - Isoniazid
  - Lithium
  - Lovastatin
  - Methyldopa
  - Oral contraceptives
  - Quinidine
  - Sulfonamides
  - Tetracyclines
  - TNF-α inhibitors
- Drug-induced subacute cutaneous lupus erythematosus
  - Hydrochlorothiazide
  - Calcium channel blockers
  - Cimetidine

- Griseofulvin
- Leflunomide
- Terbinafine
- TNF-α inhibitors

 MORBILIFORM RASHES

Symptoms
- Rash is symmetric
- Confluent erythematous macules
- Papules that spare the palms and soles
- Also known as an exanthematous eruption

Common Drug Associations
- ACE inhibitors
- Allopurinol
- Amoxicillin
- Ampicillin
- Anticonvulsants
- Barbiturates
- Carbamazepine
- Cetirizine
- Ginkgo biloba
- Hydroxyzine
- Isoniazid
- Nelfinavir
- NSAIDs
- Phenothiazine
- Phenytoin
- Quinolones
- Sulfonamides
- Thalidomide
- Thiazides
- TMP-SMX
- Zalcitabine

 PEMPHIGOUS RASHES

Symptoms
- Rash involving pruritic blisters

Common Drug Associations
- Thiols
  - Captopril
  - D-penicillamine
  - Gold sodium thiomalate

- Mercaptopropionyl glycine
- Pyritinol
- Thiamazole
- Thiopronine
- Nonthiols
  - Aminophenazone
  - Aminopyrine
  - Azapropazone
  - Cephalosporins
  - Heroin
  - Hydantoin
  - Imiquimod
  - Indapamide
  - Levodopa
  - Lysine acetylsalicylate
  - Montelukast
  - Oxyphenbutazone
  - Penicillins
  - Phenobarbital
  - Phenylbutazone
  - Piroxicam
  - Progesterone
  - Propranolol
  - Rifampicin

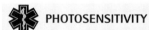 **PHOTOSENSITIVITY**

Symptoms
- Can manifest in many forms
- Usually a sunburn-like rash or dermatitis
- Occurs on sun-exposed portions of the body

Common Drug Associations
- ACE inhibitors
- Amiodarone
- Amlodipine
- Celecoxib
- Chlorpromazine
- Diltiazem
- Furosemide
- Griseofulvin
- Lovastatin
- Nifedipine
- Phenothiazine
- Piroxicam
- Quinolones
- Sulfonamides
- Tetracycline
- Thiazide

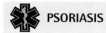 **PSORIASIS**

Symptoms
• Psoriatic rash

Common Drug Associations
• ACE inhibitors
• Angiotensin receptor antagonists
• Antimalarials
• Beta-blockers
• Bupropion
• Calcium channel blockers
• Carbamazepine
• Interferon-alpha
• Lithium
• Metformin
• NSAIDs
• Terbinafine
• Tetracyclines
• Valproate sodium

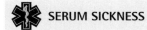 **SERUM SICKNESS**

Symptoms
• Cutaneous signs typically begin with erythema on the sides of fingers, hands, and toes and progress to a widespread eruption (most often morbilliform or urticarial)
• Fever
• Arthralgia
• Arthritis
• This is a type III hypersensitivity reaction.

Common Drug Associations
• Antithymocyte globulin for bone marrow failure
• Human rabies vaccine
• Vaccines containing horse serum derivatives

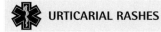 **URTICARIAL RASHES**

Symptoms
• Small wheals
• Large wheals that formed after several small wheals coalesced

Common Drug Associations
• ACE inhibitors
• Alendronate
• Aspirin/NSAIDs

- Blood products
- Cephalosporins
- Cetirizine
- Clopidogrel
- Dextran
- Didanosine
- Infliximab
- Inhaled steroids
- Nelfinavir
- Opiates
- Penicillin
- Peptide hormones
- Polymyxin
- PPIs
- Radiologic contrast material
- Ranitidine
- Tetracycline
- Vaccines
- Zidovudine

 VESICULOBULLOUS

Symptoms
- Can resemble pemphigus
- Bullous pemphigoid
- Linear IgA dermatosis
- Dermatitis herpetiformis
- Herpes gestationis
- Cicatricial pemphigoid
- Mucosal involvement commonly seen with nonthiol drugs

Common Drug Associations
- ACE inhibitors
- Aspirin/NSAIDs
- Barbiturates
- Captopril
- Cephalosporins
- Entacapone
- Estrogen
- Furosemide
- Griseofulvin
- Influenza vaccine
- Penicillamine
- Penicillins
- Sertraline sulfonamides
- Thiazides

ERYTHEMA MULTIFORME

Erythema multiforme (EM) is a cutaneous hypersensitivity reaction commonly associated with herpes simplex and *Mycoplasma* infections, but many etiologies have been reported.

Symptoms
- Viral prodrome including mild fever, malaise, sore throat +++
- Herpes simplex infection +++
- Itching and burning, followed by sudden onset of symmetric lesions over extremities ++
- Painful lip and oral blisters +++
- Other mucosal involvement: eyes, anogenital tract ++

Signs
- Target lesions: raised lesions having erythematous border with central blister, petechiae, or purpura ++++
- Lesions are symmetrically distributed, involving primarily extremities and the face. ++++
- Lip and buccal mucosal ulcers +++

Workup
- No specific laboratory testing is indicated because up to 50% of cases are idiopathic. Skin biopsy may be considered if diagnosis is not clear.

Comments and Treatment Considerations
EM is a self-limited condition and resolves in 2 to 4 weeks. Therefore, treatment should be supportive and symptom directed. Withdraw precipitating agents if known. Treatment of herpes infection with acyclovir or valacyclovir does not alter the course of EM. For severe disease, a 1- to 3-week course of prednisone (40 to 80 mg/day PO) with rapid taper is recommended.
- Limited data for treatment of recurrent or persistent EM (up to one third of cases):
  - High-dose corticosteroids
  - Acyclovir 400 mg twice a day PO for HSV-associated EM
  - Dapsone 100 to 150 mg PO daily
  - Azathioprine (100 to 150 mg PO daily), thalidomide (100 mg/day), and cyclosporine have been used for severe disease not responsive to other agents.

Scarring is uncommon, but hypopigmentation or hyperpigmentation is possible.

FUNGAL INFECTIONS

Fungal infections of the skin account for more than 6 million physician visits per year. The majority of these cases are seen by nondermatologists. Most of these infections are caused by dermatophytes, which are organisms that have acquired the ability to metabolize keratin. Accurate diagnosis is made by a combination of knowledge of the clinical presentation along with confirmatory testing. Potassium hydroxide (KOH) analysis is a confirmatory test that isolates the fungal elements under direct microscopy and is best performed when the specimen is obtained from the advancing margins of the lesion and the slide is gently heated. Various tissues can be sent for culture in Sabouraud's agar using antibiotics to suppress bacterial growth. Use of a Wood's lamp is helpful when the type of dermatophyte is *Microsporum*.

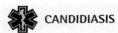 CANDIDIASIS

Symptoms
• Lesions usually pruritic but can be painful if significant skin breakdown occurs ++++

Signs
• Usually appears as erythematous macerated plaques and erosions with delicate peripheral scaling and erythematous satellite papulopustules ++++
• Typically located in areas where two skin surfaces closely oppose each other, which include the inguinal folds, axillae, scrotum, intergluteal folds, and abdominal folds (pannus) ++++

Workup
• Usually a clinical diagnosis, based on typical appearance and distribution of lesions. Can be confirmed by KOH examination, which reveals oval budding yeasts with septate hyphae and pseudohyphae (elongated, filamentous cells connected end to end) ++++

Comments and Treatment Recommendations
Effective topical treatments include nystatin, miconazole, clotrimazole, and ketoconazole creams. Use until resolution of lesions; may be used twice weekly after to prevent recurrences. Oral antifungal treatment, including fluconazole, itraconazole, and ketoconazole, can be used for extensive disease. Treatment should continue for 2 to 6 weeks.

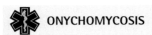 ONYCHOMYCOSIS

Symptoms
• Usually asymptomatic ++
• Can cause pain ++++

Signs

- Distal subungual onychomycosis—Begins with white, yellowish, or brownish discoloration of distal corner of nail that gradually spreads to the entire nail. Number one toenail usually affected first. Most common type causing 90% of onychomycosis ++++
- Proximal subungual onychomycosis—Affects proximal part of nail; uncommon +
- White superficial onychomycosis—Dull white spots on surface of nail plate +
- Yeast onychomycosis—Affects almost exclusively fingernails. Cause is *Candida*. +
- Mold onychomycosis—The clinical significance of nondermatophyte molds currently unclear +

Workup

- It is important to establish presence of fungus before starting antimycotic treatment because at least 50% of cases of nail dystrophy are *not* caused by onychomycosis. Other causes include trauma, lichen planus, psoriasis, and eczema.
- KOH scraping can be done but its sensitivity is variable depending on adequacy of specimen. +++
- Fungal culture of nail clippings of full thickness performed more often but sensitivity not much better than KOH; 30% of fungal cultures may be falsely negative so it is advised that if there is strong clinical suspicions repeat culture if first culture negative ++++
- For proximal subungual-type nail plate biopsy or partial/full nail removal with culture needed for confirmation ++++
- Dermatophyte test medium (DTM) can be performed in physician's office. Results available in 3 to 7 days and sensitivity/specificity similar to Sabouraud's fungal culture. ++++

Comments and Treatment Considerations

Indications for treatment are history of cellulitis of foot with ipsilateral onychomycosis, patients with diabetes mellitus, patients with discomfort/pain in infected nails, and patients' desire for cosmetic reasons (most common reason). A discussion with the patients about whether treatment is appropriate is important because onychomycosis treatment is often not effective (about 40% successful), recurrences are common, treatment may have potentially serious side effects (liver toxicity), and even when treatment is successful, nail normalization can take over 12 months after fungus is eliminated.

Topical treatments are generally ineffective. This includes ciclopirox (Penlac) in which only 7% of patients treated have complete resolution of onychomycosis. Data currently show terbinafine has greater efficacy and fewer serious side effects than other oral medications. Onychomycosis affects 8% of the population. Risk factors include older age, diabetes mellitus, tinea pedis, psoriasis, and immunodeficiency.

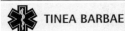 **TINEA BARBAE**

Symptoms
• Pruritus and pain in beard area of men exclusively ++++

Signs
• Limited to coarse-hair–bearing areas of beard and mustache of men
• Inflammatory—Unilateral, lesions nodular and boggy +++
• Superficial—Resembles bacterial folliculitis with pustules ++
• Actively spreading vesiculopustular border ++

Workup
• Clinical diagnosis with KOH confirmation. Culture can be done if needed. ++++

Comments and Treatment Considerations
Griseofulvin (1 g/day orally) continued for 2 to 3 weeks after clinical resolution.

 TINEA CAPITIS

Symptoms
• Asymptomatic at first ++
• If not treated can become pruritic or painful ++++

Signs
• "Black dot"—Most common type. Remnant of hair left behind in infected follicle appears as a black dot on clinical examination. ++++
• Can have various degrees of scaling, alopecia, and inflammation. The amount of alopecia and inflammation generally increases over time if not treated. +++++
• Lesions can develop rapidly into pustular folliculitis, furuncles, and kerions (intense inflammatory, boggy mass studded with broken hairs, oozing purulent material). ++

Workup
• Clinical evaluation combined with confirmatory testing, which can include KOH examination of the hair shaft (KOH scraping of the scale will *not* reveal fungus). Fungal culture can also be done for confirmation (entirely remove a few hair shafts and send to lab). ++++
• Wood's lamp is positive with *Microsporum canis* but this fungus only causes a very small percent of tinea capitis in the United States. +

Comments and Treatment Considerations
Topical treatment is futile. Griseofulvin, terbinafine, and itraconazole have currently shown equal effectiveness. When outbreaks occur it is important to identify asymptomatic carriers by cultures from hairs collected by brushing with a toothbrush and treating with selenium sulfide shampoo. It is largely a disease of childhood (4 months to 4 years). African Americans are at greater risk.

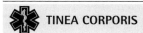 **TINEA CORPORIS**

Symptoms
• Usually pruritus ++++

Signs
• Diverse clinical presentation but begins as circular or oval erythematous scaling lesion that spreads centrifugally. Then central clearing follows, while active advancing border that is a few mm wide retains its original erythematous color and is slightly raised. +++++
• May occur throughout the body with exceptions of beard area in men (tinea barbae), groin (tinea cruris), feet (tinea pedis), or hand (tinea manuum).

Workup
• Because of the many diverse clinical presentations, KOH analysis is very helpful in confirming the diagnosis. Specimen best obtained from actively spreading border. ++++
• If vesicle or bulla sample, best obtained from roof of blister

Comments and Treatment Considerations
Usually responds very well with topical antifungals. Oral treatment may be necessary for patients who have failed topical treatment or when the infection is too extensive for topical treatment. Oral terbinafine, fluconazole, and itraconazole can be used. Avoid use of antifungal/steroid combination medications, which can make diagnosis of conditions difficult and are significantly more expensive than antifungal creams. Outbreaks occur in athletes, especially wrestlers (tinea corporis gladiatorum).

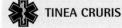 **TINEA CRURIS**

Symptoms
• Pruritus is the most common symptom, although painful if skin is macerated. ++++

Signs
• Begins as macular erythematous patch high on inner aspect of thighs opposite the scrotum, but *not* involving the scrotum. Then it spreads centrifugally with partial central clearing and slightly elevated erythematous border, which is sharply demarcated. In some cases it may extend onto perineum and perianal areas and onto the buttocks. ++++

Workup
• KOH examination of scales from active border confirmatory. Culture if needed. ++++

Comments and Treatment Considerations

Topical antifungals are usually effective. Resistant lesions can be treated with griseofulvin 250 mg three times a day for 14 days. Keeping the area dry with talcum or other desiccant powders and by wearing boxers instead of brief underwear are important in preventing recurrences. Risk factors for tinea cruris are obesity, warm climate, and concurrent tinea pedis.

 TINEA PEDIS

Symptoms
- Pruritus or pain in feet, especially between toes ++++

Signs
- Most common presentation is chronic intertriginous type in which there is fissuring, scaling, and maceration in interdigital and subdigital areas. This type is slow to progress and most commonly seen in fourth digital interspace. ++++
- Other types of tinea pedis include: (1) chronic papulosquamous pattern, a moccasin-like scaling over the soles, (2) vesicular or vesiculobullous type, and (3) acute ulcerative variant, which acutely develops maceration, weeping, and ulceration on the soles of feet. ++

Workup
- Clinical diagnosis with confirmatory KOH analysis. Culture rarely needed. ++++

Comments and Treatment Considerations

Generally all topical antifungal creams are equally effective. Interdigital tinea pedis requires only about 1 week of treatment. More involved infections may require approximately 4 weeks of treatment. Effective approach is to have patient use until skin appears normal and continue treatment for a few more days. Chronic, more extensive disease may require oral treatment (griseofulvin, terbinafine, or itraconazole). Adjunctive treatments include drying measures such as foot powders, drying feet well after bathing, and avoiding occlusive footwear when possible.

 TINEA VERSICOLOR

Symptoms
- Usually asymptomatic ++
- May have mild pruritus ++++

Signs
- Most commonly presents as scaly hypopigmented macules, but can be hyperpigmented and typically located on upper chest, upper back, and proximal extremities. Color of lesions vary (hence the name tinea versicolor) from almost white to reddish brown. +++++
- Individual lesions usually small, but often coalesce ++++

Workup
- Clinical diagnosis with KOH confirmation. Fungal culture/periodic acid–Schiff (PAS) staining if needed.++++

Comments and Treatment Considerations
Topical antifungal treatments effective for limited disease with 70% to 80% cure rates after 2 weeks of treatment. It is important to note that healing continues after active treatment stops and resumption of pigmentation can take many months. Oral treatment may be more convenient for patients with extensive disease and may be more effective in patients with recurrent infections. Most oral antifungals with the exception of griseofulvin or terbinafine may be used. Ketoconazole—400 mg single dose or 200 mg every day for 5 days—has a 90% cure rate at 4 weeks. Recurrences of tinea versicolor are very common and thus topical selenium sulfide solution applied to the body every 2 to 3 weeks can be helpful. The most common age group affected is late adolescent and early adulthood.

HENOCH–SCHÖNLEIN PURPURA

Henoch-Shönlein purpura (HSP) is the most common systemic vasculitis of childhood. It occurs between the ages of 3 to 15 years and has a incidence between 5 and 8 years of age. The annual incidence is 10 to 20 per 100,000. It has low incidence in summer months. It is more common in whites and Asians than in African Americans. Male to female ratio is 2:1. The etiology of HSP is unknown but it is thought be an IgA-mediated inflammatory vasculitis of small vessels. It can affect multiple organ systems including GI, renal, musculoskeletal, integumentary, and pulmonary.

Symptoms
- Rash—Asymptomatic +++++
- Arthralgia—Transient, oligoarticular (one to four joints). Usually localized to lower extremities ++++
- Abdominal pain, nausea, vomiting, diarrhea ++
- Low-grade fever, fatigue ++++
- Scrotal pain ++

Signs
- The clinical manifestations may develop acutely or over several days or weeks and vary in their order of presentation.

- Palpable purpura—The hallmark of the disease in 100% of patients +++++
  - Erythematous, macular, or urticarial wheals that then coalesce and progress to petechiae or palpable purpura. It usually occurs in crops, is symmetric, and lasts 3 to 10 days. Localized angio-edema may occur in buttocks or eyelids, lips, scrotum, or dorsum of the hands and feet.
  - The rash may recur intermittently for 3 to 4 months, in some cases up to 1 year from initial episode.
- Heme-positive stools ++
- Hepatosplenomegaly +++
- Lymphadenopathy ++++

Workup
- CBC to check platelet count
- Urinalysis and serum BUN/creatinine to evaluate degree of renal involvement and assess renal function +++
- LFTs, hepatitis serology and coagulation studies: hepatitis B has been reported with HSP
- Antistreptolysin O (ASO) titer to look for preceding streptococcal URI
- Antinuclear antibody (ANA), rheumatoid factor (RF), ESR, CRP to exclude SLE, RA, and check for inflammation
- Stool culture and guaiac to rule out infectious etiology and screen for occult bleeding with HSP
- Abdominal US and x-ray should be done in patients with significant abdominal pain to rule out intussusception or bowel wall perforation. Contrast enema studies cannot detect ileoileal intussusception typically seen in HSP and therefore are not helpful. +
- Chest x-ray to exclude pulmonary nodules or hilar adenopathy or lymphoma
- Skin biopsy to confirm diagnosis when in question
- Renal biopsy if proteinuria is in nephritic range
- Esophagogastroduodenoscopy: when severe GI symptoms or hematemesis present
- Colonoscopy: when severe rectal bleeding is present

Comments and Treatment Considerations
The outcome for children with HSP is excellent with 94% complete recovery. The majority of patients improve with adequate hydration, rest, and symptomatic relief of pain in the ambulatory care setting. Hospitalization is recommended for patients with symptoms.

Patients will require IV hydration and frequent monitoring of vital signs if they are unable to maintain adequate oral intake. Severe GI symptoms or bleeding will require serial abdominal examinations and may need parenteral nutrition or blood transfusions. Patients should also be monitored for possible bowel obstructions, peritonitis, or intussusception.

If the patient exhibits mental status changes, monitor for intracranial hemorrhage. For nephrotic syndrome or renal insufficiency, monitor for hypertension, check renal function, and treat accordingly. Severe joint symptoms require proper pain management.

Symptomatic treatment is required for abdominal and joint pain and includes:

- NSAIDs (such as naproxen 1000 to 1500 mg/day orally for 5-7 days), are effective in controlling joint pain and abdominal pain.
- Glucocorticosteroids—The use of steroids in HSP patients to treat abdominal pain is controversial. The role of steroids has not been evaluated in large, randomized, controlled studies. Also, glucocorticosteroids do not shorten the course of the disease or prevent recurrence. However, prednisone (1 to 2 mg/kg/day PO) may decrease inflammation and pain and may alter the course of renal involvement.

The risk of significant renal involvement is higher in adults than in children and morbidity is a result of the degree of renal disease. Recurrences appear in one third of patients and may occur up to 1 year after initial episode. Recurrences are milder, shorter, and occur more commonly in patients with nephritis, elevated ESR, or those who received glucocorticoids. Patients should be followed weekly for urinalysis and blood pressure measurements for the first 2 to 3 months after initial episode and then every 1 to 2 months for up to 1 year.

IMPETIGO

Impetigo is a common skin infection in children or in households with children. It presents equally among males and females.

Symptoms
- Fever
- Diarrhea
- General weakness
- Bullae

Signs
- "Honey-colored" crust
- Vesiculopustular lesions
- Pruritus
- Regional lymphadenopathy
- *Staphylococcus aureus*
  - Increasing incidence of MRSA in the community
- Group A streptococci
  - Decreasing incidence

Comments and Treatment Considerations
Treatment includes topical ointments (e.g., mupirocin 2%) applied to the affected area. It can also include systemic therapies including azithromycin, clarithromycin, erythromycin, or oral second-generation cephalosporins.

If patient is presenting with bullous impetigo, administer anti-methicillin-susceptible *S. aureus* agents (dicloxacillin, oxacillin, cephalexin, amoxicillin (clavulanic acid), azithromycin, clarithromycin) or anti-MRSA agents (trimethoprim/sulfamethoxazole, minocycline).

PITYRIASIS ROSEA

Symptoms
- Usually asymptomatic skin lesions ++++
- Itching—Absent, mild, or severe ++
- Preceded by a prodrome of headache, malaise, and pharyngitis in small number of cases ++

Signs
- Eruption commonly begins with a "herald" or "mother" patch, a single round or oval, pink or salmon-colored lesion on the chest, neck, or back, 2 to 5 cm in diameter. The lesion soon becomes scaly and begins to clear centrally. ++++
- A few days later oval lesions similar in appearance to a herald patch, but smaller; appear in crops on the trunk and proximal areas of the extremities +++++
- Characteristic pattern of lesions—The long axes of the lesions follow the lines of cleavage in a "Christmas tree" distribution. +++++

Workup
- Check for the "herald" patch, which can resemble tinea corporis—KOH examination of scales from the skin lesion for dermatophyte hyphae may distinguish this condition. ++++
- No lab abnormalities are found in PR. +
- The presence of "herald" patch, the characteristic exanthematous, maculopapular, red scaling eruptions and the absence of symptoms other than pruritus combine to make pityriasis rosea (PR) an easy diagnosis in most instances. ++++

Comments and Treatment Considerations
PR occurs in persons aged 10 to 35 years. Spontaneous remission occurs in 6 to 12 weeks or less. If the eruption persists for over 6 weeks a skin biopsy should be done to rule out parapsoriasis. The etiology is unknown but probably caused by an infectious agent. Relapse is unusual and infectivity is thought to be very low. In most cases of PR no treatment is necessary other than reassurance and proper patient education. The rash may persist for 2 to 3 months and new lesions may occur during this time but should disappear spontaneously.

Topical steroids can be applied two or three times daily to control itching. Topical antipruritic lotions such as Prax, Pramegel, or Sarna may also be helpful. Referral to a dermatologist for phototherapy (UVB) may be considered in patients with severe itching. A trial of erythromycin (250 mg orally four times a day for 14 days) may be useful in severe cases of PR. In one well-controlled study of 90 patients it was noted to reduce both the duration and severity of the disease. A nonrandomized single-blind trial suggested that high-dose acyclovir (800 mg orally five times daily for 7 days) may also be beneficial.

Psoriasis, secondary syphilis, tinea corporis, Lyme disease, HIV seroconversion illness, and drug eruptions must be considered in the differential diagnosis of PR.

STEVENS–JOHNSON SYNDROME AND TOXIC EPIDERMAL NECROLYSIS

Stevens-Johnson Syndrome (SJS) and toxic epidermal necrolysis (TEN) are severe hypersensitivity reactions, characterized by systemic symptoms, mucosal inflammation, and blistering and desquamation of large areas of skin.

- Drugs: Antibiotics; antiepileptics; antigout; analgesics; corticosteroids; and antiretrovirals are the most common inciting factors, with highest risk within 8 weeks of initiation.
- Viral and bacterial infections (*Mycoplasma pneumoniae,* herpes simplex, respiratory tract infection) may be more common in children.
- Risk factors: Human leukocyte antigen (HLA) B_{12}, immunosuppressed states as in HIV, SLE, and bone marrow transplant patients

 CLASSIFICATIONS

- SJS—Epidermal detachment of less than 10% body surface area
- Overlap SJS-TEN—Epidermal detachment of 10% to 30% body surface area
- TEN—Epidermal detachment greater than 30% body surface area

Symptoms
- URI-like prodrome including:
  - Fever +++
  - Sore throat
  - Chills
  - Headache
  - Malaise
  - Cough
  - Painful mucocutaneous lesions ++++
  - Involving eyes (conjunctivitis)
  - GI (oral lesions, colitis)
  - Genitourinary (dysuria)
  - Skin: painful or burning eruption on face and thorax, spreading to body ++++

Signs
- Fever: greater than 38° C in TEN, not as high in SJS +++
- Blisters, tenderness of involved skin, primarily trunk, face ++++
- Nikolsky's sign: sloughing of superficial skin layer with minimal pressure ++++
- Painful mucosal ulcerations: purulent conjunctivitis, oral ulcers ++++
- Purpuric macules; flat atypical targets may be present, becoming confluent over trunk ++++

Workup
- There are no specific laboratory tests indicated. Skin biopsy may be done to confirm the diagnosis.

Comments and Treatment Considerations

Immediate discontinuation of any suspected inciting drug(s) improves survival. Supportive care and treatment in a burn unit or ICU improve mortality, which is about 5% for SJS and 30% to 50% for TEN. Prognosis depends on age, heart rate, presence of cancer, body surface area involved, BUN, serum bicarbonate, and blood glucose; ophthalmology consultation is necessary because blindness is a potential complication.

Small series have reported mixed benefits for various treatments:
- High-dose corticosteroids for SJS
- IVIg at a dose of 0.5 to 1 g/kg/day over 3 to 5 days for SJS and TEN
- Plasmapheresis (with or without IVIg) every other day or daily for TEN
- Cyclophosphamide at 150 to 300 mg/day orally (with or without prednisone) for TEN
- Cyclosporine at 150 mg IV twice a day for TEN
- N-acetylcysteine, ulinastatin, anti-TNF-α, and pentoxifylline have limited data; thalidomide increases mortality

Recovery takes 1 to 3 weeks or longer depending on reepithelialization.

Long-Term Sequelae
- Pain, scarring, strictures of mucosal membranes (e.g., esophageal strictures, phimosis, vaginal synechiae)
- Post-inflammatory hyperpigmentation, nail growth abnormalities
- Blindness, due to dry eyes and corneal scarring
- Decreased pulmonary diffusion capacity

References

Arevalo JM, Lorente JA, Gonzalez-Herrada C, Jimenez-Reyes J: Treatment of toxic epidermal necrolysis with cyclosporin A, *J Trauma* 48:473–478, 2000.

Atherton DJ: A review of the pathophysiology, prevention and treatment of irritant diaper dermatitis, *Curr Med Res Opin* 20(5):645–649, 2004.

Auquier-Dunant A, Mockenhaupt M, Naldi L, et al: Correlations between clinical patterns and causes of erythema multiforme majus, Stevens-Johnson syndrome, and toxic epidermal necrolysis: results of an international prospective study, *Arch Dermatol* 138:1019–1024, 2002.

Bachot N, Revuz J, Roujeau JC: Intravenous immunoglobulin treatment for Stevens-Johnson syndrome and toxic epidermal necrolysis: a prospective noncomparative study showing no benefit on mortality or progression, *Arch Dermatol* 139:33–36, 2003.

Baddour LM, Wilson WR, Bayer AS, et al: Infective endocarditis diagnosis, antimicrobial therapy, and management of complication: a statement for healthcare professionals from the Committee on Rheumatic Fever, Endocarditis, and Kawasaki's disease, Council on Cardiovascular Disease in the Young, and the Cardiovascular Surgery and Anesthesia, American Heart Association: endorsed by Infectious Disease Society of America, *Circulation* 111(23):18–20, 2005.

Bakis S, Zagarella S: Intermittent oral cyclosporin for recurrent herpes simplex-associated erythema multiforme, *Australas J Dermatol* 46:18–20, 2005.

Balakrishnan R, Fleischer AB, Parathi S, Felman SR: Physicians underutilize topical retinoids in the management of acne vulgaris: analysis of U.S. national practice data, *J Dermatol Treat* 14(3):172–176, 2003.

Balfour AA, Edelman CK, Anderson RS, et al: Controlled trial of acyclovir for chickenpox evaluating time of initiation and duration of therapy and viral resistance, *Pediatr Infect Dis J* 20(10):919–926, 2001.

Bastuji-Garin S, Fouchard N, Bertocchi M, et al: SCORTEN: a severity-of-illness score for toxic epidermal necrolysis, *J Invest Dermatol* 115:149–153, 2000.

Bastuji-Garin S, Rzany B, Stern RS, et al: Clinical classification of cases of toxic epidermal necrolysis, Stevens-Johnson syndrome, and erythema multiforme, *Arch Dermatol* 129:92–96, 1993.

Behrman RE, Kliegman RM, Jenson H: *Textbook of pediatrics*, 17th ed, Philadelphia, 2004, Saunders, pp 826–828.

Chave TA, Mortimer NJ, Sladden MJ, et al: Toxic epidermal necrolysis: current evidence, practical management and future directions, *Br J Dermatol* 153:241–253, 2005.

Chuh AA: Quality of life in children with pityriasis rosea: a prospective case control study, *Pediatr Dermatol* 20:474, 2003.

Conejo-Mir JS, del Canto S, Munoz MA, et al: Thalidomide as elective treatment in persistent erythema multiforme; report of two cases, *J Drugs Dermatol* 2:40–44, 2003.

Crawford F, Young P, Godfrey C, et al: Oral treatments for toenail onychomycosis: a systematic review, *Arch Dermatol* 138:811, 2002.

Daning L, Dinguo Z, Wenwei S, Peihong J: Extensive skin candidosis in an adult: effective treatment with itraconazole, *Mycosis* 41:219, 1998.

Dedeoglu F, Kim S, Sundel R: Clinical manifestations and diagnosis of Henoch-Schonlein purpura, *UpToDate*, 2006.

Dedeoglu F, Kim S, Sundel R: Management of Henoch-Schönlein purpura, *UpToDate* 2006.

Drago F, Vecchio F, Rebora A: Use of high-dose acyclovir in pityriasis rosea, *J Am Acad Dermatol* 54:82, 2006.

Eastham JH, Segal JL, Gomez MF, Cole GW: Reversal of erythema multiforme major with cyclophosphamide and prednisone, *Ann Pharmacother* 30:606–607, 1996.

Faye O, Roujeau JC: Treatment of epidermal necrolysis with high-dose intravenous immunoglobulins (IV Ig): clinical experience to date, *Drugs* 65:2085–2090, 2005.

Fitzpatrick T, Johnson R, Polano M, et al: *Color atlas and synopsis of clinical dermatology*, 2nd ed, London, 1992, Elsevier, pp 58–60.

Fleece D, Gaughan JP, Aronoff SC: Griseofulvin versus terbinafine in the treatment of tinea capitis: a meta-analysis of randomised clinical trials, *Pediatrics* 114(5):312–315, 2004.

Forman R, Koren G, Shear NH: Erythema multiforme, Stevens-Johnson syndrome and toxic epidermal necrolysis in children: a review of 10 years' experience, *Drug Saf* 25:965–972, 2002.

Frangogiannis NG, Boridy I, Mazhar M, et al: Cyclophosphamide in the treatment of toxic epidermal necrolysis, *South Med J* 89:1001–1003, 1996.

Furubacke A, Berlin G, Anderson C, Sjoberg F: Lack of significant treatment effect of plasma exchange in the treatment of drug-induced toxic epidermal necrolysis? *Intensive Care Med* 25:1307–1310, 1999.

Garcia-Doval I, LeCleach L, Bocquet H, et al: Toxic epidermal necrolysis and Stevens-Johnson syndrome: does early withdrawal of causative drugs decrease the risk of death? *Arch Dermatol* 136:323–327, 2000.

Geraminejad P, Walling HW, Voigt MD, Stone MS: Severe erythema multiforme responding to interferon alfa, *J Am Acad Dermatol* 54:S18–S21, 2006.

Ghislain PD, Roujeau JC: Treatment of severe drug reactions: Stevens-Johnson syndrome, toxic epidermal necrolysis and hypersensitivity syndrome, *Dermatol Online J* 8:5, 2002.

Goldstein A, Goldstein B: Pityriasis rosea, *UpToDate*, 2006.

Guegan S, Bastuji-Garin S, Poszepczynska-Guigne E, et al: Performance of the SCORTEN during the first five days of hospitalization to predict the prognosis of epidermal necrolysis, *J Invest Dermatol* 126:272–276, 2006.

Gupta AK, Fleckman P, Baran R: Ciclopirox nail lacquer topical solution 8% in the treatment of toenail onychomycosis, *J Am Acad Dermatol* 43:S70, 2000.

Gupta AK, Ryder JE, Johnson AM: Cumulative meta-analysis of systemic anti-fungal agents the treatment of onychomycosis, *Br J Dermatol* 150:537, 2004.

Gupta AK, Skinner AR: Management of diaper dermatitis, *Int J Dermatol* 43:830–834, 2004.

Gupta AK: Systemic antifungal agents. In Wolverton SE, editor: *Comprehensive dermatologic drug therapy*, Philadelphia, 2001, Saunders.

Heng MC, Allen SG: Efficacy of cyclophosphamide in toxic epidermal necrolysis. Clinical and pathophysiologic aspects, *J Am Acad Dermatol* 25:778–786, 1991.

Hoffman LD, Hoffman MD: Dapsone in the treatment of persistent erythema multiforme, *J Drugs Dermatol* 5:375–376, 2006.

Huff JC, Weston WL, Tonnesen MG: Erythema multiforme: a critical review of characteristics, diagnostic criteria, and causes, *J Am Acad Dermatol* 8:763–775, 1983.

Hunger RE, Hunziker T, Buettiker U, et al: Rapid resolution of toxic epidermal necrolysis with anti-TNF-alpha treatment, *J Allergy Clin Immunol* 116:923–924, 2005.

Hurwitz S: Acne vulgaris: pathogenesis and management, *Pediatr Rev* 15:47, 1994.

Inamo Y, Okubo T, Wada M, et al: Intravenous ulinastatin therapy for Stevens-Johnson syndrome and toxic epidermal necrolysis in pediatric patients. Three case reports, *Int Arch Allergy Immunol* 127:89–94, 2002.

Johnson RW, Whitton TL: Management of herpes zoster (shingles) and post-herpetic neuralgia, *Exp Opin Pharmacother* 5:551, 2004.

Kamaliah MD, Zainal D, Mokhtar N, Nazmi N: Erythema multiforme, Stevens-Johnson syndrome and toxic epidermal necrolysis in northeastern Malaysia, *Int J Dermatol* 37:520–523, 1998.

Kim KJ, Lee DP, Suh HS, et al: Toxic epidermal necrolysis: analysis of clinical course and SCORTEN-based comparison of mortality rate and treatment modalities in Korean patients, *Acta Derm Venereol* 85:497–502, 2005.

Leaute-Labreze C, Lamireau T, Chawki D, et al: Diagnosis, classification, and management of erythema multiforme and Stevens-Johnson syndrome, *Arch Dis Child* 83:347–352, 2000.

Leenutaphong V, Jiamton S: UVB phototherapy for pityriasis rosea: a bilateral comparison study, *J Am Acad Dermatol* 33:996, 1995.

Lehmann HP, Robinson KA, Andrews JS, et al: Acne therapy: a methodologic review, *J Am Acad Dermatol* 47:231, 2002.

Lin RL, Tinkle LL, Janniger CK: Skin care of the healthy newborn, *Pediatr Dermatol* 75:25–30, 2005.

Lissia M, Figus A, Rubino C: Intravenous immunoglobulins and plasmapheresis combined treatment in patients with severe toxic epidermal necrolysis: preliminary report, *Br J Plast Surg* 58:504–510, 2005.

Martinez AE, Atherton DJ: High-dose systemic corticosteroids can arrest recurrences of severe mucocutaneous erythema multiforme, *Pediatr Dermatol* 17:87–90, 2000.

Mockenhaupt M, Kelly JP, Kaufman D, Stern RS: The risk of Stevens-Johnson syndrome and toxic epidermal necrolysis associated with nonsteroidal anti-inflammatory drugs: a multinational perspective, *J Rheumatol* 30:2234–2240, 2003.

Mockenhaupt M, Messenheimer J, Tennis P, Schlingmann J: Risk of Stevens-Johnson syndrome and toxic epidermal necrolysis in new users of antiepileptics, *Neurology* 64:1134–1138, 2005.

Mortz CG, Andersen KE: Allergic contact dermatitis in children and adolescents, *Contact Dermatitis* 41:121, 1999.

Mortz CG, Lauritsen JM, Bindslev-Jensen C, Andersen KE: Prevalence of atopic dermatitis, asthma, allergic rhinitis, and hand and contact dermatitis in adolescents. The Odense Adolescence Cohort Study on Atopic Diseases and Dermatitis, *Br J Dermatol* 144:523, 2001.

Nadalo D, Montoya C, Hunter-Smith D: What is the best way to treat tinea cruris? *J Fam Pract* 55(3), 2006.

Palmieri TL, Greenhalgh DG, Saffle JR, et al: A multicenter review of toxic epidermal necrolysis treated in U.S. burn centers at the end of the twentieth century, *J Burn Care Rehabil* 23:87–96, 2002.

Paquet P, Pierard GE, Quatresooz P: Novel treatments for drug-induced toxic epidermal necrolysis (Lyell's syndrome), *Int Arch Allergy Immunol* 136:205–216, 2005.

Rappersberger K, Foedinger D: Treatment of erythema multiforme, Stevens-Johnson syndrome, and toxic epidermal necrolysis, *Dermatol Ther* 15:397–408, 2002.

Ronkainen J, Koskimies O: Early prednisone therapy in Henoch-Schönlein purpura: a randomized, double-blind, placebo-controlled trial, *J Pediatr* 149(2):241–247, 2006.

Roujeau JC, Kelly JP, Naldi L, et al: Medication use and the risk of Stevens-Johnson syndrome or toxic epidermal necrolysis, *N Engl J Med* 333:1600–1607, 1995.

Roujeau JC: The spectrum of Stevens-Johnson syndrome and toxic epidermal necrolysis: a clinical classification, *J Invest Dermatol* 102:28S–30S, 1994.

Schofield JK, Tatnall FM, Leigh IM: Recurrent erythema multiforme: clinical features and treatment in a large series of patients, *Br J Dermatol* 128:542–545, 1993.

Sen P, Chua SH: A case of recurrent erythema multiforme and its therapeutic complications, *Ann Acad Med Singapore* 33:793–796, 2004.

Sharma VK, Dhar S: Clinical pattern of cutaneous drug eruption among children and adolescents in north India, *Pediatr Dermatol* 12:178–183, 1995.

Sharma PK, Yadav TP, Gautam RK, et al: Erythromycin in pityriasis rosea: a double-blind, placebo-controlled clinical trial, *J Am Acad Dermatol* 42:241, 2000.

Shortt R, Gomez M, Mittman N, Cartotto R: Intravenous immunoglobulin does not improve outcome in toxic epidermal necrolysis, *J Burn Care Rehabil* 25:246–255, 2004.

Tatnall FM, Schofield JK, Leigh IM: A double-blind, placebo-controlled trial of continuous acyclovir therapy in recurrent erythema multiforme, *Br J Dermatol* 132:267–270, 1995.

Velez A, Moreno JC: Toxic epidermal necrolysis treated with N-acetylcysteine, *J Am Acad Dermatol* 46:469–470, 2002.

Villiger RM, von Vigier RO, Ramelli GP, et al: Precipitants in 42 cases of erythema multiforme, *Eur J Pediatr* 158:929–932, 1999.

Weston WL, Weston JA: Allergic contact dermatitis in children, *Am J Dis Child* 138:932, 1984.

Wolkenstein P, Latarjet J, Roujeau JC, et al: Randomised comparison of thalidomide versus placebo in toxic epidermal necrolysis, *Lancet* 352:1586–1589, 1998.

CHAPTER 36

Seizures
Jennifer M. Naticchia and David M. Bercaw

Few clinical events present as dramatically as the patient with a generalized tonic-clonic seizure, nor as subtly as the patient with an *absence* seizure. The clinician's goal is to accurately and effectively diagnose and treat such patients. Clinicians should differentiate between epileptic seizures (therefore likely recurrent)—and secondary seizures (therefore possibly curable). This aids in the decision as to whether to initiate antiepileptic drug therapy. Secondary causes of seizure include infection, cerebrovascular accident, tumor, congenital injury or malformation, AVM, and others. In considering the diagnosis of seizure, the clinician must take into account the medical, social, and psychologic implications of labeling a patient as "epileptic."

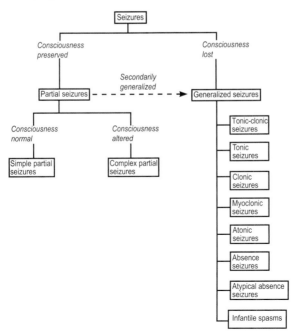

This chapter outlines the common clinical manifestations of seizures classified into three main categories: partial, generalized, and unclassified epileptic seizures. Partial seizures begin as a focal transient alteration of function compared with generalized seizures, which start with loss of consciousness and involve both sides of the body. Unclassified epileptic seizures usually have nondistinctive features presenting in neonates and infants.

ABSENCE SEIZURES

Absence seizures are a type of generalized seizure formerly known as petit mal seizures. They mainly occur in children and may occur daily, often with many episodes in a 24-hour period. These types of seizures resemble a staring spell that may be unrecognized until a teacher notes poor school performance. No postictal phase is present with these episodes. Atypical absence seizures are associated with myoclonic activity of the facial muscles or extremities. Absence seizures are associated with childhood absence epilepsy. Children with absence seizures may later develop tonic-clonic seizures and their condition is then classified as juvenile absence epilepsy.

Signs
- "Staring spell" that lasts from 4 to 20 seconds +++++
- Child resumes preseizure activity ++++
- May be associated with rolling of the eyes or flutter of eyelids
- Unresponsiveness ++++
- Partial awareness +++

Workup
- Normal lab analysis
- Normal radiologic evaluation
- EEG
- Seizure is induced with hyperventilation and characteristic spike and wave formations are noted at 1.5 to 4 Hz/sec.
- The EEG spikes are irregular in atypical absence seizures with postictal slowing.

Comments and Treatment Considerations
Ethosuximide and valproate are more commonly used for treatment. Valproate is the drug of choice if patients have tonic-clonic episodes or myoclonic jerks. Other possible therapies include lamotrigine, zonisamide, benzodiazepines, acetazolamide, levetiracetam, topiramate, and ketogenic diet.

Approximately 70% of children outgrow absence seizures, especially if the seizures start before age 10. Some may go on to develop juvenile absence epilepsy or juvenile myoclonic epilepsy. Unfavorable prognosis is associated with generalized tonic-clonic activity in the active stage of absence, myoclonic jerks, eyelid or perioral myoclonia, and atypical EEG features.

FEBRILE SEIZURES

The most common type of convulsive disorder in children younger than 5 years of age is a simple febrile seizure. Febrile seizures occur during a febrile illness and in the absence of a CNS infection, acute electrolyte imbalance, or known seizure disorder. They tend to occur within the first 24 hours of a febrile illness, and with temperatures averaging 39.8° C. The age groups most commonly experiencing febrile seizures are patients ages 6 months to 5 years, with peak occurrence in children 18 to 24 months old. Approximately 3% to 5% of children will experience a febrile seizure before age 5. A simple febrile seizure is described as a generalized seizure lasting less than 15 minutes and does not recur in 24 hours. A complex febrile seizure can have focal features, last more than fifteen minutes, and may recur within a 24-hour period. Simple febrile seizures comprise 80% of febrile seizures, carry few risks of complications, and have excellent short- and long-term prognoses. Most children who experience a simple febrile seizure do not require hospitalization. Parents should be educated and reassured about the benign nature of febrile seizures.

Symptoms
- History of fever
- Drowsiness following seizure activity

Signs
- Generalized tonic-clonic activity lasting less than 15 minutes +++++
- Rectal temperature greater than 38° C +++++
- Brief postictal phase +++++

Workup
- Thorough history and physical examination
- Laboratory tests as indicated, typically only if history or physical examination suggestive of another process (e.g., dehydration)
- If seizure occurs after the second day of febrile illness, lumbar puncture should be considered.
- If less than 1 year old, consider lumbar puncture because meningeal signs may be absent.
- CT, MRI, EEG: not indicated in simple febrile seizure with normal neurologic examination

Comments and Treatment Considerations
Treat the cause of the fever (most fevers are due to viral illness). Reduce fever with antipyretics. Anticonvulsants are not indicated in a seizure lasting less than 5 minutes. If a seizure lasts more than 5 minutes, benzodiazepines are first-line therapy.

Approximately one third of children with febrile seizures will experience a recurrence of seizure activity. In children who have their first febrile seizure before 18 months of age and a positive family history of febrile seizures in a first-degree relative, the risk of recurrence is increased. Risk of recurrence declines to zero by 5 years of age. The risk of developing epilepsy in a child with a history of febrile seizure is 1% higher than the general population. Patients with febrile seizures are not at higher risk for developing more serious bacterial illnesses. Most important, long-term consequences are rare in children who are otherwise healthy.

PARTIAL SEIZURES

All seizures are caused by abnormal electrical disturbances in the brain. Partial seizures involve electrical disturbances limited to specific areas of the brain, which may cause changes in attention, movement, and behavior. Foci in the brain tissue giving rise to these disturbances may be congenitally acquired, or they may develop following head trauma, infections, stroke, or certain other conditions. In many patients, no obvious cause can be determined. Partial seizures are subdivided into simple partial seizures and complex partial seizures.

 SIMPLE PARTIAL SEIZURES

These seizure types are classified as "simple" because consciousness is not impaired and "partial" because only part of the cortex is disrupted by the seizure.

Symptoms
- Motor
  - Single or multiple muscle jerks
  - Rhythmic jerking movements of the face, arm or leg on the side of the body opposite to the involved cortex (jacksonian seizure)
  - Spasms or rigidity of one unilateral body region
  - Eye deviation
  - Abnormal head movements
- Somatosensory
  - Unusual sensations affecting regular or special sensory symptoms (olfactory, visual, gustatory)
- Autonomic
  - Epigastric sensation
  - Nausea
  - Sweating
- Psychologic
  - Memory (e.g., déjà vu)
  - Emotional disturbance (e.g., fear)

Signs
- Single or multiple muscle jerks
- Rhythmic jerking movements of the face, arm, or leg on the side of the body opposite to the involved cortex (jacksonian seizure)

- Spasms or rigidity of one unilateral body region
- Eye deviation
- Abnormal head movements
- Normal consciousness and awareness
- Postictal focal neurologic deficit (hemiparesis or aphasia)

 COMPLEX PARTIAL SEIZURES

These seizures are classified as "complex" because consciousness is impaired, but still "partial" because only part of the cortex is involved. This type of seizure usually lasts less than 3 minutes.

Symptoms
- May be preceded by a warning or aura (auras are simple partial seizures with symptoms as described following, most commonly somatosensory, autonomic, and psychologic)

Signs
- Altered consciousness/awareness such as unresponsiveness or staring
- Repetitive behaviors (automatisms) such as lip smacking, grimacing, swallowing, picking, manipulating objects, snapping fingers, repeating words or phrases, walking, running, or undressing
- Postictal focal neurologic deficit resolving within 48 hours
- Todd's paralysis—Transient paralysis following seizure
- Postictal phase—Somnolence, confusion, headache (up to several hours)

 SECONDARILY GENERALIZED SEIZURES

Partial seizures, both simple and complex, can progress to a generalized seizure (GS). A simple partial seizure can directly evolve into a GS or, it may first evolve to a complex partial seizure, which then evolves to a GS.

Workup
- It is often difficult to diagnose a single focal seizure. A diagnosis is easier to make in patients who have recurrent, stereotyped seizures.
- Thorough history and physical examination
- Differentiate transient, provoked seizure (with an underlying cause) from epilepsy.
- Blood tests: serum glucose and electrolytes (sodium, calcium, magnesium); renal function tests; hepatic function tests if liver impairment is suspected; CBC if infection is suspected; and urine screen for drugs if abuse is suspected
- Lumbar puncture with signs that suggest CNS infection, for example, altered mental status, fever, or nuchal rigidity

- Classify type of seizure based on signs and symptoms
- EEG can show characteristic changes confirming partial (focal) seizures, and may show the focus. A normal EEG does not rule out seizures. Sensitivity is 50%; specificity is 98% to 99%.
- Neuroimaging: imaging must be performed in all patients with partial-onset seizures to identify any structural brain disease as an underlying cause and exclude an expanding mass lesion that might require acute intervention. MRI is the preferred imaging option.

Comments and Treatment Considerations

Administer first-aid measures as appropriate: protect the person from injury during the seizure and protect the airway. Treat identified underlying causes: discontinue medication and manage tumors or other brain lesions. Prescribe antiepileptic drugs (AEDs) in patients with recurrent seizures. Partial complex seizures are treated with the same AEDs used for generalized seizures (with the exception of ethosuximide used to treat absence seizure).

Follow-up includes review of the need for drugs and monitoring for side effects.

Surgery performed for refractory seizures include vagal nerve stimulator or removal of the abnormal brain cells/tissue causing seizures.

Identify and avoid and eliminate known precipitants. Studies suggest more than 60% of reported seizures are associated with certain precipitants (e.g., stress and sleep deprivation).

TONIC–CLONIC SEIZURES (GRAND MAL SEIZURES)

The seizure begins with a sudden loss of consciousness associated with a tonic phase characterized by generalized muscular stiffening of the trunk and extremities. Muscle movement or eye deviation that begins or is exhibited primarily on one side should raise the suspicion that the seizure is not truly generalized, but is focal in origin—leading to a more intense search for underlying CNS pathology. The tonic phase merges into the clonic phase, consisting of rhythmic, symmetric, and synchronous muscular jerking movements. Rarely, a generalized seizure may exhibit only a tonic phase (tonic seizure) or a clonic phase (clonic seizure), but in these cases the evaluation should be the same as for a generalized tonic-clonic event. It is followed by the recovery phase, during which there is a gradual return to consciousness that usually occurs within 40 seconds to 3 minutes from seizure onset. Finally, the seizure ends with a postictal phase characterized by confusion, stupor, sleepiness, and headache. The postictal phase may last from minutes to hours.

Symptoms
- Usually no prodromal symptoms or aura (otherwise, consider primary focal seizure that then generalizes)
- Postictal state
- Amnestic for the event

Signs
- Sudden loss of consciousness +++++
- Expiratory "scream" ++++
- Drooling, pupillary dilation, stertorous respirations
- Urinary or fecal incontinence +++
- Tachycardia and elevated blood pressure
- No focal neurologic deficits

Workup
- Inquire about withdrawal from alcohol, benzodiazepines, barbiturates
- Serum glucose and sodium
- Consider serum calcium, magnesium, complete blood count, liver function tests
- Consider toxicology screen
- Pregnancy test on women of childbearing age (may affect choice of AEDs)
- Serum drug levels (if already on AEDs)
- CT head as soon as possible if:
  - Acute intracranial process suspected
  - History of acute head trauma
  - History of malignancy
  - Immunocompromised patient
  - Fever
  - Persistent headache
  - New focal neurologic examination finding
  - Age more than 40 years
  - Focal onset before generalization
- Consider CT, or preferably MRI, in any patient with first-time seizure, even if patient is alert and has returned to baseline
- Consider lumbar puncture if:
  - Fever
  - Immunocompromised (especially if HIV positive)
  - History of malignancy known to metastasize to the meninges
  - Age less than 6 months
- Consider EEG
  - Most sensitive when performed within 24 hours of seizure (29% sensitivity)
  - If normal, consider sleep-deprived EEG (48% sensitivity)

Comments and Treatment Considerations
In acute patients, protect airway and tongue. Administer oxygen and IV access if prolonged seizure. Consider IV glucose and thiamine. Place in left lateral decubitus position. If seizure lasts longer than 5 minutes administer diazepam 0.1 mg/kg slow IV push; maximum 5 mg/min (maximum dose 5 mg in infants; 10 mg in children; 30 mg in adults), or lorazepam 1 to 2 mg IM or IV.

For status epilepticus (continuous seizure for more than 30 minutes or repeated motor seizure without recovery of baseline consciousness between attacks):
- Airway, breathing, and circulation (ABCs)
- Low threshold for intubation

- Monitor pulse oximetry
- Glucose
- IV access
- Watch for hypo- or hypertension
- Cardiac monitor
- Monitor temperature for hyperthermia
- Goal is control of seizure within 30 minutes
- Lorazepam 2 mg/min IV; maximum 10 mg
- Phenytoin 15 to 20 mg/kg up to 30 mg/kg IV at 25 to 50 mg/kg/min
- If patient is known to have been on phenytoin give 9 mg/kg IV until drug level is back
- Fosphenytoin can be given at 100 to 150 mg phenytoin equivalents per minute IV or IM.
- If seizure continues:
  - Phenobarbital 10 to 20 mg/kg IV at 100 mg/hr *or*
  - Valproic acid 15 to 30 mg/kg
- If seizure still continues:
  - Pentobarbital anesthesia 5 mg/kg IV at 25 mg/min, then 2.5 mg/kg/hr *or*
  - Diazepam 100 mg in 500 mL D_5W IV drip at 40 mL/hr
  - Lidocaine 100-mg IV bolus
  - Chloral hydrate 30 mg/kg PR
  - Isofluorane (general anesthesia)
  - Paralysis with pancuronium, with intubation
- Follow CK and creatinine for possible rhabdomyolysis
- Thiamine 100 mg IV and Mg^{++} 1 to 2 g for alcoholic and/or malnourished patients

Admit the patient to the hospital if he or she is experiencing a prolonged postictal state or drug or alcohol withdrawal, is a febrile patient, presents with expanding mass on imaging, has experienced recent trauma, presents with focal neurologic signs or status epilepticus, or has compliance issues or inadequate supervision at home.

Further treatment does not usually require a need to start AEDs if this is the first seizure and the patient has normal neurologic examination, blood work, imaging studies, and EEG. However, there may be a need to start AEDs if this is a second seizure and there is no treatable, curable, or preventable underlying cause. Appropriate therapies include phenytoin orally or IV; fosphenytoin IV or IM; carbamazepine; valproate; and phenobarbital (more side effects).

Consider the patient's occupation and public safety. You may need to notify the state department of motor vehicles, depending on state law. Consider a Medic-Alert bracelet (800-736-3342).

The physician's role in the evaluation of generalized tonic-clonic seizure is to exclude an underlying systemic cause and to determine the likelihood of recurrence. The diagnosis of epilepsy is often difficult to establish, given the low sensitivity of EEGs. Deciding whether to initiate AED therapy is often difficult and may have profound physical, psychologic, occupational, and legal implications for the patient. A complete and accurate history, combined with careful physical examination and appropriate testing, is of paramount importance in establishing the correct diagnosis. Further testing, including imaging studies, is required if the patient has any focal neurologic findings.

References

Behrman R, Kliegman R, Jenson H, editors: *Nelson textbook of pediatrics*, 16th ed, Philadelphia, 2000, Saunders, pp 1817–1825.

Betting LE, Mory SB: MRI volumetry shows increased anterior thalamic volumes in patients with absence epilepsy, *Epilepsy Behav* 8(3):575–580, 2006.

Cameron H: Neurology. In Gunn V, Nechyba C, editors: *The Harriet Lane handbook*, 16th ed, Philadelphia, 2002, Mosby.

Chan CH, Briellman RS: Thalamic atrophy in childhood absence epilepsy, *Epilepsia* 47(2):399–405, 2006.

Chen DK, So YT, Fisher RS: Use of serum prolactin in diagnosing epileptic seizures: report of the Therapeutics and Technology Assessment Subcommittee of the American Academy of Neurology, *Neurology* 67(3):544–545, 2005.

Freedman S, Powell E: Pediatric seizures and their management in the emergency department, *Clin Pediatr Emerg Med* 4:195–206, 2003.

Grosso S, Galimberti D: Childhood absence epilepsy: evolution and prognostic factors, *Epilepsia* 46(11):1796–1801, 2005.

Hirtz D, Ashwal S, Berg A, Bettis D, Camfield C, et al: Practice parameter: evaluating a first nonfebrile seizure in children, *Neurology* 55(5):616–623, 2000.

King MA, Newton MR, Jackson GD, et al: Epileptology of the first-seizure presentation: a clinical, electroencephalographic, and magnetic resonance imaging study of 300 consecutive patients, *Lancet* 352(9133):1007–1011, 1998.

Lowenstein DH: Seizures and epilepsy. In Kasper D, Braunwald E, et al: *Harrison's principles of internal medicine*, 16th ed, New York, 2005, McGraw-Hill, pp 1041–1112.

Millar J: Evaluate and treatment of the child with febrile seizure, *Am Fam Physician* 73:1761–1766, 2006.

Moljecic S, Krampf K: A mutation in the GABA receptor alpha (1)-subunit is associated with absence, *Epilepsy Ann Neurol* 59(6):983–987, 2006.

Moore-Sledge CM: Evaluation and management of first seizures in adults, *Am Fam Physician* 56(4):1113–1120, 1997.

Noebels JL, Tharp BR: Absence seizures in developing brain. In Schwartzkroin P, Cary, NC, Moshé SL, Noebels J (editors): *Brain development in epilepsy*, 1995, Oxford University Press, p 66.

Peloquin JB, Khosravani H, Barr W, Bladen C, et al: Functional analysis ca 3.2 T-type calcium channel mutations linked to childhood absence epilepsy, *Epilepsia* 47(3):655–658, 2006.

Posner EB, Mohamed K: Ethosuximide, sodium valproate and lamotrigine for absence seizures in children and adolescence, *Cochrane Database Syst Rev*, 2005, CD003032.

Posner EB: Pharmacological treatment of childhood absence epilepsy, *Exp Rev Neurother* 6(6):855–862, 2006.

Sadlier LG, Farrell MB: Electroclinical features of absence epilepsy, *Neurology* 67(3):413–418, 2006.

Segan S: *Absence seizures*. Available at www.emedicine.com/neuro/topic3.htm.

Shneker BF, Fountain NB: Epilepsy, *Dis Mon* 49(7):426–478, 2003.

Vining EP, Freeman JM: A multicenter study of the efficacy of the ketogenic diet, *Arch Neurol* 55:1433–1437, 1998.

Warden CR, Zibuleswsky J, Mace S, et al: Evaluation and management of febrile seizures in the out-of-hospital and emergency department settings, *Ann Emerg Med* 41:215–222, 2003.

Wilfong A, Schultz R: Zonisamide for absence seizures, *Epilepsy Res* 64(1–2):31–34, 2005.

CHAPTER 37

Sexual Dysfunction
Dan F. Criswell and L. Peter Schweibert

DYSPAREUNIA

Dyspareunia (literally, "painful mating") is a symptom complex characterized by persistent and/or recurrent genital pain experienced just before, during, or after sexual intercourse producing distress and/or interpersonal difficulty. The pain associated with dyspareunia involves the introitus, vulvar surfaces, vagina, and the deeper pelvic structures. Leading causes of dyspareunia are vulvar vulvodynia, infection, and endometriosis in women younger than age 50 and vulvovaginal atrophy in women older than age 50.

Symptoms
- Pain +++
- Aching: pelvic congestion
- Burning/itching

Signs
- Normal appearing introitus
- Localized discrete vulvovaginal lesions
- Erythema and hypersensitivity to touch
- Involuntary spasm on speculum examination
- Pale, dry vulvovaginal mucosa
- Vaginal stenosis
- Discharge
- Cervicitis, healed obstetric tears
- Localized tenderness or dysesthesia
- Pelvic masses
- Cystic or urethral tenderness

Workup
- Wet prep, KOH prep, gonococcal, and chlamydia probes
- Pap smear
- Complete UA
- Pelvic ultrasound
- Bladder-filling test
- Cystoscopy
- Laparoscopy
- Skin/vaginal/cervical biopsy

Comments and Treatment Considerations

Primary dyspareunia is a diagnosis of exclusion. If the onset is acute and identifiable to a specific point in time in sexually active females, infectious causes predominate. Other etiologies include endometriosis and ovarian or uterine pathology. Nongenital causes include problems in the bladder or GI tract.

In primary dyspareunia the primary goal of therapy is to diminish symptoms sufficiently to allow for successful intercourse and restoration of mutually satisfying sexual experiences. Identification of patient avoidance behaviors and development of therapeutic strategies will help her regain a degree of control over the condition. Adequate sexual arousal phase should be ensured and supplemental lubrication recommended if needed. For vulvodynia and other nondermatologic conditions associated with dysesthesia, use of nonsensitizing topical anesthetics (lidocaine 5% as needed or cromolyn cream 4% applied three times daily) may provide symptomatic relief. If pain is characterized as burning, shooting, or stabbing, gabapentin (initially 300 mg daily increasing weekly to maximum of 900 mg three times daily) and/or TCAs (nortriptyline or desipramine 25 to 75 mg at bedtime) may be helpful.

Referral is indicated when these therapeutic approaches are not beneficial or the diagnosis is in doubt. If behavioral issues predominate, if the dyspareunia is associated with posttraumatic stress disorder, or if dyspareunia is associated with personality disorders, psychiatric referral is helpful. If other organ systems are involved with dyspareunia, appropriate specialty referral may be warranted. Referral for biofeedback and physical therapy should be considered to help patients regain control of the pelvic floor musculature. Perineoplasty, flashlamp excited dye laser (FEDL), vestibulectomy, or other surgical procedures should be reserved for patients with severe and recalcitrant disease.

ERECTILE DYSFUNCTION

Erectile dysfunction (ED) is the consistent or recurrent inability to maintain penile erections sufficient to permit satisfactory sexual intercourse, for at least 3 months. Normal male sexual function consists of the following three components: desire/libido, penile erection and orgasm, which in turn depend on a complex interaction of psychiatric, hormonal, neurologic and vascular factors.

Sudden onset ED tends to be due to psychogenic, traumatic, or medication causes. Gradual onset ED tends to be vasculogenic, neurogenic, or due to or hypogonadism. Sleep-associated erections (SAEs) coupled with successful erection with a different partner or with erotic stimulus suggests psychogenic causes; absence suggests organic causes.

Symptoms
• Inability to attain or maintain erections ++++

Signs
- Lack of secondary sexual characteristics (hypogonadism)
- Postural hypotension (autonomic dysfunction)
- Absent pedal pulses (vascular)
- Testicular atrophy (hypogonadism)
- Penile corpora cavernosal plaques (Peyronie's disease)
- Abnormal bulbocavernosus reflex (neurogenic ED)

Workup
In individuals with gradual onset ED and risk factors for vascular or neurogenic causes, intracavernosal (IC) injection may differentiate. Five micrograms (suspected neurogenic) or 10 µg (suspected vasculogenic) of prostaglandin E_1 (PGE_1, e.g., alprostadil) is injected over 30 to 60 seconds into the corpus cavernosum. Erection should occur within 15 minutes and last 20 to 40 minutes. Poor or inadequate response suggests primary vasculogenic ED, whereas a satisfactory erection suggests primary neurogenic ED.
- Serum testosterone, obtained between 8 and 11 AM, is recommended in men with suspected hypogonadism.
- A fasting glucose or HbA_{1c} and lipid panel should be considered.
- Other tests to consider include TSH, CBC, serum creatinine.

Comments and Treatment Considerations
General measures to address causes/exacerbating factors of ED include weight loss if overweight, tobacco and ethanol cessation, resolution of partner conflict, and elimination (if possible) of offending drugs. For psychogenic ED, a trial of reassurance or giving permission to show intimacy in ways other than sexual intercourse (to focus on intimacy and decrease performance anxiety) is reasonable; poor response to office counseling warrants referral to a sex therapist.

Testosterone is indicated for decreased libido in men with low testosterone levels. Dihydrotestosterone (DHT) gel is dosed at 125 to 250 mg/day; the goal is to restore physiologic testosterone levels and improve symptoms (decreased libido and energy). Testosterone may worsen obstructive sleep apnea symptoms and should be avoided in men with bladder outlet obstruction. It is advisable to perform digital rectal prostate examination, prostate-specific antigen (PSA), LFTs, and lipids before initiating testosterone and again in 3 to 6 months; PSA and prostate examination should be repeated 9 to 12 months after initiating therapy, then annually if normal.

Phosphodiesterase type 5 (PDE5) inhibitors are first-line treatment for ED (Table 37-1). Side effects include headache, flushing, and dyspepsia. These drugs should not be used more than daily or with nitrates, alpha-blockers, or Class IA or III antiarrhythmics. Concurrent use with erythromycin, ketoconazole, or protease inhibitors can increase serum levels of PDE5 inhibitors.

Alprostadil (transurethral or intracavernous [IC]) is a second-line ED agent for men intolerant to PDE5 inhibitors or in whom these agents are contraindicated. Intracavernosal alprostadil is more effective than transurethral in producing erections. The starting dose for

Table 37-1. PDE5 Inhibitors in Men with Erectile Dysfunction

MEDICATION	DOSAGE STRENGTH (mg)	STARTING DOSE	MAXIMUM DOSE	ONSET (minutes)	DURATION (hr)	SUCCESSFUL INTERCOURSE RATE	
						DRUG	PLACEBO
Sildenafil	25, 50, 100	50 mg 1 hour before sex	100 mg	30-40	4	57%	14%-17%
Vardenafil	2.5, 5, 10, 20	10 mg 1 hour before sex	20 mg	30-40	4	50%-65%	32%
Tadalafil	5, 10, 20	10 mg 30 min before sex	20 mg	16-40	Up to 36	53%-70%	32%

IC alprostadil is 5 µg (neurogenic ED) or 10 µg (vasculogenic ED). Side effects include pain; 2% to 3% of men experience prolonged (>4 hours) erections with IC alprostadil.

Individuals failing the foregoing are candidates for urologic referral for possible vacuum constrictive device (VCD), microvascular bypass surgery, or implantation of a malleable/inflatable prosthesis. Other indications for urology referral are cavernosal plaques/fibrosis (Peyronie's disease) or prolonged erection (emergent referral).

References

American College of Obstetricians and Gynecologists: *Sexual dysfunction technical bulletin no. 211*, Washington, DC, 1995, ACOG.

Bodie J, Lewis J, Schow D: Laboratory evaluations of erectile dysfunction: an evidence based approach, *J Urol* 169:2262–2264, 2003.

Campbell HE: Clinical monograph for drug formulary review: erectile dysfunction agents, *J Manag Care Pharm* 11:151–171, 2005.

Godschalk MF, et al: Management of erectile dysfunction by the geriatrician, *J Am Geriatr Soc* 45:1240–1246, 1997.

Gupta M, et al: The clinical pharmacokinetics of phosphodiesterase-5 inhibitors for erectile dysfunction, *J Clin Pharmacol* 45:987–1003, 2005.

Jamieson DJ, Steege JF: The prevalence of dyspareunia, pelvic pain and irritable bowel syndrome in primary care practices, *Obstet Gynecol* 87:55, 1996.

Labbate L, Croft H, Oleshansky M: Antidepressant-related erectile dysfunction: management via avoidance, switching antidepressants, antidotes, and adaptation, *J Clin Psychiatry* 64(Suppl 10):11–19, 2003.

Latthe P, Mignini L, Gray R, et al: Factors predisposing women to chronic pelvic pain: systematic review, *BMJ* 332:749, 2006.

Lue TF, et al: Summary of the recommendations on sexual dysfunctions in men, *J Sex Med* 1:6–23, 2004.

Maas R, et al: The pathophysiology of erectile dysfunction related to endothelial dysfunction and mediators of vascular function, *Vasc Med* 7:213–225, 2002.

Morales A, et al: Endocrine aspects of sexual dysfunction in men, *J Sex Med* 1:69–81, 2004.

Tejada IS de, et al: Pathophysiology of erectile dysfunction, *J Sex Med* 2:26–39, 2005.

CHAPTER 38

Shortness of Breath
Dean Gianakos, Terry J. Thompson, Patricia Pletke,
and Sharon Diamond-Myrsten

The patient with acute shortness of breath (dyspnea) presents an immediate challenge to the family physician. Quick assessment, including a rapid airway, breathing, and circulation (ABC) check must first be done, followed by consideration of potentially life-threatening causes. Patients with severe dyspnea may present with chest pain, difficulty speaking, tachypnea, wheezing, rales, accessory muscle use, and hypoxemia. Once the patient is stabilized (i.e., airway secured, oxygen placed, IV established, and cardiac monitor applied), a more thorough history, physical, and laboratory evaluation can be performed to verify the diagnosis.

This chapter focuses on the management of six common diseases that can cause acute dyspnea, including several diagnoses often seen in children (croup and bronchiolitis). Note that there are many causes of chronic dyspnea (duration greater than 3 weeks). These include conditions such as interstitial lung disease and neuromuscular and chest wall disorders. These problems are not discussed in this chapter.

PNEUMOTHORAX

Pneumothorax is the accumulation of air between the two parietal surfaces (visceral and parietal) of the lung. If a check valve mechanism occurs in which the air cannot escape, a tension pneumothorax will develop and cause hemodynamic compromise and acute respiratory failure unless promptly treated with needle aspiration or chest tube placement. Spontaneous pneumothorax (SP) may be primary (PSP) or secondary (SSP). Primary pneumothorax occurs most commonly in tall, thin men (ages 20 to 40). SSP is a complication of diseases such as COPD, cystic fibrosis, and *Pneumocystis jiroveci* (previously *P. carinii*) pneumonia in immunocompromised patients. Iatrogenic (i.e., after central line placement) and trauma are other causes of pneumothorax.

Symptoms
- Shortness of breath +++
- Pleuritic chest pain ++++
- Cough ++
- Anxiety

Signs
- Patients with minimal pneumothoraces may have no detectable signs.
- Tachycardia (most common)
- Tachypnea
- Diminished breath sounds on affected side
- Hyperresonance to percussion
- Subcutaneous emphysema
- Neck vein distention, tracheal deviation with tension pneumothorax

Workup
- Patients with large or tension pneumothorax should be treated with needle or tube thoracostomy prior to any investigations.
- Pulse oximetry, consider ABG
- ECG monitoring, IV placement
- Chest radiograph: look for displacement of visceral line from chest wall
- CT scan may be needed to distinguish bullae from pneumothorax in COPD patients

Comments and Treatment Considerations
There is little evidence from randomized trials to support management decisions. Consensus statements (expert opinion) from American College of Chest Physicians and the British Thoracic Society are the best available evidence. Goals of therapy are to eliminate air in the pleural space and prevent recurrence.

Most patients will require subspecialty assistance from a pulmonologist or surgeon. High-flow oxygen therapy will increase resorption of pleural space air (exercise caution with COPD patients who retain CO_2). Management decisions depend on the size of the pneumothorax and clinical stability of the patient. If the patient is clinically stable and lung collapse is less than 2 to 3 cm, observation may be sufficient. Larger pneumothoraces and unstable patients often require aspiration or chest tube placement.

Patients with SSP tend to be more symptomatic, and frequently require hospitalization. Observation and oxygen therapy alone are usually not sufficient. Furthermore, aspiration is less likely to succeed in these patients—most will need chest tubes. Complicated patients with air leaks, bronchopleural fistulas, and recurrent pneumothoraces need subspecialty attention.

Most patients with PSP who have a second occurrence will require thoracoscopy or thoracotomy for prevention. Chemical pleurodesis with talc or doxycycline is considered second-line therapy. Patients with SSP may need surgical intervention after the first pneumothorax. For tension pneumothorax insert a 19-gauge needle into the second intercostal space at the midclavicular line over the superior aspect of the rib. Attach a three-way stopcock, and withdraw air with a large syringe. Then insert a chest tube after the patient is stabilized.

All patients should be encouraged to avoid or reduce risk factors, with particular emphasis on smoking cessation.

CONGESTIVE HEART FAILURE

Heart failure is classified as systolic or diastolic dysfunction. Systolic dysfunction can occur whenever changes affect heart rate, contractility, preload or afterload. The most common cause of acute systolic dysfunction is loss of contractility due to MI. Valvular disease, dysrhythmias, and severe hypertension can contribute to pump failure. Heart failure can present in the face of normal left ventricular systolic function. Diastolic dysfunction is a result of a stiff or noncompliant ventricle resulting in abnormal filling of the ventricle. This can lead to elevated diastolic pressures and a diminished cardiac output. Chronic long-standing hypertension is a common cause of diastolic dysfunction. A variety of neurohormonal and hemodynamic changes occur in response to a decrease in cardiac output that results in vasoconstriction and salt and water retention, which worsens both preload and afterload. This cycle leads to further decreases in cardiac output.

Symptoms
- Dyspnea with exertion ++++
- Fatigue
- Cough
- Angina if coexisting coronary artery disease
- Wheezing
- Orthopnea ++
- Paroxysmal nocturnal dyspnea +++

Signs
- Tachycardia
- Tachypnea
- Peripheral edema ++ (85% specific)
- Anxiety
- Frothy, blood-tinged sputum if acute pulmonary edema
- Moist rales on auscultation
- Wheezes with bronchospasm
- Jugular venous distention ++
- Murmur(s)
- S_3 gallop ++ (90% specific)
- S_4 gallop (especially in diastolic dysfunction)
- Hypoxia

Workup
- Chest radiograph
- ECG
- Pulse oximetry, consider ABG
- Chemistry (assess renal function, potassium, and liver enzymes)
- CBC
- BNP is helpful for distinguishing between pulmonary and cardiac causes in patients with coexisting CHF and lung disease.
- TSH
- Cardiac enzymes
- Echocardiogram (after stabilization)

Comments and Treatment Considerations
Preload Reduction
Diuretics have been shown to reduce both mortality and readmission for worsening heart failure symptoms (level 1A). Nitroglycerin is thought to be the fastest-acting, most effective, and predictable agent for preload reduction. Be cautions not to overdiurese patients with diastolic dysfunction or mainly right-side failure. This can cause hypotension and electrolyte derangements. Aldosterone antagonists such as spironolactone have been shown to reduce mortality, death and hospitalization from cardiac causes and death from CHF, and improved New York Heart Association (NYHA) functional class in patients with severe CHF (level 1A). Morphine sulfate's main effects are likely secondary to reduced anxiety and air hunger, which can decrease catecholamine production and thereby help reduce systemic vascular resistance.

Afterload Reduction
ACE inhibitors appear to decrease mortality in heart failure patients. They should be used with caution in patients with borderline hemodynamic status. Evidence shows that these ARBs are a good choice for patients who are ACE intolerant, and may be used in combination with ACE inhibitors. Hydralazine used either alone or with nitrates is an option in patients with renal insufficiency or ACE intolerance. One trial showed improved survival and quality of life with isosorbide dinitrate and hydralazine in African-American patients.

Beta-Blockers
Once heart failure is stabilized, beta-blockers such as carvedilol and extended-release metoprolol have been shown to decrease mortality.

Inotropic Agents
Inotropic agents may be necessary if a patient remains symptomatic. There is no survival benefit with digoxin. Digoxin can be helpful for rate control in patients with tachyarrhythmias as well. Dobutamine and dopamine are other choices for inotropic support.

Nesiritide
Human B-type natriuretic peptide, after review of evidence, needs more study. One review showed a trend toward increased mortality in acute decompensated heart failure.

CHRONIC OBSTRUCTIVE PULMONARY DISEASE

COPD is a chronic disorder associated with airflow obstruction usually caused by chronic bronchitis or emphysema. The definition of chronic bronchitis requires the presence of a chronic cough and/or production of sputum for 3 months each year over 2 consecutive years. Emphysema is characterized by abnormal, permanent enlargement of the air spaces distal to the terminal bronchioles, with destruction of the walls, and without fibrosis. Although emphysema is usually described anatomically, and chronic bronchitis is described clinically, both are often seen together. There can be airway hyperreactivity and small airway inflammation that may be partially reversible. Acute exacerbation of symptoms occurs more frequently as the disease progresses and is a common cause of acute dyspnea.

Symptoms
- Shortness of breath
- Productive cough with increase in sputum production during acute exacerbation
- Wheezing

Signs
- Tachypnea
- Tachycardia
- Accessory muscle use
- Coarse rhonchi
- Hyperresonance to percussion
- Bilateral decreased breath sounds
- Hyperinflation (barrel chest)
- Prolonged expiratory phase
- Pursed-lip breathing
- Cyanosis

Workup
- Chest radiograph
- Pulse oximetry, consider ABG
- BNP is helpful for distinguishing between pulmonary and cardiac causes in patients with coexisting CHF (level 1B).
- CBC with differential
- Serum electrolytes
- Spirometry if not done previously (FEV_1/FVC <0.70 indicates airflow obstruction)
- α_1-antitrypsin if history suggestive

Comments and Treatment Considerations
Oxygen should be used to correct hypoxia. Most cases of CO_2 retention are due to ventilation-perfusion mismatch and not depression of the respiratory center. Therefore the correction of hypoxemia should be the therapeutic preference. Oral or parenteral corticosteroids can reduce treatment failures and the need for further medical treatment.

Antibiotics reduce risk of short-term mortality by 77%, treatment failure by 53%, and sputum purulence by 44%. Inhaled bronchodilators are used routinely. The co-administration of β2 agonists and ipratropium bromide seem to be more effective than either one alone.

In patients with acute respiratory failure, noninvasive positive pressure ventilation (NPPV) can reduce likelihood of endotracheal intubation, treatment failures, and mortality. It has also been shown to reduce length of hospital stay and complications associated with treatment.

ASTHMA

Asthma is an obstructive lung disease characterized by acute, intermittent periods of tracheobronchial hyper-responsiveness to a variety of stimuli. The reversibility of the acute, obstructive attack and recurrence is diagnostic of this chronic pulmonary disease. In an acute setting, management of the acute exacerbation requires timely clinical assessment and treatment to improve airflow and decrease inflammation. Respiratory distress that is unsuccessfully managed (status asthmaticus) may lead to death. Goals of chronic asthma therapy include patient education, periodic assessment of pulmonary function, identification and avoidance of patient-specific triggers, and the use of pharmacologic agents that decrease airway inflammation and provide airway bronchodilation.

Symptoms
- Wheezing ++++
- Daytime and/or nighttime cough +++
- Shortness of breath +++
- Chest tightness
- Symptoms exacerbated by illness, exercise, or environmental exposure

Signs
- Wheezing
- Intercostal retractions and use of accessory muscles
- Prolonged expiratory phase
- Tachypnea
- Inability to speak in complete sentences
- Nasal obstruction, including nasal polyps
- Atopic dermatitis or eczema

Workup
- Peak flow meter
- Spirometry (FEV_1/FVC <0.70 indicates airflow obstruction)
- Arterial blood gas
- Chest radiograph
- Exercise spirometry

Comments and Treatment Considerations
Severity of disease varies with frequency of symptoms and FEV_1. For intermittent asthma symptoms will last 2 or fewer days per week, or 2 or fewer night awakenings per month and FEV_1 80% or more predicted value. Treat with short-acting bronchodilators as needed for acute exacerbation. Daily therapy is not indicated.

Mild persistent asthma is defined as symptoms occurring more than 2 days per week—but not daily—(or more than 2 night awakenings per month) and FEV_1 80% or more predicted value. Treatment includes short-acting bronchodilators as needed for acute exacerbation and low-dose inhaled corticosteroids for daily antiinflammatory management.

Moderate persistent asthma has daily symptoms, or more than 1 night awakening per week and FEV_1 60% or more, but less than 80% predicted value. Treat with short-acting bronchodilators as needed for acute exacerbation and daily medium-dose inhaled corticosteroids and (if required) long-acting bronchodilator.

Severe persistent asthma will have continual daytime symptoms, or nightly symptoms and FEV_1 60% or less predicted value. Treat with short-acting bronchodilators as needed for acute exacerbation. Long-term therapy should include a medium- or high-dose inhaled corticosteroid, in addition to a long-acting bronchodilator and oral corticosteroids.

Status asthmaticus has prolonged exacerbations of symptoms and fails to respond to usual treatment. Peak expiratory flow is less than 50% of predicted or best effort, oxygen saturation is less than 91% and Pao_2 less than 60 mm Hg on room air or Pco_2 greater than 42 mm Hg. Short-acting bronchodilators, inhaled ipratropium bromide, supplemental oxygen and corticosteroids are the mainstays of medical management. Hospitalize patients that do not demonstrate immediate improvement of the acute exacerbation. Consider subcutaneous and IV epinephrine for severely ill patients. A one-time bolus of intravenous magnesium sulfate may be considered for those with impending respiratory failure. Prepare to intubate any patient with progressively worsening respiratory distress, especially if patient appears to be fatiguing. However, intubation should be accomplished as a last resort because air trapping makes ventilation extremely difficult after intubation.

Other Considerations

Use of inhaled corticosteroids at the lowest effective doses offers the maximum benefit and fewest adverse effects.

Children with mild to moderate asthma demonstrate better control of their disease when using inhaled corticosteroids than with use of β-agonists as a single agent.

Although a short-term difference in growth velocity (1 cm/yr) has been observed in children with chronic use of inhaled corticosteroids, the difference does not affect final adult height.

Although written action plans for asthma management in children are recommended, there is limited evidence that symptom-based plans offer significant advantage over peak flow–based plans.

Antibiotics do not offer any benefit in the management of acute asthma exacerbation in the absence of a bacterial infection of the respiratory system.

The role of leukotriene modifiers in the chronic management of asthma is unclear. Patients with aspirin-sensitive asthma seem to derive the most benefit from this medication class.

BRONCHIOLITIS

Bronchiolitis is the most common lower respiratory tract illness of infants and very young children. It is a clinical syndrome characterized by wheezing and tachypnea. RSV causes the majority of cases; others are caused by other respiratory viruses. Peak incidence in the United States occurs in the winter and early spring. Patients at highest risk for severe disease include premature infants; infants less than 6 weeks old; those with chronic lung, heart, or neurologic disease; and those suffering from immunodeficiency.

Symptoms
- Cough
- Dyspnea
- Poor feeding

Signs
- Wheezing with or without rales
- Rhinorrhea
- Tachypnea
- Fever
- Retractions
- Nasal flaring
- Decreased oxygen saturation
- Cyanosis
- Apnea

Workup
- History and physical examination provide basis for diagnosis. Accurate assessment of severity is critical. Patients at highest risk for adverse outcomes include those with chronic lung disease, prematurity, congenital heart disease, and immunocompromise.
- Routine diagnostic studies (RSV swab, chest x-ray, cultures, or ABGs) not indicated in low-risk cases of mild severity
- Chest x-rays may be useful when diagnosis is unclear or the patient is not improving as expected.
- Rapid viral testing may be beneficial in avoidance of unnecessary testing in very young (<3 months) infants.

Comments and Treatment Considerations
Primary treatment is supportive. Consider hospitalization for infants with respiratory rates of 50 or more and/or saturations less than 95% on room air. Assess for and treat dehydration. Suctioning should be done when needed, before feeding, and prior to inhalation therapy.

Results of trials of nebulized β-agonists or racemic epinephrine have been equivocal. Many clinicians will attempt a trial of these agents early in the course of the illness. Repeated clinical assessment should be done for signs of deteriorating respiratory status. Mechanical ventilation is indicated for respiratory failure.

The use of ribavirin is controversial, its use is generally reserved for selected immunocompromised patients with severe disease. Prophylaxis with palivizumab is recommended in certain target groups, including infants with chronic lung disease, prematurity, or congenital heart disease. Antibiotics should be used only if there is clear evidence of a coexisting bacterial infection.

CROUP

Croup is a clinical syndrome seen most commonly in children between the ages of 3 months and 3 years. Croup is characterized by inspiratory stridor, a brassy or barklike cough, hoarseness, and varying degrees of respiratory distress. These symptoms are secondary to inflammation and edema of the laryngeal mucosa leading to subglottal narrowing. Bacterial tracheitis may be difficult to distinguish from croup, but typically the child with tracheitis appears more toxic. Foreign body aspiration may also present with crouplike symptoms. Acute epiglottitis and retropharyngeal abscess classically lack the barking cough of croup but may present with stridor, fever, and labored breathing.

Symptoms
- A barklike or brassy cough is a classic symptom. ++++
- Hoarseness
- Inspiratory stridor
- Symptoms worse at night
- Rhinorrhea, nasal congestion
- Irritability, poor feeding

Signs
- Inspiratory stridor
- Barklike cough ++++
- Mild to moderately inflamed pharynx
- In-drawing of chest wall with inspiration
- Respiratory rate may be increased
- Fever may be present; less likely with spasmodic croup
- Hypoxia in severe cases

Workup
- Diagnosis is clinical.
- Lateral neck x-ray may show subglottic narrowing (steeple sign).
- Pulse oximetry is normal in most, but should be used in monitoring those with more severe croup.
- Use caution in getting lab work or x-rays (if indicated) because agitation of the patient may increase respiratory distress.

Comments and Treatment Considerations
- Avoid agitation to minimize respiratory distress.
- A single dose of corticosteroids is beneficial regardless of clinical severity.
- Standard steroid treatment for croup is a single dose of dexamethasone 0.6 mg/kg PO to a maximum of 10 mg (or IM if unable to take PO).
- Inhaled budesonide is an alternative to IM dexamethasone in a vomiting child.
- Nebulized racemic epinephrine improves croup symptoms within 10 to 30 minutes, and can be repeated. Duration of improvement is about 2 hours.

- Children given one dose of steroid and a treatment of nebulized racemic epinephrine in the ED can be considered for discharge if symptoms have not recurred by 4 hours post treatment.
- Indications for hospitalization include persistent stridor at rest, hypoxemia, pallor or cyanosis, respiratory distress, depressed level of consciousness, or suspected epiglottitis.

References

ACP Journal Club: ACE inhibitors reduce mortality and hospitalization in congestive heart failure [therapeutics], *ACP J Club* 123:62, 1995.

ACP Journal Club: Isosorbide dinitrate plus hydralazine was effective for advanced heart failure in black patients [therapeutics], *ACP J Club* 142(2):37, 2005.

ACP Journal Club: Angiotensin-receptor blockers do not reduce mortality or hospitalization rates in heart failure [therapeutics], *ACP J Club* 137(2):48, 2002.

ACP Journal Club: Spironolactone reduced mortality in severe congestive heart failure [therapeutics], *ACP J Club* 132(1):2, 2000.

Agency for Healthcare Research and Quality: *Management of bronchiolitis in infants and children: evidence report/technology assessment: no. 69.* Rockville, MD. Alt. RQ Pub No. 03-E014, 2003. Available at http://ahrq.gov/clinic/epcsums/broncsum.htm (accessed September 2006).

Lieberthal A, Bauchner H, Hall C, et al: Diagnosis and management of bronchiolitis, *Pediatrics* 118(4):1774–1793, 2006.

Baumann MH, Strange C, Heffner J, et al: Management of spontaneous pneumothorax: an American College of Chest Physicians Delphi consensus statement, *Chest* 119(2):590–602, 2001.

Baumann MH: Management of spontaneous pneumothorax, *Clin Chest Med* 27(2):369–381, 2006.

Ben-Joseph R, Messonnier M, Alemao E, Gould A: A meta-analysis of the dose-response relationship of inhaled corticosteroids in adolescents and adults with mild to moderate persistent asthma, *Clin Ther* 24(1):1–20, 2002.

Bjornson C, Johnson D: Croup—treatment update, *Pediatr Emerg Care* 21:863–870, 2005.

Boushey HA, Sorkness CA, King TS, et al: Daily versus as-needed corticosteroids for mild persistent asthma, *N Engl J Med* 352:1519–1528, 2005. (abstract).

Chang AK, Barton ED: *Pneumothorax, iatrogenic, spontaneous and pneumomediastinum,* eMedicine.com, March 23, 2005.

Hunt S, Abraham W, Chin M, et al: Diagnosis and management of chronic heart failure in the adult, *J Am Coll Cardiol* 46:1116–1143, 2005.

Cincinnati Children's Hospital Medical Center: *Evidence based clinical practice guideline for medical management of bronchiolitis in infants less than 1 year of age presenting with a first time episode,* Cincinnati, OH, 2006, Cincinnati Children's Hospital Medical Center.

Database of Abstracts of Reviews of Effects Centre for Reviews and Dissemination: *Beta-blockers in congestive heart failure: a bayesian meta-analysis* (structured abstract). [Miscellaneous] Database of Abstracts of Reviews of Effects, Issue 3, 2006.

Database of Abstracts of Reviews of Effects Centre for Reviews and Dissemination: *Overview of randomized trials of angiotensin-converting enzyme inhibitors on mortality and morbidity in patients with heart failure* (structured abstract). [Miscellaneous]. Database of Abstracts of Reviews of Effects, Issue 3, 2006.

Database of Abstracts of Reviews of Effects Centre for Reviews and Dissemination: *Short-term risk of death after treatment with nesiritide for decompensated heart failure: a pooled analysis of randomized controlled trials* (structured abstract). [Miscellaneous]. Database of Abstracts of Reviews of Effects, Issue 3, 2006.

Davidson C, Ventre K, Luchetti M, et al: Efficacy of interventions for bronchiolitis in critically ill infants: a systemic review and meta-analysis, *Pediatr Crit Care Med* 5:482, 2004.

Ducharme FM, Lasserson TJ, Cates CJ: Long-acting beta$_2$-agonists versus anti-leukotrienes as add-on therapy to inhaled corticosteroids for chronic asthma, *Cochrane Database Syst Rev* 2006(4), CD003137.

Faris RF, Flather M, Purcell H, Poole-Wilson P, Coats AJS: Diuretics for heart failure, *Cochrane Database Syst Rev* 2006(1), CD003838.

Henry M, Arnold T, Harvey JE: British Thoracic Society guidelines for the management of spontaneous pneumothorax, *Thorax* 58:39–52, 2003.

Higgins JC: The crashing asthmatic, *Am Fam Physician* 67(5):997–1004, 2003.

Kleinschmidt P: COPD and emphysema, *eMedicine*, February 10, 2005.

Knutson D, Aring A: Viral croup, *Am Fam Physician* 69:535, 2004.

Management of Chronic Asthma: *Summary, evidence report/technology assessment:* no. *44.* AHRQ Publication Number 01-E043, September 2001. Agency for Healthcare Research and Quality, Rockville, MD. www.ahrq.gov/clinic/epcsums/asthmasum.htm.

McCrory DC, Brown CD: Anticholinergic bronchodilators versus beta$_2$-sympathomimetic agents for acute exacerbations of chronic obstructive pulmonary disease, *Cochrane Database Syst Rev* 3, 2006, CD003900.

McCrory DC, Brown CD: Anticholinergic bronchodilators versus beta$_2$-sympathomimetic agents for acute exacerbations of chronic obstructive pulmonary disease, *Cochrane Database Syst Rev* 2002(4), CD003900.

Mueller C, Laule-Kilia K, Frana B, et al: Use of B-type natriuretic peptide in the management of acute dyspnea in patients with pulmonary disease, *Am Heart J* 151:471–477, 2006.

Pauwels RA, Buist AS, Calverley PM: Global strategy for the diagnosis, management, and prevention of chronic obstructive pulmonary disease. NHLBI/WHO Global Initiative for Chronic Obstructive Lung Disease, *Am J Respir Crit Care Med* 163(5):1256–1276, 2001.

Ram FSF, Picot J, Lightowler J, Wedzicha JA: Non-invasive positive pressure ventilation for treatment of respiratory failure due to exacerbations of chronic obstructive pulmonary disease, *Cochrane Database Syst Rev* 2004, CD004104.

Russell KF, Liang Y, O'Gorman K, Johnson DW, Klassen TP. Glucocorticoids for croup, *Cochrane Database Systc Rev* 2011(1), CD001955.

Sahn SA, Heffner JE: Spontaneous pneumothorax, *N Engl J Med* 342:868–874, 2000.

Scarfone R: Controversies in the treatment of bronchiolitis, *Curr Opin Pediatr* 17:62–66, 2005.

Smyth R, Openshaw P: Bronchiolitis, *Lancet* 368:312–322, 2006.

The CONSENSUS Trial Study Group: Effects of enalapril on mortality in severe congestive heart failure. Results of the Cooperative North Scandinavian Enalapril Survival Study (CONSENSUS), *N Engl J Med* 316(23):1429–1435, 1987.

Zevitz ME: Heart failure, *eMedicine* , June 15, 2006.

CHAPTER 39

Sleep Disorders
Dan Sontheimer

Approximately 75% of American adults reported having had at least one symptom of a sleep problem a few nights a week or more within the past year. Sleep disorders can present across the entire spectrum of age, from children to older adults. The range of conditions that contribute to insomnia or excessive daytime sleepiness include: normal responses to lack of sleep, underlying medical conditions, and the primary sleep disorders. The key in establishing a diagnosis is gathering important historical information about the problem and the patient's risk for a given sleep disorder and using it to guide options for treatment or further testing.

INSOMNIA

Insomnia is the sleep disorder that is most prevalent in the general population. Insomnia is defined as a complaint of difficulty falling asleep, staying asleep, or sleep that is chronically perceived by the patient as nonrestorative or lacking in quality. The diagnosis of insomnia is further classified as adjustment insomnia (defined as insomnia lasting less than 3 months and due to a psychosocial stressor), insomnia due to medical disorders, insomnia due to psychiatric disorders, and idiopathic insomnia.

Symptoms
- Trouble falling asleep ++++
- Inability to stay asleep++++
- Nonrestorative sleep
- Daytime sleepiness

Signs
- Tired appearance
- Frequent yawning
- Somnolence

Workup
- Sleep history for evidence of sleep apnea, restless legs disorder, periodic limb movement disorder, inadequate sleep hygiene, or substance use
- Further testing is not necessary unless there is suspicion for another sleep disorder.

Comments and Treatment Considerations
Sleep hygiene is the mainstay of treatment and consists of regular sleep and wake times; avoiding caffeine, nicotine, and alcohol; regular exercise (not in evening hours); avoiding regular use of hypnotics; and sleeping in a quiet, relaxing environment. Treat underlying medical and/or psychiatric disorders that are disrupting sleep and administer cautious use of hypnotics for adjustment insomnia. Incorporate relaxation techniques and CBT.

NARCOLEPSY

Narcolepsy is a neurologic disorder characterized by a disturbance in the sleep-wake system in the brain that allows for the wakeful state to be interrupted by the sleep state and vice versa. It is usually identified after years of struggle and disability experienced by the patient. It is present in 1 in 2000 individuals.

Symptoms
- Excessive daytime sleepiness
- Sleep paralysis
- Cataplexy +++
- Hypnagogic hallucinations
- Hyperactivity in children

Signs
- Sleep attacks

Workup
- Combination of excessive daytime sleepiness and cataplexy nearly always is due to narcolepsy
- Polysomnography with multiple sleep latency tests is confirmatory.

Comments and Treatment Considerations
Stimulants include methylphenidate and dextroamphetamine. A wake-promoting drug, modafinil, is first-line therapy. Cataplexy may be managed with TCAs, SSRIs, or venlafaxine. Suggest regular sleep times and scheduled daytime napping.

OBSTRUCTIVE SLEEP APNEA

Obstructive sleep apnea (OSA) is diagnosed by the presence of apneic episodes and hypopneic episodes detected during polysomnography. Symptoms of sleep apnea were present in 26% of U.S. adults in a national survey. In addition, sleep apnea is also found in the pediatric population at a rate of 2% to 4% in one U.S. series.

Symptoms
- Snoring
- Witnessed apnea during sleep
- Nonrestorative sleep

- Excessive daytime sleepiness
- Headache
- Increased activity (children)

Signs
- Obesity
- Thick neck
- Somnolence
- Enlarged tonsils
- Adenoid facies
- Reduced pharyngeal volume
- Elevated BP

Workup
- Overnight polysomnography
- Overnight oximetry (suggestive, but not diagnostic)

Comments and Treatment Considerations
Continuous positive airway pressure (CPAP) is most commonly used in adults. A Cochrane Review concluded that it does reduce symptoms of sleepiness and improve quality of life for those with moderate and severe OSA. Some patients benefit from oral appliances and supplemental oxygen. Pediatric patients with evidence of enlarged adenoids or tonsils may benefit from surgical removal.

RESTLESS LEGS SYNDROME AND PERIODIC LIMB MOVEMENTS IN SLEEP

Restless legs syndrome (RLS) and periodic limb movements in sleep (PLMS) often coexist. The distinction is that in RLS the symptoms interfere with sleep initiation and in periodic limb movement disorder the symptoms lead to arousal from sleep and poor quality of sleep. Either disorder can also manifest involuntary leg movements during the day.

Symptoms
- Crawling or "pins and needles" sensation in legs, relieved only by moving the legs ++++
- Repeated leg jerks that arouse from sleep
- Excessive daytime sleepiness
- Difficulty in falling or staying asleep

Workup
- Evaluate for iron deficiency anemia, uremia, neuropathy, and peripheral vascular disease.
- Polysomnography for confirmation, if history not clear

Comments and Treatment Considerations
Dopamine agonists are generally considered first-line treatment. Ropinirole is the only FDA-approved agent available. Evidence supports the use of levodopa, levodopa-carbidopa, and pramipexole.

Anticonvulsants such as gabapentin, carbamazepine, benzodiazepines, and opiates are frequently chosen as alternative agents
for treatment. Patients with evidence of low iron stores should be
treated.

TRANSIENT DISTURBANCE IN CIRCADIAN RHYTHM

Jet lag and shift work result from alterations in a person's daily
schedule that conflict with the intrinsic circadian rhythm of the
body. Due to either a change in time zone or working at hours normally associated with sleep, the patient experiences difficulty with
wakefulness and performance.

Symptoms
- Daytime sleepiness
- Insomnia
- Loss of appetite
- Mood disturbances
- Difficulty concentrating

Workup
- Sleep history

Comments and Treatment Considerations
Take 0.5 to 5 mg melatonin around target bedtime of destination or
targeted sleep time for shift worker. Use bright light exposure in
nighttime work environment and avoid light cues during daytime
sleep hours.

References

Ancoli-Israel S, Ayalon L: Diagnosis and treatment of sleep disorders in older
  adults, *Am J Geriatr Psychiatry* 14:95–103, 2006.
Anon: Circadian rhythm sleep disorders: pathophysiology and potential
  approaches to management [Review]. *CNS Drugs* 15(4):311–328, 2001.
Giles TL, Lasserson TJ, Smith B, White J, Wright JJ, Cates CJ: Continuous pos-
  itive airways pressure for obstructive sleep apnoea in adults, *Cochrane
  Database Syst Rev* 2006(3), CD001106.
Hiestand DM, Britz P, Goldman M, Phillips B: Prevalence of symptoms and risk
  of sleep apnea in the U.S. population, *Chest* 130:780–786, 2006.
Högl B, Poewe W: Restless legs syndrome, *Curr Opin Neurol* 18(4):405–410, 2005.
International classification of sleep disorders: diagnosis and coding manual,
  2nd ed, Westchester, IL, 2005, American Academy of Sleep Medicine.
Mahowald M, Schenck C: Insights from studying human sleep disorders,
  Nature 27:1279–1285, 2005.
Herxheimer A, Petrie KJ: Melatonin for the prevention and treatment of jet lag,
  Cochrane Database Syst Rev 2002(2), CD001520.
Ohayon MM: Epidemiology of insomnia: what we know and what we still need
  to learn, *Sleep Med Rev* 6:97–111, 2002.
Rosen CL, Larkin ER, Kirchner HI, et al: Prevalence and risk factors for sleep-
  disordered breathing in 8 to 11 year old children: association with race and
  prematurity, *J Pediatr* 142:383–389, 2003.
Young T, Silber M: Hypersomnias of central origin, *Chest* 130:913–920, 2006.

Sore Throat
Roger Zoorob, Monty VanBeber, and
Ila Patel

Sore throat is a common complaint in primary care clinical practice. Although most acute pharyngitis is self-limited, the importance of its diagnosis lies in the fact that antibiotics may be needed to prevent complications of group A β-hemolytic streptococcal infection. Less common causes include GERD, allergic rhinitis, dental disease, and neoplastic causes.

Rarely, sore throat can be caused by an immediately life-threatening condition such as epiglottitis or peripharyngeal fascial space infections.

BACTERIAL PHARYNGITIS

Most sore throats are viral; however, about 20% are related to bacterial infection with the majority being group A streptococcus (GAS) in all ages, more so between 5 and 18 years old.

Symptoms
- Sore throat +++++
- Absence of cough* +++
- Fever by history* +++
- Headache
- Malaise
- Chills
- Rash

Signs
- Pharyngeal erythema
- Tonsillar exudates* +++
- Cervical adenopathy* +++
- High-grade fever
- Diffuse "sandpaper" rash (scarlet fever)
- Grayish membranes *(Corynebacterium diphtheriae)* +++
- Associated urethritis or vaginitis (gonococcal, chlamydia)

Workup
- Throat cultures are considered gold standard ++++
- Rapid streptococcal antigen test (RSAT) ++++
- If *Neisseria gonorrhoeae* is suspected, a Gram stain and throat culture on Thayer-Martin plate are required.

---

*Three out of four present equal positive predictive value for group A streptococcal pharyngitis of 40% to 60%.

Comments and Treatment Considerations
- Identification of GAS is the primary goal. If left untreated it may lead to suppurative or nonsuppurative sequelae.
- Treatment of GAS includes penicillin V 250 mg to 500 mg orally twice a day for 10 days, IM benzathine penicillin 1.2 million units once, or macrolides such as erythromycin 500 mg orally twice daily for individuals with penicillin allergy.
- *N. gonorrhoeae* is a relatively rare cause of pharyngitis. Clinicians must obtain pertinent history during the initial evaluation (oral sex, recent STD exposure, or sexual abuse). Uncomplicated infection may be treated with a single dose of ceftriaxone 250 mg IM or a fluoroquinolone such as ciprofloxacin 500 mg orally in a single dose. Resistance to fluoroquinolones is growing. Concomitant treatment of chlamydia infection is warranted.
- Diphtheria is caused by *C. diphtheriae*. Treatment includes hospitalization with close monitoring for systemic disease. Further treatment with antitoxin, IM or IV infusion, and erythromycin or penicillin orally for 2 weeks is used during the acute phase of the disease. Immunization is the key to prevention.

PERIPHARYNGEAL SPACE INFECTIONS

Infections in the peripharyngeal fascial spaces often arise from foci in the gingiva, tonsils, or sinuses, and may present as sore throat. Peritonsillar and retropharyngeal abscesses, as well as submandibular space infections (e.g., Ludwig's angina or abscesses), may all present as a sore throat. Most infections are polymicrobial, and usually involve aerobic and anaerobic bacteria.

Symptoms
- Extreme sore throat ++++
- Neck pain
- Dysphagia

Signs
- Drooling
- Muffled voice
- Fever
- Erythematous pharynx
- Trismus
- Asymmetry of tonsils and contralateral deviation of uvula (peritonsillar abscess)
- Cervical adenopathy ++++
- Submandibular and/or neck swelling

Workup
- Culture of drained pus
- CBC
- US, CT, or MRI

Comments and Treatment Considerations

- In peritonsillar abscess if there is no airway compromise, needle aspiration and outpatient treatment with antibiotics can often be accomplished.
- In most other peripharyngeal space infections, aggressive airway evaluation and management, IV antibiotics, and evaluation for surgical intervention are necessary.
- Complications of peripharyngeal abscesses include septic thrombosis, brain abscess, airway obstruction, and carotid artery involvement.

EPIGLOTTITIS/SUPRAGLOTTITIS

Epiglottitis is an acute, severe, life-threatening condition resulting from an inflammation of the supraglottic structures. It is a cellulitis of the epiglottis, aryepiglottic folds, and other adjacent tissues. Although it occurs in children more than adults, peak incidence in adults is the 35- to 39-year age group.

Symptoms

- Sore throat ++++
- High fever +++++
- Dysphagia +++-++++
- Drooling
- Respiratory distress
- Stridor
- Toxic appearance
- Muffled speech

Signs

- Erythematous "cherry red" and edematous epiglottis +++++
- Stridor
- Cervical adenopathy
- Minimal cough
- Toxic appearance
- Increased respiratory effort

Workup

- Blood cultures
- CBC may show leukocytosis and left shift.
- Lateral soft tissue neck x-rays show "thumb sign" ++++ -+++++
- Chest x-ray to rule out pneumonia and for tube placement if intubated

Comments and Treatment Considerations

- Emergency inpatient hospital evaluation with intubation equipment at bedside. Keep a child calm in parent's arms. Ensure respiratory and cardiac monitoring.
- Nasotracheal intubation is the preferred way to stabilize the airway but preparing for tracheotomy is warranted.

- Avoid throat examinations and direct attempts to visualize epiglottis because this increases respiratory effort and anxiety and may lead to further airway obstruction.
- Empiric treatment with broad-spectrum antibiotic therapy such as ceftriaxone 50 to 75 mg/kg orally per day in addition to an antibiotic active against MRSA, such as clindamycin or vancomycin is recommended.
- Steroids and racemic epinephrine mixture inhalation are of no benefit.
- Preventive measures include *Haemophilus influenzae* vaccine to all children and rifampin prophylaxis (20 mg/kg/day orally) for 4 days for household and daycare contacts.

VIRAL PHARYNGITIS

Nasal symptoms, such as sneezing, watery nasal discharge, or postnasal drip tend to precede throat symptoms.

Symptoms
- Nasal symptoms
- Throat soreness +++++
- Fatigue
- Malaise ++++
- Nonproductive cough
- Myalgia
- Odynophagia

Signs
- Fever
- Pharyngeal edema
- Pharyngeal erythema
- Pharyngeal exudates or vesicles
- Conjunctival injection
- Palatal petechiae
- Hoarseness
- Tender lymphadenopathy
- Mucosal ulcers
- Splenomegaly (EBV, HIV)

Workup
- Diagnosis is clinical.
- Atypical lymphocytosis more prominent in infectious mononucleosis, acute CMV infection, and acute retroviral infection (such as HIV)
- Rapid streptococcal antigen test and bacterial cultures are negative.
- Heterophil antibody test (EBV)
- PCR techniques can be used for specific virologic diagnosis if required.

Comments and Treatment Considerations
Symptomatic relief is the mainstay of treatment. Rest, fluids, and saltwater gargles are used for soothing effect and symptomatic

relief. Analgesics and antipyretics are prescribed for relief of pain or pyrexia. Ibuprofen and acetaminophen are preferred drugs for symptomatic relief in children and adults along with anesthetic gargles and lozenges containing phenol or menthol. If odynophagia is intense, IV hydration may be necessary. Antibiotics neither hasten the recovery period nor reduce bacterial superinfection.

- Influenzavirus: Pharyngitis and sore throat are present in about 50% of type A influenza. It is a self-limited disease usually resolving within 3 to 4 days. It does not warrant antiviral therapy in healthy individuals. Rimantadine or amantadine can decrease duration of symptoms if administered within 48 hours of onset of illness. Oseltamivir and inhaled zanamivir are newer neuraminidase inhibitors active against both A and B strains. They decrease duration of illness in severely ill patients if administered within 30 hours of onset of symptoms.
- Coxsackieviruses and other enteroviruses cause herpangina and hand, foot, and mouth disease. Treatment is symptomatic.
- HIV: HIV pharyngitis is one of the presenting symptoms of acute retroviral syndrome. It may present as an infectious mononucleosis-like syndrome; 40% to 80% of these individuals develop a generalized maculopapular roseola-like or urticarial-type rash.
- Infectious mononucleosis

Corticosteroids may be indicated in severe tonsillar hypertrophy or impending airway obstruction. Avoidance of contact sports is highly recommended for approximately 6 weeks post infection.

GASTROESOPHAGEAL REFLUX

Chronic pharyngitis may be associated with GERD. Patients may present with a long history of a sore throat and a lump sensation in their throat. Most common symptoms are heartburn, regurgitation, and dysphagia.

Symptoms
- Heartburn
- Chronic sore throat
- Choking with swallowing
- Chest pain
- History of aspiration pneumonia
- Regurgitation
- Dysphagia
- Laryngitis
- Chronic cough

Signs
- Erythematous pharynx

Workup
- Therapeutic trial of H_2-blocker or PPI
- Barium swallow

- Esophageal pH monitoring
- Endoscopy

Comments and Treatment Considerations
- Lifestyle modifications: There is evidence showing improvement with elevation of head of bed and weight loss.
- Diet modifications (chocolate, high-fat foods, alcohol, tobacco, coffee) may be effective.
- Start with H_2-blockers followed by PPIs (more effective); if unsuccessful, patient may require surgery.

NEOPLASM

Tonsillar and oropharyngeal cancer is a rare cause of sore throat. It should be considered in the older adult or younger patient presenting with prolonged history of sore throat or unilateral swelling of one tonsil.

Symptoms
- Hemoptysis
- Difficulty in swallowing
- Pain referred to the ear
- Lump in the neck
- Hoarseness
- Progressive unilateral increase in tonsillar size

Signs
- Hard swelling of the tonsil
- Ulceration
- Cervical lymphadenopathy
- Neck mass
- Tonsillar asymmetry

Workup
- CBC
- Laryngoscopy
- Chest x-ray
- CT scan
- Biopsy

Comments and Treatment Considerations
Management of squamous cell carcinoma of the tonsil and oropharynx is most frequently surgical.

TRAUMA

Trauma is due to physical causes such as penetrating trauma or retained foreign body. Other causes are due to vocal abuse, which may result from shouting. Environmental trauma includes smoke or dry air exposure leading to irritative pharyngitis, or burns from hot or cold liquids.

Symptoms
- Sore throat +++++
- Hoarseness
- Fever
- Respiratory distress
- Cough
- Dysphagia or odynophagia

Signs
- Quality of patient's voice (coarse, rough, weak, wet, or irregular)
- Vocal cord paralysis or nodule on examination

Workup
- Complete examination of laryngopharynx
- X-rays to rule out foreign body
- CT scan or MRI
- CBC
- Biopsy if necessary

Comments and Treatment Considerations
- Avoiding exposure to smoke and air humidification may help in environmental trauma.
- Refer to an ear, nose, and throat (ENT) specialist in case of foreign body or physical trauma.
- Patients with hoarseness for more than 2 weeks should have complete examination of laryngopharynx. CT scans and radiography are not a substitute for direct visual examination.

ALLERGIC RHINITIS/POSTNASAL DRIP

Allergic rhinitis is associated with multiple nasal symptoms. Common allergens that cause seasonal allergic rhinitis are trees, grass, and weed pollen. Indoor allergens caused by dust mites, pets, fungi, and other household items are usually associated with year-round symptoms.

Allergic rhinitis and secondary postnasal drip manifest as sore throat due to chronic irritation to the pharyngeal mucosa.

Symptoms
- Nasal congestion
- Postnasal drip +++
- Pruritus of nose, eyes, and palate
- Sneezing
- Rhinorrhea
- Cough

Signs
- Bluish or reddish discoloration of nasal turbinates +++ - ++++
- Erythematous pharynx
- Sinus tenderness
- Transverse nasal crease

- Allergic shiners
- Postnasal discharge

Workup
- CBC with differential
- Nasal endoscopy
- Nasal smear for eosinophils ++++ - +++++
- IgE levels
- Allergen skin testing +++ -++++
- Sinus x-rays or CT

Comments and Treatment Considerations
- Patients are instructed to locate triggers and limit exposure. Recommendations include using allergy covers on mattresses and pillows, discouraging house pets, limiting smoking exposure, and avoiding use of perfumes.
- Next tier of therapy is pharmacotherapy. Newer second-generation antihistamines are recommended in combination with nasal steroids to treat allergic rhinitis. Some relief may come with mast cell stabilizers or leukotriene modifiers for patients with severe symptoms.
- Immunotherapy is recommended for patients failing both avoidance of allergens and pharmacologic treatment.

References
American Academy of Pediatrics: *Haemophilus influenzae* infections. In *2003 Red Book: Report of Committee of Infectious Diseases*, 26th ed, Elk Grove Village, IL, 2003, American Academy of Pediatrics, p. 293.

Bisno AL, Gerber MA, Gwaltney JM, Jr, et al: Practice guidelines for the diagnosis and management of group A streptococcal pharyngitis, *Clin Infect Dis* 35:113–125, 2002.

Brietzke SE, Jones DT: Pediatric oropharyngeal trauma: what is the role of CT scan? *Int J Pediatr Otorhinolaryngol* 69:669–679, 2005.

Brunton S, Pichichero M: Considerations in the use of antibiotics for streptococcal pharyngitis, *J Fam Pract* July, S9–S16, 2006.

Candy B, Hotopf M: Steroids for symptom control in infectious mononucleosis, *Cochrane Database Syst Rev*, 2006, CD004402.

Centers for Disease Control and Prevention: *Infectious mononucleosis*. Available at www.cdc.gov/ncidod/diseases/ebv.htm (accessed Oct 14, 2006).

Craig FW, Schunk JE: Retropharyngeal abscess in children: clinical presentation, utility of imaging and current management, *Pediatrics* 111:1394–1398, 2003.

DeVault KR, Castell DO: Updated guidelines for the diagnosis and treatment of gastroesophageal reflux disease, *Am J Gastroenterol* 100:190, 2005.

Ebell MH: Epstein-Barr infectious mononucleosis, *Am Fam Physician* 70: 1279–1287, 2004.

Faden H: The dramatic change in the epidemiology of pediatric epiglottitis, *Pediatr Emerg Care* 22:443–444, 2006.

Frew AJ: Advances in environmental and occupational diseases 2003, *J Allergy Clin Immunol* 113:1161, 2004.

Gerber MA, Shulman ST: Rapid diagnosis of pharyngitis caused by group A streptococci, *Clin Microbiol Rev* 17:571–580, 2004.

Hafidh MA, Sheahan P, Keogh I, Walsh RM: Acute epiglottitis in adults: a recent experience with 10 cases, *J Laryngol Otol* 120:310–313, 2006.

Holsinger F, McWhorter A, Menard M, et al: Transoral lateral pharyngectomy for squamous cell carcinoma of the tonsillar region: I. Technique, complications, and functional results, *Arch Otolaryngol Head Neck Surg* 131:583–591, 2005.

Jefferson T, Demicheli D, Rivetti D, et al: Antiviral agents for influenza in healthy adults: systemic review, *Lancet* 367:303–313, 2006.

Kaltenbach T, Crocket S, Gerson LB: Are lifestyle measures effective in patients with gastroesophageal reflux disease? An evidence-based approach, *Arch Intern Med* 166:965–971, 2006.

Martin Campagne E, del Castillo Martin F, Martinez Lopez MM, et al: Peritonsillar and retropharyngeal abscess: a study of 13 years, *Ann Pediatr (Barc)* 65:32–36, 2006.

McIsaac WJ, Kellner JD, Aufricht P, et al: Empirical validation of guidelines for the management of pharyngitis in children and adults, *JAMA* 291:1587–1595, 2004.

Neuner JM, Hamel MB, Phillips RS, et al: Diagnosis and management of adults with pharyngitis: a cost effective analysis, *Ann Intern Med* 139:113–122, 2003.

Park SY, Gerber MA, Tanz RR, et al: Clinician's management of children and adolescents with acute pharyngitis, *Pediatrics* 117:1871–1878, 2006.

Price D, Bond C, Bouchard J, et al: International Primary Care Respiratory Group (IPCRG) Guidelines: management of allergic rhinitis, *Prim Care Respir J* 15:58–70, 2006.

Quillen DM, Feller DB: Diagnosing rhinitis: allergic vs nonallergic, *Am Fam Physician* 73:1583–1590, 2006.

Rafei K, Lichenstein R: Airway infectious disease emergencies, *Pediatr Clin North Am* 53(2):215–242, 2006.

Reveiz L, Cardona A, Ospina E: Antibiotics for acute laryngitis in adults, *Cochrane Database Syst Rev*, 2005, CD004783.

Sataloff RT, Spiegel JR, Hawkshaw MT: History and physical exam of patients with voice disorders. In Rubin JS, Sataloff RT, Korovin GS, Gould WJ, editors: *Diagnosis and treatment of voice disorders*, New York, Tokyo, 1995, Igaku-Shoin.

Schraff S, McGinn JD, Derkay CS: Peritonsillar abscess in children: a 10-year review of diagnosis and management, *Int J Pediatr Otorhinolaryngol* 57: 213, 2001.

Sniboski C, Schmidt B, Jordan R: Tongue and tonsillar carcinoma, *Cancer* 103:1843–1849, 2005.

Stokes JR, Csale TB: Allergy immunotherapy for primary care physicians, *Am J Med* 119:820–823, 2006.

Syrjanen N: HPV infections and tonsillar carcinoma, *J Clin Pathol* 57:449–455, 2004.

Van Pinxterin B, Numans ME, Bonis PA, Lau J: Short-term treatment with proton pump inhibitors, H_2-receptor antagonists and prokinetics for gastro-oesophageal reflux disease-like symptoms and endoscopy negative reflux disease, *Cochrane Database Syst Rev*, 2006, CD002095.

Vincent MT, Celestin N, Hussain AN: Pharyngitis, *Am Fam Physician* 69: 1465–1470, 2004.

CHAPTER 41

Substance Abuse
Robert Mallin and D. Todd Detar

ALCOHOL

Alcohol, the third leading cause of preventable death, is a chronic disease with genetic, psychosocial, and environmental factors influencing its development and manifestations. About 100,000 deaths annually are associated with alcohol abuse and dependence.

The DSM-IV defines alcohol abuse as maladaptive pattern with one or more of the following:
- Failure to fulfill work, school, or social obligations
- Recurrent substance use in physically hazardous situations
- Recurrent legal problems related to substance abuse
- Continued use despite alcohol-related social problems

The DSM-IV defines alcohol dependence as maladaptive pattern with three or more of the following:
- Tolerance
- Withdrawal
- Substance taken in larger quantities than intended
- Persistent desire to cut down or control use
- Time is spent obtaining, using, or recovering from the substance.

Symptoms
- Increased tolerance, blackouts, and memory lapses
- Sleep disturbances, tremors
- Quick drinking and gulping first drink
- Use of alcohol for stress relief
- Frequent thoughts about drinking
- Tardiness or absence from work
- Motor vehicle accident with alcohol involved
- Family problems related to alcohol
- Erectile dysfunction

Signs
- Hypertension
- Cognitive defects
- Peripheral neuropathy
- Cirrhosis of the liver
- Cardiomyopathy
- Pancreatitis
- Wernicke-Korsakoff syndrome

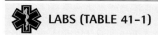 **LABS (TABLE 41-1)**

Table 41-1. Lab Values

ABNORMALITY	DIAGNOSTIC CHARACTERISTICS
Serum AST>ALT (ratio >2:0, both usually <300 IU/L, and almost never >500	Sensitivity and specificity not well studied, but may vary with the magnitude of the ratio
Elevated carbohydrate-deficient transferrin (CDT)	Sensitivity ~60%-70%, specificity 80-90%
Elevated serum AST	Sensitivity 50%, specificity 82%
Elevated ALT	Sensitivity 35%, specificity 86%
Elevated GGT	Sensitivity 70%, specificity 60%-80%

ALT, Alanine aminotransferase; *AST,* aspartate aminotransferase; *GGT,* gamma-glutamyl transpeptidase.

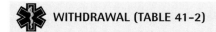 **WITHDRAWAL (TABLE 41-2)**

Table 41-2. Withdrawal

SYNDROME	CLINICAL FINDINGS	ONSET AFTER DRINK
Minor withdrawal	Tremulousness, anxiety, headache, diaphoresis, palpitations, anorexia, gastrointestinal upset	6-36 hours
Delirium tremens	Delirium, tachycardia, hypertension, agitation, fever, diaphoresis	48-96 hours
Seizures	Generalized, tonic-clonic, status (rare)	6-48 hours
Alcoholic hallucinosis	Visual, auditory, and/or tactile hallucinations	12-48 hours

Workup
- CAGE questionnaire: two positive answers are about 85% sensitive, 90% specific
  - Have you felt the need to **C**ut down on your drinking?
  - Have people **A**nnoyed you when they criticize your drinking?
  - Have you ever felt bad or **G**uilty about your drinking?
  - Have you ever had a drink first think in the morning (**E**ye opener) to steady your nerves or help with a hangover?

Comments and Treatment Considerations

For treatment of inpatient acute withdrawal, the first dose of benzodiazepine should achieve sedation without respiratory compromise; drugs then are tapered daily as long as withdrawal symptoms are stable. The combination of alcohol and benzodiazepines when coingested can be fatal, so counseling and careful patient selection are required. Inpatient treatment for withdrawal/delirium tremens (DTs) may require very large doses of benzodiazepines.

Outpatient treatment choices include:

- Chlordiazepoxide 25 to 100 mg PO/IM up to three times daily
- Diazepam 5 to 20 mg PO/IM/IV up to three times daily
- Lorazepam 1 to 4 mg PO/IM/IV every 2 to 6 hours as needed; lorazepam preferred in older adults, severe liver disease, or for IV drip
- Phenobarbital 60 to 120 mg PO/IM/IV three or four times daily may be safer in pregnancy
- Nalmefene, newer opioid antagonist, IV in U.S., odds ratio for relapse was 2:4.
- Magnesium sulfate 1 g IM/IV every 4 to 6 hours (especially if history of DTs or withdrawal seizure)

 ## OUTPATIENT MANAGEMENT

- Naltrexone 50 mg once daily, an opioid receptor antagonist, decreases relapse and rates of withdrawal from treatment (good in primary care setting)
- Carbamazepine 800 mg/day for 7 days with good outpatient outcomes
- Gabapentin 400 mg three times daily for 3 days, 400 mg twice daily for 1 day, 400 mg once for 1 day; good results for outpatient management for withdrawal
- Topiramate up to 300 mg daily, fewer days of heavy drinking
- Acamprosate 666 mg three times daily – evidence of efficacy is unclear

 ## ADJUNCTS TO DETOXIFICATION

- Beta-blockers for tachycardia
- Clonidine 0.1 to 0.2 mg PO three times daily for autonomic hyperactivity
- Haloperidol for psychosis, agitation

 ## ADJUNCTS TO REHABILITATION

- Thiamine 100 mg PO/IV every day (first dose IV)
- Folic acid 1 mg PO/IV every day

- Multivitamin PO every day
- Motivational Enhancement Therapy (Project Match) has equivalent outcomes to CBT and a 12-step program (Alcoholics Anonymous) at 12 weeks.
- Studies of brief intervention and multicontact interventions show approximately 10% to 20% reduction in usage
- Alcoholics Anonymous—per person treatment cost significantly lower than outpatient treatment groups. Best long-term option.

COCAINE DEPENDENCE

In 2004, 34.2 million Americans ages 12 and over reported lifetime use of cocaine; 5.6 million reported annual use of cocaine; and 2 million Americans reported current use of cocaine. There were 1 million new users of cocaine in 2004 and most were ages 18 or older although the average age of first use was 20 years. Cocaine or stimulant intoxication can cause significant physical symptoms (Table 41-3).

Cocaine is generally not considered to cause a physical withdrawal syndrome, although there are some predictable symptoms associated with abrupt discontinuation of cocaine use.

Symptoms
- Dysphoric mood
- Fatigue, malaise

Table 41-3. Symptoms and Health Problems Associated with Cocaine Intoxication

ORGAN SYSTEM	SIGNS/SYMPTOMS	DIAGNOSES
Psychiatric	Anxiety, hallucinations, mania	Substance-induced psychosis
Neurologic	Headache, mydriasis, tremor, hyperreflexia, movement disorders, seizures, neurologic deficits	Cerebral edema, intracerebral hemorrhage, infarcts
Cardiopulmonary	Chest pain, dyspnea, syncope, hemoptysis, cough, wheezing	Cardiac ischemia, dysrhythmias, pulmonary edema, asthma, barotrauma
Gastrointestinal	Abdominal pain, nausea, vomiting	Mesenteric ischemia, bowel perforation
Renal	Polyuria, dark urine, oliguria, anuria	Acute renal failure
Other	Fever, stiffness, myalgias	Rhabdomyolysis, malignant hyperthermia

- Vivid unpleasant dreams
- Sleep disturbance
- Increased appetite
- Psychomotor retardation

Comments and Treatment Considerations

Pharmacologic treatment for cocaine addiction is widely used, despite little evidence to support its efficacy. Numerous treatments have been evaluated in large clinical trials with disappointing results.

As with other addictions, patients addicted to cocaine are more likely to remain abstinent if they complete a drug rehabilitation treatment program, including aftercare, and attend 12-step recovery groups.

HALLUCINOGENS AND DISSOCIATIVE DRUGS

Hallucinogens are the third most frequently abused class of drugs in high school students, after alcohol and marijuana (Table 41-4). Intoxication with hallucinogens causes complications that are both serotonergic and stimulant in etiology (Table 41-5).

Treatment of acute hallucinogen intoxication includes reassurance, use of benzodiazepines for the treatment of undue anxiety and agitation, and if necessary high-potency neuroleptics to treat persistent or severe symptoms of psychosis.

Symptoms
- Depression
- Memory impairment
- Anxiety
- Suicidal or homicidal ideation
- Hallucinations

Table 41-4. Commonly Abused Hallucinogens and Their Street Names

HALLUCINOGEN	STREET NAME
Lysergic acid diethylamide	LSD, acid, blotter
Phencyclidine (PCP)	Angel dust
Psilocybin	Mushrooms, magic mushrooms, shrooms
Mescaline	Peyote, cactus
3,4-Methylenedioxymethamphetamine (MDMA)	Ecstasy, X
Ketamine	Special K
Tetrahydrocannabinol (marijuana, hashish)	Mary Jane, pot, weed, dope, grass, ganja, herb

Table 41-5. Physiologic Effects of Hallucinogen Overdose

Neurologic	Mydriasis tremor, hyperreflexia, movement disorders, seizures, neurologic deficits	LSD, PCP, MDMA
Cardiopulmonary	Chest pain, dyspnea, syncope, tachycardia, elevated blood pressure	LSD, marijuana, PCP
Gastrointestinal	Nausea, vomiting	LSD, MDMA, PCP
Renal	Polyuria, dark urine, oliguria, anuria	LSD, MDMA, PCP
Other	Stiffness, myalgias, rhabdomyolysis	MDMA, PCP

Signs
- Psychosis
- Mania
- Disorientation
- Delirium

INHALANT ABUSE

Volatile substances that produce psychoactive effects, inhaled by sniffing, snorting, bagging, huffing, or spraying directly into the mouth are dangerous. In 2002 and 2003, an annual average of 718,000 youths ages 12 to 13 had used an inhalant.

 TYPES

- Solvents—Paint thinners, dry cleaning fluids, gasoline, glue, felt pens
- Nitrites—Amyl nitrite, butyl nitrite
- Aerosols—Whipped cream containers, deodorant, and cleaning sprays
- Gases—Nitrous oxide, ether, chloroform

Symptoms
- Euphoria
- Dizziness
- Hallucinations
- Tinnitus
- Headache
- Vivid dreams

Signs
- General effects—Chemical odors on breath, intoxication
- Pulmonary—Hypoxia, pulmonary edema, pneumothorax

- Cardiovascular—Dysrhythmia, myocarditis, myocardial infarction, bradycardia
- CNS—Slurred speech, ataxia, disorientation, hallucinations, agitation, violent behavior; all have some brain damage, seizures, coma, neuropathy
- GI—Vomiting, nausea, abdominal pain
- Renal—Metabolic acidosis, calculi, nephritis
- Hematologic—Bone marrow suppression, malignancy, methemoglobinemia
- Dermatologic—Eczematoid dermatitis, erythema, pruritus
- Pregnancy and postnatal—Spontaneous abortion, premature delivery, fetal malformation
- Other—Falls, drowning, motor vehicle accidents

Workup
- CBC, BMP, ECG and cardiac monitoring
- Drug screen
- Chest x-ray
- Methemoglobin levels if nitrites suspected

Comments and Treatment Considerations
Remove the patient from the inhalant. Supplement with oxygen. Monitor for toxic effects and treat cardiac and pulmonary symptoms according to standard protocols. Recommend addiction counseling specifically for inhalants, and consider neuropsychologic testing.

MARIJUANA ABUSE

Marijuana is the most frequently used illicit drug in the United States and may predict use of harder drugs later on. The effect after smoking is short, lasting 3 to 4 hours. Chronic use may cause lung problems, cancer, reproductive effects, cognitive dysfunction, increased risk of schizophrenia, and depression.

Symptoms
- Palpitations
- Anxiety
- Depression
- Shortness of breath
- Dry mouth
- Increase in appetite
- Short-term memory loss
- Paranoia
- Reduced libido
- Galactorrhea

Signs
- Tachycardia
- Elevated BP
- Elevated respiratory rate

- Orthostatic hypotension
- Conjunctival infection
- Agitation
- Gynecomastia

WITHDRAWAL SYNDROME

Withdrawal from marijuana is not life threatening, but frequently uncomfortable, and patients may present with insomnia, agitation, tremor, or depression. COPD, cognitive dysfunction, and increase in psychiatric illness have been reported.

Workup
- Urine drug screen—Unreliable for acute intoxication
- O_2 saturation
- Chest x-ray
- ECG

Comments and Treatment Considerations
Rarely requires medical treatment. Treat psychosis if needed. Drug treatment center referral may be of benefit.

METHAMPHETAMINE

Methamphetamine is an addictive stimulant that releases high levels of dopamine, enhancing mood and body movement. Speed, meth, chalk, ice, crystal, glass, and tina are some street names. In 2004, 6.2% of high school seniors reported lifetime use of methamphetamine, unchanged from 2003. In 2008, lifetime prevalence of methamphetamine use among 18-49 year olds was 8.6%. Addiction, psychotic behavior and brain damage are effects of methamphetamine.

Rhabdomyolysis, seizures, stroke, acute coronary syndrome, ventricular dysrhythmias, and death are some of the complications.

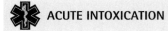 **ACUTE INTOXICATION**

Symptoms
- Dizziness
- Palpitations
- Hot flashes

Signs
- Tremor
- Restlessness
- Tachycardia ++++
- Hypertension
- Euphoria or irritability
- Seizure

CHRONIC INTOXICATION

Symptoms
- Depression
- Fatigue
- Poor concentration

Signs
- Tremor
- Hypertension
- Nasal symptoms (discharge, bleeding, sniffles)

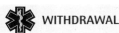 **WITHDRAWAL**

Abstinence syndrome: "Crash" or drastic reduction of mood and energy starts 15 to 30 minutes after cessation of binge.

Work up
- Lab work based on symptoms
  - CBC, CK, and myoglobin levels for rhabdomyolysis
  - Troponin for suspected cardiac involvement
  - Chest x-ray, CT brain scan for altered mental status

Comments and Treatment Considerations
Abrupt discontinuation: Monitor for marked depression after one-week and treat accordingly. No medications help with withdrawal or abstinence.

OPIOID DEPENDENCE

As many as 1 million people in the United States are dependent on opioids. From the IV use of heroin to prescribed narcotic analgesics, these drugs are highly reinforcing and cause physical dependence in a matter of weeks, and addiction in those vulnerable just as quickly. Opioid dependence is highly correlated with criminal activity, HIV, viral hepatitis, and depressive disorders.

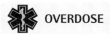 **OVERDOSE**

Signs
- Obtundation +++++
- Hypotension +++
- Hypothermia
- Miosis
- Bradypnea +++++
- Respiratory failure

Immediate death from opioid abuse is often due to respiratory depression secondary to overdose. Increasing tolerance brings the patient closer to respiratory depression, each time the dose is increased to overcome tolerance.

Comments and Treatment Considerations
Administer naloxone 0.2 to 0.4 mg IV; repeat every 2 to 3 minutes as necessary, along with IV fluids, respiratory, and blood pressure support. Alternatively, airway management may be required.

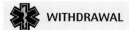 **WITHDRAWAL**

Symptoms
- Dysphoric mood ++++
- Drug craving
- Insomnia
- Asthenia
- Nausea
- Anorexia, abdominal pain

Signs
- Mild elevations in pulse rate, respiratory rate, BP, and temperature
- Piloerection (gooseflesh)
- Lacrimation or rhinorrhea
- Mydriasis, yawning, diaphoresis
- Vomiting, diarrhea

Comments and Treatment Considerations
- Methadone: a pure opioid agonist restricted by federal legislation to inpatient treatment, or specialized outpatient drug treatment programs. Methadone 15 to 20 mg orally for 2 to 3 days then tapered with 10% to 15% reduction in dose daily, guided by patient's symptoms and clinical findings. Methadone maintenance for opioid dependence must be carried out in a federally licensed methadone clinic.
- Clonidine: an α-adrenergic blocker, 0.2 mg orally every 4 hours to relieve symptoms of withdrawal may be effective. Hypotension is a risk and sometimes limits the dose. It can be continued for 10 to 14 days, and tapered by the third day by 0.2 mg daily.
- Buprenorphine: this partial mu receptor agonist can be administered sublingually, in doses of 2, 4, or 8 mg every 4 hours for the management of opioid withdrawal symptoms.
- Naltrexone/clonidine: a rapid form of opioid detoxification involves pretreatment with 0.2 to 0.3 mg of clonidine followed by 12.5 mg of naltrexone (a pure opioid antagonist). Naltrexone is increased to 25 mg on the second day, 50 mg on day 3, and 100 mg on day 4, with clonidine given at 0.1 to 0.3 mg three times daily.

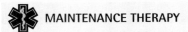 **MAINTENANCE THERAPY**

Because abstinence-based approaches have had little success in opioid dependence maintenance, therapy with methadone and now buprenorphine and naloxone combinations is often recommended.

Buprenorphine/naloxone has been approved for use in primary care clinics, and physicians who have been trained in its use may prescribe it for treatment of opioid dependence.

TOBACCO

With more than 440,000 deaths per year attributed to smoking in the United States, tobacco is the most deadly substance in our society. Tobacco is a "gateway" drug, leading adolescents to use alcohol and other addictive substances. Nearly 70% of smokers want to quit, but only 7% will be successful on their own. With counseling and medication rates increase to 35% to 40%.

The Five A's of smoking cessation (Table 41-6) is a strategy for intervention in patients with tobacco use disorders.

ASK your patient if he or she uses tobacco. When tobacco use is included as a vital sign, providers are three times more likely to discuss smoking with their patients.

ADVISE your patient to quit with a clear, strong, personalized message. Example: "As your physician I must tell you that stopping smoking is the most important thing you can do for your health. Cutting back will not be enough. Your symptoms (cough, shortness of breath, etc.) will improve when you quit."

ASSESS your patient's willingness to make a quit attempt. Using the stages of change (Table 41-7) and the principles of motivational interviewing help your patient become ready to make a quit attempt.

ASSIST your patient by helping him or her to:
- Set a quit date
- Make a list of triggers
- Make a list of alternative behaviors
- Make a list of support persons
- Provide educational literature
- Prescribe appropriate pharmacotherapy (Table 41-8)

ARRANGE for close follow-up care and monitoring.

Table 41-6. Five A's of Smoking

Ask	Every patient if they smoke
Advise	Every patient to quit
Assess	Each patient's willingness to make a quit attempt
Assist	Patients with counseling and pharmacotherapy
Arrange	Follow-up and support

Table 41-7. Stages of Change Example

Precontemplation	"I don't have a problem with smoking."
Contemplation	"I know I need to quit but am not ready."
Preparation	"I want to set a quit date."
Action	"I quit smoking."
Maintenance/relapse	"I stopped 6 months ago/I started smoking again."

Table 41-8. Pharmacotherapy for Smoking Cessation

DRUG/ DELIVERY	INITIAL DOSE	MAINTENANCE DOSE	DURATION OF THERAPY	APPROXIMATE COST/MONTH
Nicotine				
Gum 4 mg	10-15 pieces/day	5-8 pieces/ day	8 wk-5 yr	$90
Patch	21 or 14 mg daily depending on number of cigarettes smoked	Taper to next lowest dose in 4-6 wk	8-12 wk	$115
Inhaler	4 puffs/day	4/day taper	8-12 wk	$120
Nasal spray	5 sprays/hr	8-80 sprays/ day	8-12 wk	$100
Bupropion	150 mg every day × 3 days	150 mg bid	7-12 wk	$90
Varenicline	0.5 mg every day × 3 days 0.5 mg bid × 4 days	1 mg bid	12 wk	$100

References

American Psychiatric Association: *Diagnostic and statistical manual of mental disorders*, 4th ed, Washington, DC, 1994, American Psychiatric Association.

Anderson CE, Loomis GA: Recognition and prevention of inhalant abuse, *Am Fam Physician* 68:869–887, 2003.

Bell H, Tallaksen CM, Try K, Haug E: Carbohydrate-deficient transferrin and other markers of high alcohol consumption: a study of 502 patients admitted consecutively to a medical department, *Alcohol Clin Exp Res* 18(5): 1103–1108, 1994.

Cami J, Farre M: Drug addiction, *N Engl J Med* 349(10):975–986, 2003.

Center for Substance Abuse Treatment: Treatment Improvement Protocol (TIP) Series 24 (HHS Publication No (SMA) 97-3139), Rockville, MD: Substance Abuse and Mental Health Services Administration; 1997a. A Guide to Substance Abuse Services for Primary Care Clinicians.

Crider RA, Rouse BA: Epidemiology of inhalant abuse: an update, NIDA Research Monograph 85, Rockville, MD, 1988.

Durell TM, Kroutil LA, Crits-Christoph P, Barchha N, Van Brunt DL: Prevalence of nonmedical methamphetamine use in the United States, *Subst Abuse Treat Prev Policy* 25(3):19, 2008.

Enoch MA, Goldman D: Problem drinking and alcoholism: diagnosis and treatment, *Am Fam Physician* 65(3):441–448, 2002.

Fiore MC, Bailey WC, Cohen SJ: *Smoking cessation.* Clinical practice guideline no. 18, Rockville, MD, 1996, U.S. Dept of Health and Human Services.

Gorelick DA: Pharmacologic management of cocaine addiction, *Einstein Q J Biol Med* 16:61–69, 1999.

Harder S, Reitbrock S: Concentration-effect relationship of delta-9-tetrahydrocannabinol and prediction of psychotropic effects after smoking marijuana, *Int J Clin Pharmacol Ther* 35(4):155–159, 1997.

Hubbard JR, Franco SE, Onaivi ES: Marijuana: medical implications, *Am Fam Physician* 60:2583–2592, 1999.

Johnston L: *Monitoring the future study*, University of Michigan, Ann Arbor, 1998, National Institute of Drug Abuse.

Kenna GA, McGeary JE, Swift RM: Pharmocotherapy, pharmacogenomics, and the future of alcohol dependence treatment, part 1, *Am J Health Syst Pharm* 61:2272, 2004.

Kosten TR, O'Connor PG: Management of drug and alcohol withdrawal, *N Engl J Med* 348(18):1786–1795, 2003.

Krambeer LL, Von Mcnelly W, et al: Methadone therapy for opioid dependence, *Am Fam Physician* 63:2404–2413, 2001.

Matching alcoholism treatments to client heterogeneity: Project MATCH three-year drinking outcomes, *Alcohol Clin Exp Res* 22:1300–1311, 1998.

Mersy DJ: Recognition of alcohol and substance abuse, *Am Fam Physician* 67(7):1529–1532, 2003.

National Institute on Alcohol Abuse and Alcoholism: Highlights from the Tenth Special Report to Congress on Alcohol and Health, *Alcohol, Research and Health* 24(1):2000.

Substance Abuse and Mental Health Services Administration: *Results from the 2005 national survey on drug use and health: national findings* (Office of Applied Studies, NSDUH Series H-30, DHHS Publication No. SMA 06-4194), Rockville, MD, 2006.

Substance Abuse and Mental Health Services Administration Office of Applied Sciences: *preliminary results from the 2001 national household survey on drug abuse.* DHHS No. (SMA) 02-3759, Rockville, MD, 2002, SAMHSA.

Toomey R, Lyons MJ, Eisen SA, et al: A twin study of the neuropsychological consequences of stimulant abuse, *Arch Gen Psychiatry* 60:203, 2003.

Weaver MF, Schnoll SH: Stimulants-amphetamines, cocaine. In McCrady BS, Epstein EE, editors: *Addictions: comprehensive guidebook*, New York 1999, Oxford University Press, p 105.

Wilkins NW, Mellot KG, Markvista R, Gorelick DA: Management of stimulant, hallucinogen, marijuana, phencyclidine and club drug withdrawal. In Graham AW Schultz TK, editors: *Principles of addiction medicine*, Chevy Chase, MD, 2003, American Society of Addiction Medicine.

Wyse D: Deliberate inhalation of volatile hydrocarbons: a review, *Can Med Assoc J* 108(1):71–74, 1973.

CHAPTER 42

Urinary Problems
Travis Stephensen

Disorders of the urinary tract are ubiquitous in primary care practice. Appropriate detection, diagnosis, and treatment of these common conditions will minimize morbidity and prevent the development of complications.

ACUTE CYSTITIS

Symptoms
- Dysuria ++++
- Frequency ++++ (dysuria and frequency without vaginal discharge or vaginal irritation increases probability of UTI to >90%)
- Urgency +++
- Suprapubic pain ++
- Hematuria ++
- Urethritis +
- Vaginitis +
- Nausea, vomiting + (suggests upper UTI)

Signs
- Fever +
- Suprapubic pain ++
- Costovertebral angle tenderness +
- Pelvic examination if urethritis or vaginitis +

Workup
- Urinalysis—Instruct on proper urine collection technique to avoid vaginal contamination. 10^5+ WBCs/mL in a urinalysis is both sensitive (95%) and specific (71%) for UTI. Bacteria seen on microscopy is 50% sensitive and 90% specific. WBC casts indicate an upper UTI. Hematuria is associated with UTIs, kidney stones, and menstrual bleeding, but is not generally associated with vaginitis or urethritis.
- Urine cultures—Not routinely necessary with uncomplicated UTIs because infectious organisms are well known and symptoms are likely to resolve or worsen prior to result availability. Cultures are indicated if a complicated UTI is suspected, or if symptoms persist or recur less than 1 month after previous antimicrobial therapy for a UTI.

- Urine dipstick—Leukocyte esterase (sensitivity 75% to 96%, specificity 94% to 98%); nitrite is specific for enterobacteriaceae. However, it does not detect low-count UTIs, or other species, and can be falsely positive if using OTC phenazopyridine, or if eating beets.

Comments and Treatment Considerations
- Postcoital voiding—Flush urethra regularly with adequate hydration to increase voiding frequency. Consider postcoital vitamin C or cranberry juice to acidify the urine and to hydrate the patient sufficiently to result in nocturia, to prevent prolonged duration between voiding. Avoid spermicide use. Consider intravaginal estrogen if postmenopausal.
- Antibiotics—If local *Escherichia coli* resistance to TMP-SMX is less than 20% and the patient has no sulfa allergy, then TMP-SMX 160/800 mg orally twice a day for 3 days. If local *E. coli* resistance rates are greater than 20% or the patient has a sulfa allergy, then nitrofurantoin 50 to 100 mg PO every 6 hours for 7 days or fosfomycin 3 g single dose. Alternative is ciprofloxacin 250 mg orally twice a day for 3 days, extended release ciprofloxacin 500 mg orally daily for 3 days; levofloxacin 250 mg orally daily for 3 days. Do not use moxifloxacin or gemifloxacin.

Add phenazopyridine if the patient has dysuria: 100 to 200 mg PO three times a day for 2 days.

BENIGN PROSTATIC HYPERPLASIA

Benign prostatic hyperplasia (BPH) is a disorder affecting males that increases in frequency with age. It affects roughly 25% of men ages 41 to 50, 40% to 50% of men ages 51 to 60, 70% of men ages 61 to 70, and more than 80% in men older than age 80. Untreated BPH can cause acute urinary retention, recurrent urinary tract infections, hydronephrosis and rarely, renal failure. BPH develops in the periurethral transitional zone of the prostate. No causal relationship between BPH and prostate cancer has been established.

Symptoms
Measure symptoms with the American Urologic Association symptom score. Scores range from 0 (never present) to 5 (almost always present). Total the symptom scores: mild BPH, 0-7; moderate, 8-19; severe, 20+.
- Frequency (0-5)
- Nocturia (0-5)
- Hesitancy (0-5)
- Urgency (0-5)
- Weak urinary stream (0-5)
- Intermittence (0-5)
- Incomplete emptying (0-5)

Signs
- Digital rectal examination: assess prostate size, consistency, nodularity, firmness, and/or asymmetry, which suggests prostate cancer. The transitional zone of the prostate, which surrounds the urethra, cannot be felt on digital rectal examination.

Workup

- Urinalysis—Urinary tract infections can cause similar symptoms
- Serum creatinine—Renal etiologies, but also bladder outlet obstruction
- Serum PSA
  - If the patient has obstructive symptoms, the specificity of PSA is lower than in asymptomatic men.
  - Consider that PSA levels may be affected by digital rectal examination or ejaculation prior to testing.
  - Results should be interpreted with age, race, and perhaps weight-based norms.
- Maximal urinary flow rate
- Postvoid residual volume can be determined by a postvoid in-out catheter.
- Rule out:
  - Neurogenic bladder
  - Prostatitis
  - Urethral stricture (any history of urethral instrumentation)
  - Bladder neck contracture
  - Prostate cancer
  - Bladder cancer
- Anticholinergic drugs impairing bladder function
- Sympathomimetic drugs that increase outflow resistance

Comments and Treatment Considerations

Treatment is generally indicated when the symptoms of BPH begin to interfere with the patient's quality of life, or if he develops upper or lower urinary tract complications. Medical treatment is usually based on symptom progression as measured by the American Urologic Association symptom score and, when indicated, urine flow rate studies.

The α-adrenergic antagonists (terazosin, doxazosin, tamsulosin, and alfuzosin) act on the physiologic and reversible component of the obstructive symptoms. They are effective in the short term. The 5-alpha-reductase inhibitors (finasteride, dutasteride) act on the fixed obstructive component by reducing the size of the prostate gland.

PYELONEPHRITIS

Uncomplicated pyelonephritis is a kidney infection in a healthy person who does not have comorbid conditions that could complicate treatment.

Complicated pyelonephritis includes patients with renal calculi, diabetes mellitus, pregnancy, a neurogenic bladder, obstruction, urinary tract diverticula, fistula, urinary diversions, vesicoureteral reflux, an indwelling catheter, a ureteral stent, a nephrostomy tube, renal failure, renal transplant, immunosuppression, and multidrug-resistant organisms.

Symptoms

The first two are more frequent in pyelonephritis than a UTI; the remainder may be found in both.

- Flank pain +++
- Nausea/vomiting ++
- Dysuria ++++
- Urgency, frequency ++++
- Suprapubic pain ++
- Hematuria ++

Signs

- Fever (>37.8° C)
- Costovertebral angle tenderness ++

Workup

- Pyuria is present in a large percentage of women with pyelonephritis. WBC casts indicate the infection is from an upper urinary tract source. Most have elevated WBC count and usually elevated ESR and CRP.
- Consider pelvic examination because pelvic inflammatory disease is commonly mistaken for pyelonephritis. Look for evidence of vaginitis, urethral discharge, herpetic lesions, cervical motion tenderness, and ectopic mass, and strongly consider cervical cultures and pregnancy testing.
- Bacteremia (blood cultures are positive in 10% to 20% of women with acute uncomplicated pyelonephritis); blood cultures may be limited to patients who need hospitalization. Nitrite should not solely be relied on because it does not detect non-nitrate–reducing organisms such as *Staphylococcus*.

Comments and Treatment Considerations

- Indications for hospitalization: nausea and vomiting to an extent that preclude oral hydration and oral medications; concerns about patient compliance, unclear diagnosis, or marked illness with high fevers, pain, or debilitation; also if there is any concern for complicated pyelonephritis
- The advent of the fluoroquinolones, which have the similar bioavailability IV or orally, has increased the number of patients who can be managed as outpatients. If outpatient management is attempted the patients should be called or seen after 2 to 3 days of therapy to ensure improvement and defervescence. Also this is usually the point when urine or blood cultures with sensitivities become available and may change treatment.
- In complicated pyelonephritis a repeat urine culture should be obtained 1 to 2 weeks after completed antibiotic therapy. In uncomplicated pyelonephritis it is not generally necessary to repeat urine culture.
- Imaging: routine imaging is not indicated unless the patient has a second episode of pyelonephritis, or symptoms persist more than 48-72 hours. At that time CT or US may be used to look for renal calculi, perinephric abscess, or anatomic abnormality.

URETERAL CALCULUS

An estimated 12% of men and 8% of women will develop kidney stones by age 70. There is a 15% chance of recurrence within 1 year, 35% to 40% chance by 5 years, and 80% chance by 10 years. Approximately 80% of stones are calcium oxalate or calcium phosphate; the remainder are uric acid, struvite (magnesium ammonium phosphate), and cystine. Risk factors include a history of stones, hypercalciuria, hyperuricosuria, hypocitraturia, low dietary calcium intake, low fluid intake, family history of kidney stones, short bowel syndrome, diarrhea, obesity, dehydration, and frequent UTIs.

Symptoms
- Renal colic (usually lasts 20 to 60 minutes) ++++
- Atraumatic, unilateral flank pain ++++
- Passage of "gravel" or small stones in urine ++++
- Hematuria ++++
- Difficulty urinating +++
- Groin pain +++
- Urgency (typically occurs when the stone has entered the bladder) +++
- Dysuria (typically occurs when the stone has entered the bladder) +++
- Vague abdominal pain ++
- Acute abdominal pain ++
- Nausea ++

Workup
- Urinalysis (looking for hematuria and evidence of urinary tract infection)
- hCG to rule out ectopic and/or minimize fetal radiation exposure
- Noncontrast helical CT (sensitivity 95%, specificity 98%)
- Use US in patients who should avoid radiation (i.e., pregnant patients).
- Strain for stones to determine stone composition, which may suggest means to prevent recurrence, or need for further workup.

Comments and Treatment Considerations
Uric acid stones are radiolucent. Stones may be missed that are smaller than the width of the CT scan slices (standard cuts are generally 8 mm). A dilated ureter may represent a recently passed stone. Approximately 95% of stones less than 2 mm are passed on their own in an average of 8.2 days, with 95% passed within 31 days; 83% of stones 2 to 4 mm are passed on their own in an average of 12.2 days, with 95% of stones passed in 40 days; and 50% of stones 4 to 6 mm are passed on their own in an average of 22 days, with 95% passed in 39 days.

Urology should be consulted if there is evidence of UTI, acute renal failure, anuria, or intolerable or protracted pain.

Pain medications should include NSAIDs and opioids. NSAIDs decrease ureteral smooth muscle tone, but exercise caution in patients with renal disease. Indomethacin and ketorolac have been studied in renal colic and are effective.

Increase water intake to 2 L/day.

URETHRITIS

Urethral inflammation generally has three possible causes: a sexually transmitted infection—specifically *Neisseria gonorrhoeae* and *Chlamydia trachomatis*—a urinary tract infection, or a vaginal infection.

Symptoms
- Urethral discharge ++++
- Dysuria ++++
- Urgency +++
- Frequency ++
- Vaginal discharge ++
- Genital ulcers ++

Signs
- Urethral discharge ++++
- Genital lesions +++
- Cervical motion tenderness +++
- Epididymitis ++

Workup
- Urinalysis
- Pelvic examination, to include vaginal sample with wet mount and KOH to assess for bacterial vaginosis, trichomonas, or yeast infections
- Consider STD screening—Include gonorrhea/chlamydia

Comments and Treatment Considerations
UTIs can cause urethral irritation and dysuria, but they do not commonly cause urethral discharge. Vaginal inflammation from a yeast infection, bacterial vaginosis, trichomonas, or other causes could masquerade as dysuria when the voiding of urine contacts vulvar tissue.

Most gonorrheal infections in men produce a thin to thick mucoid urethral discharge that prompts evaluation. Urethritis that is not caused by *N. gonorrhoeae* is called nongonococcal urethritis (NGU), and is caused primarily by *C. trachomatis* and *Ureaplasma urealyticum*. It is not possible to differentiate among these infections based solely on urethral discharge, and they may be concurrent.

Treatment should be directed toward the organism. Please see the section on urinary tract infections for recommendations for that disorder. For gonorrhea, a one-time dose of ceftriaxone is effective. For chlamydia a 7-day course of doxycycline or a one-time dose of azithromycin are recommended. For vaginal infections see the respective sections for treatment guidelines.

URINARY TRACT INFECTION (UTI)

A woman's lifetime risk for having a UTI is approximately 50% to 60%. A young woman's risk is approximately 0.5 episode per person year; 25% of women get recurrent episodes, with an average of 2.6 episodes per year. Causative organisms include *E. coli* (80% to 85%) and *Staphylococcus saprophyticus* (5% to 15%); the remainder are enterococci and other uropathogens.

A complicated UTI includes:
- Pregnancy
- Upper UTI
- Antibiotic-resistant organisms
- Male gender
- Older adult
- Hospital acquired
- Indwelling urinary catheter
- Anatomic abnormalities
- More than 7 days of symptoms at time of presentation
- DM
- Recurrent infections
- Immunosuppression

If a UTI is complicated this may change the type and duration of antibiotics used.

 RISK FACTORS

- Sexual intercourse
- Spermicide containing contraceptives (presumably by killing normal vaginal flora)
- A history of greater than six UTIs
- Insulin-dependent DM

References

Barry JM, Fowler FJ Jr, O'Leary MP, et al: The American Urological Association Symptom index for benign prostatic hyperplasia, *J Urol* 148:1549, 1992.

Berry SJ, Coffey DS, Walsh PC, et al: The development of human benign prostatic hyperplasia with age, *J Urol* 132:474, 1984.

Bossens MM, Van Straalen J, De Reijke TM, et al: Kinetics of prostate specific antigen after manipulation of the prostate, *Eur J Cancer* 31A:682, 1995.

Broghi L, Meschi T, Amato F, et al: Urinary volume, water and recurrences in idiopathic calcium nephrolithiasis: a 5-year randomized prospective study, *J Urol* 155:839, 1996.

Burnett AL, Wein AJ: Benign prostatic hyperplasia in primary care: what you need to know, *J Urol* 175:s19, 2006.

Coe FL, Parks JH, Asplin JR: The pathogenesis and treatment of kidney stones, *N Engl J Med* 327:1141, 1992.

Cole RS, Fry CH, Shuttleworth KE: The action of the prostaglandins on isolated human ureteric smooth muscle, *Br J Urol* 61:19, 1988.

Coley CM, Barry MJ, Fleming C, et al: Early detection of prostate cancer. Part I: prior probability and effectiveness of tests, *Ann Intern Med* 126:394, 1997.

Coll DM, Varanelli MJ, Smith RC: Relationship of spontaneous passage of ureteral calculi to stone size and location as revealed by unenhanced helical CT, *AM J Roentgenol* 178:101, 2002.

Cordell WH, Larson TA, Lingeman JE, et al: Indomethacin suppositories versus intravenously titrated morphine for the treatment of ureteral colic, *Ann Emerg Med* 23:262, 1994.

Cordell WH, Wright SW, Wolfson AB, et al: Comparison of intravenous ketorolac, meperidine, and both (balanced analgesia) for renal colic, *Ann Emerg Med* 28:151, 1996.

Curhan GC, Willett WC, Rimm EB, Stampfer MJ: Family history and risk of kidney stones, *J Am Soc Nephrol* 8:1568, 1997.

Dailrymple NC, Verga M, Anderson KR, et al: The value of unenhanced helical computerized tomography in the management of acute flank pain, *J Urol* 159:735, 1998.

Fairley KF, Carson NE, Gutch RC, et al: Site of infection in acute urinary tract infection in general practice, *Lancet* 2:615, 1971.

Gillen DL, Worcester EM, Coe FL: Decreased renal function among adults with a history of nephrolithiasis: a study of NHANES III, *Kidney Int* 67:685, 2005.

Hoebe C, Rademaker C, Brouwers E, et al: Acceptability of self-taken vaginal swabs and first-catch urine samples for the diagnosis of urogenital *Chlamydia trachomatis* and *Neisseria gonorrhoeae* with an amplified DNA assay in young women attending a public health sexually transmitted disease clinic, *Sex Transm Dis* 33(8):491–495, 2006.

Hooton TM, Stamm WE: Acute pyelonephritis: symptoms, diagnosis, and treatment, *UpToDate* January 2005.

Johnson CM, Wilson DM, O'Fallon WM, et al: Renal stone epidemiology: a 25-year study in Rochester, Minnesota, *Kidney Int* 16:624, 1979.

Marberger MJ, Andersen JT, Nickel JC, et al: Prostate volume and serum prostate-specific antigen as predictors of acute urinary retention. Combined experience from three large multinational placebo-controlled trials, *Eur Urol* 38:563, 2000.

Morgan TO, Jacobson SJ, McCarthy WF, et al: Age-specific reference ranges for serum prostate-specific antigen in black men, *N Engl J Med* 335:304, 1996.

Morré S, Rozendaal L, van Valkengoed IG, et al: Urogenital *Chlamydia trachomatis* serovars in men and women with a symptomatic or asymptomatic infection: an association with clinical manifestations? *J Clin Microbiol* 38:2292–2296, 2000.

Oesterling JE, Jacobsen SJ, Chute C, et al: Serum prostate specific antigen in a community-based population of healthy men: establishment of age-specific reference ranges, *JAMA* 270:860, 1993.

Pienta KJ, Esper PS: Risk factors for prostate cancer, *Ann Intern Med* 118:793, 1993.

Pinson AG, Philbrick JT, Lindbeck GH, Schorling JB: Fever in the clinical diagnosis of acute pyelonephritis, *Am J Emerg Med* 15:148, 1997.

Rohr HP, Bartsch G: Human benign prostatic hyperplasia: a stromal disease? *Urology* 16:625, 1980.

Sheafor DH, Hertzberg BS, Freed SK, et al: Nonenhanced helical CT and US in the emergency evaluation of patients with renal colic: prospective comparison, *Radiology* 217:792, 2000.

Tchetgen MB, Song JT, Strawderman M, et al: Ejaculation increases the serum prostate-specific antigen concentration, *Urology* 47:511, 1996.

Teichman JM: Clinical practice. Acute renal colic from ureteral calculus, *N Engl J Med* 350:684, 2004.

Uribarri J, Oh MS, Carroll HJ: The first kidney stone, *Ann Intern Med* 111:1006, 1989.

CHAPTER 43

Vaginal Discharge
Karl E. Miller

One of the most common presenting complaints in a family physician's office is vaginal discharge. This symptom can represent a variety of infections ranging from relatively benign vaginal fungal infections to severe infections causing PID. The underlying cause of vaginal discharge can usually be determined by a patient's symptoms, visualization of the type and characteristics of the discharge, and the microscopic examination of the discharge. Other symptoms can be present in addition to the vaginal discharge. These include external genital itching or discomfort, bleeding after intercourse, painful intercourse (dyspareunia), pelvic or abdominal pain, fever, chills, sweats, nausea, and vomiting.

Patients describe vaginal discharge color and texture, if an odor is present with the discharge, and what type of odor (i.e., "fishy") and if it is causing other symptoms. Physical findings (Table 43-1) include a description of the discharge, any odor, if the discharge originates from the cervical opening or posterior vaginal vault, and the presence or absence of changes in the cervix or external genitalia. Testing on the discharge can include pH, "whiff test," and microscopic examination of the discharge using wet preparation and KOH.

BACTERIAL VAGINOSIS

Bacterial vaginosis occurs when the normal vaginal bacteria flora is replaced by a high concentration of anaerobic bacteria, usually *Gardnerella vaginalis*. This is the most common cause of vaginal discharge. In most women this is an annoying disease process, but in pregnant women it has been associated with adverse outcomes.

Symptoms
- Majority have no symptoms ++++
- Usually a malodorous (fishy) discharge +++
- Discharge is thin, homogeneous grayish white
- No external genitalia symptoms

Signs
- Discharge is homogeneous grayish white from vaginal vault ++++
- Discharge coats vaginal wall
- Cervix appears normal ++++

Table 43-1. Clinical Characteristics of Vaginal Discharges

	NORMAL	BACTERIAL VAGINOSIS	CANDIDIASIS	CHLAMYDIA/ GONORRHEA	PID	TRICHOMONIASIS
Symptoms	None, mild, transient	Malodorous, thin, homogeneous white discharge	Thick white discharge, external pruritus, no odor	Many with few or no symptoms	Pelvic or abdominal pain, fever, dyspareunia	Diffuse, malodorous discharge that may increase after menses
Signs	None	Discharge coats vaginal wall, cervix is normal	Inflamed external genitalia, cottage cheese–like discharge	Cervix appears inflamed and yellow cloudy discharge from cervix	Cervical motion tenderness, uterine/adnexal tenderness	Copious, yellow-green or gray, frothy discharge, inflamed cervix (strawberry)
Vaginal pH	3.0–4.5	>4.5	Normal	Normal	Normal	pH >5.0
Microscopic wet preparation	Squamous cells are prominent	Clue cells	Loss of bacteria	Increased WBCs	Increased WBCs	Increased WBCs, mobile trichomonads
KOH examination	Negative	Negative	Budding yeast or hyphae	Negative	Negative	Negative
"Whiff" test	Negative	Positive	Negative	Negative	Negative	Negative
Comments		DNA probe for *Gardnerella vaginalis* if diagnosis uncertain	Recurrent infections need to be assessed for other causes	NAAT test can be performed on endocervical or urine sample	CDC recommends treatment if one of the signs is present	Cultures only indicated if diagnosis is uncertain

CDC, Centers for Disease Control and Prevention; *KOH*, potassium hydroxide; *NAAT*, nucleic acid amplification test; *PID*, pelvic inflammatory disease; *WBCs*, white blood cells.

Workup
- Clue cells are present on microscopic examination. These are epithelial cells that are coated with bacteria. +++
- Vaginal pH is greater than 4.5 (normal pH is 3 to 4). ++++
- Positive whiff test—A fishy odor is released when KOH is added to the sample of the vaginal discharge ++++
- Culture of discharge is usually not necessary.
- If diagnosis is in doubt, DNA probe for *Gardnerella vaginalis* can be performed.
- If three of four are present, meets Amstel's criteria for bacterial vaginosis ++++

Comments and Treatment Considerations
The CDC has recommended various treatment regimens. Treatment options include oral and intravaginal regimens that have been proven to provide equal cure rates. Recommended regimens include metronidazole 500 mg orally twice per day for 7 days, metronidazole gel 0.75%, one applicator intravaginally once per day for 5 days, or clindamycin cream 2%, one applicator intravaginally at bedtime for 7 days. Clindamycin cream is oil based and could weaken latex condoms or diaphragms.

Alternative regimens include metronidazole 2 g orally in a one-time dose, clindamycin 300 mg orally twice per day for 7 days, or clindamycin ovules 100 g intravaginally once at bedtime for 3 days. Bacterial vaginosis has been associated with premature rupture of membranes, preterm labor, preterm birth, and postpartum endometritis. Treatment of all pregnant women with bacterial vaginosis has had inconsistent results in reducing these adverse events. Current CDC guidelines recommend that women who are at high risk for preterm delivery (i.e., prior preterm delivery) should be treated. Metronidazole and clindamycin can be used during pregnancy.

CANDIDIASIS

Vulvovaginal candidiasis is one of the most common causes of vaginitis. The usual etiology is *Candida albicans* but can also be caused by *C. tropicalis* or *C. glabrata*. Risk factors for developing this infection include recent antibiotic use, diabetes mellitus, pregnancy, oral contraception use, receptive oral sex, or a sexual partner with candidiasis.

Symptoms (see Table 43-1)
- Thick white discharge
- No odor
- Intense external and internal genitalia pruritus distinguishes this from other discharges. +++

Signs
- External genitalia is red, inflamed, and edematous.
- Odorless, thick cottage cheese–appearing discharge in vaginal vault
- Cervix is normal ++++

Workup
- Discharge pH is 4.0 to 4.5 ++++
- Examining secretions after adding potassium hydroxide shows budding yeast or hyphae. ++++
- Recurrent candidiasis infections need to be evaluated for other causes such as diabetes mellitus and HIV infection.

Comments and Treatment Considerations
Many effective antifungal treatments are available OTC. In cases that may be resistant terconazole (Terazol) 0.8 or 0.4% vaginal cream in a 3- or 7-day course respectively can be used. One oral treatment regimen is available using fluconazole (Diflucan) 150 mg in one dose.

Both intravaginal and oral treatment regimens have similar cure rates. The oral regimen has more adverse effects. In complicated cases of vulvovaginitis the treatment regimen my need to be expanded to 10 to 14 days for the vaginal preparations. If oral treatment is used, a fluconazole dose can be repeated in 3 days.

CHLAMYDIA AND GONORRHEA CERVICITIS

Infections with *Chlamydia trachomatis* and *Neisseria gonorrhoeae* are the most common sexually transmitted infections. These infections can cause few or no symptoms but also can cause significant infection resulting in PID (see Table 43-1).

Symptoms
- Vaginal discharge +++
- Dysuria
- Abnormal vaginal bleeding
- Pelvic or abdominal pain ++
- Pleuritic right upper quadrant abdominal pain +

Signs
- Cervix appears inflamed (chlamydia and gonorrhea) +++
- Yellow or cloudy discharge from the cervix (chlamydia and gonorrhea) +++
- Cervix may be friable and bleed easily (chlamydia)
- No vaginitis present (chlamydia and gonorrhea)
- Cervix may appear normal (gonorrhea)

Workup
- Nucleic acid amplification test available for both ++++
- Can be performed on either endocervical or urine sample
- Culture can be performed but is difficult to transport

Comments and Treatment Considerations: Chlamydia
- Azithromycin 1 g orally in a single dose
- Doxycycline 100 mg orally twice daily for 7 days
- Both are equally effective.

Alternative Treatment: Chlamydia
- Erythromycin base 500 mg orally four times daily for 7 days
- Erythromycin ethylsuccinate 800 mg orally four times daily for 7 days
- Ofloxacin 300 mg orally twice daily for 7 days
- Levofloxacin 500 mg orally once daily for 7 days

Comments and Treatment Considerations: Gonorrhea
- Cefixime 400 mg orally as a single dose
- Ceftriaxone 125 mg IM as a single dose
- Ciprofloxacin 500 mg orally as a single dose*
- Levofloxacin 250 mg orally as a single dose*
- Ofloxacin 500 mg orally as a single dose*

PELVIC INFLAMMATORY DISEASE

Women who have infections in the lower genital tract may develop an ascending infection that causes acute inflammation in the fallopian tubes or endometrium called pelvic inflammatory disease. Symptoms can vary and usually develop during menses or during the first 2 weeks of the cycle (see Table 43-1). Women who develop PID are at higher risk for infertility.

Symptoms
- Vaginal discharge +++
- Pelvic pain +++
- Abdominal pain ++
- Intramenstrual bleeding
- Fever, chills, sweats ++
- Nausea/vomiting
- Dyspareunia (painful sexual intercourse)

Signs
- Cervical motion tenderness +++
- Uterine/adnexal tenderness +++
- Abnormal cervical discharge
- Oral temperature greater than 101° F (>38.3° C) ++
- Abdominal tenderness +++

Workup
- PID is primarily a clinical diagnosis and no specific tests are required.
- CRP is elevated ++++
- Sedimentation rate is elevated +++
- Saline preparation of vaginal secretions shows significant WBCs

---

*These antibiotics should not be used in individuals who live in Asia, the Pacific Islands, or in California or may have contracted the infection while visiting these areas. Also they should not be used during pregnancy or in men who have sex with men.

- CBC; elevated WBCs
- Nucleic acid amplification tests for chlamydia and gonorrhea +++
- Endometrial biopsy, transvaginal ultrasound, MRI, or pelvic laparoscopy indicated if diagnosis is uncertain or pelvic abscess may be present

Comments and Treatment Considerations

Hospitalization for IV therapy if any of the following criteria present:
- Unresponsive to oral antibiotic therapy
- Pregnancy
- Severe illness (i.e., vomiting, nausea, high fever)
- Unable to follow-up as an outpatient
- Surgical emergencies cannot be excluded.
- Tubo-ovarian abscess present
- Oral and parenteral treatment regimens are equally effective.

Combined Parenteral/Oral Regimen (Treatment for 14 Days)

- Ceftriaxone 250 mg IM once or cefoxitin 2 g IM plus probenecid 1 g PO in a single dose concurrently plus doxycycline 100 mg PO twice daily for 14 days
- Metronidazole 500 mg orally twice daily for 14 days (consider adding to regimen if clinically indicated)

Parenteral Regimen

- Cefotetan 2 g IV every 12 hours
  or
- Cefoxitin 2 g IV every 6 hours
  and
- Doxycycline 100 mg IV or orally every 12 hours
- Change to oral regimen when clinically stable
- Doxycycline should be given orally as soon as possible because the IV form can cause sclerosis of the vein.

TRICHOMONIASIS

Trichomoniasis is caused by the protozoan *Trichomonas vaginalis* and is considered a sexually transmitted infection. The incubation period is 3 to 21 days after exposure. Because of pH changes around menses, women are more susceptible to this infection during this portion of their cycle (see Table 43-1).

Symptoms

- Most have no symptoms +++
- Diffuse malodorous vaginal discharge
- Vaginal soreness
- Dyspareunia
- Vaginal discharge may increase immediately after menses.

Signs
- Copious vaginal discharge
- Discharge is yellow-green or gray, frothy, and malodorous
- Cervix may be inflamed and have a "strawberry" appearance

Workup
- Vaginal pH 5 or greater +++
- Mobile trichomonads visible on microscopic examination of vaginal discharge +++
- Microscopic examination: 10 WBCs per high-power field ++++
- Cultures only indicated if diagnosis is uncertain

Comments and Treatment Considerations
- Metronidazole 2 g orally in a single dose
- Alternative is metronidazole 500 mg orally twice daily for 7 days
- If persists or recurs use metronidazole 500 mg orally twice daily for 5 days
- Treatment failures should be given metronidazole 2 g orally once daily for 3 days.
- It is important to treat the sexual partner as well.

References
Centers for Disease Control and Prevention: Screening tests to detect *Chlamydia trachomatis* and *Neisseria gonorrhoeae* infections, *MMWR* 51(RR-15):1–38, 2002.

Forna F, Gulmezoglu AM: Intervention for treating trichomoniasis in women, *Cochrane Database Syst Rev*, 2003, CD000218.

Hanson JM, McGregor JA, Hillier SL, et al: Metronidazole for bacterial vaginosis: a comparison of vaginal gel vs. oral therapy, *J Reproduct Med* 45:889–896, 2000.

Landers DV, Wiesenfeld HC, Heine RP, et al: Predictive value of the clinical diagnosis of lower genital tract infection in women, *Am J Obstet Gynecol* 190:1004–1010, 2004.

McDonald H, Brocklehurst P, Parsons J: Antibiotics for treating bacterial vaginosis in pregnancy, *Cochrane Database Syst Rev*, 2005, CD000262.

Ness RB, Soper DE, Holley RL, et al: Effectiveness of inpatient and outpatient treatment strategies for women with pelvic inflammatory disease: results from the Pelvic Inflammatory Disease Evaluation and Clinical Health (PEACH) randomized trial, *Am J Obstet Gynecol* 186:929–937, 2002.

Watson MC, Grimshaw JM, Bond CM, et al: Oral versus intravaginal imidzole and triazole anti-fungal agents in the treatment of uncomplicated vulvovaginal candidiasis (thrush): a systematic review, *Cochrane Database Syst Rev*, 2001, CD002845.

Workowski KA, Levine WC: Sexually transmitted diseases treatment guidelines 2002. Centers for Disease Control and Prevention, *MMWR* 51(RR-6):1–80, 2002.

CHAPTER 44

Generalized Weakness
Deborah S. Clements

This chapter focuses on selected causes of generalized weakness. Although many causes of weakness exist, the differential diagnosis will be considerably narrowed if care is taken to differentiate between weakness and fatigue or asthenia. Fatigue is the inability to continue performing a task following multiple repetitions. A sense of weariness or exhaustion without demonstrated muscle weakness is asthenia. Asthenia may lead to muscle weakness over time because of deconditioning. True weakness is the inability to perform the first repetition of a task.

Symptoms of weakness can be seen in a wide variety of conditions. These include infectious, neurologic, and genetic problems.

AMYOTROPHIC LATERAL SCLEROSIS

Also known as Lou Gehrig's disease, amyotrophic lateral sclerosis (ALS) is a progressive neuromuscular condition that affects about 30,000 people in the United States. The disease is most commonly seen in men between 30 and 60. Patients become severely disabled over a period of months to years with death occurring typically within 5 years of diagnosis.

Symptoms
- Dysphagia
- Dysarthria
- Muscle weakness in limbs and bulbar muscles ++++

Signs
- Asymmetric muscle weakness
- Hyperreflexia
- Fasciculations
- Muscle atrophy ++++
- Normal sensory examination
- Normal mental status

Workup
- The clinical diagnosis of ALS is characterized by a combination of both upper and lower motor neuron lesions, with evidence of progression and the absence of an alternative diagnosis.

- Nerve conduction studies and electromyography may be performed.
- Neuroimaging and blood and cerebrospinal studies may be helpful to exclude alternative diagnoses.

Comments and Treatment Considerations

Management involves aggressive relief of symptoms and prevention of complications such as aspiration pneumonia, spasticity, and contractures. The only agent currently considered for treatment is riluzole, 50 mg orally twice daily. Riluzole reduces release of presynaptic glutamate and may slow progression. Muscle spasticity may improve with use of baclofen or diazepam. Depression is common in ALS and should be treated appropriately. Supportive care is essential and may include the coordination of multiple services including physical therapy, speech therapy, occupational therapy, speech pathology, and nutrition.

BOTULISM

Diagnosis is based on a history of recent ingestion of home-canned, smoked, or reheated foods and demonstration of toxin in serum or food. In infants younger than 1 year, botulism may be associated with the consumption of honey.

Symptoms
- Diplopia
- Dry mouth
- Dysphagia
- Dysphonia
- Muscle weakness

Signs
- Loss of accommodation
- Ptosis, cranial nerve palsies
- Impairment of extraocular muscles
- Fixed, dilated pupils
- Normal sensory examination
- Normal mental status examination
- Constipation

Workup
- In the acute setting, diagnosis is most commonly clinical.
- EMG testing may be helpful in supporting the diagnosis.
- Botulinum toxin present in patient's serum or stool

Comments and Treatment Considerations

Rapid identification and treatment are essential because of the high fatality rate associated with respiratory paralysis. In foodborne botulism, enemas or cathartics may be helpful. In wound botulism, debridement and antimicrobial therapy should be considered. All cases should be reported to the local public health authorities.

The CDC should be contacted immediately when botulism is suspected for assistance with obtaining antitoxin and assays for identification of toxin. Because botulinum toxin is destroyed at high temperatures, home-canned foods should be boiled during preparation.

CEREBROVASCULAR ACCIDENT/TRANSIENT ISCHEMIC ATTACK

CVA or acute stroke is a sudden neurologic deficit caused by vascular compromise in the brain. Strokes are ischemic as the result of a thrombotic, embolic, or hemorrhagic occlusion. If neurologic symptoms resolve spontaneously within 24 hours, the diagnosis of TIA is appropriate.

Symptoms
- Weakness or paralysis +++
- Dysarthria
- Visual change
- Loss of consciousness
- Headache
- Seizure

Signs
- Paralysis or paresis
- Upper motor neuron lesion
- Hemianopsia or other defined visual finding
- Nystagmus

Workup
- Head CT differentiates between ischemic and hemorrhagic stroke.
- MRI and MRA may be helpful if available.
- Obtain ECG, chest x-ray, CBC, renal function, PT/INR, and serum electrolytes.
- Other tests may include carotid Doppler studies and echocardiogram.

Comments and Treatment Considerations
Initial management includes stabilization and evaluation for potential complications. Medical therapy, including antiplatelet therapy, should begin as soon as possible after imaging studies. Hyperglycemia, fever, and hypertension are associated with poor prognosis. Hypertension should be treated cautiously to prevent the risk of reducing cerebral perfusion. In selected patients presenting within 3 hours of symptom onset, thrombolysis may be appropriate (see Chapter 19 for more information).

GUILLAIN-BARRÉ SYNDROME

Patients present with an acute, progressive radiculoneuropathy resulting in ascending, symmetric weakness. The condition often ensues following an acute infection, surgical procedures, or immunizations. An association with the syndrome is sometimes seen with *Campylobacter jejuni* gastroenteritis.

Symptoms
- Weakness of variable severity ++++
- Proximal, symmetric symptoms
- Dysphagia
- Numbness and tingling
- Palpitations
- Flushing
- Encopresis due to loss of sphincter control

Signs
- Tachycardia
- Cardiac dysrhythmias
- Hypotension or hypertension
- Absent or depressed deep tendon reflexes

Workup
- CSF demonstrates a normal cell content and high protein concentration.
- Nerve conduction studies and needle electromyography are helpful in making the diagnosis.

Comments and Treatment Considerations
Several variant forms of Guillain-Barré syndrome exist. Up to 30% of patients require intubation and ventilatory support. Vital capacity and negative inspiratory force should be measured regularly. Patients may not be able to clear secretions or swallow. Dysautonomia may require management with pressors, fluids, and other agents. IVIg and plasma exchange are equivalent in efficacy. Most patients eventually recover over a period of several months; 10% to 20% have some residual deficit.

MULTIPLE SCLEROSIS

Multiple sclerosis is one of the most common neurologic causes of muscle weakness. About 300,000 patients are affected in the United States with the highest incidence in young adults between 20 and 40 years of age and a twofold predominance in women. The disease is thought to have an autoimmune basis.

Symptoms
- Numbness or tingling in a limb
- Gait disorder
- Lower or upper extremity weakness
- Diplopia
- Urinary urgency or hesitancy
- Sudden loss of vision or blurring in one eye

Signs
- Absent abdominal reflexes
- Hyperreflexia
- Lower extremity ataxia
- Impaired vibratory sensation
- Impaired rapid alternating movements
- Nystagmus
- Intention tremor
- Spasticity
- Dysarthria
- Impaired pain or temperature sensation

Workup
- Diagnosis is based on symptomatology as well as laboratory and imaging. Cases are classified as "possible MS, MS, or not MS" based on the McDonald criteria.
- CSF shows slightly increased protein, mild lymphocytosis, and positive oligoclonal bands.
- MRI of the brain and cervical spinal cord may demonstrate multiple white matter lesions.
- Evoked potential testing may provide further diagnostic information.

Comments and Treatment Considerations
Partial recovery from acute episodes is common but predicting relapse is difficult. High-dose prednisone, 60 to 80 mg/day, for 1 week hastens recovery from acute episodes but will not provide long-term benefit or prevent relapse. Incomplete remissions eventually lead to spasticity, ataxia, impaired vision, and urinary incontinence. Relapses are more common in the first months following pregnancy.

In patients with progressive disease, daily injections of glatiramer acetate may reduce frequency of exacerbations. Cyclophosphamide, azathioprine, methotrexate, cladribine, and mitoxantrone have been used with variable success in delaying secondary symptoms. During acute episodes, excessive fatigue should be avoided. Although disability is likely to eventually occur, up to half of all patients are without significant permanent disability even 10 years after onset of symptoms.

MUSCULAR DYSTROPHY

The muscular dystrophies are an inherited group of disorders causing progressive muscle weakness and wasting. The inheritance pattern, age of onset, muscle pattern distribution, and prognosis are variable depending on the specific dystrophy (Table 44-1). Patients may also have accompanying skeletal deformities and contractures.

Workup
- Serum creatinine kinase may be elevated, especially in Duchenne and Becker dystrophies.

Table 44-1. Signs and Symptoms of the Muscular Dystrophies

DISORDER	INHERITANCE	AGE AT ONSET	DISTRIBUTION OF WEAKNESS	PROGNOSIS
Duchenne	X-lined recessive	1-5 years	Pelvic, shoulder girdle then limb and respiratory muscles	Rapid; death within 5 years of onset
Becker	X-lined recessive	2-25 years	Pelvic, shoulder girdle	Slow; may have normal life expectancy
Erb	Autosomal recessive	10-30 years	Pelvic, shoulder girdle	Variable; severe disability in mid to later life
Fascioscapulohumeral	Autosomal dominant	Any	Face and shoulder, later pelvis and legs	Slow; usually normal life expectancy
Emery-Dreifuss	X-linked recessive or autosomal dominant	5-10 years	Humeroperoneal or scapuloperoneal	Variable
Ocular	Autosomal dominant	5-30 years	External ocular muscles; some mild weakness of arms, neck, and face	Slow

- EMG may confirm myopathic weakness.
- Genetic carrier detection is an important component of the evaluation of patients and their families.

Comments and Treatment Considerations
No specific treatments are recommended for the muscular dystrophies. Contractures and deformities are worsened by bed rest, so patients and their families should be encouraged to lead as normal a life as possible. Physical therapy and orthotics may be helpful in preventing disuse sequelae.

MYASTHENIA GRAVIS

In myasthenia gravis autoantibodies bind to the acetylcholine receptors of the neuromuscular junction resulting in fluctuating weakness and fatigability of voluntary muscles. This condition may be fatal when respiratory muscles are affected. Symptoms may occur at all ages and can be associated with thymic tumors, thyrotoxicosis, SLE, or RA. Exacerbations may occur with the use of anesthesia, sedatives, or narcotics.

Symptoms
- Diplopia
- Ptosis
- Dysphagia
- Fluctuating weakness ++++

Signs
- Cranial nerve palsies
- Normal papillary responses
- Muscle weakness increases with sustained activity and improves with rest. +++
- Normal sensation ++++
- Preserved deep tendon reflexes

Workup
- Elevated serum acetylcholine receptor antibodies
- Chest CT to determine presence of thymoma
- Edrophonium challenge with a dose of 2 mg, IV, initially followed by 8 mg about 30 seconds later if tolerated. Improvement typically lasts about 5 minutes.
- EMG studies indicate a disturbance of neuromuscular transmission.

Comments and Treatment Considerations
Anticholinesterase medications such as neostigmine and pyridostigmine provide symptomatic relief but do not alter the course of the disease. Immunomodulating agents, such as corticosteroids, azathioprine, and cyclosporine may be used. Plasma exchange or IVIg therapy are often considered as "bridge" therapy. Thymectomy should be considered in all patients younger than age 60. Spontaneous remissions can occur.

POLIOMYELITIS

Poliomyelitis (polio) is caused by an enteroviral infection of the lower motor neurons. Infection occurs predominantly by the fecal-oral route. Although rare in the developed world, polio remains common across the globe and has been targeted for eradication by the World Health Organization. Prevention is effective with the use of a parenteral inactive vaccine in children.

Symptoms
- Headache
- Sore throat
- Stiff neck
- Abdominal pain
- Weakness ++++

Signs
- Fever
- Muscle pain and spasm
- Meningismus
- Lower motor neuron paresis or paralysis, commonly asymmetric

Workup
- CSF reveals lymphocytosis.
- Viral culture, serum titers

Comments and Treatment Considerations
Treatment is mainly supportive. For every 1 person with paralytic polio, an estimated 200 subclinical cases exist; 15% to 30% of adults who contract paralytic polio die from the illness.

RABIES

Rabies is caused by a rhabdovirus infection transmitted to humans by bites from animals with infected saliva. Although cases are rare in the United States, the most common vectors are bats, raccoons, skunks, foxes, and coyotes. Prevention includes immunization of household cats and dogs and avoidance of animals associated with rabies.

Symptoms
- Pain at the site of the animal bite
- Fever
- Nausea
- Headache
- Muscle weakness and confusion
- Hydrophobia

Signs
- Delirium
- Painful laryngeal spasms

- Paresis
- Coma

Workup
- Diagnosis is confirmed by fluorescent antibody testing of the animal's brain.
- The risk of infection must be carefully evaluated based on the type of exposure, circumstances surrounding exposure, and the evidence of a bite.
- Consultation with the local or state health department may be necessary to determine the need for prophylaxis.

Comments and Treatment Considerations
In previously unvaccinated patients exposed to rabies, rabies immune globulin (RIg) is administered once to provide immediate antibodies. Postexposure prophylaxis after contact with bats may be appropriate even if a bite, scratch, or mucous membrane exposure is not obvious because data suggest bats can transfer the virus through minor or unrecognized bites. All wounds should be thoroughly cleansed with soap and water and irrigated with an agent such as povidone-iodine solution. As much RIg as possible should be administered at 20 IU/kg by infiltrating around the wound. Any remaining volume can be given IM at a site distant from vaccine administration. Rabies vaccine 1 mL, IM, should be given in the deltoid area on days 0, 3, 14, and 28 after exposure in previously unvaccinated patients. Rabies vaccine 1 mL IM should be given in the deltoid area on days 0 and 3 for patients previously vaccinated. The rabies vaccine should not be given in the gluteal region because of resulting lower neutralizing antibody titers.

References
Berge E, Sandercock P: Anticoagulants versus antiplatelet agents for acute ischaemic stroke, *Cochrane Database Syst Rev*, 2003, CD003242.

Calabresi PA: Diagnosis and management of multiple sclerosis, *Am Fam Physician* 15;70(10):1935–1944, 2004.

Centers for Disease Control and Prevention: Poliomyelitis prevention in the United States: introduction of a sequential vaccination schedule of inactivated poliovirus vaccine followed by oral poliovirus vaccine. Recommendations of the Advisory Committee on Immunization Practices (ACIP), *MMWR Morb Mortal Wkly Rep* 46:1–25, 1997 [Published erratum in *MMWR Morb Mortal Wkly Rep* 46:183, 1997.]

Centers for Disease Control and Prevention: Human rabies prevention—United States, 1999: Recommendations of the Advisory Committee on Immunization Practices (ACIP), *MMWR Morb Mortal Wkly Rep* 48(RR-1):12, 1999.

Cox N, Hinkle R: Infant botulism, *Am Fam Physician* 65(7):1388–1392, 2002.

Hankins DG, Rosekrans JA. Overview, prevention, and treatment of rabies. Available at http://www.bt.cdc.gov/ncidod/dbmd/diseaseinfo/botulism_a.htm (accessed October 29, 2006).

Hughes RA, Cornblath DR: Guillain-Barre syndrome, *Lancet* 366(9497):1653–1666, 2005.

Hughes RA, Wijdicks EF, Barohn R, et al: Practice parameter: immunotherapy for Guillain-Barre syndrome: Report of the Quality Standards Subcommittee of the American Academy of Neurology, *Neurology* 61(6):736–740, 2003.

Keesey JC: Clinical evaluation and management of myasthenia gravis, *Muscle Nerve* 29:284, 2004.

Murray TJ: Diagnosis and treatment of multiple sclerosis, *BMJ* 332(7540):525–527, 2006.

Newsanger DL, Warren CR: Guillain-Barre syndrome, *Am Fam Physician* 69(10): 2405–2410, 2004.

Querfurth H, Swanson PD: Vaccine Associated Paralytic Poliomyelitis. Regional Case Series and Review, *Arch Neurol* 47(5):541–544, 1990.

Solenski NJ: Transient ischemic attacks: diagnosis and evaluation, *Am Fam Physician* 69(7):1665–1674, 2004.

Vincent A: Unravelling the pathogenesis of myasthenia gravis, *Nature Rev Immunol* 2:797–804, 2002.

Wagner KR: Genetic diseases of muscle, *Neurol Clin* 20:645–678, 2002.

Walling AD: Amyotrophic lateral sclerosis: Lou Gehrig's disease, *Am Fam Physician* 59(6):1489–1496, 1999.

Whitley RJ, Gnann JW: Viral encephalitis: familiar infections and emerging pathogens, *Lancet* 359(9305):507–513, 2002.

Williams DB, Windebank AJ: Motor neuron disease (amyotrophic lateral sclerosis), *Mayo Clin Proc* 66:54–82, 1991.

CHAPTER 45

Weight Change

Samuel N. Grief, Shailendra Kapoor, Yves-Mario Piverger, and Jamila Williams

Weight loss is one of the most common symptoms associated with malignancies.

CANCER

Eighty percent of cancer patients in advanced stages experience weight loss and as many as 40% report weight loss at the time of initial presentation. Weight loss in a cancer patient is particularly concerning and indicates severe malnutrition if there is greater than 2% weight loss per week, 5% or more weight loss in the previous month, 7.5% or more weight loss over the previous 3 months, or 10% or more weight loss over the previous 6 months.

Weight loss in cancer patients is important because it may result in poor response to cancer treatments, increased predisposition to secondary infections, poor prognosis, and shorter survival times.

Symptoms
- Cachexia
- Anorexia ++++
- Fatigue
- Mood disturbances

Signs
- Decreasing serial body weights
- Muscle wasting
- Dehydration
- Anemia

Workup
- CBC
- Serum albumin
- Serum prealbumin
- Serum cholesterol
- BUN
- Creatinine
- Electrolytes
- Glucose

Comments and Treatment Considerations

Treatment options for treating weight loss in cancer patients include increasing protein intake. To maintain lean body mass cancer patients require at least 1.5 to 2.0 g of protein/kg daily. Isoleucine, valine, and leucine (branched chain amino acids [BCAAs]) are particularly effective in increasing lean body mass. Ideal sources of protein include lean fish and chicken. Whey-based protein powders may be used to supplement meals.

Dietary modifications should also be encouraged. Eat small, frequent meals. Keep snacks such as ice cream within easy access. Include foods in meals that the patient enjoys the most. Eat more when one feels the hungriest. Drink liquids such as juices if unable to tolerate solids. Try cool or frozen foods/beverages.

Consume omega-3 fatty acids. Fish oils are rich in omega-3 fatty acids especially eicosapentaenoic acid (EPA). Significant increases in lean body mass and weight gain have been noted in studies using EPA. Omega-3 fatty acids are readily available as OTC supplements.

Consider using medications such as ondansetron, dolasetron, granisetron or aprepitant to not only treat nausea and vomiting but also prevent it.

Steroids act by inhibiting the synthesis of cytokines, decrease nausea, and improve appetite. However, most studies have demonstrated beneficial effects of steroids up to 1 month only. Extended use of steroids can lead to osteoporosis, immunosuppression, glaucoma, and psychiatric side effects.

Megestrol in a dosage of at least 320 mg/day orally has successfully produced weight gain in cancer patients. Megestrol use has been associated with decreased cytokine levels in some studies. Patients are usually started on a dosage of 160 mg daily in divided doses. The daily dose can be increased to 800 mg daily depending on the clinical response.

Weight gain might even be noticed after megestrol is stopped. Side effects include edema, constipation, and delirium. Megestrol is also associated with an increased incidence of thromboembolic events. Megestrol should not be used in patients with heart disease or thromboembolic disease.

Cyproheptadine has antihistaminic properties and has been shown to increase appetite in cancer patients. A controlled trial showed that cyproheptadine increased appetite in cancer patients although it did not decrease weight loss. Side effects include drowsiness and dizziness.

Dronabinol is a synthetic version of tetrahydrocannabinol (THC), the active ingredient in marijuana. Side effects include somnolence, confusion, and dizziness. Megestrol is more effective than dronabinol.

Depression plays a significant role in cancer-related weight loss. Mirtazapine (Remeron), an atypical antidepressant, has been shown to treat depression and induce weight gain.

Oxandrolone, ornithine, and anabolic steroids may be used to increase lean body mass in cancer patients. Somatotropin (recombinant human growth hormone) may also be considered to treat wasting syndromes.

Consider tube feeding or TPN for patients in whom these measures are ineffective. Addition of BCAAs to TPN significantly improves albumin synthesis. Percutaneous endoscopic gastrostomy (PEG) or J-tubes are surgical alternatives in patients in whom medical therapy has failed and no surgical contraindications exist.

Exercise helps to rebuild lost lean body mass. Exercise options include doing gentle weight training such as lifting light weights several times a day and low-impact aerobic exercise such as walking.

Thalidomide, pentoxifylline, interleukin 15 (IL-15), antimyostatin antibodies, gherlin, and ubiquitin ligase inhibitors are some of the other treatment modalities currently being investigated for treatment of weight loss in cancer.

EATING DISORDERS

Eating disorders are behaviors characterized by abnormal eating patterns, cognitive distortions related to food and weight, and have adverse effects on health status and function. More than 5 million Americans suffer from eating disorders with a female-to-male ratio of 5:1.

Eating disorders are the third most common chronic illness in adolescent women. Over the past decade there has been a documented increase among American female adolescents in eating and weight-related problems and unhealthy weight control practices such as self-induced vomiting; laxative, diuretic, and diet pill misuse; and excessive exercise.

Types of eating disorders according to the DSM-IV include:
- Anorexia nervosa (AN): voluntary restriction of caloric intake accompanied by the obsession to be thinner and the delusion of being fat
- Bulimia nervosa (BN): voluntary episodes of ingesting large amounts of food followed by "purging" behavior (i.e., exercise, diuretics/laxatives, vomiting, fasting)
- Binge eating disorder
- Compulsive eating disorder

Symptoms
- Amenorrhea
- Cold intolerance
- GI problems
- Lack of energy
- Depression +++

Signs
- Weight loss or failure to gain weight (in AN:BMI ≤17.5) +++++
- Weight fluctuations (especially in BN)
- Osteoporosis
- Dysrhythmias
- Hypotension
- Hypothermia

- Electrolyte abnormalities
- Dry skin
- Hair loss

Workup
- Screening questions
  - Has there been any change in your weight?
  - How do you feel about your appearance?
  - What did you eat yesterday?
  - How much do you exercise in a typical week?
  - Have you ever used laxatives, vomiting, or medications to lose weight or compensate for overeating?
  - BMI and weight documentation
  - Initial assessment should focus on exploration of the underlying factors.
  - Is weight loss intentional and desired or related to an organic process?
  - Are weight-control habits excessive or unhealthy?
  - What is the patient's desired goal weight?
- Record energy intake
  - Seven-day food diary
- Labs: focus on detecting underlying medical conditions
  - Thyroid disease—TSH
  - Diabetes—Fasting blood sugar (FBS)
  - Anemia—CBC with differential

Comments and Treatment Considerations
The four elements of successful treatment include recognizing the disorder and restoring physiologic stability early in its course; establishing a trusting, therapeutic relationship with the patient; involving the family in treatment; and using an interdisciplinary team approach to include family, psychiatrist/psychologist, nutritionist, school officials, physician, and dentist.

Pharmacotherapy: SSRI (fluoxetine) is used in both BN and AN.

FAILURE TO THRIVE

Failure to thrive (FTT) is diagnosed within the first 2 years of life in an infant or child whose physical growth is significantly less than that of his or her peers. FTT is often divided into two categories: organic failure to thrive (OFTT) and nonorganic failure to thrive (NOFTT).

OFTT implies an illness resulting in FTT. Organic FTT is marked by an underlying medical condition (Table 45-1).

NOFTT indicates a psychosocial issue (includes child abuse and neglect, behavioral issues) resulting in FTT. NOFTT is the most commonly seen in primary care.

Signs
- Weight below 5th percentile on more than one occasion ++++
- Low weight for height

Table 45-1. Underlying Medical Conditions Causing Organic Failure to Thrive

SYSTEM	CAUSES
Gastrointestinal	Gastroesophageal reflux, celiac disease, pyloric stenosis, cleft palate/cleft lip, lactose intolerance, Hirschsprung's disease, milk protein intolerance, hepatitis, cirrhosis, pancreatic insufficiency, biliary disease, inflammatory bowel disease, malabsorptions
Renal	Urinary tract infection, renal tubular acidosis, diabetes insipidus, chronic renal insufficiency, acute renal insufficiency
Cardiopulmonary	Cardiac diseases leading to congestive heart failure, asthma, bronchopulmonary dysplasia, cystic fibrosis, anatomic abnormalities of the upper airway, obstructive sleep apnea, chronic aspiration, respiratory insufficiency
Endocrine	Hypothyroidism, diabetes mellitus, adrenal insufficiency or excess, parathyroidism disorders, pituitary disorders, growth hormone deficiency
Neurologic	Mental retardation, cerebral hemorrhages, degenerative disorders, cerebral palsy
Infectious	Parasitic or bacterial infections of the gastrointestinal tract, tuberculosis, HIV, or AIDS
Metabolic	Inborn errors of metabolism
Congenital	Chromosomal abnormalities, congenital syndromes (fetal alcohol syndrome), perinatal infections, congenital immunodeficiency syndromes, cleft palate
Miscellaneous	Lead poisoning, malignancy, collagen vascular disease, recurrently infected adenoids and tonsils, prematurity, low birthweight

AIDS, Acquired immunodeficiency syndrome; *HIV,* human immunodeficiency virus.
Adapted from Behrman R, Kliegman R, Jenson H: *Pocket companion to accompany Nelson textbook of pediatrics,* 2nd ed, Philadelphia, 2001, Saunders.

- Diminished rate of weight gain so that there is a decrease in weight of two or more major percentile categories over time
- Weight less than 80% of ideal weight for age on standard growth charts
- Rate of daily weight gain less than expected for age

Workup
- FTT evaluation should include assessing the following four dimensions of the child and family: medical, nutritional, developmental or behavioral, and psychosocial.

- Most infants with FTT secondary to malnutrition resulting from inadequate caloric intake, malabsorption, or altered metabolism, typically have normal head circumference, and weight is reduced out of proportion to height.
- Laboratory examination for suspected FTT should be based on history and physical examination findings. Basic laboratory studies to be obtained in all or most cases should include:
  - CBC
  - Electrolytes and kidney functions
  - Tuberculin skin test
  - Urinalysis and culture
  - Stool studies for *Giardia* antigen.

Further studies, such as a radiologic bone age may be considered, especially if indicated by history or physical examination.

Comments and Treatment Considerations

Whether the cause of FTT is organic or nonorganic, establishing an appropriate feeding atmosphere at home is important. Children with severe malnutrition must be re-fed carefully to avoid potential complications. For children with organic FTT, the underlying medical condition should be treated.

Outpatient treatment of FTT includes weekly visits to check weight, height, head circumference, and physical assessment until weight has reached the 5th percentile. Schedule monthly visits until adequate weight and height gain have been achieved and maintained for at least 3 consecutive months.

Support parents with referral to the Women, Infants and Children (WIC) program, nutritionist, social worker, Medicaid office, and support groups, as needed. Involve mental health professionals for families with concerns of psychologic or psychiatric disorders, substance abuse, or family dysfunction.

Indications for hospitalization include severe malnutrition, need for further diagnostic laboratory evaluation, and lack of catch-up growth, despite outpatient treatment.

References

American Psychiatric Association: *Diagnostic and statistical manual of mental disorders*, 4th ed rev, Washington, DC, 2002, APA, pp 588–595.

Argiles JM, Meijsing SH, Pallares-Trujillo J, et al: Cancer cachexia: a therapeutic approach, *Med Res Rev* 21(1):83–101, 2001.

Behrman R, Kliegman R, Jenson H: *Pocket companion to accompany Nelson textbook of pediatrics*, 2nd ed, Philadelphia, 2001, Saunders.

Comerci GD: Eating disorders in adolescents, *Pediatr Rev* 10(2):37–47, 1988.

Fox J: *Primary health care of infant,s children, and adolescents*, 2nd ed, St Louis, 2002, Mosby.

Gale T: Position of the American Dietetic Association: nutrition intervention in the treatment of anorexia nervosa, bulimia nervosa, and eating disorders not otherwise specified, *J Am Diet Assoc* 7:810, 2001.

Graef J: *Manual of pediatric therapeutics*, 6th ed, Philadelphia, 1997, Lippincott Williams & Wilkins.

Grimble RF: Nutritional therapy for cancer cachexia, *Gut* 52(10):1391–1392, 2003.

Hay WW: *Current pediatric diagnosis and treatment*, 15th ed, Norwalk, CT, 2001, Appleton & Lange, p 250.

Kelleher KJ, Casey PH, Bradley RH, et al: Risk factors and outcomes for failure to thrive in low birth weight preterm infants, *Pediatrics* 92(1):190, 1993.

Kotler DP: Cachexia, *Ann Intern Med* 133(8):622–634, 2000.

Kreipe R, Yussamn S: The role of the primary care practitioner in the treatment of eating disorders, *Adolesc Med* 14(1):133–147, 2003.

Olsen EM: Failure to thrive: still a problem of definition, *Clin Pediatr* 45(1):1–6, 2006.

Powers P: Initial assessment and early treatment options for anorexia nervosa and bulimia nervosa, *Psychiatr Clin North Am* 19(4):639–655, 1996.

Raynor P, Rudolf MC: Anthropometric indices of failure to thrive, *Arch Dis Child* 82(5):364–365, 2000.

Shah MD: Failure to thrive in children, *J Clin Gastroenterol* 35(5):371–374, 2002.

Tisdale MJ: Cachexia in cancer patients, *Nat Rev Cancer* 2(11):862–871, 2002.

Wilensky DS, Ginsberg G, Altman M, et al: Jerusalem Child Development Centre, Ilan Child Guidance Clinic: a community based study of failure to thrive in Israel, *Arch Dis Child* 75(2):145–148, 1996.

Wright C, Birks E: Risk factors for failure to thrive: a population-based survey, *Child Care Health Dev* 26(1):5–16, 2000.

Wright CM, Callum J, Birks E, Jarvis S: Effect of community based management in failure to thrive: randomized controlled trial, *Pediatrics* 91(5):941–948, 1993.

Index

A

AAAs (abdominal aortic aneurysms), 22–24. *See also* Aneurysms.
Abdominal conditions
  aneurysms. *See also* Aneurysms.
    AAAs, 22–24
    ruptured, 277
  pain, 1–25
    cardiovascular, 22–24
    etiology/epidemiology of, 1
    GI, 1–22
Abnormal conditions
  platelet function, 123–130, 125*t*, 126*t*, 128*t*
    etiology/epidemiology of, 123
    medication-related, 127, 128*t*
    vWD, 126*t*, 127–130
  vaginal bleeding, 26–34
    etiology/epidemiology of, 26
    prepubertal, 26–27
    in reproductive years, 27–33
Abscesses
  breast, 155–157. *See also* Breast masses.
  TOA, 423–424
Absence seizures, 476*f*, 477. *See also* Seizures.
Abuse
  child, 196–200
    assessments of, 197–200
    differential diagnosis for, 199
    documentation for, 198
    etiology/epidemiology of, 196
    histories for, 197–198
    legal considerations for, 200
    management strategies for, 199
    physical, 196–197
    physical examinations for, 198
    prevention of, 200
    sexual, 197

Abuse *(Continued)*
  domestic violence and, 295–298
  substance, 514–526
    alcohol, 514–517, 515*t*. *See also* Alcohol abuse.
    cocaine dependence, 517–518, 517*t*
    dissociative drugs, 518–519, 518*t*, 519*t*
    hallucinogens, 518–519, 518*t*, 519*t*
    inhalants, 519–520
    marijuana, 520–521
    methamphetamines, 521–522
    opioid dependence, 522–524
    tobacco, 524, 524*t*, 525*t*
    withdrawal syndrome, 521
Accidents
  CVAs. *See* CVAs (cerebrovascular accidents).
  water, 292
Achilles tendinopathy, 86. *See also* Tendinopathy.
Acne, 434–436, 435*f*
  acne vulgaris, 439–440
  etiology/epidemiology of, 434
  mild, 435*f*, 437
  nodulocystic, 434, 435*f*
Acne vulgaris, 439–440. *See also* Acne.
ACS (acute coronary syndrome), 170–177
Acute conditions
  ACS. *See* ACS (acute coronary syndrome).
  blood loss, 52–53
  vs. chronic. *See* Chronic conditions.
  cystitis, 527–528
  depressive disorders, acute phases of, 242–247

Entries followed by *"b"* indicate boxes; *"f"* figures; *"t"* tables.